Occupational Therapy and Physical Dysfunction

Occupational Therapy and Physical Dysfunction

Principles, Skills and Practice

Edited by

Ann Turner TDipCOT
Senior Lecturer, St Andrew's School of Occupational Therapy, Northampton

Margaret Foster TDipCOT CertEd
Senior Lecturer, Derby School of Occupational Therapy, Institute of Health and Community Studies, Derbyshire College of Higher Education

Sybil E. Johnson TDipCOT CertHSM
District Occupational Therapist, Sheffield Health Authority

Foreword by

Mavis Wallis TDipCOT
Principal, Essex School of Occupational Therapy

THIRD EDITION

CHURCHILL LIVINGSTONE
EDINBURGH LONDON MELBOURNE NEW YORK AND TOKYO 1992

CHURCHILL LIVINGSTONE
Medical Division of Longman Group UK Limited

Distributed in the United States of America by Churchill
Livingstone Inc., 650 Avenue of the Americas, New York,
N.Y. 10011, and by associated companies, branches and
representatives throughout the world.

First edition 1981
Second edition 1987
Third edition 1992
   Reprinted 1993
   Reprinted 1994

ISBN 0-443-04307-8

British Library Cataloguing in Publication Data
A catalogue record for this book is available from the
British Library.

Library of Congress Cataloging in Publication Data
A catalogue record for this book is available from the
Library of Congress

Produced by Longman Singapore Publishers (Pte) Ltd
Printed in Singapore

For Churchill Livingstone

Publisher: Mary Law
Project Editor: Dinah Thom
Copy Editor: Anne Marie Todkill
Production Controller: Nancy Henry
Design: Design Resources Unit
Sales Promotion Executive: Hilary Brown

Foreword

It is a great honour to be asked for a second time to write the foreword for the new edition of what has often been known as 'Ann Turner's book', and I take the opportunity to commend this text to therapists and students.

The contributors, working under the careful guidance of Ann Turner and the two new co-editors, Margaret Foster and Sybil Johnson, have produced a wealth of new material, exploring issues and techniques further than is indicated by the title. Part 1 is relevant to all occupational therapists, wherever they practise, as it explores the roots, philosophy and key skills of the profession. Having spent many hours extricating similar material from various sources, I am grateful for an authoritative British text which presents a coherent and readable introduction to occupational therapy.

In conferring with the fifth cohort of in-service students shortly to qualify from the Essex School about their opinions of 'Turner' (second edition), which they have used throughout the course, favourable comments arose spontaneously about the clear lay-out and diagrams and the ease of use for quick reviews and references. These aspects, which make the book particularly user-friendly, have been retained and enhanced in the third edition.

One comment, 'It's British and easy to read', was very telling, as it reflects the problem that exists with the necessity to use texts from across the Atlantic to supplement the few home-produced texts; the terminology and methods of health care delivery are often very different from familiar British customs. Now we have a text that integrates theory with practice, identifies frames of reference, explains the application of models of practice and explores issues in the delivery of health and social care in Britain.

Students regard the second edition as 'a good starting point', which is a great compliment to a basic text, hence the feeling that 'no bibliography is complete without it'. In the third edition we have a book that should be kept within easy reach on every occupational therapist's bookshelf. The new chapters illuminate and inform current practice, while the up-dated chapters explore, justify and define standards of care. An emphasis throughout on the psychological and social aspects of physical impairment reinforces the holistic approach that is inherent in occupational therapy.

But, far from being a dry, theoretical treatise, the text is readable and it focuses on people, their problems and the measures relevant to the provision of high quality therapy.

From my privileged position of reading a proof copy, I am confident that this new edition will remain 'the first book students turn to' and that it will become an integral part of their lives as therapists, retaining the affection that earlier editions have achieved as 'the student's friend'.

Essex, 1992   M.A.W.

Preface

Since the first edition of this book was published in 1981 the practice of occupational therapy has grown and developed in many ways, reflecting the healthy state of a lively and expanding profession. In embarking on this new edition, we looked carefully at how occupational therapy has changed: the result is virtually a new book, with a new title and a radically revised contents.

What have been the most important developments in occupational therapy over the past decade? We have observed three main areas of change.

The first and perhaps the most encouraging change has been the realisation by most occupational therapists that their practice must be firmly grounded in the profession's philosophy and theory base. Gone are the days when carrying out a prescriptive programme of departmental activities was considered the epitome of good practice. Today's occupational therapist must base her intervention on a firm theoretical base, consider her treatment priorities based on her holistic knowledge of the person she is helping, and reflect upon and evaluate her intervention in order to ensure it remains as effective as possible.

Secondly, the profession's methodology, always willing and able to move with the times, has encompassed many new fashions and techniques in order to provide the most effective treatment media. However, occupational therapists have not merely abandoned media that have proven their worth over the years: many therapists are using tried and tested techniques alongside those which are still being developed.

Lastly, changes in the organisation and financing of care have had an effect on *all* the health and social care professions, including occupational therapy. Today's therapist must be able to manage resources efficiently, define the profession's boundaries and explain her role and function to employers, colleagues, students and the general public. Complacency is fatal in the prevailing economic climate, and no profession can take its position for granted. Rather, therapists must be confident of their unique contribution to health and social care and able to articulate their beliefs clearly to others.

Developments in education have kept pace with these changes. The majority of occupational therapy programmes have moved, or are in the process of moving, from diploma to first degree status. Many practising therapists are enhancing their knowledge by further study at first and higher degree level and through a wide variety of post registration courses.

Changes in the content of most education programmes have been a predictable and a most welcome development. It is now generally accepted, for example, that a solely biomedical practice paradigm will no longer satisfy the profession's needs. The occupational therapist's concept of health extends beyond the somatic dysfunctions studied by traditional medical practice and, consequently, a greater knowledge of a person's psychological, sociological and environmental context is essential for assessing needs and priorities.

A textbook for the 1990s must reflect all these

changes and developments. It must emphasise the *principles* which link the occupational therapist's approach to various fieldwork situations, and it should reflect a sound philosophy translated through a variety of frames of reference and models into effective methodology.

This third edition, therefore, has been completely rewritten to meet these requirements. As indicated by the main title, *Occupational Therapy and Physical Dysfunction*, the new edition continues to deal primarily with the physical side of treatment. However, throughout the text, careful attention has been paid to the psychological and social issues of therapy, reflecting the occupational therapist's belief in holistic care. It should also be noted that much of the information included in the book, especially in Part 1, is relevant to *all* therapists, in all areas of practice.

The division of the book into three parts is an innovation for this edition. The subtitle, 'Principles, Skills and Practice', alludes to these three main sections: *Part 1* discusses the profession's philosophical, historical and psychosocial base; *Part 2* gives information on the core skills required by all occupational therapists; *Part 3* shows how this knowledge base can be applied in practice.

The clinical conditions in Part 3 are not treated as separate entities but are divided into groups whose principles and approaches are linked. Each of these subsections in Part 3, therefore, is introduced by a chapter which sets the scene for the way in which the conditions may be considered. The clinical chapters in Part 3 are nearly all written by practising senior occupational therapists, while Parts 1 and 2 have been written by those whose experience lies in education and management. As editors, we would like to pay tribute here to the work of all the contributors, whose knowledge and experience are so amply illustrated in the quality of each chapter.

There is, of course, continuity between this edition and those that preceded it. Readers of previous editions will be pleased to see that we have retained many features of the past, such as clear headings, attractive page layout and copious illustrations. The importance of these features cannot be overemphasised, since they help to make the book readable and easy for the student — especially the new student — to use and to retain the information presented.

Finally, a word about the editorship of this new edition. The expansion of knowledge and skills in occupational therapy made it obvious that the task of editing could no longer be handled successfully by one individual. The original editor (Ann Turner) is therefore especially indebted to the new co-editors, Margaret Foster and Sybil Johnson, for lending their time and skills to this project. We have worked well together as a team and feel the book has been strengthened by having three editors, whose collective experience spans the fields of general hospital medicine, community work, education and management. It also provided the very practical benefit of sharing the labour, and it is not too much of an exaggeration to say that the third edition of this book could not have been produced without the creation of this editorial team.

Northampton, 1992   A. T.
                                           M. F.
                                           S. E. J.

Acknowledgements

The editors would like to thank the following people, without whom this edition could not have been written:

- all our contributors for sharing their expertise
- our objective readers
- our colleagues for their tolerance
- our families — Peter, Matthew and Louisa; Graham, Alex and Nick; and Rodney — for their love and support.
- the staff at Churchill Livingstone for their encouragement and guidance.

In addition we should like to thank: Anne Ashby for her objective reading of, and comments on the chapter on Management; Eunice Batchford for her typing; Richard Body for his advice concerning speech therapy for people with Parkinson's disease; Sue Hirst and Avril Bagshaw for their assistance with Chapter 14 Introduction to neurology; the basic grade occupational therapists in Sheffield who commented on the Appendix; and the occupational therapy staff at the Psychiatric Unit, Northern General Hospital, Sheffield, for their permission to use photographs.

Contributors

Kate Abbott DipCOT
Senior Hand Therapist, Derbyshire Royal
Infirmary

Susan Beresford DipCOT
Senior Occupational Therapist, Cynthia Spencer
House, Manfield Hospital, Northampton

Maryanne Cook DipCOT CertEd(FE)
Occupational Therapist, Warwickshire County
Council

Jean Colburn MSc BOT DipCOT
Senior Lecturer, Dorset House School of
Occupational Therapy

Rosemary Cooper DipCOT
Head Occupational Therapist, Pinderfields
General Hospital, Wakefield

Glenys R. H. Crooks DipCOT
Head Occupational Therapist, Derbyshire Royal
Infirmary, Derby

Louise Cusack DipCOT
Head Occupational Therapist and Specialist in
HIV/AIDS, Westminster and St Stephen's
Hospitals, London

W. JoAn Davies TDipCOT
'Relate' Counsellor; Former Tutor, St Loye's
School of Occupational Therapy, Exeter and
Dorset House School of Occupational Therapy,
Oxford

Margaret Foster TDipCOT CertEd(FE)
Senior Lecturer, Derby School of Occupational

Therapy, Institute of Health and Community
Studies, Derbyshire College of Higher Education

Jenny Goulter DipCOT
District Senior Occupational Therapist, Dorset
Social Services, West District

Jane Henshaw DipCOT
Head Occupational Therapist, Duke of Cornwall
Spinal Treatment Centre, Odstock Hospital,
Salisbury

Sue Hirst BA DipCOT
Senior Occupational Therapist, Royal
Hallamshire Hospital, Sheffield

Vivienne Ibbotson DipCOT
Senior Occupational Therapist, Disablement
Services Centre, Northern General Hospital,
Sheffield

Jane James DipCOT
Principal Assistant, Disabled Persons Services,
Leicestershire Social Services

Sybil E. Johnson TDipCOT CertHSM
District Occupational Therapist, Sheffield
Health Authority

Jenny C. King DipCOT
Honorary Head Occupational Therapist
(Research), Cardiac Department, Charing Cross
Hospital, London

Ruth Larder DipCOT
Senior Occupational Therapist, Nether Edge
Hospital, Sheffield

Annette C. Leveridge DipCOT
Head Occupational Therapist, Mount Vernon
Hospital, Northwood, Middlesex; Head of
Occupational Therapy Service to Regional Burns
and Plastic Surgery Unit; Chairman of British
Association of Hand Therapists

Charlotte V. MacCaul BSc DipCOT
Secretary, National Occupational Therapy
Special Interest Group in Microcomputers; Head
Occupational Therapist, Psychiatric Services
(Swale), Keycol Hill Hospital, Sittingbourne,
Kent

Steve McWilliams BA(Hons) DipCOT
Senior Occupational Therapist, Oakwood
Cheshire Home, Stockport; Former Senior
Occupational Therapist, Head Injury
Rehabilitation Centre, Sheffield

Louise Phillips DipCOT
Former Senior Occupational Therapist in
AIDS/HIV, Westminster and St Stephen's
Hospitals, London

Lorraine L. Pinnington BA MSc DipCOT
Former Lecturer, Derby School of Occupational
Therapy, Institute of Health and Community
Studies, Derbyshire College of Higher
Education; currently undertaking postgraduate
research in psychology and rehabilitation
robotics, University of Keele

Patricia M. Riley DipCOT
Head Occupational Therapist, Leeds General
Infirmary, Leeds

Pauline Rowe DipCOT CertEd
Lecturer, Derby School of Occupational
Therapy, Institute of Health and Community
Studies, Derbyshire College of Higher Education

Doreen Rowland DipCOT
Head Occupational Therapist, Atkinson
Morley's Hospital and Wolfson Medical
Rehabilitation Centre, London

Ruth Sampson DipCOT
Senior Occupational Therapist, Derbyshire
Royal Infirmary

Elke Small DipCOT
Head Occupational Therapist, The Royal
National Hospital for Rheumatic Diseases, Bath

Helen E. Stoneley DipCOT
Peripatetic Tutor, Derby School of Occupational
Therapy, Institute of Health and Community
Studies, Derbyshire College of Higher Education

Ann Turner TDipCOT
Senior Lecturer, St Andrew's School of
Occupational Therapy, Northampton

Jenny Wilsdon BSc(Hons) DipCOT
Lecturer in Biological Sciences and Professional
Studies (Paediatrics), St Andrew's School of
Occupational Therapy, Northampton

Contents

Part 1
Principles

The splendour of its vision goes far beyond rating it as an idea conceived once in a lifetime or even once in a century. Rather it falls in the class of one of those great beliefs which has advanced civilisation. Its magnificence lies in the optimistic vote of confidence it gives to human nature. It implies that there is a reservoir of sensitivity and skill in the hands of man which can be tapped for his health. It implies the rich adaptability and durability of the central nervous system which can be influenced by experiences. And more than all this, it implies that man, through the use of his hands, can creatively deploy his thinking, feelings and purposes to make himself at home in the world and to make the world his home.

Mary Reilly 1962 Occupational therapy can be one of the great ideas of 20th century medicine. *American Journal of Occupational Therapy* 16: 1–9

1

The philosophy of occupational therapy

Ann Turner

INTRODUCTION

Although occupational therapy is one of the fastest-growing paramedical professions, the number of occupational therapists is still comparatively small. This fact, together with the ever-changing and varied nature of occupational therapy practice, perhaps helps to explain why the underlying aims and values of the profession are not always clearly understood.

The outside observer may be forgiven if, following the occupational therapist in the course of her★ professional activities, he is unable to discern an underlying rationale for her actions. Whilst the purpose of ordering a wheelchair or making an orthosis might be plain enough, what is he to make of her use of such diverse activities as cookery or carpentry, planting daffodil bulbs or singing a song? He may well wonder exactly what the therapist is aiming to achieve, and what these wide-ranging activities have in common.

In order to answer this question the observer would have to look beyond the activities themselves to the reasons why they have been chosen. For the occupational therapist, activity is the

---

★ Throughout the book, 'he' has been used to refer to the patient/client and 'she' to the occupational therapist.

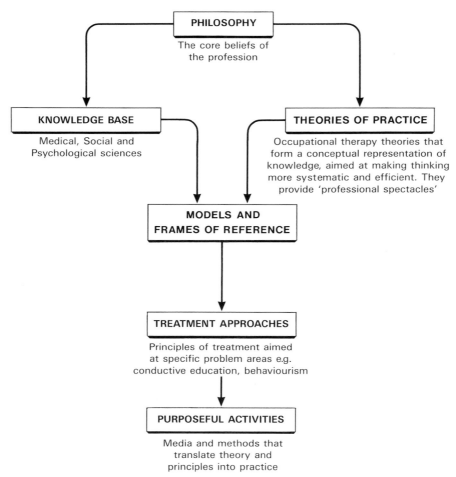

Fig. 1.1 A hierarchy for practice.

medium through which she works with the person she is treating. Her choice of activities is made in accordance with the various principles and theories upon which she bases her practice. These principles and theories are linked to the medical, psychological and social sciences, which inform her of how the healthy individual, his family and his society function, and provide insight into how this functioning can be disrupted by ill health and disability. However, underpinning these bodies of knowledge, from which the therapist will choose to suit her particular area of practice, lie the fundamental beliefs upon which the therapist bases all her professional practice.

This chapter reviews several definitions of occupational therapy that have been put forward over the years in order to draw from them these fundamental beliefs and assumptions that all occupational therapists hold and which together might be called the 'philosophy of occupational therapy' — that is, the profession's 'view of the nature of its existence'. This philosophy guides and gives meaning to the occupational therapist's activities. It is a set of core beliefs, values and principles — a creed that shapes the thinking of the profession, forming a basis for practice and for the acquisition of knowledge, skills, principles and methods.

DEFINITIONS OF OCCUPATIONAL THERAPY

Whilst occupational therapy has been established in the United Kingdom only since the Second World War, some of its basic principles are rooted in the medical practice of ancient times (see Ch. 2). More than 100 years before Christ, Aesclepiades was reputed to recommend activity for his patients. In AD 172, Galen maintained that 'Employment is nature's best physician and is essential to human happiness' (cited in MacDonald et al 1970). In modern times, definitions of occupational therapy have echoed this idea, whilst, at the same time, expanding the thinking that underlies the profession's holistic ideas.

One of the earliest definitions of occupational therapy came from the Board of Control in England in a 1933 memorandum, which stated that 'Occupational therapy is the treatment, under medical direction, of physical or mental disorders, by the application of occupation and recreation, with the object of promoting recovery, of creating new habits and of preventing deterioration.'

In 1945 J. H. C. Colson, author of *The Rehabilitation of the Injured*, defined occupational therapy as 'the use of any occupation which is prescribed and guided for the purpose of contributing to, and hastening the rehabilitation of the unfit'. In 1946, Howarth and MacDonald, early pioneers of occupational therapy in Britain, published *The Theory of Occupational Therapy*, where they defined occupational therapy as 'any work or recreational activity, mental or physical, definitely prescribed and guided, for the distinct purpose of contributing to, and hastening, recovery from disease or injury'.

'An active method of treatment with a profound psychological justification' was the definition put forward by Clark in 1952, followed, in 1955, by O'Sullivan, an English doctor specialising in physical medicine, who wrote in *The Textbook of Occupational Therapy* that he favoured the definition that occupational therapy was 'the treatment, under expert medical supervision, of mental or physical disease, by means of suitable occupation, whether mental, physical, social or recreational'.

As occupational therapy practice continued to expand and gain credibility, various definitions of the profession appeared in order to explain and consolidate the basis upon which occupational therapists practised. More modern definitions have endeavoured to either give a fully comprehensive idea of the scope of occupational therapy — namely, this Definition for Licensure from the Minutes of the 1981 AOTA Representative Assembly: 'Occupational therapy is the use of purposeful activity with individuals who are limited by physical injury or illness, psychosocial dysfunction, developmental or learning disabilities, poverty and cultural differences or the aging process in order to maximise independence, prevent disability and maintain health'; and this, written in *Current Occupational Therapy Practice* by a group of occupational therapists working in the North East Thames Regional Health Authority in 1987: 'Occupational therapy is the assessment and treatment of people of all ages with physical and mental health problems, through specifically selected and graded activities in order to help them reach their maximum level of functioning and independence in all aspects of daily life. These aspects will include their personal independence, employment, social, recreational and leisure pursuits and their interpersonal relationships.'

Alternatively, the profession has tried to provide a short, readily understood and easily remembered definition such as this European definition published in the *British Journal of Occupational Therapy* in May 1989: 'Occupational therapists assess and treat people using purposeful activity to prevent disability and develop independent function'; or this World Federation of Occupational Therapy definition (also May 1989): 'Occupational therapy is the treatment of physical and psychiatric conditions through specific activities in order to help people reach their maximum level of function and independence in all aspects of daily life.'

FUNDAMENTAL BELIEFS

Whilst probably none of these statements would claim to be definitive, they serve as excellent starting-points for an examination of the philosophy of occupational therapy. Throughout the definitions there appear to run several underlying thoughts and common links. These are:

1. That the individual is in a state which he wishes to improve

Words and phrases such as 'physical and mental disorder', 'unfit', 'hastening recovery', 'mental or physical disease', 'illness', 'dysfunction', 'disabilities' and 'problems' imply that the person is not in a state of well-being. This unfitness has traditionally been defined and studied in medical terms. Whilst occupational therapists need to be aware of the effect of illness on the individual in order to understand and predict the likely passage of that person through his various treatments, they have come to recognise with more confidence in recent years that whilst medical illness is often a catalyst for dysfunction or disability, its wider-ranging implications for the person's social, work and recreational roles are just as important. Therefore, whilst it is vital for the occupational therapist to have a sound theoretical background in those areas of medical illness that are most likely to cause prolonged disability, it is equally important that she study the psychological, social, economic and recreational aspects of the healthy and unhealthy individual.

With this understanding it is easier to see that, whilst many occupational therapists are 'hospital-based' (for hospital, after all, is the focal point of treatment in the acute stages of illness or disability), equally as many are now based in areas where people who have passed through the acute stages of treatment are gaining support from both society and professionals in order to learn to live their lives to the fullest.

2. That the therapist uses activity as the medium for this improvement

There is frequent use, in the definitions above, of words such as 'employment', 'occupation' and 'activity'. Throughout, it is emphasised that the activity used should be 'selected' and 'purposeful', that is that the activity is not used for its own sake but it is directed and chosen for a specific need of the individual. Hinojosa et al, writing in the American Journal of Occupational Therapy on 'Purposeful Activities' in 1983, stated that 'Purposeful activity can be defined as tasks or experiences in which the individual actively participates. Engagement in purposeful activity requires and elicits co-ordination between one's physical, emotional and cognitive systems. An individual who is involved in purposeful activity directs attention to the task itself, rather than to the internal processes required for the achievement of the task'.

Activity, therefore, is a means to an end (see Ch. 6). It is not always the particular *nature* of the activity that is important (other than the fact that it should encourage the participation of the individual), but rather the *purpose* for which it was selected and the *aim* it hopes to achieve. In 1955, O'Sullivan wrote in *A Textbook of Occupational Therapy* that 'The curative aspect [of activity] is to occupational therapy what the soul is to the body. It is the vital principle which gives life, and without which the treatment is no longer treatment . . . . The soul, or therapy, is gone and the lifeless body, or occupation, is all that remains.' This principle is exactly reflected in the words of an anonymous patient:

Here I sit at this great big loom,
Making God knows what for God knows whom.

The use of activity also implies that the individual is *active*, that is that he participates in the occupation or task that is being used. It reflects the belief that man is an inherently active animal who, when in a state of well-being, will normally work, play and take care of himself. Occupational therapists believe, therefore, that the use of this natural state of activity in order to restore the status quo is one that draws upon the individual's inherent nature. As we have seen, although the purpose of activity may be the acquisition of a long- or short-term goal which will help, in part, or wholly, to restore a state of well-being, the activity used should also be appropriate to the individual, reflecting his interests, skills, culture and age. In other words, the activity itself, in order to bring its own rewards, should be one with which the individual can identify. For example, the therapist may be seeing two people, both of whom require activity to encourage the use of an injured and unsightly hand. For one person cookery may provide the medium through which he will be encouraged to work whilst the other will be more inclined to use a computer or word processor.

Participation and achievement in activity does, in itself, bring reward, which may be reflected in the individual's willingness to continue. There are many activities in which humans participate which have developed beyond the satisfaction of basic needs. Why else, for instance, do we spend hours decorating a cake or planning a surprise party when a simple sandwich would satisfy hunger or a hug and a kiss would say 'I love you'? One explanation may be that participation in the (goal-directed) activity brings satisfaction in its own right. Similarly, humans derive pleasure from participating in art, social and musical activities, and the pleasure and sense of achievement gained from such activities can also be used to advantage by the therapist.

3. *That the individual is aiming for the restoration, or achievement, of the skills required for daily life and that he has the capacity to change in order to achieve this.*

The definitions talk of 'creating new habits', 'rehabilitation', 'recovery', 'maximis[ing] independence', 'reach[ing a] maximum level of functioning and independence' and helping the individual to 'restore function'. This reflects the therapist's belief that the individual wishes to acquire skills that will enable him to return to, or reach, a level of function in everyday tasks which will enable him to perform his daily activities to the best of his abilities. It also reflects the belief that humans in a normal state of well-being wish to function autonomously. Whilst 'no man is an island' capable of existing without interaction with others, the individual's desire to be able to take care of himself and his family, to work and play and make decisions in a manner which he finds acceptable, is a normal and natural one, and it is this state which the therapist aims to help him achieve.

There is also a basic assumption within this that individuals are capable of change. Keilhofner (1980), in depicting the human being as an 'open system' (see p. 373), acknowledges this ability of the individual to react to, and be changed by, his environment. With a basic belief in the ability of the individual to embrace change, be it at the level of performance, habituation or volition (Keilhofner 1980), the occupational therapist can establish a programme of intervention with each individual on the understanding that he has the ability to change in response to it. Without this fundamental belief the possibility of establishing new habits, ideas and functions could not be acknowledged.

In *Occupational Therapy in Rehabilitation* (MacDonald et al 1970) these beliefs are aptly reflected in the statement that 'even as techniques and aspects change, the basic philosophy and principles of treatment remain very much the same as they have been throughout history. The primary needs of man are still for acceptance, recognition and security in home and job.' Or, as Betty Yerxa, an American professor of occupational therapy says, we 'elevate the commonplace' — we attach importance to, and help restore, everyday skills, however mundane they may appear to be.

4. *That each person is an individual and inherently different from any other*

This belief is also fundamental to the principles discussed so far. Why else, for example, should the therapist be concerned that the activity, task or occupation chosen should reflect the interests and skills of the individual? Why else should skills be achieved that enable the individual to function within his own culture and environment?

This belief is also reflected in the fact that the therapist works *with* the person in order to decide which areas of function are lacking and which of these the person feels should be given priority. It also behoves the therapist to acquire knowledge of social, cultural, occupational and physical functioning so that, as well as gaining as thorough an understanding of the other person's way of life as possible, she may be able to establish these priorities temporarily for the person should he not be capable of doing so for himself (see Ch. 3).

It is interesting to note Licht's observation in the *Occupational Therapy Source Book* (1948) that 'the concept of occupational therapy . . . goes back to the time of Cicero but its practical application was not possible until men regarded other men as equal.' This statement has interesting implications. Within it lies the fact that occupational therapists respect and treat others as individuals in their own right. They accept that people differ from one another, and, indeed, from the therapist herself, in their beliefs, needs, standards and aspirations, but that none of these is 'right' or 'wrong'. Whilst a therapist may need to discuss the concept of whether a behaviour is acceptable or not within society, this does not imply that she should inflict standards and beliefs on others.

OCCUPATIONAL THERAPY AND MEDICINE

It is also interesting to follow the development of beliefs related both to those who are 'sick' and to the growth of occupational therapy as it relates to the medical profession. Historically, occupational therapy has grown up under the wing of medicine. For whatever reason, be it a desire to gain respectability, recognition or confidence, or a lack of adequate resources to carry out its 'holistic' philosophy independently, occupational therapy has traditionally been linked to the medical model. Early texts reflect this position. In *An approach to Occupational Therapy* (1960) Mary S. Jones writes: 'On admission the occupational therapist stresses to the patient that "the work is planned to fulfil the doctor's aims of treatment"' and that 'It is the medical officer's responsibility to place the emphasis of treatment where it is of most value to the individual patient.' Howarth and MacDonald state in *The Theory of Occupational Therapy* (1946) that 'The occupational therapist carries out her treatment on prescription from the medical officer only. No case should be dealt with without this prescription.' The use of words such as 'patient', 'prescription' and 'case' signals that the setting is certainly a medical one. The implication of this, i.e. that the medical officer takes overall responsibility for the treatment, certainly reflects that both the therapist and patient were well and truly under the doctor's thumb and that the treatment prescribed wholly reflected the doctor's rather than the patient's view of his needs. How different from the practice of today, in which, as Eileen

Bumphrey (1987) states, 'The emphasis is on the therapist working *with* the disabled person to achieve what he or she wants to do.'

But medicine and occupational therapy have always been rather uneasy bedfellows (see Table 1.1). Their beliefs are fundamentally different, even opposing, and whilst occupational therapy may have gained much in confidence and succour from medicine during its developmental years its status as a Profession Supplementary to Medicine is not one that rests entirely happily on its shoulders. This growing confidence in the therapist's policy of working *with* the individual and increasingly, in locations other than hospitals, perhaps heralds the emergence of a more widely-based professional practice.

Table 1.1 A comparison of the values underlying the practices of occupational therapy and medicine (from Kielhofner 1983)

Occupational therapy	Medicine
Essential humanity of patient, obligation to provide life satisfaction for severely disabled	Freedom from threat of death, responsibility limited to illness
Maintain and enhance health, support healthy aspects of person	Eradicate disease, pathology, confer the sick role
Self-directedness and responsiblity of patient	Of patient compliance to orders, moral authority
Generalist, integrated view of patient	Specialist, reductionistic emphasis on organ systems
Therapeutic relationship of mutual cooperation with patient; shared and sapiental authority of physician	Therapeutic relationship of activity of physician, passivity of patient; Aesculapian and sapiental authority of physician
Patient acts on environment rather than determined by it	Patient as determined by environment and 'body machine'
Faith in patient's potential	Faith in science and healer's competence and charismatic authority
Patient productivity and participation	Patient relieved of all responsibilities except getting well
Play, leisure activities as essential components of balanced life	Recovery from illness, freedom from disease as major concern
Understand subjective perspectives of patient	Emphasis on objectivity, analysis, observation and diagnosis

CONCLUSION

In conclusion, therefore, we can summarise the beliefs of the occupational therapy profession. Occupational therapists believe that:

- Occupation (purposeful activity) is central to normal human existence and that its absence or disruption is a threat to health.
- When health is disrupted, selected occupation is an effective means of recouping normal behaviour and function.
- There is inherent value in activity; experiencing the 'doing process' is what brings results. This involves active participation and effort on the part of the individual, and selection of the appropriate activity, occupation or task by the therapist.
- All individuals have value. Each individual has his own skills, problems, needs and motives, and social and cultural heritage. The individual needs to work *with* the therapist in determining the priorities for the restoration of function.

Perhaps a final word can come from Jean Edwards, principal of the Dorset House School of Occupational Therapy in Oxford until 1989, who, in 1980, said: 'The uniqueness of occupational therapy does not lie in individual parts of its theory but in the particular combination of knowledge, skills and experience the occupational therapist brings to her/his work.'

ACKNOWLEDGEMENT

My thanks to Betty Collins, former principal of the Dorset House School of Occupational Therapy, Oxford, for helping in the formulation of the thinking behind this chapter.

REFERENCES

British Journal of Occupational Therapy 1989 May: 52:5, OT News
Bumphrey E 1987 Occupational therapy in the community. Woodhead-Faulkner, Cambridge
Colson J H C 1945 The rehabilitation of the injured. Cassell, London
Howarth N A, MacDonald E M 1946 The theory of occupational therapy, 3rd edn. Baillière Tindall & Cox, London
Hinojosa J, Sabari J, Rosenfeld M 1983 American Journal of Occupational Therapy 37: 805–6
Jones M S 1960 An approach to occupational therapy. Butterworth, London
Kielhofner G 1983 Health through occupation. F. A. Davis, Philadelphia

Licht S 1948 Occupational therapy source book. Williams & Wilkins, Baltimore
MacDonald E M, MacCaul G, Murrey L 1970 Occupational therapy in rehabilitation, 3rd edn. Baillière Tindall & Cassell, London
Minutes of AOTA Representative Assembly 1981 American Journal of Occupational Therapy 35: 798–9
O'Sullivan E 1955 Textbook of occupational therapy. H K Lewis, London
Punwar A 1988 Occupational therapy principles and practice. Williams & Wilkins, Baltimore
World Federation of Occupational Therapy 1989 British Journal of Occupational Therapy. May: 52:5, OT News
Young M 1984 Models of practice for occupational therapy. British Journal of Occupational Therapy 381

2

The history of occupational therapy

Ann Turner

INTRODUCTION

As has been seen in the previous chapter, occupational therapy aims to help people with disabilities to regain the highest possible level of functioning through the use of selected, purposeful activity. Although the profession of occupational therapy is relatively young, the idea of using activity as a means of helping the 'sick' is by no means new. This chapter follows the use of activity as therapy from antiquity to modern times in order to provide a historical context for present-day theory and practice.

It will be seen that the use of therapeutic occupation in previous centuries was applied to the treatment of mental illness. In our own century, immediately following the Second World War, it also found application in the treatment of physical disability. The influence of the 'medical model' of treatment upon occupational therapy in the post-war period is considered, along with the subsequent — and rather unfortunate — division of the discipline into 'diversional' and 'therapeutic' branches.

The rapid expansion of medical knowledge in recent decades has also had a profound impact upon the profession, leading occupational therapists to re-examine their role. The last section of the chapter briefly outlines the search by occupational therapists for an invigorated philosophy and for sound models of practice, a search which has led towards the more overtly holistic approach that characterises the practice of occupational therapy today.

ROOTS FROM ANCIENT TIMES

Whilst there is no historical reference to occupational therapy as such until the present century, Egyptian writings dating from as long ago as 2000 BC tell of temples where 'melancholics' congregated in large numbers to seek relief. 'Games and recreations' were instituted, and everyone's time 'was taken up by some pleasurable occupation' (Pinel, *Nosographic Philosophique* 1803, cited in Howarth & MacDonald 1946). The classical god of healing, Aesculapius, was reputed to have quietened delirium 'with songs, farces and music' (Le Clerc, *History of Physick* 1699, cited in MacDonald et al 1970). Aulus Cornelius Celsus (AD 14–37), a Roman encyclopaedist whose writings included an account of surgical practice, also recommended 'music, conversation, reading, exercise to the point of fatigue, travel and a change of scenery' to ease troubled minds (Licht 1948). The celebrated Greek physician, Galen (AD c. 130–200) advocated treatment by occupation, suggesting digging, fishing, housebuilding and shipbuilding. Galen also felt that 'Employment is nature's best physician and is essential to human happiness' (cited in MacDonald et al 1970).

Little development of the idea of using occupation therapeutically seems to have been recorded in the Dark Ages, although the fifth-century author, Martianus Capella, recommended music for the treatment of 'disturbance of the mind and disease of the body' (Licht 1948) and Caelius Aurelianus, a physician whose writings date from the fourth or fifth century, emphasised that the patient should share the effort of rehabilitating himself.

THE 18TH AND 19TH CENTURIES

Our modern understanding of the nature and treatment of disease has its roots in the nineteenth century. Prior to that time, it was felt that the key to the treatment (of lunatics) lay in fear, and that the best means of producing fear was by punishment. Deriving from the practices of the Dark Ages, many forms of cruel and torturous 'treatments' were devised. Lunatics were not regarded as having rights and needs, but as deserving only ridicule, confinement and punishment. The French physician, Philippe Pinel (1745–1826), took a more enlightened view and instituted reforms in the treatment of the mentally ill, the most famous of which was to release asylum inmates from their shackles. He 'prescribed physical exercises and manual occupations', believing that 'rigorously executed manual labour is the best method of securing good morale and discipline' (Pinel, *Treatise in Insanity* 1806, cited in Licht 1948). He wrote of a Spanish hospital which received patients of all ranks, pointing out that the recovery rate was higher amongst the lower classes, who were employed in the work of the hospital, than amongst the 'idle grandees'. But the idea of patients being 'put to work' met with resistance in private hospitals, where it was thought that those who paid for treatment should not be expected to work.

In the same period, the English Quaker and philanthropist William Tuke (1732–1822) established The Retreat in York, where special emphasis was placed on 'spiritual occupation' for the treatment of the mentally ill. Many physicians followed Tuke, and the 19th century saw more widespread acceptance of occupation and activity for the treatment of the mentally ill in particular. A Dr Cleaton of Liverpool, in a report to the Lunacy Commission, said: 'The most important recent improvement . . . is the extent to which occupation is adopted' (cited in Licht 1948).

THE 20TH CENTURY

By the beginning of the 20th century the idea of using activity, occupation or work in the treatment of the mentally ill had become quite widely established. At this time, it was becoming more socially acceptable for women to take up careers and to join the professions. Their traditional role, therefore, as carers of the sick, could now incorporate the expanding knowledge related to that care, and this role became more 'respectable'. According to

MacDonald (1970), however, the acceptance of treatment through activity suffered fluctuating popularity, partly because of its apparent simplicity and partly because too much depended on the enthusiasm of particular doctors to use and prescribe it. One might be tempted to ask, cynically, 'What has changed?!', for MacDonald's complaint could be echoed today, particularly by occupational therapists based in hospitals, and perhaps epitomises the difficulties of many of the professions supplementary to medicine.

The term 'occupational therapy' was first coined in the 19th century by George Barton, an American doctor. The first English training school for occupational therapists was set up at Dorset House, Bristol, a treatment centre for neurotic and early psychotic patients, by Dr Elizabeth Casson in 1930 (Fig. 2.1) and the first English conference on occupational therapy was held in 1934. Shortly thereafter, in 1936, the English Association of Occupational Therapists was formed (its active membership rising to 120 by 1944) and in 1938 the first public exams in occupational therapy were held (see Box 2.1).

(a)

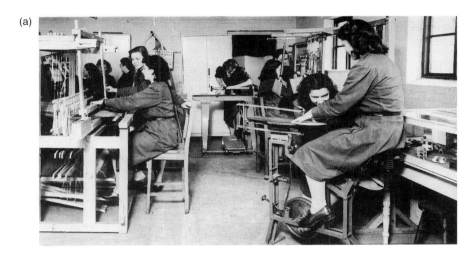

(b)

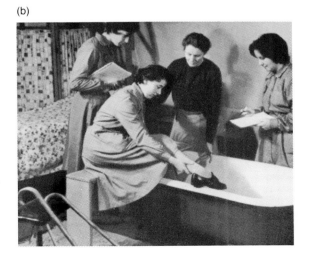

(c)

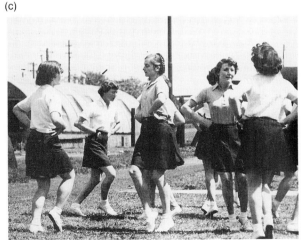

Fig. 2.1   Students training in the early days of the Dorset House School. **(a)** In the workshop. **(b)** In Activities of Daily Living. **(c)** In recreational activities. (Reproduced by kind permission of the Dorset House School of Occupational Therapy, Oxford.)

Box 2.1 Case examples

The following case histories, published in the *Lancet*, were written in 1941 by Dr Elizabeth Casson, Medical Director of the Dorset House School of Occupational Therapy, to draw attention to occupational therapy. (Reproduced by kind permission of the Dorset House School of Occupational therapy, Oxford.)

CASE 1.

A woman of 23 with arthrodesis of tuberculous hip. After operation she had developed a functional disease of the knee-joint. She was lacking in self-confidence and was too conscious of her disability. Her inability to sit at an ordinary table seemed the chief cause of her unhappiness and also her inability to return to her work as a shorthand-typist. She was taught to weave on a small loom with hand controls in order to interest her in the subject without referring to her leg. She was then promoted to a foot-power loom in which the warp was raised or lowered by flexing the knee-joint. While using the hand-loom she had become so keen on the texture and pattern of the material she was weaving that she was glad to perform the necessary movements, and was soon able to realise that her knee was quite capable of being bent to a more aesthetic posture. Her gait improved at the same time. She asked to stay on for a few weeks to finish the length of material she was weaving and then returned to her office work.

CASE 2.

A man of 53, suffering from the after-effects of acute infective polyneuritis. He had been completely paralysed for several months but had recovered sufficiently to walk, and by several trick movements he could feed himself. Treatment began with weaving a rug on a frame threaded with a warp of string. The patient's deltoid and exterior muscles were weak and could not bear the weight of his arms so his arms and hands were slung in canvas loops from brackets extended from the top of the frame. He had a spasmodic contraction of the shoulder muscles which relaxed when his arms were suspended. Improvement became evident in the first few days, since the patient enjoyed the work. The next stage was to support the wrists only on an adjustable slat placed across

the frame, again leaving the fingers free to weave and to push the threads into place, thus getting active extension of the fingers and wrists. As the muscles improved in tone and strength, new crafts were prescribed, such as knotting dog leads, stool-seating and woodwork. The dart-board for a few minutes each day helped in the cure.

CASE 3.

A man, aged 61, who had had a compound fracture of the radius from a conveyor-belt accident. His shoulder had been strained, and he had arthritis of shoulder, elbow and wrist with much residual disability of shoulder, arm and forearm. Mental depression was pronounced. Treatment was first given in the form of easy weaving on small hand-loom; at this time the therapist was making friends with the patient and gaining his confidence. Later he made a warp on the 'mill', encouraged by the knowledge that the warp was needed for another patient's work. An occupation had to be chosen that could be carried out at a level which gave easy abduction of the upper arm to begin with; this was increased gradually by raising the height of the mill without the patient noticing that he was doing more. As soon as he realised that his angel of abduction had increased his confidence was aroused and he then willingly cooperated in carrying out the changes in his work that increased the effort needed. His recovery was completed by getting him to sand-paper and paint screens raised to a level above his shoulder and to drill holes in a solitaire board, which exercised flexion and extension of wrist. Finally he did weaving on a large foot-loom which enabled him to get larger movements; easy supination was achieved by throwing and catching the shuttle.

CASE 4.

A left-handed man with compound fracture of left proximal phalanx of ring finger and simple fracture of little finger. Even passive extension of these fingers was impossible. Treatment was by joinery, which was his hobby; first he did planing with fingers extended as far as possible on the plane, and then sawing and generalised movement, with various tools, to ensure complete movement and suppleness. The patient was entirely cooperative and the fingers became almost normal.

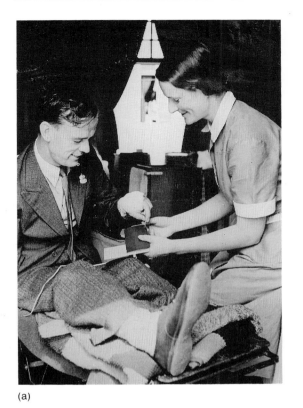

(a)

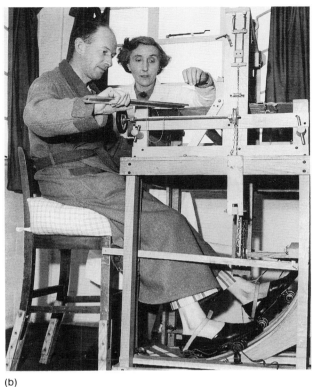

(b)

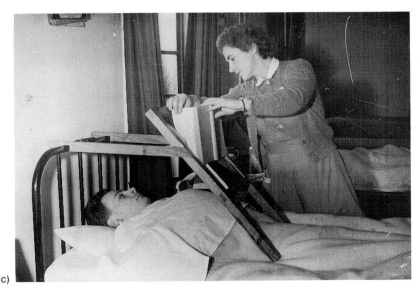

(c)

Fig. 2.2 Early days in physical occupational therapy. **(a)** A one-handed air-raid casualty learning to use his left hand. **(b)** Weaving on a loom adapted to encourage flexion and extension of the knees. **(c)** Providing a book to read for a tuberculosis sufferer on long-term bed rest. (Reproduced by kind permission of the Dorset House School of Occupational Therapy, Oxford.)

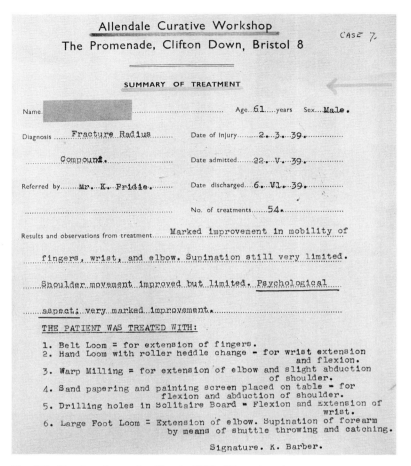

Fig. 2.3 Treatment report written in 1939. (Reproduced by kind permission of the Dorset House School of Occupational Therapy, Oxford.)

The Second World War has often been seen as the herald of the expansion of occupational therapy, especially in the field of treatment of the physically injured. Many young men who suffered appalling physical and psychological trauma during the war needed rehabilitation, particularly in relation to their 'occupational' or work needs (Fig. 2.2).

The influence of the medical model

Occupational therapy at this time was firmly established within the medical model. Colson, in 1945, defined the aims of occupational therapy in purely physical terms. He said that they were:

Conservation of muscular function,
Strengthening of weak muscles,
Mobilising of stiff joints,
Re-education of neuromuscular co-ordination in the hand, and,
Teaching the normal use of the affected part.

In deference to the holistic approach buried deep within the philosophy of occupational therapy Colson did, lastly, say that it also aimed 'To encourage the patient' (see Fig. 2.3).

A year later, in 1946, Howarth and MacDonald wrote that the occupational therapist carried out her treatment on prescription from the medical officer only. They emphasised that no case should be dealt with without his prescription. In the same year, presumably in an effort to deal with the vastly increased numbers of people requiring the services of occupational therapy, they divided the discipline into two branches. These they defined as:

1. General: This was where some form of occupation was necessary, for example where a patient has to remain in bed for a long period, in order to prevent depression and to maintain his morale
2. Special: This, by contrast, was carefully selected and prescribed treatment which had some remedial purpose in view.

One can see the separation of occupational therapy into 'diversional' (general) and 'therapeutic' (special) branches, a division which has plagued occupational therapists ever since. As 'special' occupational therapy was to be restricted to the 'curative workshops' and 'general' occupational therapy was to be restricted to long-term, bed-bound patients (Fig. 2.4), it is easy to see that the diversional side of occupational therapy is the one that was more on public view in the wards and, therefore, the one that became firmly established as the main component of occupational therapy in the eyes of other patients and hospital staff. Additionally, as many conditions involved protracted bed treatment (two years bed-rest was not exceptional for people with tuberculosis) and as, due to 'trade prejudice' it was not possible to use 'more realistic occupations', thus limiting activities the field of crafts, 'the wrong emphasis [was given to] the occupational aspect of treatment' (MacDonald et al 1970). It is clear why present-day occupational therapists have had to work hard to dispel the idea that they are mainly involved in keeping people occupied with craft activities.

However, although we have inherited some negative legacies from the immediate post-war period we are also indebted to many active pioneers who set up excellent departments during this time, based on the specific therapeutic use of a wide range of both craft and non-craft activities. Jones (1960) describes the setting-up of the Farnham Park Rehabilitation Centre (Fig. 2.5). The occupational therapy department included in its treatment programmes the repair of old

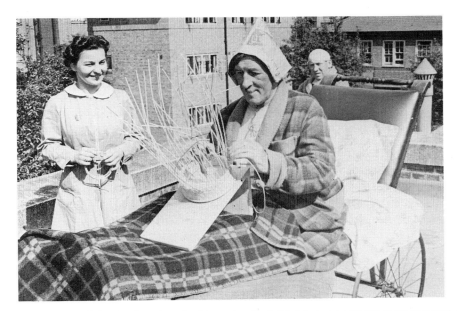

Fig. 2.4 Basketry (and sun hat!) for the long-term bed-bound patient, St John's and St Elizabeth Hospital, London, circa 1940. (Reproduced by kind permission of the Dorset House School of Occupational Therapy, Oxford.)

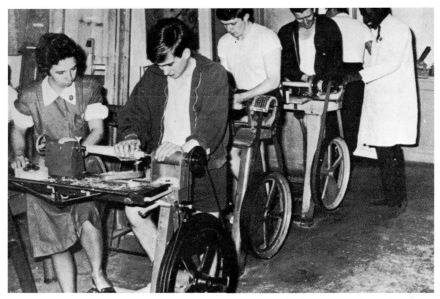

Fig. 2.5 Occupational therapy at Farnham Park Rehabilitation Centre, as depicted in the Association of Occupational Therapists' publicity brochure, 1960. (Reproduced by kind permission of the College of Occupational Therapists.)

lawnmowers and other equipment which was then used for the benefit of the department. Tool-makers and engineers helped to work out 'Heath Robinson' ideas for the first specifically designed therapeutic machinery. Those requiring brick-laying as part of treatment built the woodstore and the occupational therapy office and 'bicycle fretsaws and filing machines [were] designed and made up in the OT workshops from angle iron'. Jones reflects that there was little difficulty in arousing cooperation, as almost all the patients had been in the services. One can envisage from her account the comradeship and military heritage inherent in the establishment and functioning of Farnham Park. It is also interesting to read that, where the occupational therapists were treating people with hemiplegia, they were advised to abandon treatment in order to make way for others if improvement did not make itself evident. Clearly this was the heyday of the biomechanical approach to treatment and the future of those who did not fit readily into this legacy of World War II was not given priority. The treatment of (basically) fit young men with orthopaedic or other biomechanical problems was the order of the day in the physical field.

Following this surge of occupational therapy practice came the establishment of the World Federation of Occupational Therapists (WFOT) in 1951. In 1960 occupational therapists became State Registered under the Professions Supplementary to Medicine Act. The Council for the Professions Supplementary to Medicine was established in 1961 and the Registration Board for occupational therapists in 1962.

Re-establishing the basic philosophy

Around this period occupational therapy seemed to 'lose its way' somewhat. The basic philosophy, though unchanged, was battered by a change in expectations and attitudes, and by a vast increase in medical knowledge which left occupational therapists wondering exactly where their role lay and to which areas they should give priority. Treatment became somewhat recipe-like and occupational therapists appeared to jump on the bandwagon of whatever expanding body of knowledge was in fashion. Training schools crammed their syllabi full of 'essential' medical knowledge that the luckless student was obliged to take on board, and this academic emphasis often took place at the expense of the more practical 'activity' side of training, which was squeezed,

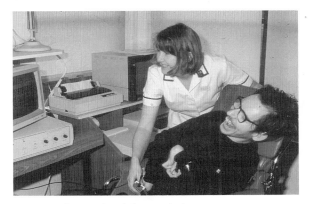

Fig. 2.6 Occupational therapy today.

somewhat, into second place. The basic philosophy of occupational therapy was rarely mentioned and students, rather than being educated into the role of problem-solvers, were instructed in the use of rather rigid treatment programmes for differing diagnoses.

Despite changing demands, occupational therapists working in the physical field still saw the problems of their patients in mainly physical, medical and biomechanical terms. Most situations were treated using specifically designed or adapted equipment such that the complexity and importance of the adaptation or equipment frequently obscured the activity it was designed to perform. Equipment was, on occasion, used for its own sake entirely and the activity was forgotten, or felt to be unnecessary or too time-consuming to organise. Lip service was paid to 'psychological problems'. 'Boosting morale' or asking about leisure activities was felt to be important but the bulk of the treatment emphasis lay in the restoration of physical function. Occupational therapists were still being asked to 'occupy' patients. They complained of occupational therapy departments being used as 'dumping grounds' where bored or long-stay patients were sent (often without reference to the occupational therapist) to 'make something' or to 'occupy their minds'. Occupational therapists, who had an increasing lack of professional confidence and virtually no managerial expertise, did not know how to correct this appalling misuse of their services. They frequently tried to cover all requests on their time, spreading their skills so thinly that they became ineffectual. It became

increasingly obvious that all was not well, that the profession had lost its way and that many occupational therapists, when challenged about what they actually did or what their philosophy was, found the question very hard to answer.

As a reaction to this, several people began hunting for a sound philosophical basis for the profession. Alongside this, the changing demands and treatments within the Health Service, the increased turnover of 'beds' within hospitals and the implementation of the Chronically Sick and Disabled Persons' Act in 1970, which heralded the influx of occupational therapists towards community care, forced occupational therapists to look back at their roots to discover and redefine the bases of their profession. From this re-examination sprang new concepts upon which occupational therapists began to be able to base their practice. These ideas, drawing upon the basic philosophy of occupational therapy, were conceptual representations aimed at organising the therapist's knowledge and making more effective and systematic her thinking and approach to the individual and his problems (see Ch. 12). 'Activities therapy', first presented by Anne Cronin Mosey in the early 1970s and the 'model of human occupation' developed by Gary Kielhofner in the 1970s and 80s are examples of such concepts.

Alongside these concepts, the first to be exclusive to occupational therapy, developed a series of approaches to specific functional problems. As previously mentioned, most intervention in the physical field was based upon the biomechanical approach. This approach viewed treatment in terms of strengthening muscles and increasing ranges of movement. As knowledge increased, however, there developed approaches to problems caused by neurological dysfunctions. Practitioners (not necessarily occupational therapists) such as Ayres, Bobath, Brunnstrom, Peto and Rood were instrumental in developing approaches to these particular problems, and their ideas were readily adopted in principle (and adapted in practice) by occupational therapists.

Additionally, occupational therapists worked increasingly in fields where preventative and prophylactic approaches were appropriate. These areas, which include coronary care, rheumatology and back care, are continually developing and implementing their approach and reflect the philosophy that the individual must take increased responsibility for his own health and well-being and work together with the therapist, who acts as a facilitator and teacher, in order to achieve this. Equally, as occupational therapists looked back to their professional roots and gained more confidence in their identity, they rediscovered the real meaning of a holistic approach to an individual and his problems. No longer are 'physical' occupational therapists averse to recognising that relaxation techniques, counselling, or behavioural regimes may be appropriate approaches to use with an individual that they are helping. Indeed, the use of educational and support groups and of perceptual and cognitive techniques are commonplace in what was once a rigid 'physical' approach to treatment.

CONCLUSION: THE FUTURE OF OCCUPATIONAL THERAPY PRACTICE

As concepts developed they increasingly encompassed the occupational therapists' basic belief in the uniqueness of the person and reflected more clearly the fact that inability to perform an activity can lie beyond the realm of pure medical science.

Thereafter came the ever-changing methods of practice. The activities used by occupational therapists as the medium through which to carry out their programmes inevitably continue to change, expand and vary depending on a wide number of influences, including (though not exclusively) fashion, technology, finances, facilities and the knowledge and interests of the therapist and the individual.

Thus has developed the hierarchy of thought, knowledge and method upon which we base our practice today (see Fig. 1.1). As we approach the 21st century occupational therapy seems to be consolidating its professional boundaries of practice. It has re-established its roots, is developing its own knowledge base and is increasingly regaining its professional identity and confidence. Clearly, occupational therapy will have much to offer in the future. Swayed and moulded as their profession will be by changing policies, fashions, knowledge and demands, occupational therapists of the future will continue to be able to offer a service to those in need of help to improve their level of functional ability.

ACKNOWLEDGEMENT

My thanks are extended to Sally Croft, Librarian at the Dorset House School of Occupational Therapy, Oxford, for all her help in compiling material for this chapter.

REFERENCES

Colson J H C 1945 The rehabilitation of the injured. Cassell, London
Howarth N A, MacDonald M 1946 The theory of occupational therapy. Baillière Tindall, London
Jones M S 1960 An approach to occupational therapy. Butterworths, London
Keilhofner G 1985 A model of human occupation. Williams and Wilkins, Baltimore

Licht S 1948 The occupational therapy source book. Williams and Wilkins, Baltimore
MacDonald M, MacCaul G, Murrey E M 1970 Occupational therapy in rehabilitation. Baillière Tindall, London
O'Sullivan E 1955 A textbook of occupational therapy. Lewis, London
Reed K, Sanderson S 1980 Concepts of occupational therapy. Williams and Wilkins, Baltimore

3

Using psychology in the treatment of physical disability

W. JoAn Davies

INTRODUCTION

This chapter aims to provide the occupational therapist with a framework within which the psychological and physical development of individuals may be understood. Beginning with a discussion of the problematic concept of 'normality', the first sections of the chapter emphasise that stress, disability and illness are not 'abnormal' but, rather, virtually inevitable challenges of human life. In seeking to set and meet his own goals for self-fulfilment the disabled person is particularly disadvantaged by the general perception that he is not like 'normal' people, whereas his needs — for security, self-esteem, understanding, and so on — are fundamentally the same as everyone else's.

Next, the chapter considers the effect that particular factors such as social context, bonding, play and role expectations have upon psychological development and well-being.

The middle sections of the chapter are devoted to Summaries of Development through Different Age Groups. Following Erik Erikson's theory of developmental stages, these trace the physical and psychological changes that occur over the course of a person's lifetime.

The remaining sections of the chapter consider the responses that the occupational therapist might expect from someone whose life-course has been seriously disrupted by disability, illness or some other significant loss. The components of bereavement — loss of self-esteem, loss of earlier roles, etc. — are described and the stages of mourning, through which the individual's initial reactions of numbness, guilt, anger and denial are replaced by acceptance and optimism, are laid out. This is followed by a description of the impact of emotions, attitudes and motivations upon the disabled individual's adjustment to his changed circumstances.

In the concluding section of the chapter, the relationship between the therapist and the individual is considered, giving special emphasis to the holistic approach that the therapist must adopt when entering into a rehabilitative partnership with the disabled person.

NORMALITY, STRESS AND STIMULATION

An understanding of the normal, or usual, physical, psychological and social events in the lives of human beings is important for us as therapists as we deal with people in varying situations and at different points along the continuum of what we call 'normality'. Such an understanding provides a point of reference from which any particular situation can be measured. But the old question, 'What is normality?', arises, and while this is no place for a full debate on this concept there are some important points that need to be borne in mind.

● Luke, now 18 months old, is a happy, lively and boisterous little boy who has been walking unaided since he was 15 months old. He's a non-stop chatterer but has only about six words that the rest of us use. His favourite pastime is putting things into other things or emptying every container in sight. He has 16 teeth and enjoys feeding himself, and is beginning to keep his spoon from turning over. Sometimes he prefers to be helped as it seems to be quicker.

● Amanda was walking at 12 months and at 18 months has a large vocabulary of about 40 words.

She's a quieter, shyer child whose favourite occupation seems to be 'reading' her books. She has 8 teeth and tries to feed herself though she cannot yet prevent her spoon from turning over. At present she is very determined to do it all herself, and so gets very frustrated.

● Adam is a bright, friendly little boy of 16 months who uses his 20 words or so as often as he can with everyone he meets. He may sit quietly, playing on his own for almost an hour, though sometimes he enjoys making lots of noise with his favourite toys — cars and aeroplanes. Adam is still not walking without holding on and has just 4 teeth. He feeds himself quite well without making too much mess.

These three children are all different, having reached their own, differing stages of development. Each of them can be described as a normal, healthy toddler.

When we think of normality as a continuum we can see that what is normal for one person may not be so for another. In the first place, we have to guard against our tendency to make assumptions about another's life events or experiences in terms of normality. When involved in treatment we need to start by assessing not only the individual's physical situation but also his social and psychological background (see p. 52). Secondly, it is important that we examine our own attitudes to what people call 'illness' or 'disability'. Why, for instance, is there a prevalent idea in society today that these are abnormal states, with the result that people labelled 'ill' or 'disabled' are somehow placed in a different category from others, who then become labelled 'normal'? A common assumption, it seems, is that anything of a stressful nature is bad and provides an abnormal situation to be coped with.

NORMALITY AND STRESS

Stress, to a certain degree, is essential to our development as healthy human beings, keeping us mentally alert and helping us to find and use appropriate methods for coping. In normal circumstances none of us is without stress; stress is inevitably provided by the demands of daily life.

However, we all know when these small stresses begin to come too thick and fast and we may say 'I can do without all this hassle.' On the other hand, we also know that when nothing seems to challenge us or to require us to make decisions we feel bored and set out to look for excitement because the stress level is too low. Stress helps to satisfy the need for stimulation, particularly in the

THE HOLMES AND RAHE SOCIAL READJUSTMENT RATING SCALE	
Life event	Mean value
1 Death of spouse/child	100
2 Divorce	73
3 Marital separation from mate	65
4 Detention in jail or other institution	63
5 Death of a close family member	63
6 Major personal injury or illness	53
7 Marriage	50
8 Being fired at work	47
9 Marital reconciliation with mate	45
10 Retirement from work	45
11 Major change in the health or behaviour of a family member	44
12 Pregnancy	40
13 Sexual difficulties	39
14 Gaining a new family member	39
15 Major business readjustment (e.g. merger, reorganisation, bankruptcy, etc.)	39
16 Major change in financial state	38
17 Death of a close friend	37
18 Changing to a different line of work	36
19 Major changes in the number of arguments with spouse	35
20 Taking on a mortgage greater than ...? (the maximum possible — author.)	31
21 Foreclosure on mortgage or loan	30
22 Major change in responsibilities at work	29
23 Son or daughter leaving home	29
24 In-law troubles	29
25 Outstanding personal achievement	28
26 Wife beginning or ceasing to work outside the home	26
27 Beginning or ceasing formal schooling	26
28 Major change in living conditions	25
29 Revision of personal habits	24
30 Trouble with the boss	23
31 Major change in working hours or conditions	23
32 Change in residence	20
33 Changing to a new school	20
34 Major change in type and/or amount of recreation	19
35 Major change in church activities	19
36 Major change in social activities	18
37 Making a large purchase, (e.g. TV, car, freezer etc.) or getting a small mortgage	17
38 Major change in sleeping habits (amount of time)	16
39 Change in number of family get-togethers	15
40 Change in eating habits	15
41 Vacation	13
42 Christmas	12
43 Minor violations of the law	11

Fig. 3.1 The Holmes and Rahe Social Readjustment Rating Scale. (From: Holmes & Rahe 1967)

young, for whom coping is often learnt through play, and for the elderly, for whom the mental and physical activity involved in coming to terms with stress can provide motivation and an interest in life. Helping older people to sort out *all* their problems in an attempt to relieve them of stress is in fact doing them a disservice. Too much boredom and general lack of stimulation for many old people can contribute to both depression and a lessening of intellectual abilities. On the other hand, it must be remembered that too much stress is not good either, and can be linked with physical as well as psychological ill health (see also Yerkes–Dodson Law, p. 47). When the magnitude of life events exceeds a person's ability to cope, he suffers what we call 'stress'.

In general, the excess of stress experienced today by many people is due to 'hassle' factors, although individual life events such as those listed in Figure 3.1 increase the strain experienced. A glance at Figure 3.1 will reveal that there is in fact a good deal of stress involved in pleasant and enjoyable life events as well as in difficult and traumatic ones. Possibly the most important point about challenging events is that they involve change, and change is rarely easy. Yet another assumption we tend to hold is that the change and adjustment occasioned by pleasant life events will be easier than that demanded by painful ones. We assume that it is easier for Everyman to adjust to marriage than to bereavement, or to being made well again than to remaining an invalid. This is not necessarily so.

Illness and accidents are to some extent inevitable and cause varying degrees of stress through which we come to learn something about coping with subsequent ill health. Trauma — the severe accident — and long-term illness may lie towards one extreme of our normality continuum but they are not outside it. They may be shocking, frightening and depressing, they may make us resentful and angry, and drastically upset our equilibrium, but they are not abnormal.

Nor are these emotions 'bad' or 'good' — another commonly-held assumption. In fact, all emotions are a part of our humanity. As we have fingers and toes, so we have emotions, and the emotion an individual displays can give the therapist insight into his psychological condition. There is nothing to be gained from expecting a person's emotions to be other than they are, or from telling him that he ought to be feeling other than he is. It is what a person does with his emotions that is important, and much of a therapist's work, in any field, relates to helping him to adjust emotionally; any other approach will be counter-productive (see p. 47).

A person does not have to strive towards a mid-point of normality set out for him by society, since normality for him relates to his need to establish and maintain a comfortable fitting-together of his past with his present, so that he can face his future with confidence. It is the role of the therapist to help him to achieve this.

In order to be able to do this a person needs to have fairly high self-esteem, an ability to form affectionate bonds with others, a fair knowledge of himself and his capabilities, an ability to see what is possible and what situations he has to accept, and an ability to exercise control over himself and his life. A person with these abilities is likely to move positively towards readjustment, identifying alternative possibilities and exercising choices. However, most people would need some help, not least in the area of self-esteem. This is discussed in more detail later on (see p. 29).

DIFFERENT LIFE STAGES

It is relevant here to look at some of the usual experiences a person might have had in the past which have helped to equip him to face severe illness or disability. In order to do this, aspects of personality will be looked at in more detail, and Summaries of Development through different age groups are set out between p. 31 and p. 42 for the reader's reference.

The concept of Life Stages is a useful one in that it helps to make the point that it is the sequence in which development takes place rather than the age at which events occur that is of importance. Any new stage of physical, psychological or social development builds on the last one and is itself a prerequisite for the next stage. To take an example from physical development, a child cannot walk unless he is first able to balance and stand. Further, no amount of trying to make him walk will enable him to do so until he is ready. This is the general rule concerning development, although there are individual differences. For example, some children will be slower in learning to crawl and others may miss out this stage altogether. It is, of course, essential that therapists have expert knowledge of human physical development, from the early responses of infants to the symptoms and processes of old age, but it is not in the brief of this chapter to dwell on these.

In the psychological area of development, Erik Erikson's theory is particularly relevant since he acknowledges the importance of conflict and the stress resulting from it, emphasising the way in which individuals develop through, and indeed because of, the presence of conflict (Erikson 1963). The way in which conflicts at any one stage are dealt with by the individual sets the scene for his encounter with the conflicts of the succeeding stage. Erikson believes that the ability of children to pass through each stage successfully is largely dependent on their parents and those who care for them. However, he acknowledges that in later years a person has free will and can to some extent be responsible for himself. Further comment on his theory is to be found in the Summaries of Development.

Abraham Maslow (1954) approaches the idea that we struggle to overcome stress in a slightly different way. He says that people have various needs that have to be satisfied. He does not consider these to occur at different stages through life but to be relevant and present for all ages. He suggests that a person's main motivation in life is to satisfy his needs, which are inborn and the same for everyone, although the ways in which people satisfy them are learned and different. It is the way in which people learn and then apply their learning to coping with and satisfying their needs that results in each person being different from every other. The needs of individuals as perceived by Maslow can be summarised as a hierarchy (Fig. 3.2). He shows that until the needs in the lower part of the hierarchy are satisfied those higher up cannot benefit from attention. Thus, when a per-

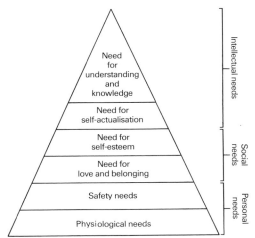

Fig. 3.2 Maslow's hierarchy of needs. (After Dworetzky 1988.) Who needs what? The patient, the family and the therapist all have their individual needs.

son is very ill he needs to have everything done for him by others — he needs security and safety. He does not at this stage care whether he is loved by others and is not concerned with self-esteem. As his physical condition improves and the lower needs are sufficiently satisfied he will be motivated to satisfy higher needs (see p. 51). When he is ill all aspects of his personality will regress so that his needs are more basic than when he is well.

Erikson helps us to see crises as a normal part of life and Maslow helps us to recognise the importance of motivation in the attainment of satisfaction. Thus we can see reinforcement for the idea that stress, illness and disability are normal and that the objective for the therapist is to help the person find the motivation to meet the challenge to cope, to find solutions, to reduce stress, and continually to adjust and reestablish equilibrium.

THE SOCIAL CONTEXT

Each aspect of development is important to, and interacts with, every other aspect. For example, the presence, and then the absence, of early physical reflexes are a basis for further physical development, but if these do not develop as expected then there will be implications for both the child's psychological development and for his social environment. How will parents cope with a child who does not do things when he 'should'? Will they reject him or give up spending time with him? How in turn will this affect his intellectual development? Will he in fact need more stimulation and attention, and if given this, what will be the effect on other children in the family? What sort of a bond will be formed between parents and the child? And, of great importance, what will the self-esteem and coping ability of the individual be as he grows into adulthood?

The term *individual differences* is one that is used to describe the differences between people in their intellectual functioning and in their personalities. While to some extent both of these depend on innate, genetic factors, the context in which development of the genetic and innate occurs is provided by the environmental setting and the experiences people have. Opportunities to learn and use certain skills, and the acquisition of learning strategies, together with what Sarason (1972) calls 'happenstance' — the chance events that occur throughout life and which can profoundly affect the individual — all form part of this environment.

Thus the environment provides the social setting for the development of individual differences, both physical and intellectual. This is the context within which a person gains his perceptions of life, of others and of himself. It is here, too, that whatever self-esteem and self-confidence he has is nurtured or stunted. In addition, what may be the 'happenstance' of trauma or illness occurs within a social setting and will have implications for a great deal of change and loss, and also will help to direct his development along lines that had not been expected.

BONDING

The socialisation of the individual begins within the family group, and it is here that there is the opportunity for the formation of the vital, close relationships between the infant and his carers which we call 'bonding'. It is these earliest relationships that first give the infant the opportunity to experience, and consequently to learn about, love and trust. It is here, too, that the infant gains the foundation for thinking and feeling

well about himself, that is, for his future self-esteem. This in turn will better enable him to cope with future strains and stresses. The importance of early bonding cannot be over-emphasised. Without it the individual may at best develop into a very insecure person greatly lacking confidence in others and in himself. At worst, if he has not learned to love, he may behave antisocially, having a total disregard for others, and being apparently unable to feel with or for them. The failure of early bonding is likely also to have a detrimental effect on intellectual development. It has been found that if for any reason this early bond is not made (sometimes due to the parents' inability to love but sometimes due to other factors) it is far more difficult to make other bonds in the future.

Factors which will influence bonding and the overall development of the child are the culture, attitudes, values and financial circumstances of his family; his sex; his birth order within the family; the expectations that others have of him; the intellectual stimulation that he is given, and so on. Each of these will have a bearing on every other factor, and it is worth making a few comments on those areas relevant to our work as therapists.

PLAY AND LEISURE

One of the most important ways in which much of our learning takes place is through play. Play helps physical development. In childhood, balance and coordination are gained from such activities as jumping, running and climbing trees. In adult life many skills are practised and learnt through leisure activities. The implications that play and leisure have for physical development and rehabilitation have always been recognised by occupational therapists. Play, however, is also essential for learning in other areas. Childhood play increases perception through the exploration and manipulation of objects. This in turn encourages creativity and originality in later years. Concepts are formed and revised, and language is encouraged through interaction with others.

Moreover, play helps a child to acquire moral codes of behaviour; through play, he learns that there are some rules that have to be kept. He learns to socialise. He learns about other people's reactions to his behaviour and about what sort of a person he is. Herein lies the basis for his self-esteem (see p. 29).

Play is not easy to define. In part this may be due to the two-sided nature of play. On one side of the coin is the way the child views play. From his point of view it is non-serious and full of enjoyment; he involves himself in it wholeheartedly. On the other side of the coin are the more serious aspects of play — these are what the educator and the therapist look at (see Fig. 3.3). Here are learning, exercise, relaxation, competition, rehabilitation, an acting-out of anxieties, and practise for future, adult events.

All these are important both in childhood play and adult leisure, and are relevant, in particular, to motivation. If a child does not want to play he will withdraw from the situation or spoil it for himself and others, and adults will not involve themselves in activities if they see them as pointless or unenjoyable. Finally, just as the two sides of the coin are still only one coin so it is important that the child's view of play dovetail with the purposes held by the therapist.

Play and leisure are important parts of life and, like all activities, take place within a sociological context. Various backgrounds and cultures will result in very different play opportunities. An impoverished child in India may be too ill or hungry to have energy even to make his own play as more fortunate children do; the rich Western child may be so accustomed to having lots of expensive toys that he soon becomes bored with them. Most young children will be happy with something so simple as a tin with a stone in it that rattles, as long as it provides opportunities for experimentation and observation.

Children who have had little opportunity for play are likely to have difficulty in adult life, particularly in their relationships with others, but it is neither the wealth nor the culture of the family that is decisive in determining the conditions for play but the attitude to play of those around the child.

Childhood play and adult play — leisure — are both important for overall health; accordingly, play and leisure are considered throughout the Summaries of Development.

CULTURE

In our country there are many people who come from other cultural backgrounds. Some have been born here, and are second or third generation British. Others have come more recently and may have brought a whole way of life from their native country. The tendency of the latter group is to live alongside others from the same cultural back-

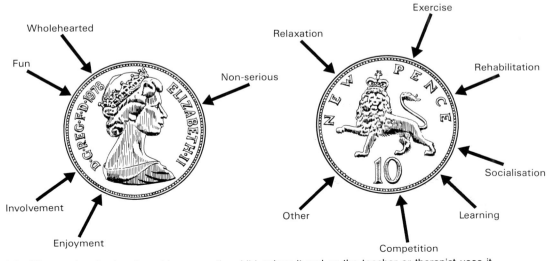

Fig. 3.3 Like a coin, play has two sides — as the child enjoys it and as the teacher or therapist uses it.

ground and to integrate very little with those of their adopted country. However, when it comes to illness it is the system of the adopted country that finds itself coping with those with different beliefs and habits and therefore with different expectations. It is not so much the colour of a person's skin that makes him different as the beliefs and attitudes fundamental to his culture. Many of these arise from religious beliefs. Moslems and Hindus often practice their religion more strictly than do people in Western society; their beliefs may be reflected in the preparation of food and the practice of fasting, the attitude to alcohol, the treatment of women and in views concerning education. In Western societies, education is geared towards the acquisition of knowledge and skills. For the Hindu or Moslem, education is geared towards 'becoming a good person'. Inevitably, these differences in education are going to have far-reaching cultural and social implications.

Culture and sickness

In a Moslem culture illness or accidents will be seen as 'the Will of Allah' and there will be a degree of passive acceptance. This also occurs in pagan societies where belief in spirits is paramount and where people may live or die according to what the 'medicine man' might say. Such attitudes sometimes inhibit recovery because the person tends to give up. It is here that the therapist may be tempted to become frustrated or even angry with one who 'will not try'. Realising that this attitude is based in a person's religion might help her to see things from his perspective, and to take his point of view rather than her own expectations as a starting-point. It is essential, always, that the therapist aims to 'meet' a person where he is rather than where she would like him to be.

Behaviour regarding illness is also different. People from many other countries expect to be fed by their relatives in hospital. Instead they find they have to eat foreign food, which is sometimes 'unclean' by their religious standards. They expect to be able to support each other in times of stress or illness by sitting with them for long hours, even sleeping on the floor alongside — a practice hardly acceptable to Western society. In Western society, those in hospital will probably be left on their own for long hours, particularly at night. When such deprivation has to be faced by people used to the constant presence and support of their family it must be devastating, and add an unacceptable degree of fear to the situation. Fortunately, most hospitals are ready and able to accommodate the particular needs of other cultures more easily now than in past years.

The religious quest for wholeness is also relevant to the experience of pain. In Western cultures we go to the doctor and try to describe particular symptoms and pains, but in Asia, for example, a person will say he is not functioning very well and has pain everywhere. Pain and illness are recognised by him as affecting his whole being and way of life, and so he experiences the pain as being 'everywhere'. His concern with wholeness also leads to a reluctance with respect to post mortems and transplants.

ROLES

Our cultural background also provides the setting in which we develop various roles, in particular those relating to family membership. The role of a mother or of a wife in a Western family will be different from that of a Chinese wife or mother.

The perceptions we have of others and of ourselves to a great extent depend on the roles that people occupy in life since, 'role' refers to expected patterns of behaviour associated with positions in society.

Our gender role seems to be established early in life, probably in part due to learning to identify with the behaviour of those of our own sex at home, at school and wherever we are seen to be dressed as members of one or the other sex. The role of wife or mother mentioned above will be based on learning that complies with the cultural expectations of the female sex. There may well be biological reasons, as well, for our gender identification, but whatever the reasons it is certain that being able to identify with one or the other sex is one of the fundamental points of reference for the perception we have of ourselves.

Our role identification also relates to the job we do and in life we have to switch between various roles according to differing situations. A woman may be mother and wife at home, a solicitor at work, a good athlete with her hockey team and a valued member of the church in her home town. All these together help to build her self-image and self-esteem. Others, however, will see her in only one or two of these roles — as the mother and wife or the solicitor, and so their perception of her will inevitably be different.

The sick role

When a person is in hospital he does not suddenly change his own behaviour or become a different person. It is the situation that has changed and seems to require him to be a different person. In hospital he is seen initially as 'a patient', since those treating him will know little or nothing else about him. As he enters the hospital, he brings with him the person he perceives himself to be, but soon realises that the role he is now expected to adopt is that of 'patient'. It must sometimes feel as though he has been asked to leave his real self at home, just as might happen when a man enters prison and has all of his own clothes taken away from him (see Fig. 3.4). In hospital he loses his autonomy. He sits or lies down to converse with others, is told what has to be done for him — in which decision he probably has little choice — and is literally pushed around by other people.

There is also a role expectation for the position of being 'disabled' which tends to belittle the person, who is now not expected to be able to do anything much and nothing terribly well. Everyone, including the disabled person, needs to take responsibility for himself and his progress towards fulfilment. His attitudes and motivation are very important aspects of this. If subjectivity alone were relevant the disabled person might be able to cope with the practical aspects of his life, with or without the help of the appropriate therapist. But although he may learn to adapt, he has to be very strong to break out from the role inflicted on him, which verifies rather than negates his position as a disabled person. This is considered further when attitudes are discussed in relation to slow progress towards recovery (p. 50).

SELF-ESTEEM

Self-perception and self-esteem have been mentioned so far only in passing, but it is hoped that already it is apparent just how important they are, not least in illness — short or long term — and disability.

Self-esteem relates directly to the image a person has of himself; in accordance with his self-image he will value himself more, or less, highly. The individual learns to develop a self-image when he is very young and during his teenage years; in this he is influenced both by adults, who will tell him whether or not they like his behaviour, and by his peers, particularly when at play or engaged in informal activities. To some extent his own personality is relevant. For example, a sensitive person may pick up more messages (verbal and non-verbal), and may even read more into them than was intended, than

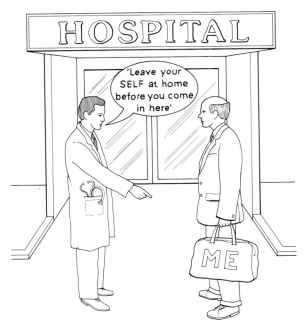

Fig. 3.4 It must feel as if he's been asked to leave his real Self at home.

would someone less sensitive. But it is the interpretations of the messages that have a great effect on the resulting perception and, therefore, on the self-esteem which a person develops. A child who is praised, encouraged and approved of and who is helped to face and come to terms with stresses and conflicts in his early years will grow up to think well of himself and to have confidence in his ability to face the future, whatever it brings.

A child who is much criticised, ridiculed and shamed is likely to grow up having low self-esteem and to be lacking in confidence. Equally, a child who has not been helped to face up to his childhood problems but has had them all solved for him has indeed been 'spoilt', since he will find it difficult to face up to life's crises in adulthood.

Low self-esteem and a lack of self-confidence may well be seen in the way a person tries to put others down, to criticise and even to bully, since in so doing he strives (in vain, as it happens) to raise himself up, by comparison. He needs to behave like this because it feels to him as though he is unloved and unappreciated and that life is not fair. He has brought the opinions of others from childhood into adult life where, it seems, he is stuck with them. This is the person who will tell you he is as good as the next man, but only because, deep down, he does not actually feel that this is so; in fact, he possibly believes he is not worth bothering with or that he hasn't got the physical or emotional strength to survive the situation. Such a person will not have good coping ability for facing the crisis of his illness or accident and its future implications. This is the person who needs help to realise that much of what he was blamed and criticised for, as a child, lies far in his past and is not relevant to his adult life. Possibly (and there are many people who have suffered much misunderstanding and cruelty as children) much of what he was led to believe about himself never, in fact, was true.

However well or poorly the person is equipped to cope, the fact remains that the crisis that his illness or disability has faced him with is not going to be easy to adapt to. He is going to need all the help that the therapist has to offer him.

SUMMARIES OF DEVELOPMENT THROUGH DIFFERENT AGE GROUPS

All human growth takes place within a developmental framework and it is necessary for us to take this framework into consideration in our work as occupational therapists. To help in this, the various events that take place throughout life have been summarised below, along with the physical changes and developments that occur at each stage of life and the effect all these have on a person's psychology as he grows and changes.

It will be seen that the summary of the development of the young child is set down in slightly different form from the other four, which cover adolescence, young adulthood, the middle years and old age.

Reference has been made throughout the Summaries to Erik Erikson's (1963) stages of psychosocial development; the age groupings are his. There is a summary of each stage as seen by Erikson, together with the new strength or 'basic virtue' which, in Erikson's view, a person will gain from that stage if all goes well. Erikson suggests that each stage of development can be summarised in terms of one particular conflict or 'crisis'. The virtue a person is able to gain from each crisis becomes the foundation on which he is able to face the next stage and a new crisis. As a cumulative theory, Erikson's helps to stress the importance of each stage for the development of a balanced and healthy person; as a holistic theory, it has great value in relating each aspect of the person to every other.

It is worth repeating that in any area of life it is not the events themselves that are of greatest importance, but the ability of a person to overcome, and with the help of others, to take something positive from the unfortunate events, and to make the most of the good experiences in order to help build a fulfilling future.

Finally, because play is a feature of development of great importance for the individual from childhood to old age, regular comments on play and leisure are made throughout the summaries.

STAGE 1: CHILDHOOD
(BIRTH–11/12 YEARS)

PHYSICAL DEVELOPMENT

It goes without saying that a child grows and changes from the moment of conception. It is important that therapists are aware of the processes involved in this growth and change. As there are many books that discuss child development the subject will not be explored here, but Illingworth (1983) sets out some basic principles which need to be remembered. These are summarised below.

The basic principles of physical development

- It is a continuous process from birth to maturity.
- The sequence involved is the same for all but the rate of progress varies.
- It is related to maturation, e.g. all nerve cells are present at birth but pathways develop and muscles are used with increasing skill.
- Mass activity is replaced by specific responses, i.e. the use of gross movements is followed by the ability to use fine movements.
- Development is cephalocaudal, i.e. it takes place from the head downwards. (Control of the head preceeds that of the arms and hands, which preceeds that of the legs.)
- Primitive reflexes have to be lost before voluntary control is acquired. For example, a neonate supported in the standing position will carry out walking movements with his legs ('placing'). These disappear, to occur later under gradually increasing voluntary control.

The following are also of importance:
- Prenatal factors adversely affecting growth and development, such as drugs, smoking, diet, etc.
- The possible effects of birth trauma, e.g. anoxia or brain damage.
- Postnatal care to avoid such problems as phenylketonuria, congenital hip dislocation, etc.

- 'Sensitive periods' (when development is most likely to take place).
- Inherited and environmental factors influencing physical and psychological development.
- The holistic nature of development. It takes place physically in relation to psychological development, and within a specific social setting.

Readers will find it helpful to have easy reference to *From Birth to Five Years: Children's Developmental Progress* by Mary Sheridan (1975), which offers further insight into these areas.

SOCIAL DEVELOPMENT

The most important early relationship is experienced in *bonding* — the forming of a close emotional relationship between the infant and his primary carer or carers. Bonding can take place with more than one person — perhaps with up to five who are very familiar to the infant. Through bonding the child is thought to learn to love and trust others because of his experience of being loved himself. Privation or deprivation of bonds is likely to affect, adversely, the adult personality.

Play: 0–1 year

Interactions with others develop through play. At first the child plays on his own, but responds to adults.

Erikson's stage of Trust versus Mistrust (0–1 year)

Trust provides the beginning of Ego Identity. The *basic virtue* at this stage is *hope*. This grows out of trust; the child has been given a feeling of constancy, which he expects to continue in the future.

Play: 9 months–2 years

The child watches others playing and learns about objects. The use of imagination begins.

Play: 2–3 years

The child plays alongside others. Pretend play begins (e.g. using a banana as a telephone).

Erikson's stage of Autonomy versus Shame and Doubt (1–3 years)

The child is learning new muscular skills — climbing, pushing, pulling, holding on and letting go. He also learns that he has the control to make choices, e.g. to have a battle (let go in rage) or to let the matter pass.

The *basic virtue* resulting from this is *will*, which helps the child develop autonomy and make his own choices.

Play: 3–4 years

The child borrows from other children. Fantasy and imagination continue to be important for coping with painful experiences and trying out forbidden activities.

Erikson's stage of Initiative versus Guilt (3–4 years)

In this stage there is rivalry with the parent of the same sex for the attentions of the parent of the opposite sex. If this is well handled the child acquires a moral sense of what is and is not permissible. The child is being helped to develop a Superego.

The *basic virtue* is *purpose*, which arises from initiative and gives the child the courage to pursue goals.

Play: 4–7 years

The child learns to cooperate with others. Play is to some purpose. The child learns about rules, and that others have rights. Play is more constructive than before.

Play: school age

The child plays mostly with his own sex 'against' the opposite sex. He learns about adulthood, e.g. making tree houses and model aeroplanes, cooking, sewing, etc. He uses reasoning and manipulative skills.

Erikson's stage of Industry versus Inferiority (4/5–11 years)

The child is exposed to situations/pressures outside the home. He learns about working, and uses concentration.

The *basic virtue* is *competence*, which comes from industry and encouragement and constructive guidance from adults. If the child's attempts are ridiculed or he is scolded in relation to his efforts he is likely to feel inferior and inadequate. Competence carries him forward to pursue greater creativity and forms the foundation for his self-concept.

PERCEPTUAL AND INTELLECTUAL DEVELOPMENT

Perception refers to the ability to experience the outside world through the senses, discriminating between different sensations and conceptualising them. By 'conceptualising' is meant organising stimuli, understanding them, forming concepts and finally reaching some conclusion. The ability to understand and form concepts increases as intelligence develops, and in relation to the individual's experiences. D. O. Hebb's (1966) definition of intelligence puts this into context:

- Intelligence consists of:
  — Intelligence A: the innate potential, and
  — Intelligence B: the interaction between Intelligence A and the environment.

At birth, perception is limited since the nervous system is still immature, but a neonate is sensitive to varying intensities of light at 5 days old and can begin to follow movement of objects within 48 hours of birth, when he tends to scan his surroundings about 5–10% of his waking time. He can distinguish the primary colours by 3–4 months. The ability to focus increases rapidly in the first 6 months and may be perfected between 6 months and 1 year, though some children do not achieve this until they are 11 years old. It is thought that depth perception may be present at birth.

Readers are advised to refer to the work of Jean Piaget on intellectual development (Piaget 1952; see also Isaacs 1974), but a few general points can be made here.

- A stimulating environment is essential in the early formative years.

- Play is an important medium for intellectual development. Through play,
  — new perceptions are experienced
  — concept formation is supported and new concepts learnt
  — rules are learnt — intellectual and interpersonal
  — concentration is encouraged
  — language is practised
  — memory is stimulated
  — children are motivated to seek new goals, in a relaxed and happy environment.
- Childhood is a 'sensitive' period for intellectual development.
- Intelligence reaches its peak around the age of 18 years. Formal learning becomes more difficult as age increases.
- The development of intelligence is cumulative, each stage forming an essential foundation for the next.
- Probably most people function at Piaget's 'Concrete Operations' stage and find problem-solving, in any area of life, to be easier if based on practical activity rather than on theory (as in 'Formal Operations').
- Morality is based in part on cognitive ability and the child sees things as right or wrong in different ways according to his ability to reason.

Erikson's stage of Industry v Inferiority (4/5–11 years) is relevant here in terms of the need for encouragement and guidance rather than criticism.

PERSONALITY DEVELOPMENT

'Personality' refers to:

The more or less stable and enduring organisation of a person's character, temperament, intellect and physique — in part innate, and in part having developed in relation to his unique environment — which determines his individual response to the world around him. (Adapted from H. J. Eysenck, 1953)

There are many theories of personality, varying from those suggesting that the personality is moulded or determined by others, to those maintaining that a person has free will and is in charge, at least to some extent, of his own developing personality. 'Humanistic' psychologists add to this the crucial value of the individual as a person of 'worth' who, as such, is able to be responsible for himself. Some, such as Maslow, consider motivation as the fundamental concept in personality development, while Freud and the Psychoanalysts lay great stress on the power of the unconscious to influence development. Such theories, and others, are not mutually exclusive; for example, Freud believed in the power of motivation though he considered much of this to be unconscious. Each of these approaches has something to offer the therapist as she attempts to understand why people develop and behave as they do.

The word 'personality' derives from the Latin 'persona', which refers to the masks used by actors in the Greek theatre of long ago. The personality is portrayed by its owner in an acting-out of various parts to suit differing situations. The person seems to put on public faces for others to see. This is important since not only is each person different from every other, but in different situations — when he adopts different roles — he shows other people a different aspect of himself. One very important reason for this is that it is necessary for the individual to show himself in a light that serves his purpose best, i.e., that helps maintain his self-esteem and an equilibrium concerning his values and attitudes which provides, overall, a best fit between the situation and the person he perceives himself to be. To this end he will employ varying mechanisms that will, he hopes, defend his 'self' — the most important part of any individual.

Most theorists would acknowledge the existence and use of such 'defence mechanisms' but the concept was first introduced by Freud and relates closely to his three-part personality theory of the Id, the Ego and the Superego. This theory will not be discussed here but the characteristics of defence mechanisms can be found in Box 3.1. According to Freud (Schultz 1976) everyone needs to use such mechanisms, since life could not be borne if we had to face up to absolute truths about ourselves or certain situations. Some mechanisms are inappropriate and do not serve the person well. Thus, if (possibly as a result of psychotherapy) these unconscious mechanisms are brought into consciousness — in which case they can no longer defend the self — then another set of more ap-

Box 3.1 Characteristics of defence mechanism

- They are a normal method of defending the Self, used by everyone in the course of everyday life, but may also be very crippling if the mechanisms are extreme.
- They help the person to cope with any situation he finds difficult.
- They are distortions of reality.
- They are unconscious. If they appear to be conscious, as for example when we know we are rationalising, they are not serving to defend the self.
- They involve displacement of reaction from one problem onto another object, person or idea.

propriate defences must be allowed. For example, if a man is faced with the fact that he is violent towards his wife because he is basically angry with himself (i.e. he blames her for his accident when really it was his fault), he first needs to accept this realisation. Then it is necessary to help the man find other, more acceptable ways of expressing his anger. It is dangerous and wrong to 'strip a man of his dirty clothes and to leave him naked to face the world'.

On the other hand, Carl Rogers (1967) a Humanist, said that defence mechanisms cripple the personality and that with empathy and warmth

Box 3.2 A few defence mechanisms relevant to the work of the therapist with physically ill and disabled persons

- *Repression* — Pushing down into the unconscious the thoughts or memories that seem too hard to bear. Thus they are 'forgotten'. (If a person is consciously trying to forget something he is in fact rehearsing the memory and therefore making it harder to forget.) It is important that repression be avoided if possible because it leads to an unrealistic pattern of life for the person and those around him.
- *Denial* — The refusal of the mind to recognise unpleasant facts of life, with the result that the person behaves as if they were not true. (For example, a person has been told he has a terminal illness and books a holiday for a year ahead.) To the onlooker such reactions seem unreasonable and extreme, but to the person concerned the situation is quite clearly as he perceives it.
- *Regression* — The reverting to an earlier stage of development. As occurring in everyday life this can be seen in childish weeping or foot-stamping or going home to mother when things go wrong. It is also seen in children when a new sibling arrives. When a person is ill — at home or in hospital — it may be seen in over-demanding behaviour, in an inability to recover due to enjoyment of being the centre of attention, or in the way the person expresses his emotions. If the person seeks attention he may well need it but he should not be treated as if he were a child.
- *Fixation* — The person remains at the stage to which he has regressed. For example, the ill

person unconsciously does not want to return to an independent life and continues for years as an invalid.
- *Projection* — The attributing of the person's own undesirable traits to others. Commonly, people blame others if, for example, they knock over a vase. More seriously it is seen in the man mentioned earlier who is angry with his wife, blaming her for his accident because he is unable to take responsibility himself and face the implications of being responsible. This is often seen in hospital wards when a person — or his relatives — continually blames the medical staff for not doing their best.
- *Rationalisation* — A common mechanism used by everyone to give logical reasons for impulsive or inappropriate actions. The observer sees this as making excuses. The person will believe it to be a genuine reason. A clear example would be if a person has been told by a hypnotist to dance a jig on the table at 12 noon. When asked why he did it he might answer, 'Someone needed to liven up the place.'
- *Dissociation* — One manifestation of this is *Excessive theorising*, i.e. talking a lot about what one is going to do but never actually doing it. This might be seen in patients who feel (unconsciously) that they have not got the courage to take an important step towards health and fitness and so talk about it instead. It probably enables them to feel that at least something is being done.

extended to him the person would be able to cope with his environment without using defences.

In any event, there are many mechanisms that people use when under threat and stress. A few common ones are to be found in Box 3.2 and these may help the reader to think again when she finds a patient to be behaving in a way that she does not think is conducive to health and independence.

STAGE 2: ADOLESCENCE (12–18 YEARS)

This is a time of great change. As with all the stages there is no fixed age for this group but adolescence starts around the age of 12 years and may extend into the early twenties. Many aspects of the adolescent are developing and causing him certain problems at the same time, so it is a time of stress and adjustment as well as of growing independence.

Nicholson (1980) says: 'Maturity starts in Biology and ends in Culture'. In the adolescent stage the person tries to fit his biology into the cultural demands set for him. Because he is physically mature, parents and others tend to have unrealistically high expectations of him. He is at the same time neither child nor adult, yet in part he is both. Thus at times he tends to live up to one expectation that adults have, i.e. that he will be 'difficult'. There is no doubt that adolescents can be a great problem to their parents in our present society with its changing (but not necessarily worsening) standards of behaviour.

In retrospect, adolescents say that this stage was, on the whole, not too bad.

Erikson's Stage of Identity versus Role Confusion

This is a crucial stage when the basic identity must be met and resolved. For the child, it is a difficult and anxious time, a sort of marking-time period of experimentation and self-determination, the satisfactory outcome of which will be the attainment of a strong sense of identity. He then will know himself and how he fits in with his world and consequently will be able to face adulthood with self-confidence and high self-esteem.

Difficulty in achieving identity — the *identity crisis* — leads to 'Role Confusion'. The person does not know who he is or how he fits in with others and society. As a result he may drop out of the accepted life sequence (e.g. education — job — marriage) and accept an alternative pattern of life. Sometimes this is a 'negative identity' in which he may be delinquent or enter the drug scene, etc. This is still an identity and better than no identity at all.

Nowadays it seems more acceptable for the adolescent to take longer and to experiment more widely in order to find his identity. In fact he should be able to take all the time he needs, even though parents may find this a worrying time.

The *basic virtue* from this stage, which is carried forward as a foundation for the next stage, is *fidelity*, which grows out of Ego Identity and is marked by loyalty, a sense of duty, sincerity and genuineness.

Table 3.1 Adolescence (cont'd overleaf)

Physical aspects	• Physical/sexual maturity reached.
	• Sexual differences: perhaps due to different needs and goals
	—Boys: want quick arousal and immediate satisfaction. Feelings for opposite sex less committed. Tend to be aggressive physically
	—Girls: slower arousal but of greater significance. Have more sexual fantasies and relationships with opposite sex are more committed.
	• In the main are healthy, but anorexia in girls is not uncommon. If pushed too hard may have breakdown; seem vulnerable at this time. Prone to accidents due to experimenting (e.g. on motorbikes, etc.).
	• *Early maturers*: girls who mature earlier (i.e. are taller and more sexually developed) tend to be less popular.
	• *Late maturers*: boys who mature later are less popular.
Perception/ intelligence	• Ability at its peak at approximately 18 years and for next 10 years.
	• Some can operate at Piaget's Formal Operations stage; many, satisfactorily at Concrete Operations stage.

Table 3.1 Adolescence (cont'd)

Perception/ Intelligence (cont'd)	• Academic goals sometimes set by parents. If these are reasonably achievable and acceptable to the adolescent he can settle and do well. If not, low self-esteem and/or psychological problems may result. • Self-perception is important for Ego Identity. • Adolescent tends to be egocentric as he tries to find what fits with his ideal self. • *Early maturers*: seem to have slightly higher cognitive intelligence. Greater intelligence tends to enhance self-esteem, but this may not lessen anxiety. • *Late maturers*: better at visual and tactile skills than at cognitive ones.		best socially. He tries out differing behaviour, also to help him find his 'best fit'. • Sexuality: there is conflict between sexual desires and the norms of society. • *Early maturers*: girls seem less popular if too well developed physically. • *Late maturers* are generally more sociable and prefer to be one of a crowd.
		Attitudes	• Ego Identity: earlier, internalised attitudes are re-examined and possibly changed as the person tries to establish his own, rather than other, adults', identity. • Attitudes on the whole more conservative than they appear; e.g. research shows basic agreement with statements like 'Hard work is good.' Adolescents tend to comply with parents' views on important issues but agree with peers on everyday matters, e.g. dress, hairstyle. • Peer groups very important as point of reference for present and future attitudes and behaviour.
Motivation	• Is towards achieving in all areas. Main goal is to find Ego (Self) Identity. This provides framework for motivations and perceptions. • *Late maturers* are more concerned to behave in order to enhance self-esteem. Goals are often set by parents. If parents take an active interest, offspring will gain higher self-esteem, probably because they get more reinforcement. Permissive parents seem to have children of lower self-esteem. • Adolescents are more highly motivated as a result of discussion than through enforcement of set rules.		
		Morals	• Considerably altruistic, tending to fight for just causes, but still somewhat confused since this behaviour itself possibly hurts others (e.g. causing parents considerable anxiety by getting into trouble with the police while fighting for Greenpeace).
Emotions	• Maturity comes at this age but many mood swings are experienced and emotions are strongly expressed. • Anxiety concerning various conflicts shows in rebellious/ aggressive behaviour, as the person strives for self-identity. • Main struggle is dependency v. independence as feelings vacillate. Parents are still needed but the adolescent wants to feel valued as independent. • Sexuality: emotionally confused. Focus shifts from own to opposite sex. Anxious re peer attachments to same or opposite sex. All this relates in part to establishing identity. • *Late maturers* are more emotionally dependent on others; even at, say, 33 years they seem less confident and more neurotic	Main stresses	• Stresses relate to establishing self as a mature, independent person. These are many as the adolescent feels himself to be pulled in all directions, e.g.: —coping with powerful and stirring emotions —sorting out ambitions —coping with academic pressures, which are usually considerable at this period —coping with conflicting loyalties to parents, peers and self.
		Play/leisure	• Much leisure is social in nature with one friend or in a group. It often involves sport. Boys tend to go around in gangs. Adolescents seem concerned to be with others who are like themselves rather than involving themselves with and appreciating others with different gifts and attitudes. The most enjoyed activity seems to be spending long hours talking.
Socialisation	• Ego Identity: interactions with peers and adults help the adolescent to see where he fits in		

STAGE 3: YOUNG ADULTHOOD
(18–35 YEARS)

For most, this stage starts with a launch into complete independence and ends in the stability that can mark the onset of the middle years. There is a considerable change in relationships, and most in this age group want to settle down both at work and in their leisure to a more steady life-style. During this time married couples start their young families.

Erikson's stage of Intimacy versus Isolation

This exciting time is when the person becomes in-dependent of parents and institutions and starts functioning as a mature, responsible adult. He wants to settle into a lifetime commitment to a job and to relationships. One of these may be with his sexual partner but his quest for intimacy is not restricted to sexual relationships. Intimacy involves caring, commitment and loyalty openly displayed and expressed without fear of upsetting the sense of identity. In other words, now the individual is not going to be overly influenced by the attitudes and behaviour of others.

Those who fail to establish such intimacy function in isolation, avoiding, rejecting and even fearing others because of the threat to their own selves.

The *basic virtue* at this stage is *love*, derived from intimacy. This is the greatest of the virtues and refers to finding and losing oneself in others.

Table 3.2 Young adulthood (cont'd overleaf)

Physical aspects	• Full maturity has been established and there tend to be few health problems for most in this age group.		agreement concerning common goals.
Perception/ intelligence	• This age often sees the summit of achievement and abilities. • The person selects and pursues his own objectives. • Though the intellectual peak was reached some years earlier, the person is able to continue to achieve due to motivation.	Emotions	• Security is important for self and family, therefore many by about 40 do not feel able to change jobs with great confidence. • Still have strong ties with parents, who are usually still needed by this age group. • The unemployed experience considerable feeling of inadequacy and guilt due to their inability to fulfil the required role in society. The concept of bereavement is relevant to the unemployed and to those faced with redundancy. • Tends to be a loss of the romance of earlier years with partner. Some couples need help adjusting to new feelings that they cannot explain.
Motivation	• This is directed mainly towards establishing an independent life. By 30 many are married and starting their own families, who become the centre of their lives. • Economic independence is important. For some there is considerable struggle, especially in times of unemployment and high mortgages. Motivation lessens when a person is unable to get a job. This negates the high expectations the person had held for this stage and nothing seems worthwhile. • All of Maslow's Needs are relevant for self and for family. • By 40 most know what sort of success they will make of their work and are often considered too old for promotion by this time. • Want to work hard at marriage; this requires tolerance, cooperation, mutual respect, and	Socialisation	• If the self-identity is established social perceptions can turn to seeing others, (e.g. own parents and children) as being of central importance. Sometimes this leads to this age group not giving enough time and value to themselves. • 80% of this group married by 30 (90% in all marry at some time). Also very high divorce rate in 30–40 age group, with separations before the 4th anniversary. Usually divorce follows within the next 2 years.

Table 3.2 Young adulthood (cont'd)

Socialisation (cont'd)	• Friendships involve smaller groups of firmer friends with greater commitment to them. Few school friends last a lifetime. • Parents take on new role, at best as friends. Alternatively, the generations lose touch, or never change the original parent/child relationship. • Can be a lonely time for young mothers, confined to home and the care of children. Some husbands want to come home to relax and the wife feels excluded. Other husbands very involved in sharing child care and rearing.		this to themselves and to their relationships.
		Main stresses	• Most young adults cope very well with this time when many adjustments are being made. This can give them increased confidence for the future. • Sometimes considerable stress for single people who would like to be married. • Job pressures and responsibility for young family. • Social isolation may be a new and difficult experience for some mothers. • Unemployment extremely stressful. • Possibly a more difficult time for women who have to give up careers and friends, and change roles if having a family. Men do not have to do this and are sometimes unable to appreciate the wife's problem.
Attitudes	• May be conflict between career and marriage/family so attitudes to these need clarifying. Many unmarried by this time feel they have missed out. • Attitudes to elders now moderated with increased insight into adulthood. • Some prejudices will remain but, generally, attitudes mellow as the person becomes more tolerant.		
Morals	• Responsibilities increase towards others so there is less time to be concerned with their own wishes. Spouses and children are central but their own parents may be beginning to need care. • Very important for this group to acknowledge they themselves need to be considered. They owe	Play/leisure	• Few adults carry on with very strenuous sport. Some get so involved in work that there is little time for leisure, which mainly takes the form of going out with friends or watching TV. • Women may find little time to relax due to presence of young children. • Evening classes are favoured by this group to give mental and/or physical stimulation.

STAGE 4: THE MIDDLE YEARS (35–50 YEARS)

The middle years (Middlescence) are reached after young adulthood. It is important to be wary of generalisations with regard to any age group because chronological age is not an accurate guide to the well-being of the individual. Middle age is not a period of life like a fixed plateau between youth and old age, but a time of continuing physical, psychological, social and behavioural adaptation.

Erikson's stage of Generativity versus Stagnation

Erikson suggests that the age range for this group is 35 to 50 years, but for purposes of our dis-

cussion it is suggested that the events of this stage occur over a much wider age span.

In middle age a person needs more intimacy with others and to be actively involved in guiding and teaching the next generation. This need is different from the concern of parents or teachers for their children. The concept is a broader, more long-range one extending to future generations and is related to the kind of society in which we live. It concerns a sort of involvement in history in which the person wants to pass on his learning and a part of himself to future generations. Erikson says that all institutions of learning reinforce and safeguard the expression of 'generativity' in that they establish a fund of knowledge and methods to guide future generations. This can be done in many different ways.

If this need is not met the person is overwhelmed by a feeling of 'stagnation, boredom and interpersonal impoverishment' (Erikson 1963) resulting in regression to a stage of pseudo-intimacy in which he indulges in childlike behaviour aimed at satisfying only his own needs. He may become a physical or psychological invalid because of his total obsession with himself and his own needs and comforts. As a result he makes it very difficult for anyone trying to help him.

The *basic virtue* of this stage is *care*, emerging from satisfactory generativity — the broad concern for others, shown in the need to guide and help others. Generativity serves in part to fulfil a person's own identity.

Table 3.3 The middle years (cont'd overleaf)

Physical aspects	• Senses become less acute and sensory motor activity slows down. Heart efficiency is reduced. • Menopause in women with possible accompanying symptoms, e.g. headaches, hot flushes or general lack of well-being. The beginnings of osteoporosis may occur. • Sexual desire *may* lesson. • Changes, due to gradual slowing down of cell regeneration, to general 'wear and tear' and to an increasingly sedentary life-style, will begin to have their effect. • Nearly everyone over 40 will have aches and pains of some sort, often rheumatic in nature, and many people will have experienced illness and operations of some kind by this time in their lives.		• Considerable time and energy may be spent on considering religious beliefs and life after death.
		Emotions	• This is a time of positive feelings and contentment or feelings of depression. Probably some alternating between the two. • High divorce rate in this group makes this an exceedingly difficult and painful time for many. • Own physical changes may be seen as depressing. Anxiety over spouse's and own health. • Freedom from own children gives time for deepening relationship with spouse. There may be a need for other emotional ties, especially if those with spouse are not good. • Elderly parents may now need more care, so this age group could feel buffeted by older and younger generations, with freedom from children not being complete and the demands of the parents being added. • Possible bereavement due to children leaving home or parents dying.
Perception/ intelligence	• Learning ability remains high with reasoning and vocabulary increasing as memory shows little sign of decline. • Some older people take up academic studies again. • Cognitive flexibility and reaction time tend to slow down, in part due to the ageing process but also because of the lessening acuity of the senses. • Any possible loss of intellectual capacity is well compensated for by high motivation.		
Motivation	• Both sexes have reached the height of their careers, probably finding fulfilment here. Wife may want to return to work or spend more time on her career. • Both sexes concerned with generativity if feelings are positive, but may lose interest and become self-centred if feelings are negative. • Great satisfaction is possible from areas of a) jobs, and b) grandchildren, to give two examples. • Motivation closely linked with the emotion causing it or caused by it. The needs (of Maslow) relate to satisfying self-esteem and fulfilling potential since offspring are no longer of all-absorbing importance.	Socialisation	• Social factors change as own children leave home but are still a cause for concern. • Interactions with spouse and new friends possible as own children become increasingly independent. • High divorce rate can make for social isolation. • May get involved in social activities in church or clubs; may do voluntary work. • May be greatly involved with grandchildren. • Certain amount of role change in this age group; e.g. wife and mother may become grandmother and professional woman. • There is a certain role expectation of this age group in relation to dress and behaviour. Society will exert pressure for people to adopt these roles.

Table 3.3 The middle years (cont'd)

Attitudes	• Attitudes were acquired when young and consolidated in adolescence; thus they are fairly set and may be a cause of difficulty with younger generations whose attitudes will inevitably differ to some extent. Thus this age group is often thought to be rigid. • There is a need to reconsider attitudes in order to relate well with children and grandchildren. Increasingly, people in this age group are able to do this, so younger people find them approachable and dependable. • Alternatively they may become even more rigid. This depends on their perceptions of the world and their own self-esteem.		to anxieties re sex, drugs, inappropriate companions, etc. causing friction between the generations. Fortunately, some parents and children are good friends, but this is rarely an easy time. • Children leaving home very stressful for some. • Elderly parents can cause concern. Extra attention needed by them can limit and frustrate. Their physical illness and general increasing weakness can be upsetting: 'He's not the person he was.' • Own physical aches and pains may begin to cause concern.
Morals	• The morals of younger generations may cause concern, suggesting that a re-evaluation of own attitudes might be of benefit to all. • At this age thoughts of death cause many to reconsider religious beliefs and the purpose of life. • Helping behaviour may be greater, in part due to above, in part to more available time and less need for a high income.	Play/leisure	• All sorts of activities. For the 'sporty' it may be badminton rather than squash. Also intellectual activities like crosswords and bridge. • Person has opportunity to take up activities that he finds rewarding to himself — sometimes quite new activities such as painting or woodwork. • Often activities are related to keeping healthy, e.g. jogging. • Leisure of considerably more relevance to some in this group, but others who lead a busy and satisfying life with work of various sorts feel that leisure is even more distant.
Main stresses	• Physical and psychological changes around menopause, and general realisation of getting older. • Older children's behaviour may add		

STAGE 5: OLD AGE (50/60 YEARS AND ONWARDS)

There are great individual differences between people and certainly the elderly are no exception. Old age can be beautiful to see and happy for the person, or it can be very sad and ugly.

The environment will have considerable influence on both the physical and psychological well-being of the individual in old age, as will his general health and his own personality. It seems that the extroverted person who goes out to find stimulation will do better than the introvert who does not particularly want much company. This, however, is a generalisation and there is a tendency for older people to disengage socially — that is, to withdraw from the activities and concerns of society. At the same time there is a tendency for society to disengage from the elderly, since now other, younger people have become the centre of all that is going on. The considerable research being done in this area indicates that it is important for the elderly to be helped at this stage to find stimulation and variety for an active old age.

Erikson's final stage of Ego Integrity versus Despair

This is a time for the individual to look back and reflect on his past life and measure its outcome. It is the way in which he perceives his past that will result in Ego Integrity or in Despair.

Ego Integrity is achieved when the person can look back feeling that he has had a reasonably good life and has been able to do and achieve most of what he wanted, and is now left with few regrets about what he has not done. Thus he has a sense of fulfilment and a feeling that he has adjusted to life's successes and failures.

Despair is felt when the person looks back with discontentment and frustration — perhaps even with rancour or anger — at missed opportunities, regretting mistakes which he cannot rectify and resenting or blaming others for his lack of success. He is now disgusted with life, contemptuous of others and bitter about what might have been.

This final attitude to life has a great influence on the sort of old age the person will have and on the relationships others will have with him through this stage.

The *basic virtue* of old age is *wisdom*, which arises out of Ego Integrity and relates to a contented concern with the wholeness of life. With this the person can convey to the next generation the wholeness of life integrated with experience, which Erikson calls 'heritage'.

Table 3.4 Old age (cont'd overleaf)

Physical aspects	• Senses become less acute resulting in reduced ability to carry out daily functions, e.g. washing up and cleaning the house, to a high standard. • There is a general dislike for starting to use aids, e.g. hearing aids, to help the senses. It is much harder to get used to using these later in life. This can also apply to the use of emergency 'necklaces', etc. • Body functions are wearing out. The back is more bent and knees permanently flexed. Osteoporosis may cause considerable deformity in women. • Cardiovascular system functions less well. • This age group often complains of sleepless nights, but sleep briefly and often during the day. • Less able to maintain body heat, so is vulnerable to hypothermia at times when younger people do not realise it is cold enough for this to happen. • Psychologically, depression is quite common among the elderly but is often not recognised. Symptoms vary, but can often be identified by the fact that behaviour seems different from before.		• New skills not so easy to learn. Old ones have been perfected to high standard so remain good until allowed to lapse. • Build-up of knowledge over the years enables person to have good judgement and wisdom to hand on to others. This, called 'crystallised intelligence' by Cattell (1971), remains good whereas 'fluid intelligence' — the ability to make use of knowledge and experience in meeting challenges and problems — lessens over the years.
		Motivation	• In Maslow's terms the greatest need may be for personal safety and the satisfaction of physiological needs, but many old people have these well catered for and so the need for love, belonging and self-esteem is the main motivation. There are of course many very able and fit old people who will be motivated to higher, intellectual needs. Some tend to want a lot of attention for themselves, and compete with others for this, resenting it if they feel they are not getting enough. This is usually when they have little in the way of their own interests.
Perception/ intelligence	• Less intellectual agility, possibly due to physical/perceptual problems, e.g. reduced hearing. • Not so good with number problems. Shapes and patterns now more confusing. • Takes in information more easily verbally than visually. Some need to use both when communicating. • Long-term memory is good, short-term gets poorer due, possibly, to proactive interference.	Emotions	• Seem to adjust very well to increasing number of sorrows with friends and relatives dying. • Some find themselves more emotional than in earlier years. • Anxiety often a strong emotion, usually over apparently trivial things while coping with seemingly greater problems very well. Considerable anxiety — even fear — about dying for some but this fear is not often shared with others.

Table 3.4 Old age (cont'd)

Emotion (cont'd)	• Depression quite common. Helpers need to watch for this so it does not become an illness.		hand there is sometimes a relaxation in the judging of others at this stage.
Socialisation	• Main factor is 'disengagement' due to social and physical factors. • Bereavement also helps to cut a person off from interactions. • Retirement also can lead to less contact with others, but can lead to exploration of new interactions. • Relationships with own children not always easy. The old person may feel he is a trouble and a bother to the young, or may be over-demanding. • Relationships with grandchildren often very good indeed, but in some cases they may find little in common.	Main stresses	• Pain is often considerable for old people and is very tiring. Also causes worry about the future and being able to cope • Social isolation and boredom hated by some. • Many psychological changes, in part due to physical deterioration, can cause confusion both within and as a result of having to move house or go into hospital, etc.
Attitudes	• Often these are fixed and relate to the person's own frame of reference. Some may then appear to be old-fashioned and narrow-minded. However, a lot of people happily tolerate the attitudes of others, even if those attitudes are not appropriate for themselves. • Some may become self-centred (see Motivation). • Coming to terms with death and the possibilities for an afterlife causes considerable problems for some while others have made their peace with God, or are content not to have done so.	Play/leisure	• Stimulation is the greatest need here for physical and mental alertness and health. • Even emotions need stimulating and a little anxiety is no bad thing especially if it can prove to the person that he can cope. • Intellectually, stimulation can help the person to be more 'with it', which is important for his continuing development. He is not now on a run down towards death but needs to be helped to keep very much alive. • Activities tend to be based on skills learned and enjoyed when young, since basic techniques have already been learnt and practised. These can be rewarding.
Morality	• There is going to be little change in the moral outlook of this age group, although they may find it increasingly difficult to accept the morality of others. On the other		• Group activities often more beneficial from a therapeutic point of view than for the personal enjoyment of the old person, who would often prefer to sit quietly rather than be treated as one of many or as though he were a child.

REACTIONS TO ILLNESS AND LOSS

A person coming to terms with severe illness or disability is faced with a crisis. He must cope with great psychological turmoil as realisation of his situation strikes him with a staggering blow that sends him reeling. Although this may be more sudden and shocking for someone with an acute illness or sudden disability, there are going to be times when the chronically ill person is also struck by the implications for his future. How will he react to his illness? How can he cope with his fears, his shattered hopes, his deflated self-image and the inevitable loss of previous roles? Will he ever be able to find that there is still a worthwhile life ahead of him?

Although he may not be able to verbalise such vast questions, a person who becomes severely ill or disabled will experience at some stage many fears and doubts concerning his future. Unvoiced questions will rush through his mind:

• 'Will I ever be able to walk again?'
• 'How will the kids feel having a cripple for a father?'
• 'My colleagues won't respect me now.'

- 'How can we pay the mortgage?'
- 'How humiliating it all is not being able to do anything for myself.'
- 'I don't want to die so young.'
- 'I don't think I can cope; life's not worth living.'
- 'God, I'm frightened.'

Along with such thoughts and feelings there will also be swings of mood from extreme helplessness to some degree of hopefulness. These concerns are psychological rather than physical; moreover, the person is going to have to come to terms with his present and his future within a social setting and, as we have seen, it is the social environment of his early years that may or may not have equipped him with the ability to cope through these times of stress and strain.

LOSS AND BEREAVEMENT

One of the difficulties for the therapist as she learns to deal with these psychological factors is that each individual is just that — he is different from everyone else. It is hard for her to know, therefore, whether she is doing the right and best thing for any particular person. There are, however, some guidelines to be found both in what has been written so far, and in the following consideration of the experiences that most people have when facing similar situations. Serious illness and disability involve 'loss' in the physical and psychological sense.

Loss is also an important experience when a person has to leave a job through retirement or redundancy. Unemployment, too, is accompanied by loss, in the sense of something being missing. These and other such events can be the cause of severe ill health, and most people go through a kind of bereavement when any sort of loss is experienced.

BEREAVEMENT

Bereavement is the inevitable cost of commitment to living. Few of us would wish to avoid this commitment and in truth most of us can find that the price was worth paying. Apart from the joy that we experience as we find, to our surprise, that we can adjust to an unforeseen future, the experience of 'grief work' can make us kinder and wiser people and more aware of the needs of others who suffer.

'Bereavement' refers to the forcible loss of something that is precious — usually of another person, but also of anything that is central to a person, such as his job or his home and independence. 'Grief' refers to the resulting emotional experience of being bereaved, while 'mourning' refers to a set of learned responses which are determined by the norms and customs of the person's particular culture.

For purposes of clarity we will consider bereavement in terms of the loss of a loved one, but everything that is said here will apply also to other great losses — not least to the loss of health or a limb, and the psychological losses that result from these. It is worth considering first what these psychological losses are.

Loss of independence and self-esteem

Independence relates in part to being able to work and support one's self and family; having the freedom to go where one wants, when one wants; having privacy; and having the ability to look after oneself. If these things — and others specific to the individual — are lost, then self-esteem is also damaged, since without them a person may not value himself or expect others to do so. The degree to which the loss is felt will depend on personality, previous self-confidence and attitudes towards disability. Research has indicated that the greater the level of disability the more negative is the self-concept, while on the other hand:

A patient with a realistic yet positive self concept oriented towards the future, stands a far better chance of recovery than one who disparages himself.
(Burns 1980)

Loss of earlier roles

It is probable that a person whose health has been seriously affected will have to adjust or change some of his previously occupied roles and abandon some of the expected behaviour of former days. For example, a man with a serious heart condition may be unable to work any more or do such things as carrying the logs for the fire or digging the garden. This he could experience as 'loss'. The gender role is also of importance, and if it is affected because of difficulty in carrying out the sexual act, the loss may be considerable.

Family members also have their expectations for the disabled person. They may assume that earlier roles may be taken up again after a short break, or that they will never be resumed. Either assumption may be wrong. Relatives and friends also have to adjust to the loss, which is in part theirs too. Part of the therapist's role must concern the rehabilitation of the whole family since, to a greater or lesser extent, a disabled person creates a disabled family.

GRIEF AND GRIEF WORK — STAGE ONE

Grief is natural and healthy even though it is very stressful. Grieving occupies an intermediate period between the anticipation or experience of loss and some ultimate reorganisation in the individual's pattern of life. This involves a gradual process of adjustment — of letting go and of sorting out what aspects of the loved one can, psychologically, be kept and internalised and so stay with the person for ever, and of finding new inner strengths which may never have been tapped before or which might now be used to greater advantage in the face of a new and unanticipated future. All this involves hard work and the expressing of many different and often seemingly contradictory emotions. But grief is itself an emotion and like all the others it is natural and normal and should be allowed expression.

The hard work that is involved is called 'grief work'. It begins when a person knows that a loved one is going to die, possibly weeks or even years before the loss actually takes place (except when the person tries to defend himself from the pain by denying that the loss will ever take place). If some of the grief work can be done in anticipation, it is thought to be of benefit in that there will be

less to be done after the actual loss. There is also the opportunity for the saying of good-byes — and there is as much need to do this to a limb that will be amputated as to a person who is going to die. After all, a leg has been a good friend for many years.

On the other hand, there may be long weeks and months of anxiety, fear, false hope and, possibly, difficult nursing, which all make for an extremely stressful time.

When a loved one dies suddenly there is, in addition to the grief, a very great shock that will probably upset the physical and psychological equilibrium of the survivor more extremely than will the shock of an expected loss.

The experience of loss

Grief work does seem to involve certain recognisable stages which may follow one after the other but are equally likely to alternate and to come and go with varying intensity. Sometimes there is a predominant emotion. Again, the experience of each person will be different.

Numbness

There is a feeling of emptiness, numbness, being stunned. It seems that — to use an attractive phrase — 'God's anaesthetic' is at work. This is probably very necessary because if the person is totally aware and responsive to all his emotions at this time he will be unable to cope. There is for the person a real awareness of emptiness, with the result that there is an almost mechanical 'cut-out' or 'shut-down' of mental processes. This lasts for about a week — often until the funeral is over — after which time, so often, the bereaved person is left on his own. This is a time when it is not necessarily a good thing for the person to be taken away to stay with relatives, since he will only have to face the empty house later. It is a time when, if possible, it is good for the person to have someone staying with him.

Guilt

This seems to be an almost inevitable accompaniment to bereavement, and at times it is justified.

There really are sins of omission and of commission. Usually, however, the guilt is a projection of the person's disappointment, anger and general resentment. It seems that he seeks out something for which to condemn himself. Possibly he feels guilty for still being alive. Perhaps he is unconsciously doing penance — for, in all honesty, no loved one left behind has ever behaved perfectly towards the loved one lost. So in a sense, this is a suitable form of self-punishment and may bring about a catharsis, if that is what is sought. The person may have no other way of putting things right.

As with the other emotions, the guilt reaction is perfectly normal and if the person were helped to forgive himself he would he tempted to find a new reason for feeling guilty. Both the helper and the bereaved person might cope better by accepting that guilt seems to be part of the process, not something to be tackled, and that with time it will pass.

Anger

We tend to get angry when something is taken away from us, whether it be a play-thing or a job, so it is not suprising that anger is experienced here.

The anger may be directed at the loved one for deserting the person, at the doctors or nurses, at other relatives or at oneself for not trying harder or doing something different. The anger may be towards God; but as Lily Pincus (1976) comments, 'That's all right, God can take it.' The question underlying much of the anger is 'Why did this happen to me?'

Searching and Denial

Many years ago I lost a gold pencil that had been given to me as a present. It took me many years to give up hope that it might turn up one day. We all hate losing things, and the sense of disbelief that something — or someone — is really gone is very strong. In any case we don't want the person or object to be lost to us.

Searching can take the literal form of going round the home, into the bedrooms, the garage, the workshop or wherever, to see if, perhaps, really, after all, the lost loved one is there. Part of the bereaved person knows that he is not . . . but there is still this little bit of hope. Perhaps as a cause of his searching or as a result of it the bereaved person often feels the loved one to be very close indeed. He may have very vivid dreams and may even have realistic and meaningful experiences that the rest of us might call hallucinations. Along with this there is a tendency for the person to forget momentarily that the loved one has gone and to start to behave as if he were still there, and then to be upset because he feels he has been 'stupid'.

The desire to hang on to the bereaved person is one reason why it is considered of great importance for people that they actually see the person after death: the body is the actual evidence. This is important for children too. They may not necessarily have to see the person but they need to have it made very clear that he is no longer there and is not coming back, and to be included in the mourning process rather than being sent away to stay with friends.

Searching is a part of the deep-seated wish to negate the reality of the loss. Such denial is a mechanism which guards the person from the shock and somehow helps to delay the impact of the situation allowing time to accept what is so unwelcome (see Defence Mechanisms, p. 34).

THE STAGE OF ACCEPTANCE — STAGE TWO

These emotional responses will continue for varying lengths of time after the bereavement, but usually for about six months to a year and possibly longer than this. Gradually the anger will burn itself out, the searching cease and the denial subside in the face of unavoidable reality. The peak of the grief is usually experienced a few weeks (but it may be months) after bereavement and then gradually subsides, but as has been said, everyone is different. Many people find that after a period when they feel they are beginning to adjust something — often not in itself very significant — will throw them off-balance so they feel their pain as acutely as ever (Fig. 3.5).

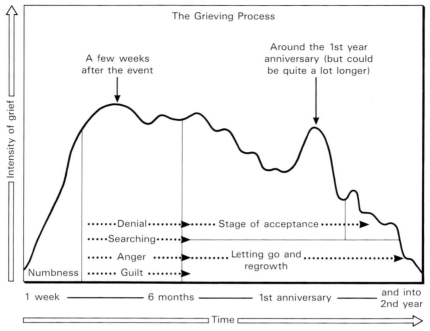

Fig. 3.5 The possible intensity of grief over a period of time.

LETTING GO: THE STAGE OF REGROWTH — STAGE THREE

Now the stage of renunciation and rehabilitation can start. A new life has to begin and while grief and all it involves is still present the person begins to look towards the future. This may begin after about six months, sometimes coinciding with an anniversary of some sort. The first anniversary of the loss is often significant, providing an important milestone. Birthdays and Christmas may be difficult times but can also be times for looking forward in a positive way, and may be real turning-points.

Depression and grief

It is often difficult to differentiate between depression as a part of grief and depression as an illness. The first may lead into the second if it is turned inwards and not expressed or if it is delayed or inhibited or denied altogether. If grief appears to last longer than about two years there is sometimes need for help through psychotherapy

but, again, some people may just need a little longer. However, any talk of suicide should always be taken seriously and advice taken.

THE EFFECTS OF CULTURE ON MOURNING

Western society has tended to adopt an attitude towards mourning of 'Let's get it over and done with as soon as possible.' This has lead to some inappropriate haste so that instead of grieving some people smother their emotions. This results in a need to grieve at a later date, perhaps years later, sometimes necessitating professional psychiatric help. Grieving cannot be hastened. The mourning customs of any culture should enable a person to reflect upon what faith he has, and should provide comfort for him by allowing grief to be expressed through acceptable modes of behaviour. The hospice movement is playing an increasing part in helping to change attitudes and behaviour in this direction. Other cultures could teach us much about coping with loss in the way people support each other and do not avoid expressing their feelings.

HOW CAN OTHERS HELP?

There is no easy answer, but a few comments might help.

- Stay close to the person and share what you can of his experience, but never say 'I know how you must be feeling.' No one person can ever know what another is experiencing; your experiences might have similarities but are never the same.
- Encourage the person to talk of his anger, resentment or guilt; to share his feelings. Reassure him that these are normal and are allowed. It is important that the grief be overtly expressed rather than turned inwards, which might lead to psychological problems later on. The 'stiff upper lip' is not the appropriate response to loss and some people need to be encouraged not to be too 'wonderful' but to allow others to do things for them.
- Accept that depression is part of the bereavement situation. There is bound to be a certain inability to sleep, restlessness or inertia, sighing and sadness. None of these indicates mental illness and if possible sedatives should not be encouraged as they cause the person to avoid or delay the grief work which will have to be gone through at some time as an important part of his readjustment to the future.
- At this time the bereaved person is not really able to see his situation realistically and decisions would be better delayed until he has been able to re-establish some sort of equilibrium. He may need gentle persuasion in this.

Above all, do nothing that may discourage the natural expression of the grief.

THE PROCESS OF DYING

What has been written here has been linked with the loss of another, but also has important implications for the one who is actually dying. Faced with the prospect of his own death, the person undergoes a mourning process similar in many ways to that experienced upon the death of another. This important area will not be examined at this point, other than to mention that a great deal of emotion is involved here also. The five stages that the individual passes through when facing death are:

1. Denial and isolation
2. Anger against God and man: 'Why me?'
3. Bargaining for more life
4. Depression
5. Acceptance — sometimes even triumph.

EMOTIONS, ATTITUDES AND MOTIVATION

These three psychological aspects of a person have special relevance to physical illness and disability and so are given consideration here.

EMOTIONS

Emotions are the affective part of our motivation and behaviour. They are what a person feels. Clearly, positive emotions are conducive to maintaining good health, but the therapist is likely to have to help in combating more negative feelings, not least anxiety.

Anxiety is an ongoing state of apprehension or foreboding, and it is thought to affect the physiological processes which control emotions. If, for example, a person is constantly anxious he will be unable to sleep, and this will affect him physically and psychologically. Such a state of arousal is counter-productive to rehabilitation.

Anxiety usually concerns the unknown. This shows how emotions are closely related to our cognitions, and suggests that if the therapist keeps her patient well informed about his situation, his chances of recovery, and the alternatives for treatment, his anxiety will be reduced. He will then be more relaxed and gain more from therapy.

The Yerkes–Dodson Law (Yerkes & Dodson 1908) is relevant here. It states that there is an optimum but differing level of arousal for all behaviour. If emotional arousal is too high or too low (as when there is too much 'hassle' or too much boredom, see p. 23) the performance will

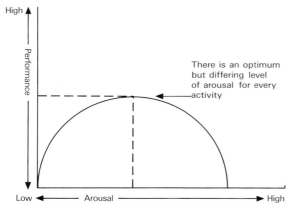

Fig. 3.6 The Yerkes–Dodson law. There is an optimum but differing level of arousal for every activity.

be less than optimal (Fig. 3.6). A person's inability to sleep, as already mentioned, is an example of over-arousal, but there are times when it may be necessary for the therapist to help stimulate the level of arousal (and so encourage motivation) for the maximum benefit to rehabilitation. Reference might be made here to the section on play and leisure and to the Summaries of Development to see the relevance of stimulation for health.

Wolpe (1964) put forward the theory of Reciprocal Inhibition, which states that two opposing emotions cannot exist at the same time. So, staying with anxiety, a person cannot be anxious and relaxed at the same time. Wolpe's theory, which lies at the basis of much behaviour modification, has great relevance to helping the ill and the disabled, since while mental relaxation helps the body to relax, anxiety tends to tense the muscles so that the patient may be unable to carry out the movements required of him. His state of apprehension is also likely to interrupt his concentration.

The 'stiff upper lip' can make things very difficult for the therapist. Even if she asks a person about his feelings he may not feel able to share them. The therapist requires a considerable level of skill to be able to identify what is the true situation from what the person says, from his behaviour and from his non-verbal cues, such as tone of voice, frowning, and lack of eye contact (see Fig. 3.7). She will also need to build up a partnership of trust to encourage the person to express more freely the way he feels.

Being an integral part of behaviour, emotions are relevant to the discussions of attitudes and motivation that follow.

ATTITUDES

This term is used loosely by professionals and the public alike. If someone is asked what he means by the term his answer is usually vague. A clearer understanding of the notion of 'attitudes' could, however, equip the therapist with a set of useful tools to use in her work.

An attitude can be defined as:

A reaction to, a belief about and a behavioural tendency towards or away from a particular object, concept or situation. (Wheldall 1975)

Thus there are three components that need consideration (see Fig. 3.8). If a person holds certain attitudes to, say, disability, then he may *feel* compassion and a longing to help, or he may feel pity and revulsion. At the same time he will hold certain *beliefs* about disability. He may think it also

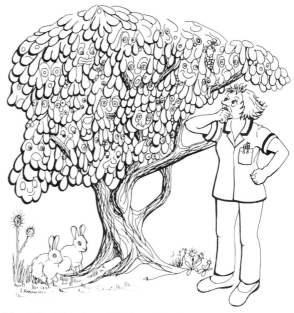

Fig. 3.7 It is often difficult to identify a person's true feelings.

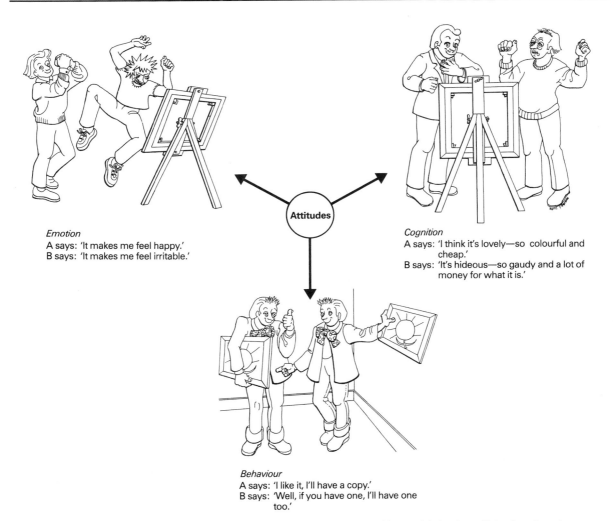

Emotion
A says: 'It makes me feel happy.'
B says: 'It makes me feel irritable.'

Attitudes

Cognition
A says: 'I think it's lovely—so colourful and cheap.'
B says: 'It's hideous—so gaudy and a lot of money for what it is.'

Behaviour
A says: 'I like it, I'll have a copy.'
B says: 'Well, if you have one, I'll have one too.'

Fig. 3.8 Attitudes are the combination of three components: emotion, cognition and behaviour. Behaviour is not necessarily in keeping with the other two.

involves mental handicap or impairment; or that it is a sign of weakness and the person should 'try harder'; or that the disabled person is really the same as everyone else; or that the government should do more to help such people. Feelings and beliefs tend to complement each other so that negative beliefs are accompanied by more unpleasant feelings, while more positive ideas are accompanied by more comfortable feelings.

This combination predisposes the holder to *behave* accordingly, so that the person with negative feelings and beliefs may speak only to the person's companion ('Does he take sugar?'), generally ignoring or patronising the person himself. On the other hand, if others around him behave differently he may conform to their behaviour and be friendly in a manner that is in keeping not with his own attitude, but with the behaviour of others who influence him. The behavioural part of attitudes does not always back the other two components and the observer could be misled by this. When such contradiction occurs there is a certain degree of discomfort for the individual concerned, since he is being pulled in different directions. Festinger (1957) called this 'cognitive dissonance'.

Attitudes and slow progress towards readjustment

A person who has become disabled may himself have held negative attitudes to disablement when he was fit. So what does he do now? He is in an even worse state of dissonance since his attitudes do not fit in with his particular situation. In order to reduce the dissonance he has either to change his behaviour, and thus act as a weak, mentally incompetent person in order to conform to his attitudes, or else he must change his attitudes in order to adopt behaviour that enables him to maintain his self-esteem. Cognitive dissonance is very common in everyday situations but adds another problem to disability since people cannot be at peace mentally with such contradictions in their lives. Cognitive consonance, therefore, is necessary and the acquiring of it is part of the person's adjustment to his changed situation. This will involve shuffling his attitudes (because attitudes are not held in isolation but dovetail with one another to form a whole value system) to make them fit him comfortably. This is no easy task and will need time and help from the therapist; the person has to sort out not only his situation but has to come to terms with the attitudes of a society in which there is still a considerable degree of stigma attached to disability. These factors may account in part for slow progress towards recovery.

As the disabled person struggles to adjust to his changed situation there may be times when his behaviour makes it difficult for others who are also trying to adjust to his disability. On the one hand, he wants his independence and so shrugs off offers of help. On the other, he needs the love, presence and attention of others but finds they do not seem to enjoy visiting him. Probably they do not know how to behave in order to help him most. Alternatively, family members or carers may encourage the person to remain an 'invalid' as they try to use him to help meet needs of their own. For example, a mother may have been unable to cope with the fact that her children have grown up and left home so she treats the person as her needy child. Or a man may feel guilt for the way he has treated his wife over the years and now tries to make it up to her by doing everything for her. In many ways,

then, disabled people and those close to them have a powerful effect on each other, and can make or mar the adjustment process. The struggle for adjustment may not always progress as society would like it to.

Another reason for slow progress might be that the person considers his disability to be God's punishment which, for some reason, he deserves. In time this may turn to a 'playing the martyr' syndrome through which he gains increased attention from everyone. Basically, the person comes to a point where he does not want to get better since gaining increased attention and sympathy may itself be seen as preferable to being well. The fact that needs to be understood and catered for by the therapist is that the person has — or believes he has — a need for this increased attention, even if it is not always possible to give it to him.

It is difficult to know whether lack of progress leading ultimately to the person becoming institutionalised could be due to such attitudes, or to 'learned helplessness' (see p. 52), or to various other factors. Whatever the causes of slow adjustment or non-adjustment, it is, in the end, the patient who becomes the loser since:

. . . empathy turns to sympathy, and beyond that to pity, eventually becoming irritation and loss of patience if the sick person is not coming up with a suitably rapid recovery. (Shapiro 1981)

All this makes it fairly evident that the therapist needs to have consideration for the whole family. Her understanding of the interaction of Wheldall's three components, as discussed above, will help to address the psychological needs of the disabled person since she will know that she has three possible channels through which she might help. She can approach the emotional component by helping the person to *feel* better about his disability and himself. She can help him to *understand* his situation by keeping him fully and honestly informed not only about his own disability and progress, but also about the various choices that are available to him in terms of his changing life-style. Finally, she can help him to try out different *behaviour* patterns and styles to see what 'fits' him most comfortably. The best behavioural fit will also be the one he *thinks* to be best and with which he *feels* most comfortable. This work towards attitude change is one area in which a number of people in reasonably similar circumstances might help and learn from each other in a group situation, and where the use of counselling skills by the therapist will be invaluable.

MOTIVATION

Motivation refers to a movement or striving towards certain incentives, goals or needs. It implies that a person is moving towards his own, not another's, goals (Fig. 3.9). Thus it is not appropriate for one person — in particular, a therapist — to try to inflict her own motivations onto another. Although therapists are frequently heard to complain 'I don't know how to get him motivated' it is a fact that normally extrinsic and social motivators such as money or a cup of coffee have to be internalised before they can spur a person on: coffee will not help if a person only drinks tea. When a person has become ill or disabled and the bereavement process is taking place, motivation is at a very low ebb, so all that others can do is be available to provide incentives and choices for exploration when he is ready.

Theories of motivation indicate that what a person strives for in life relates to the sort of person he is. Much has been said and written about the importance of motivation in relation to behaviour and rehabilitation, but the therapist would do well to consider Maslow's hierarchy of needs here. This has been explained in relation to the motivation that is necessary for satisfying needs and reducing stress through life (see Summaries of Development and Fig. 3.2).

Motivation and learning theory

Learning has been defined by Atkinson et al (1987) as:

a relatively permanent change in behaviour that occurs as a result of practice or experience.

Learning involves perception, attention and memory and is highly dependent on motivation and attitudes. All the various theories of learning are relevant for the therapist as she helps a disabled or seriously ill person to lead a new life. One concept that is of particular importance is that of *reinforcement*.

Giving positive reinforcement in the form of realistic encouragement is an essential part of the helping process and is itself a very strong motivator. It is important to concentrate on the person's abilities, on the things that he does well, and on his strengths; to look at his ability to function rather than on his disability, weakness and dysfunction. To concentrate on the dysfunction might have the effect of making things seem worse, and thus be interpreted by him as punishment or as the reinforcement of his disability. This

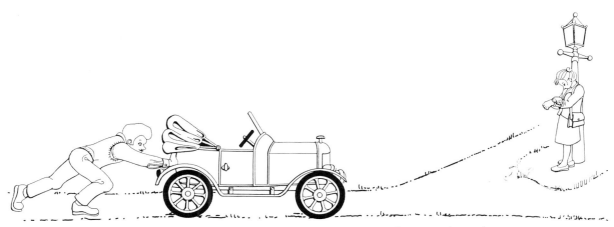

Fig. 3.9 Motivation implies that a person is moving towards his own, not another person's, goals.

could in turn help him to feel an increased degree of hopelessness and eventually helplessness. Such 'learned helplessness' results from his feeling powerless to have any effect through his own efforts on his perceived, dreadful situation, so that he gives up trying.

In the early days of treatment the person may think he has very limited choices, in spite of much reinforcement in the guise of encouragement, and he may expect what so often happens, namely that others will make decisions for him. Gradually, though, as he is encouraged to take on responsibility for himself and look at the choices before him, and as he gains new insights, it is likely that his motivation will increase and that he will move quickly towards mental as well as physical readjustment.

The occupational therapist's role as one of the helpers in this process must fit in with her view of her role as therapist; the reader is directed to the discussion of the philosophy of occupational therapy in Chapter 1.

CONCLUSION: THE RELATIONSHIP BETWEEN THE THERAPIST AND THE DISABLED PERSON

Any model that concerns helping a person towards maximum functioning in relation to his illness or disability must be set within a developmental framework if it is to be truly 'holistic', that is, relating to all aspects of the person. It is generally accepted that development is a continuous process from conception until death. Disability or serious illness can therefore be seen as a blocking of the

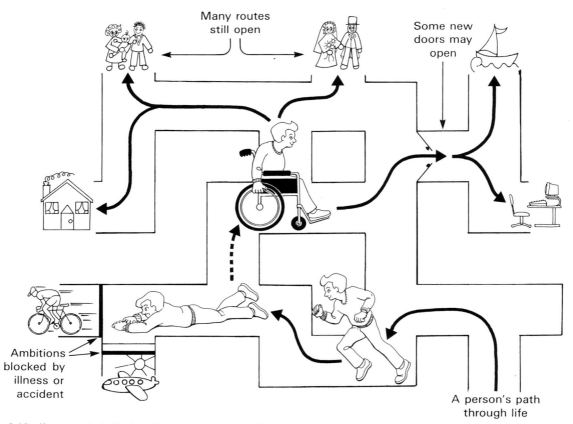

Fig. 3.10 If one route is blocked there are a number of alternative paths.

way forward. If one thinks of a map, there are a number of routes that could lead to the same end-point (see Fig. 3.10). So in life if certain routes are blocked there still remain other paths that his life could follow, for even the most severely disabled person. There are still choices that can be made, and it is the role of the therapist to assist the disabled person in the making of those choices.

Thus occupational therapy is not merely a means of helping a person to achieve his maximum potential in spite of his disability, but a way in which the therapist works with the person who is ill or disabled in selecting and trying out alternative choices for a changed but nevertheless full life. This process involves physical and psychological considerations within the individual's social setting (see Fig. 3.11).

The therapist's approach has to be a holistic one throughout since, for example, where a physically disabled person is concerned, it may be that his psychological needs are not only equal to but greater than his physical ones — he may need considerable time offered to him for talking about his feelings, for example — or it may be that considerable changes are needed in his social

surroundings. These might vary from adaptations in the home to a change of where or with whom he lives. Realistically, there is no way in which the occupational therapist can justifiably avoid involving herself in the needs that become apparent in every aspect of the person's life. This should involve assessment and the setting of long-term goals and immediate objectives for all aspects of the whole person so that a sequence is followed that leads towards health and 'functioning' from the initial illness or 'dysfunction' (Keilhofner 1985).

To this end the therapist acts as facilitator. Everything she does must work towards helping the person to ultimate independence. Initially, when possibly the person may be physically ready for treatment but is still unable to handle the situation psychologically, it is suggested that the therapist act 'in loco personae' — in place of the person. Because, at this stage the person is not able to take responsibility for himself, she will have to consider choices and alternatives that seem to her to relate best to what she knows about his normal way of life and his motivations. Such a position implies that it is because of her knowledge and skills as a therapist that she is able to take on

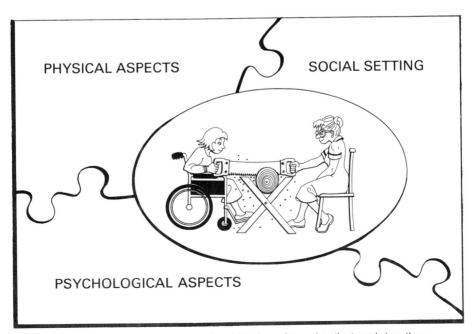

PHYSICAL ASPECTS   SOCIAL SETTING

PSYCHOLOGICAL ASPECTS

Fig. 3.11 Occupational therapy: a way in which therapist and patient work together.

this role as a temporary measure. She will always remember, however, that in so doing she is taking upon herself a responsibility for the person — for his 'self' — since he is the 'prime person' in relation to his own recovery and to the re-establishing of his equilibrium in the new situation.

The second stage involves the therapist and disabled person working together in partnership as soon as the latter is ready, physically and psychologically, to enter that partnership. This may not always be easy since disability, as we have seen, can sometimes serve unconscious purposes for the person concerned and these are not conducive to rehabilitation (for example, a regressive wish to be looked after or a fear of facing the future resulting in denial of the fact that improvement is taking place). For the therapist to be *'in loco personae'* places on her the responsibility of gradually refusing to adopt that role once the person is ready to take it up for himself, even if he is still unwilling to do so.

It might justifiably be asked 'when is a person ready?' and there is of course no simple answer to this. It is possible that the difficulty involved in reaching this decision has led to many therapists avoiding the consideration of psychological aspects of their patients' condition and making judgements solely on the measurable, physical factors. It is suggested, however, that a thorough understanding of psychology by the therapist will enable her skilfully to use the principles involved as she sets out to assess and help him. As her understanding of human nature grows she will become increasingly skilled in drawing out her patient, in listening to him and ultimately in being able to sense his needs. The aim of this chapter has been to help her in this.

Once the partnership is in operation, the disabled person and the therapist work together towards the easing of stress and solving of conflicts until, gradually, the individual is able to take over responsibility for himself. In this way the person's development can continue towards a positive future that will eventually enable him to say, 'I have had a reasonably good life and have achieved something that is worthwhile without having too many regrets, in spite of — perhaps even because of — my disability.'

REFERENCES

Atkinson R L, Atkinson R C, Hilgard E R 1987 Introduction to psychology, 9th edn. Harcourt Brace Javonovich, New York

Burns R B 1980 Essential psychology. MTP Press, Lancaster

Cattell R B 1971 Abilities: their structure, growth and action. Houghton Mifflin, Boston

Erikson E 1963 Childhood and society. Norton, New York

Eysenck H J 1953 The structure of human personality. Methuen, London

Festinger L 1957 A theory of cognitive dissonance. Harper & Row, New York

Hebb D O 1966 Textbook of psychology, 2nd edn. Saunders, London

Holmes T H, Rahe R H 1967 The social readjustment rating scale. Journal of Psychosomatic Research 11: 213–218

Illingworth R S 1983 The development of the infant and young child: normal and abnormal, 8th edn. Churchill Livingstone, Edinburgh

Isaacs N 1974 A brief introduction to Piaget. Schocken Books, New York

Kielhofner G 1985 A model of human occupation. Williams & Wilkins, Baltimore

Maslow A 1954 A theory of human motivation. Psychological Review 50: 370–396

Nicholson J 1980 Seven ages. Fontana, London

Piaget J 1952 The origins of intelligence in children. International Universities Press, New York

Pincus L 1976 Death and the family. Faber, London

Rogers C 1967 On becoming a person. Constable, London

Sarason I G 1972 Personality: an objective approach, 2nd edn. John Wiley, London

Schultz D 1976 Theories of personality. Brooks Cole, Monterey, California

Shapiro D A 1981 Crisis, stress and the sick role. In: Dunkin F N (ed) Psychology for physiotherapists. Macmillan, London

Sheridan M D 1975 From birth to five years: children's developmental progress. NFER/Nelson, Windsor

Wheldall K 1975 Social behaviour. Methuen, London

Wolpe J 1964 The comparative clinical status of conditioning therapies and psychotherapies. In: Wolpe J, Salter A, Reyna L J (eds) The conditioning therapies and psychotherapies. Holt, Rinehart and Winston, New York

Yerkes R M, Dodson J D 1908 The relation of strength of stimulus to rapidity of habit formation. Journal of Comparative Neurology and Psychology 18: 458–482.

REFERENCES AND FURTHER READING FOR SUMMARIES OF DEVELOPMENT

General

Bee H L 1989 The developing person: a lifespan approach, 2nd edn. Harper & Row, New York
Erikson E 1963 Childhood and society. Norton, New York
Lowe G 1972 The growth of personality from infancy to old age. Penguin, London
Nicholson J 1980 Seven ages. Fontana, London
Rapaport R, Rappaport R 1980 Growing through life. Harper & Row, London
Schuster C S, Ashburn S S 1980 The process of human development — a holistic approach. Little, Brown & Co, Boston
Sze W C 1975 Human life cycle. Jason Aronson Inc, New York

Childhood and adolescence

Bee H 1978 The developing child, 5th edn. Harper & Row, New York
Burns R B 1986 Child development: a text for the caring professions. Croom Helm, London
Conger J 1979 Adolescence. Generation under pressure. Harper & Row, London
Illingworth R S 1983 The development of the infant & young child. Normal & abnormal. Churchill Livingstone, Edinburgh

Richards M 1980 Infancy world of the newborn. Harper & Row, London
Rutter M 1981 Maternal deprivation reassessed, 2nd edn. Penguin, London
Sandstrom C 1979 the psychology of childhood and adolescence. Penguin, London
Santrock J W 1989 Life span development, 3rd edn. William C Brown, Dubuque, Iowa
Sheridan M D 1975 From birth to five years: children's developmental progress. NFER/Nelson, Windsor
White S, White B N 1980 Childhood. Pathways of discovery. Harper & Row, London

Adulthood and old age

Bromley D B 1974 The psychology of human ageing. Penguin, London
Carver V, Liddiard P 1978 An ageing population. Hodder & Stoughton, Sevenoaks
Fiske M 1979 Middle age. The prime of life? Harper & Row, London
Kastenbaum R 1979 Growing old. Years of Fulfilment. Harper & Row, London
Stott M 1981 Ageing for beginners. Basil Blackwell, Oxford

FURTHER READING

Atkinson R L, Atkinson R C, Smith E E, Bem D J 1990 Introduction to psychology, 10th edn. Harcourt Brace Javonovich, San Diego, California
Burns R B 1979 The self concept. Longman, London
Carter L, Willson M 1984 Attitudes and attitudinal change. In: Willson M (ed) Occupational therapy in short-term psychiatry, 1st edn. Churchill Livingstone, Edinburgh
Chapman A J, Gale A (eds) 1982 Psychology and people. Macmillan, London
Goffman E 1963 Stigma and social identity. In: Boswell D M, Wingrove J M 1974 The handicapped person in the community. Tavistock, London
Grellier D 1988 Physical dysfunction. In: Willson M (ed) Occupational therapy in short-term psychiatry, 2nd edn. Churchill Livingstone, Edinburgh
Gross R D 1987 Psychology: the science of mind and behaviour. E Arnold, London
Hart N 1985 The sociology of health medicine. Causeway Press, Ormskirk
Jay P 1984 Coping with disability, 2nd edn. Disabled Living Foundation, London, ch 14
Kubler-Ross E 1975 Death: the final stage of growth. Prentice Hall, New York
Mandelson M 1981 The role of the clinical psychologist in the physical rehabilitation unit. British Journal of Occupational Therapy 44 (12) 379–381

Morgan M, Calman M, Manning N 1985 Sociology: approaches to Health Medicine. Croom Helm, Beckenham
Nichols K A 1984 Psychological care in physical illness. Charles Press, Philadelphia
Parkes C M 1976 Bereavement. Penguin, Harmondsworth
Patrick D L, Scambler G 1986 Sociology as applied to medicine, 2nd edn. Ballière Tindall, London
Pedretti L, Zoltan B 1985 Occupational therapy, 3rd edn. Mosby, St. Louis, Missouri
Pincus L 1976 Death and the family. Faber, London
Portilo R 1984 Health professional/patient interaction, 3rd edn. W B Saunders, London
Rogers C 1967 On becoming a person. Constable, London
Series C, Lincoln N 1978 Behaviour modification in physical rehabilitation. British Journal of Occupational Therapy 41 (7) 222–224
Stewart A 1988 Stress and the vulnerable personality. In: Willson M (ed) Occupational therapy in short-term psychiatry, 2nd edn. Churchill Livingstone, Edinburgh
Versluys H P 1989 Psychosocial accommodation to physical disability. In: Trombly C A, Scott A D (eds) Occupational therapy for physical dysfunction. Williams & Wilkin, Baltimore

4

The occupational therapy process

Margaret Foster

INTRODUCTION

A process is a 'series of actions or stages for a particular purpose' (Heinemann English Dictionary). Many different approaches and techniques are used by occupational therapists but the process is essentially the same in most areas of practice and consists of four distinct stages (Fig. 4.1):

1. gathering and analysing information
2. planning and preparing for intervention
3. implementing intervention
4. evaluating outcomes.

The success of each stage is dependent on the thoroughness and accuracy with which the previous one is carried out. In this chapter the main concerns and aims of the occupational therapist at each stage are described, along with key concepts that provide a theoretical underpinning for intervention.

The occupational therapy process follows a logical sequence, for which the therapist's initial collection and analysis of information provides the foundation. The first section of the chapter describes the process by which the therapist identifies the individual's problems and prioritises them in the context of his disability, attitude, environment and aspirations. This assessment is carried out in cooperation with the individual,

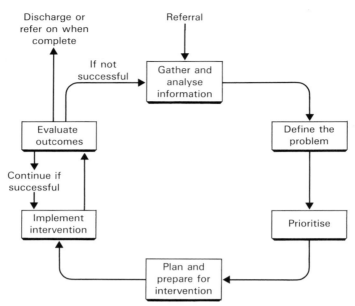

Fig. 4.1 The occupational therapy process.

and is guided by the therapist's skills in clinical reasoning, which are based on her scientific knowledge, a holistic understanding of the individual, and in her own personal strengths.

Second, the planning and preparation of intervention is described. The distinction between 'aims' and 'goals' is discussed and a framework within which these might be selected in cooperation with the individual is outlined. General considerations that the therapist should bear in mind when choosing specific activities and solutions are discussed: these include the therapist's preferred model of practice, the inclinations of the individual and his carers, the range of the therapist's expertise and the resources available to her.

Third, the implementation stage is outlined. As in the planning stage, the therapist must consider practical constraints upon time and physical resources. Her liaison with other members of the treatment team will help to ensure that all available services are being used with maximum efficiency and effectiveness.

The occupational therapy process is often cyclical in nature, particularly where the impairment has progressive or long-term implications. Thus,

the therapist may find that the outcome of the fourth stage, evaluation, prompts a return to the first stage, gathering information. The concluding section of the chapter discusses the therapist's responsibility in discerning areas of her programme which should be continued, adapted or abandoned. She may find that the individual will now benefit from referral to another professional, or that he is ready to leave the treatment programme altogether. As always, the therapist's ability to make a sound judgement will depend upon her clinical expertise, her past experience and, above all, on her holistic approach to meeting the individual's needs.

GATHERING AND ANALYSING INFORMATION

Although procedures for information gathering are more fully explored in Chapter 7, we might first consider this area of practice in the context of the entire process of occupational therapy. Information gathering for the purpose of assessment occurs early in the sequence to form a basis on which to plan intervention. It may be repeated throughout the process and at the end to evaluate progress and plan further intervention or support. Wade et al (1985, p. 69) state:

There must always be a clear reason for doing the assessment; this is by far the most important underlying principle. Assessments are performed by individuals upon individuals; it is vital that the assessor knows the purpose of the tests she is doing, and it is preferable that the patient does too. Routine collection of information for no purpose is a waste of time and effort; it is unlikely to be accurately recorded, it destroys morale and it devalues the tests.

Information gathering aims to provide a basis on which to identify the person's problems and establish his needs. This is a two-stage process: the acquisition of the information followed by its interpretation. The sequence and methods by which the information is gathered will be determined by the model of practice to which the therapist subscribes; for example, information concerning volition will be of prime importance in the application of the Model of Human Occupation (Kielhofner 1985).

Information gathered should be appropriate, valid and reliable, and should be recorded accurately and concisely. Analysis of the dysfunction will extend beyond the person's present impairments and disability to include the progression of the disease and its possible prognosis. This prognosis will be influenced by the individual's aspirations and degree of motivation, the support he is receiving, or is likely to receive, the health care and treatment location, the therapist's own skills, and the resources available to her.

The knowledge base, experience and skill of the assessor will in part determine her view of the importance of particular information for the individual. The neglect of a vital area of need or an unrealistic programme of intervention could result from misinterpretation of information.

Defining the problem (Fig. 4.2)

Problems are the difficulties which occur for a particular individual as the *result* of a combination of factors. They may be stated in terms of the disabilities and handicaps which result from impairments. Problems may vary greatly from person to person, depending on personality, life aspirations, needs and social setting.

The individual's own perceptions and definition of a problem will influence its severity. One person may perceive the inability to perform a particular task as a major problem, while another may dismiss it as a minor inconvenience which can easily be overcome.

There may be additional factors which should be considered in the identification of a person's true problems (the hidden agendas which may influence the outward presentation of the problem).

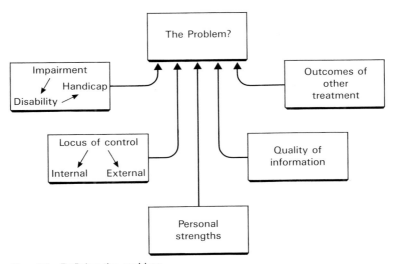

Fig. 4.2 Defining the problem.

These may be linked to the efficiency of the assessment process itself, the quality of the information gained, or to the degree of success of other interventions.

Impairment, disability and handicap

When identifying problems it is important to understand the precise meaning of these terms, which the World Health Organization (1980) defines as follows:

- *impairment* — any loss or abnormality of psychological, physiological or anatomical structure or function
- *disability* — any restriction or lack of ability (resulting from impairment) to perform an activity in the manner or within the range considered normal for a human being
- *handicap* — a disadvantage for a given individual, resulting from an impairment or disability, that limits or prevents the fulfilment of a 'survival' role that is normal (depending on age, sex, social and cultural factors) for that individual.

In simple terms, impairment is the loss or limitation of ability, disability is the effect such loss or limitation has on functional performance, and handicap is the restriction these limitations place on the person's life-style.

Problems are therefore the disabilities or handicap which result from impairment. Many impairments may contribute to a single problem. For example, the person who suffers a stroke may have impaired vision, poor muscle strength and coordination and limited sensory awareness. These impairments may all contribute to the problem of reduced mobility, which in turn may handicap the person in the role of housewife. In order to appreciate the extent of the problems experienced by someone in this situation the therapist should identify the person's family and home environment and the value she places on housewifely duties. Two people with the same impairments may have totally different problems. One may have considerable domestic support, live in an apartment or bungalow and place little value on the housewife role. This person's problems may

have more to do with mobility outside the home, compared to those of the dutiful housewife living in two-storey accommodation, because of social circumstances and personal values.

Locus of control

Studies of locus of control by Rotter may also assist the occupational therapist by providing another framework for understanding a person's problems (Rotter 1966, Rotter 1975, Lau 1982). People differ in their beliefs about how much control they can exert over their lives. The person who believes that control is located outside the self may feel that outcomes are dependent on fate, or may feel he is actively controlled by others. Such a person may show ready compliance with any suggestions made by the therapist because he perceives her as representing 'powerful others'; he may not even attempt to strive for success because 'his fate is already sealed'. Through increased understanding the person may be encouraged to exercise more control over his situation and the illness may then be positively affected by an active coping style. The therapist should therefore endeavour to educate him about his situation and involve him in making choices and initiating ideas at all stages of the programme.

Individuals who see control as lying within their own realm of responsibility are more likely to contribute their own ideas and to be more evaluative about others' suggestions. They are usually more motivated to overcome difficulties, provided that the goals are realistic in view of the person's perceived needs and wishes, and that emphasis is given to choice and personal responsibility.

Personal strengths

There is often a tendency for the occupational therapist to address the most obvious areas of deficit. The therapist's broad knowledge base and experience should ensure that associated areas of difficulty are not overlooked — in other words, that she approaches the individual holistically.

The basis of problem-solving is the identification of the individual's true problems. Frequently, therapists tend to focus on loss of function: impairment and disability. However, it is equally if not more important to identify strengths and skills; these will be the foundations on which to build the future and base the programme. Particularly in the early intervention, when successful outcomes are important in maintaining the person's motivation to continue, the employment of these strengths and skills to achieve success, however small, will boost morale. They may be the means by which a problem is overcome or minimised in the long term. An example may be seen in the individual who is able to minimise problems, despite substantial disability, by maintaining a willing support team to assist with daily needs by virtue of his strength of character and engaging personality.

Quality of information

Despite a wealth of information gained from case notes, interviews, observations and specific assessments, the true extent of a person's problems may not be clearly defined. This may be the result of the limited quality of the information gathered. The individual and his carers may, for whatever reason, not wish to reveal their real concerns. Language difficulties, limited understanding and other communication problems may restrict the exchange of information.

Identification of problems may rest with the therapist's appraisal of the quality of information gathered. She may be able to identify areas of difficulty which have not been addressed, or in some cases recognised, by the individual or his carers by utilising her understanding of the physical, psychological, social and clinical facets of the person's disability and environment. A person who has difficulty rising from a chair is also likely to have problems getting up from the toilet, bath, bed or car seat. The therapist's understanding of movement from her learning in biological sciences, together with her awareness of living skills and environmental design, will enable her to identify those tasks which are likely to cause problems. Her clinical science base will assist her in planning the most appropriate approach to the problem in light of the pathology and prognosis of the person's impairment. Additionally, understanding

of interpersonal dynamics and behavioural processes, together with astute observation, can help the therapist to identify whether the person is physically able to perform a given activity, or whether he is prevented from attempting to do so by, for example, an over-anxious or over-protective carer. The person may not be motivated to perform independently because of the secondary gains of disability (i.e. the attention provided by the carer may compensate for loneliness, when there is no real physical need for assistance) or because the activity is not perceived as personally valuable.

Outcomes of other treatments

Other intervention and treatment the person is receiving, or has received in the past, should also be considered when identifying the extent of his problems. The interrelation of other treatments with occupational therapy can be a significant factor in success. Both physiotherapy to improve mobility and speech therapy to increase communication will affect the occupational therapist's programme to reintegrate a person into school, work, the family and the social environment. Progress in other treatments will favourably influence the progress of the occupational therapy intervention; a lack of progress may indicate the depth and extent of the person's problems.

Prioritising (Fig. 4.3)

Once the therapist and the individual have jointly identified the problems that must be addressed, the next task is to establish their relative importance and urgency. Since it is unlikely that all problems can be dealt with simultaneously, it is important to prioritise them in this way before planning the treatment programme. Factors contributing to priority include:

- the wishes of the individual and his own perspective on his most vital needs
- the nature of the dysfunction
- the culture of the individual and the social climate in which he lives
- the complexity of the tasks which the person wishes to be able to perform.

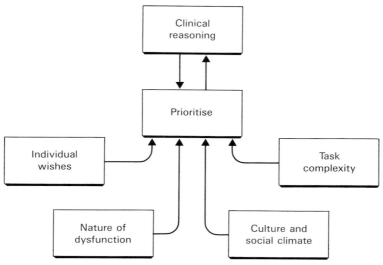

Fig. 4.3 Prioritising.

The wishes of the individual

These are often referred to in American texts as 'personal causation' and 'volition' and are closely linked to aspirations and personal drives. Factors that determine a person's drives include:

- past individual life-style experiences
- locus of control
- life-style needs and social pressures.

The occupational therapist's belief in the autonomy, dignity and personal potential of the individual should lead her to take time to identify each person's desires and drives. She should not be tempted to interpret the range of a person's problems solely in terms of her *own* priorities and values. Similarly, care must be taken in the application of theoretical models to individual cases. Maslow's hierarchy of needs (1968), for example, identifies a structure of values which applies to many people — basic personal needs requiring satisfaction before higher, intellectual ones — and may help the therapist to understand human nature and personal preferences. However, like all psychological models, it must not be rigidly applied to every individual.

Every individual who is faced with a problem will bring to the situation his own personality and drives, and his particular understanding of locus of control. Therapists have seen individuals who have overcome tremendous difficulties in order to succeed, and those who will not even attempt the first hurdle. These personality factors may contribute to the choice of priorities for activity. Those who appear to have a low level of drive, or a belief in an external locus of control, need to be involved in the choice of activity and to achieve success. Early intervention may involve the performance of small, simple tasks which are relatively unimportant in the total context of needs but whose successful outcome will foster self-respect and encourage the person to tackle more demanding or complex activities.

Identifying personal wishes may be relatively easy with some people. An individual with arthritis may be able to express a particular need in a daily living activity. However, where cognitive or communication skills are impaired — for example, following stroke or head injury — or where the person has no previous life experience on which to base judgements — as in the case of cerebral palsy in childhood — identification of personal drives may be more difficult. Observation of the individual's non-verbal responses to suggestions or levels of enthusiasm when participating in particular activities may give an indication of personal inclinations.

Many personal wishes are based on previous life

experiences or life roles — parent, partner, bread-winner and independent being. Life-style needs and social pressures will almost certainly contribute to priorities. A person who lives alone may perceive mobility and safety in self-care activities as his most vital need. The breadwinner may rate gaining competence in work-related tasks in order to retain employment over achieving independence in all aspects of personal and domestic care.

The nature of the dysfunction

The therapist's knowledge of the clinical features of the disorder, together with an understanding of the anatomical, neurological and physiological processes of recovery, will help to determine her choice of approach and treatment plan. For example, when recovery or improvement is anticipated following motor neurone damage, priority will normally be given to achieving active mobility and strength in the proximal joints and to preventing secondary complications in distal joints until recovery commences.

Where disability is likely to persist or deteriorate, priority will be given to maintaining function and facilitating life-style adjustments. Many people are eager to find ways of retarding the deterioration and welcome advice on methods of maintaining function whilst recognising that they will not be able to return to previous levels of attainment. Education and practice in joint preservation techniques for the person with rheumatoid arthritis, and energy conservation programmes for people with multiple sclerosis are two examples of interventions appropriate to long-term disability.

Where deterioration is inevitable a person may strive to maintain ability in one particular task, and assistance to achieve this aim may be the prime focus of intervention. This is often particularly evident when the illness causes severe impairment and achievement of a particular goal is the main priority. This goal may be as diverse as learning to play a musical instrument or to use a computer, or may involve completion of a task or plan already in hand. The person's energy and attention may be totally directed towards achieving success in the chosen task, while assistance is readily accepted in other areas of living.

If physical recovery is anticipated the occupational therapist's chosen approach will aim to promote such progress. However, where there is likely to be residual deficit, or deterioration, a compensatory rehabilitative approach may be more appropriate. Similarly, the psychosocial implications of the dysfunction may influence the therapist's choice of approach in order to holistically address the person's needs for return to an optimum community life-style. For example, the therapist may use a combination of neurodevelopmental and behavioural or cognitive techniques to overcome the effects of hemiplegia with behavioural or learning difficulties following head injury.

Culture and social climate

The therapist should make herself aware of the main beliefs and practices of the person's culture if she is not to risk offending him or his carers. In some cultures personal independence may not be highly valued because of the recognised duty of care within the extended family. Assisting a person to strive to perform self-care skills may in this context even be viewed as cruel.

Recognition of cultural or religious practices may be impeded by the therapist's lack of experience or knowledge and may be further complicated by language barriers. In some religions accepted hand dominance for personal activities (i.e. the right hand is the clean hand used for feeding and greeting others, and the left hand for personal cleanliness) is vitally important and should be respected, if the person is not to be ostracised from his own community as unclean. Personal cleansing may take priority over feeding or toileting because of its importance to religious practice. The therapist should inform herself about such cultural beliefs and respect them in planning intervention.

The social climate — the general attitudes or feelings of those with whom we come into contact — may also influence priorities. This may be related to social roles or may be determined by poverty or affluence.

The individuals' social role in the family or local community may be an important personal driving factor. For example, for the person who is accustomed to the role of leader, organiser, extrovert or active participant, cognitive, communicative and motor skills may assume prime importance.

Where poverty exists basic needs such as shelter, communication, food and toileting may take priority, along with financial concerns.

Complexity of the task

Some tasks are simple to perform, requiring only a relatively basic level of skills in limited areas of function. For example, switching on a light requires upper limb mobility, coordination and some dexterity in conjunction with visual and cognitive skills in locating and recognising the light switch. Putting on a round-necked jumper is a much more complex task, requiring a greater degree of upper limb motor skills and considerable ability in visual and cognitive functions to identify the correct parts of the garment — which is the front and which is the back — and to remember and follow the appropriate sequence for dressing.

The therapist's skills in activity analysis will enable her to identify the component parts of a task and to determine the particular skills required to perform each part in a successful sequence. By linking these requirements to the person's strengths and weaknesses she can judge the probable difficulty he will have in completing the task.

It is usual for the sequence of activities in a therapeutic programme to reflect this progression of activity complexity — commencing with activities which are less demanding and building up to those which require a particularly high level of skill in one or more areas of ability. Where there is a likelihood of deterioration the reverse procedure may be suitable, provided that the downgrading of the activity is managed sensitively.

However, when prioritising activities the therapist should bear in mind that for reasons of safety or particular need it may be preferable or even essential for the person to become competent in a relatively complex task early in the intervention programme. In such a case the task may be broken down into component parts, each part

analysed in detail, and a range of options for successful completion of the task explored. After all the components of the activity are analysed, a simple programme may be developed to reflect the person's present skill level. For example, a person living alone who needs to be independent in making a hot drink might be provided with an instruction chart to assist with cognitive sequencing and modified equipment which he can safely handle. Alternative methods, such as using a thermal jug might be explored.

In conclusion, prioritising is itself a complex activity which is dependent on a number of factors. When determining the intervention sequence the occupational therapist may guide the discussions concerning the range of options but the wishes of the person and his carers should be respected when the final choice is made.

Clinical reasoning

The therapist's skills in clinical reasoning are vital to the sound analysis of information and to the planning and preparation of intervention.

Clinical reasoning (or clinical inquiry) is the thinking which guides the occupational therapist's analysis and helps her to work with the individual to come to a clinical judgement — an opinion or decision on the pertinent facts.

Rogers (1983, p. 601) sums this up in her statement that 'the goal of clinical reasoning is a treatment recommendation issued in the interests of a particular patient.' Rogers maintains that clinical reasoning has three basic aspects — scientific, ethical and artistic — and that 'without science clinical inquiry is not systematic; without ethics it is not responsible; without art it is not convincing'.

The scientific component of clinical reasoning is founded in the therapist's knowledge base. This includes knowledge she may have gained from theoretical learning and from previous experience and practice, as well as the knowledge acquired through the information gathering stage of the occupational therapy process.

The ethical component is based in the therapist's philosophy of valuing human dignity and is used in clinical reasoning to decide what option should be chosen from a range of possibilities. It is founded in the therapist's recognition of and respect for the person's own values and is reflected in the cooperative manner in which the determination of priorities and activities for therapy is made.

The artistry lies in the way in which the therapist uses her own personal skills to perfect her information gathering and analysis, and in her ability to impart values and guide decisions without imposing her opinions. Rogers (1963, p. 601) states that 'the artistry of clinical reasoning is exhibited in the craftsmanship with which the therapist executes the series of steps that culminates in a clinical decision.'

Clinical reasoning is therefore based on the therapist's understanding of the value and reliability of information, her knowledge of possible options and their merits and limitations, her positive humanistic values and her own personal strengths.

PLANNING AND PREPARING FOR INTERVENTION

Once the person's problems have been identified and prioritised, the next stage is to determine the aims and goals to be achieved. When these have been decided on it will be necessary to consider a range of ways of attaining them, the approaches and media to be used, and individual responsibilities for specific aspects of the intervention.

Setting aims and goals

It is important to understand the difference between aims and goals as well as their relative value in the total process. An *aim* is a general statement of the situation one hopes to attain, usually in the long term. *Goals*, sometimes called *objectives*, are much more concise descriptions of specific outcomes, usually written in positive terms on the part on the participant. Goals state the activity the person will perform, under specified conditions and to a particular degree of success. The activity is described in assessable, observable terms. The conditions are the particular circumstances in which the person will perform the activity; the

degree of success is the acceptable level of performance. It is usual for a progressive sequence of goals to be prerequisite to the attainment of an aim.

An example of an aim may be: Mrs Jones will achieve maximum independence in dressing.

A specific goal towards this aim may be: Mrs Jones will be able to dress the upper half of her body every morning, sitting on the chair beside her bed, without manual assistance or verbal prompts, by the end of one month.

Goals should be appropriate and specific to the individual. They should be measurable and attainable.

The benefits of incorporating aims and goals into the intervention process may be outlined as follows:

- Because they require a clear identification of strengths, weaknesses and needs in order to be specific, they encourage accurate assessment
- They make completion of the total task less onerous by tackling the problem in small attainable steps
- By considering each short-term step, they make the programme flexible, reflecting specific needs or skills at each stage of intervention
- They can be applied to many areas of activity and practice and therefore provide a consistent method for planning in a variety of situations
- They encourage consistency in care and increase understanding of the reasons for particular practices by presenting a systematic, ordered approach which can be understood by staff from various disciplines, as well as by the individual and his carers
- They help to identify the intervention activity and the learning methods
- By providing opportunities to measure achievement, they allow the success of the intervention to be clearly evaluated.

It is usual to include a number of aims, some of which may be addressed simultaneously, in the intervention programme. Similarly, the achievement of one specific goal may involve the acquisition of

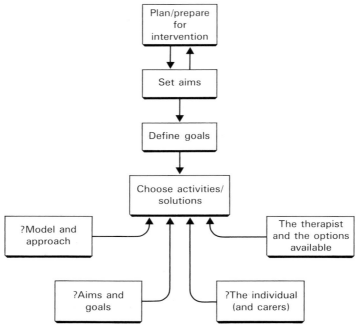

Fig. 4.4 Planning and preparing for intervention.

a particular skill which contributes to more than one aim. For example, achievement of a goal concerning a specific mobility task may contribute to long-term aims related to self-care, work activities or leisure pursuits.

The value of the therapist's skill in determining particular strengths and needs and developing these into specific aims and goals in partnership with the person cannot be underestimated. Aims and goals provide the foundation for clear, concise, accurate, individual intervention, in which the person is an active participant. They provide a system which may be understood by everyone, thereby promoting liaison and cooperation among all concerned.

Identifying suitable solutions

As long ago as 1960, E. M. Macdonald stated in her book *Occupational Therapy in Rehabilitation* that 'almost *any* activity can be used. What matters is the *aim* of its use, and whether it achieves, or is suitable to achieve, the purpose for which it is employed.' This statement is still true today,

despite advances in the range of activities available to the therapist, the changes in health care, and the evolving needs of disabled persons and their carers.

Having identified aims and goals the choice of activities by which they can be achieved is the next logical step. This choice will depend on:

- the model of practice and the approach chosen
- the aims and goals of rehabilitation
- the wishes and motivations of individual (and carers where appropriate)
- the therapist's skills and the options available to her.

Model and approach

In the selection of appropriate activities for a therapeutic programme, much will depend upon the model of practice and the treatment approach adopted by the therapist. It is also necessary, in choosing activities, to consider the person's priorities and aspirations, his situation and needs, the likely progression of his dysfunction, and the setting of the therapeutic intervention.

In many instances the therapist's choice of model will have been made early in the intervention process and will have determined the way in which she has gathered and analysed information. For example, assessments that are based upon the Model of Human Occupation (Kielhofner 1985), will reflect the hierarchical structure of subsystems, commencing with volition and culminating in performance, set out in that model. The solutions and activities that are subsequently chosen will attempt to provide ways of meeting the person's needs in accordance with that hierarchy, such that activities which stimulate performance but also meet volitional and habituational requirements will be considered more favourably than those which merely improve performance.

Where recovery is anticipated but has not yet commenced, a predominately rehabilitative approach will initially be appropriate in facilitating successful achievement in some essential activities. As recovery commences, other approaches may assume greater significance. For example, a neurodevelopmental approach may be used with someone who has experienced a cerebrovascular accident, and a biomechanical approach with someone who has suffered a hand injury. When maximum improvement is achieved any residual deficit may necessitate a return to the humanistic rehabilitative approach to compensate for long-term loss.

In some instances the sequencing of activity will also be determined by the approach. When a cognitive approach is employed to teach or re-teach a skill, the activity will be graded according to the learning methods and the nature and complexity of the task itself. For example, when learning to prepare food it is usual to start with a simple drink and snack before embarking on the preparation of a full meal. In some approaches the progression will follow the process of expected recovery; for example, in the neurodevelopmental approach activities to improve sitting balance and posture will precede those which promote hand control and dexterity.

The therapist's abilities in identifying the person's interests, strengths and needs, and her skills in analysing and modifying activities will enable her to identify how a particular activity

which the person values and enjoys may be used in a number of different approaches to meet the aims and goals specified.

Aims and goals

Having identified general aims, the therapist must plan her intervention in the context of achieving a particular goal. A range of options may be available and it is frequently necessary to implement a number of these to identify which is most helpful in achieving the desired goal. This may be illustrated by the different ways by which independence in toileting may be attained, i.e.: through the use of specific activity to improve strength and mobility in order to perform transfer techniques independently; by adapting clothing, either in choice of design or modification of fastenings; through the use of assistive equipment such as seat raises, rails, frames or commodes; or through alterations to the environment to provide an accessible toilet. Through discussion of the merits and constraints of each option, the individual, his carers and the therapist can decide upon the solution most suitable for all concerned.

The individual and his carers

Choice of activity must be realistic in view of the life-style and needs of the individual, taking into account his personal, domestic, work and leisure experiences as well as his sociocultural environment. Activity should be chosen in light of the person's previous physical, cognitive and social competence, but should be graded according to his present strengths and deficits. This will be based on thorough baseline assessment and knowledge of activity analysis, application and grading.

Activities should be appropriate to the person's age, sex and culture, but care should be taken to ascertain suitability *in each case* and not to impose sexist, chronological or cultural boundaries as a matter of course. Activities involving the use of modern technology, such as computing, may be more appropriate for the person wishing to return to paid employment, whilst cookery or creative craft activity may have more appeal to the elderly housewife. However, such assumptions should not be made without due consultation with the person concerned, as the elderly housewife may be an enthusiastic computer user from contact with her grandchildren. Such enthusiasm may motivate her to pursue computing and thereby gain cognitive skills or fine motor functions in excess of those acquired through cookery or other creative craft activity.

In many instances the needs of the carer will have equal consideration in the choice of activity. If a carer is willing to continue assistance with dressing, but is at risk of personal injury through helping with lifting or transfers, creative activity to strengthen the disabled person's limbs and develop balance for independent transfers may be more appropriate than daily dressing practice. Assistance with dressing, if given out of a genuine desire to help, may be the basis of secure friendship and trust, while the risk of personal injury through lifting may cause the carer anxiety and make him or her reluctant to continue. Practice with mechanical hoists may overcome the carer's risks, but such equipment offers less flexibility than the acquisition of personal skill, and is expensive to provide.

While many technical factors may be considered in the choice of activity the therapist should not overlook the purely emotive aspect of personal interests. An activity chosen predominantly for pleasure and interest may be the driving force in motivating the person to pursue the treatment programme despite some discomfort and considerable effort. However, choice of an activity in which the person has had a previously moderate level of skill should be considered with care, as the negative effects of reduced capability because of impairment may only serve to reinforce a sense of loss.

The therapist's skills and the options available

Occupational therapists are recognised for their holistic and flexible approach to problem-solving. However, the therapist herself is an individual with particular skills which extend or limit her own capability and expertise. Individual differences between therapists may be the result of previous learning and experience, and of personal

preferences with regard to areas of interest. Some therapists prefer to specialise in particular treatment approaches, activities, or areas of disability and may develop in-depth knowledge and skill in these areas, often at the expense of other facets of practice.

The depth and range of the therapist's skills will be of vital importance in her choice of activities for an intervention. She may have specialist knowledge in the area of need and be the ideal person to assist the individual. She may have a number of skills available to her and she should use her clinical judgement, in consultation with the individual, in identifying the range of suitable options and making the most appropriate choices. On the other hand, she may have limited expertise in the area of need. In this situation she should consider the choices available. Is there someone else in the department or team who may be more appropriate and who is available to assist? Will other skills the therapist possesses be likely to achieve the same aims for the individual in the same time-scale? If the therapist feels that she lacks expertise in a given area it is important for her to recognise this, discuss options with the person and his carers, identify where such skills may be available and take steps to make the appropriate contacts and referrals.

The therapist should not see this as a shortcoming on her part, particularly where the person's needs are very specialised. Her knowledge of the expertise offered by a broad range of disciplines in the hospital and the community is a support in itself. The therapist's skills in recognising needs, and her communication and liaison with outside disciplines is a vital part of her role in facilitating the most appropriate solution.

Where the person has a long-term regular need for support, it is unlikely that this will be provided by the occupational therapist. Referral to others who are able to provide such support, for example the community nurse or a day centre, earlier rather than later in the therapy intervention, will enable this contact to be developed while the therapist is still involved and able to evaluate the adequacy of the provision for the person's needs.

Occasionally no one is available to help with a particular problem. This should be acknowledged with the individual and possible alternative coping strategies considered which, while not ideal, will minimise the handicap in the short term in an acceptable way until such support becomes available. Take, for example, the case of a young woman with cerebral palsy who wishes to live independently and requires a modified living environment and considerable practice in domestic and life skills. The accommodation is not available at present and a place in a skills training programme will be available in three months' time. The therapist is not able to provide regular domestic or skills training but she may be able to assist the person and her carers in developing ways of gradually increasing her responsibilities and skills in the home and the community until such outside support becomes available. The therapist's contribution as facilitator and educator is thus no less important than the provision of direct treatment in the intervention process.

To summarise, choosing a solution is a complex task which depends upon many aspects of the individual's personal needs, experiences and drives, the environment in which he lives, the nature of the dysfunction and the services that are available. The therapist's skills in clinical reasoning will be vital in guiding selection.

Choice of activity should be realistic. That is, it should be geared to the person's requirements and wishes in accordance with the facilities and resources available. The activity should present a challenge which is valued and the goal should be perceived to be achievable. The part any activity plays in attaining a broader solution or aim should be clearly understood by all concerned.

IMPLEMENTING INTERVENTION

An intervention plan should set out *how* to meet short-term goals in the most appropriate way for a particular person. It will state the approaches and methods to be used and identify the therapeutic activity, chosen from the range of options that has been identified.

Choices of *where* the activity should take place will be important. This may be the ward, the therapy department, the person's home, a day centre or some other suitable location. Obviously, if therapy is to occur away from the person's residence (whether home or hospital) the distance to travel and the method of transport should be anticipated, and the impact travel may have on the person's performance and gains should be considered.

Factors to consider

Time

The programme plan should also take into account the optimum length of time for each therapy session, and how frequently sessions should occur.

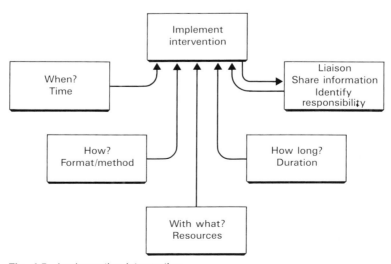

Fig. 4.5 Implementing intervention.

This may be based on the disability, its cause, course and prognosis, and the advantages gained by regular intervention.

There may be particular times during the day when therapy is more advantageous. Activities to improve physical performance for the person with an arthritic disorder characterised by morning stiffness may be more successful in the afternoon. Similarly, in situations where the person has an increasing level of fatigue through the day, activities in the morning may be especially successful. However, it will be necessary for the therapist to observe some self-maintenance activities performed when the person is at the worst stage during the day, in order to consider methods by which he can cope successfully in the daily routine. When the person has cognitive problems, particularly those affecting orientation in time or place, the timing and location of self-care and domestic activities should equate, as far as possible, with his 'normal' daily routine.

Format

The intervention should be carried out in the most suitable therapy format: on a one-to-one basis or in a group. The occupational therapist's basic philosophy of recognising individuality, together with the variations among different persons' goals, will demand that much of the intervention be on a one-to-one basis, particularly in the initial stages. Some goals, especially those related to the development of social and communicative skills, may be more readily achieved by participation in group activities. The format will also be affected by the choice of activity medium and the amount of direction or guidance required by the person to safely succeed in achieving the desired goal.

Resources

Having considered her plan for intervention in relation to the person's needs, the therapist should also consider whether the programme is realistic and achievable in practical terms. In an ideal world all things might be attempted. In reality, limitations of the therapist's knowledge and skill, together with constraints on practical resources such as staff, a suitable location, transport, tools, materials, equipment and finance may restrict the intervention programme. Demands made upon the therapist's time by her entire caseload and the inavailability of support may limit the frequency and duration of therapy. The therapist should weigh the ideal quantity or extent of her interventions against the need for quality assurance. She should also endeavour to ensure that the goals of those in greatest need are met. In many situations, excessive case overloads leading to the risk of unsatisfactory outcomes for all have led to the use of priority ratings for therapy intervention.

Duration

In some instances it may also be necessary to identify the anticipated total length of the intervention and the pattern of contact for purposes of caseload planning and clinical budgeting. For example, where the intervention aims to promote physical improvement, identification of an anticipated length of treatment may serve as a time framework for the evaluation of outcomes. This evaluation should be consistent with the aims and goals of the programme, and may provide a basis for consideration of the continuation or termination of therapy. It may be found that further goals remain to be achieved, or that discharge or referral to other sources is now indicated. While an estimate of programme duration is valuable for intervention planning and for caseload and staff management, care should be taken to ensure that rigid time criteria are not applied at the expense of genuine benefit from further therapy.

Where major home adaptations are planned the occupational therapist's pattern of intervention may not be regular. It will often extend over a considerable period of time — from initial assessment of need, through planning and the monitoring of progress, to successful completion. At some stages the person's needs will be urgent and particularly time-consuming for the therapist.

Liaison with the team

The personnel with whom the occupational therapist should liaise may vary, depending on the nature of the problem, the choice of solutions and plan for intervention, and the setting of the therapy.

In the hospital environment

The therapist may need to liaise with the medical and nursing staff and others in the rehabilitation team. She may also have to liaise with others outside the hospital, in addition to the family or carers, depending on the person's needs and the choice of activity. This may involve personnel in social services departments, the community occupational therapist, or other community resource personnel — for example, members of voluntary organisations, or staff from community health care, employment, education or leisure facilities.

Outside the hospital environment

Therapists may need to liaise with similar personnel in both the hospital and the community. They will be particularly involved with personnel outside the hospital environment in the majority of instances. Liaison with staff from local authority departments, particularly housing and social services, plays an important part in work in the community.

Why is liaison important?

● To ensure that the programme of intervention is cohesive. Liaison is a two-way process of giving and receiving information. The therapist should inform herself of other support or treatments the person is receiving and of the aims and goals of these. She should gain information on the frequency and timing of other activities, in addition to the details of the methods used. The therapist should also give information on her proposals. Any divergence or overlap should be discussed and outcomes negotiated to achieve optimum benefit for the person and the carers in the most appropriate format.

● To identify responsibilities. It is important to ensure that all members of the team clearly understand their duties and that attention to any area of need is not overlooked or duplicated. This promotes efficiency on the part of the team in terms of time and effort, and the best utilisation of individual skills. The clear delineation of responsibilities is likely to encourage a greater sense of duty and a desire for achievement, which in turn promotes quality of care.

When discussing the range of possible solutions with the individual, his own responsibilities should be negotiated with the therapist. When identifying the responsibilities of the provider — the therapist or carer — the demands these may make in terms of skills, knowledge and time should be discussed and agreed on.

Frequently, there is some role overlap among members of the multidisciplinary rehabilitation team. In some instances it may be more advantageous for one person to take the key worker role, thus preventing confusion and the duplication of effort. Conversely, in some situations which involve learning a particular skill, repetition by more than one person may promote or consolidate learning, provided the teaching is consistent.

When identifying needs and planning for intervention it will have been necessary to consider a wide range of factors. If these have been identified and fully explored with all concerned, the therapist, the individual and his carers should be well prepared for the programme of intervention.

In many cases intervention may proceed according to the chosen plan but there may be unforeseen factors, such as an alteration in the person's health or social situation, or in the facilities or resources available, which necessitate a change of course. The therapist should be prepared to modify her plans accordingly. This may prompt a total reappraisal of the intervention, or only a minor modification, or a delay or advancement of an activity already included in the programme.

The therapist needs to retain a flexible, positive approach to such changes to accommodate the needs of the individual and others in the team, in line with her duties of employment.

EVALUATING OUTCOMES

The aim of evaluation is to appraise and monitor the effectiveness of the intervention programme.

This may be considered in terms of its success and limitations for the person concerned. Such information may also form part of an analysis of occupational therapy in the wider context of researching the value of specific strategies for a particular group in a given situation.

Evaluation may be carried out formally through specific tests, measurements and assessments or informally through observation and conversation with the person, his relatives, and others concerned in the intervention programme.

Why evaluate?

- *To measure progress* (or the lack of it) in order to determine whether the treatment should be continued or whether a change of activity or strategy is needed. This type of evaluation should occur at regular intervals throughout the programme and is usually made with reference to the specific goals identified when the intervention strategy was planned.
- *To plan for discharge or referral* to others for further intervention. This usually occurs at the end or in the later stages of the programme in order to measure the *extent* of the progress and identify any residual deficits which have not been overcome. It is based on the aims identified in the plan and is usually carried out through a formal assessment. Frequently this is a repetition of some or all of the initial assessments performed before planning the intervention.

A final evaluation carried out at the end of the programme provides a valuable record for future reference in the event of the person's re-referral to occupational therapy or another discipline at a later date. Information gained will also form part of the basis for the therapist's referral of the person to other sources to meet his residual needs.

- *To monitor or measure efficacy.* Information may be gained through evaluation of part or all of the intervention to identify the value of specific activities or the interrelation of a number of techniques in the total programme. Such information may be useful to the therapist in her justifications to others, such as management staff. It may also form a valuable resource for reflection on and analysis of practice and may lead to the development of new intervention strategies or therapeutic activities.

Evaluation is therefore a means for determining continuation or change — both for the individual and for the therapist. It confirms that intervention is progressing at the anticipated level and alerts the person and the therapist to any particular need for change. This illustrates the cyclical nature of the occupational therapy process: the earlier stage of analysis of information is returned to, in the reappraisal of priorities and the adjustment of preparation and planning. Gillette (1988, p. 211) writes:

Evaluation serves the purpose of keeping the therapist's work current, for it is a spiral building

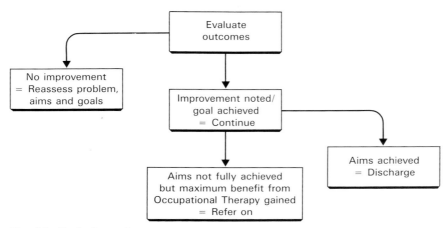

Fig. 4.6 Evaluating outcomes.

process. Each treatment session should be assessed, and each target area should be reviewed in order to determine the effectiveness of the activity process and to revise the objectives as they are mastered or found to be unreachable. Treatment should not persist in a straight line. It is the system of evaluation that is built into the treatment process that ultimately determines the effectiveness of treatment.

Evaluation is also one of the major bases on which research is founded, promoting wider change or development in professional practice. Evaluations of outcomes may provide evidence that helps to confirm or refute theories, ideas or beliefs about particular practices. Further investigation or analysis may identify the reasons behind the outcomes. Successful investigations in this area lead to an increased understanding which may be the basis for objective continuation or cessation of particular techniques, or may promote totally new thinking which enhances professional enquiry and development.

CONCLUSION

The practice of occupational therapy must follow a clearly identified process if the treatment it offers is to be organised, systematic and successful. As this process must aim to realistically and sensitively meet human needs in a wide variety of situations it will inevitably be somewhat complex.

The complexity of the process lies in the identification of needs, the recognition of individuality and the variety of options available for implementation. The greatest effort and detail are required in the investigative and preparatory stages. If these stages are managed correctly, the treatment programme based on their outcome should run smoothly. Evaluation, ideally, will provide confirmation that all is well, and may give rise to new ideas for future development.

None the less, the therapist may find that a particular action has failed to meet a person's needs or to respond to changes in circumstance. In such a case, the ultimate success of her intervention will depend upon her objectivity, flexibility, 'artistry' and holistic understanding of the individual as she finds alternative strategies to help him meet his evolving goals.

REFERENCES

Gillette N 1988 Occupational therapy and mental health. In: Hopkins H L, Smith H D (eds) Willard and Spackman's occupational therapy, 7th edn. J B Lippincott, Philadelphia
Kielhofner G 1985 The model of human occupation. Williams & Wilkins, Baltimore
Lau R R 1982 Origins of health locus of control beliefs. Journal of Personality and Social Psychology 42(2): 322–334
Macdonald E M 1960 Occupational therapy in rehabilitation. Baillière Tindall & Cox, London
Maslow A H 1968 Toward a psychology of being, 2nd edn. Van Nostrand Reinhold, New York
Rogers J C 1983 Clinical reasoning: the ethics, the science and art. American Journal of Occupational Therapy 37(9): 601

Rotter J B 1966 Generalised expectancies for internal versus external control of reinforcement. Psychological Monographs 80(1) No. 609. American Psychological Association
Rotter J B 1975 Some problems and misconceptions related to the construct of internal versus external control of reinforcement. Journal of Consulting and Clinical Psychology 43: 56–67
Wade D T, Langton-Hewer R, Skilbeck C E, David R M 1985 Stroke — a critical approach to diagnosis, treatment and management. Chapman & Hall, London
World Health Organization 1980 International classification of impairments, disabilities and handicaps. WHO, Geneva

Part 2
Skills

If only we knew what we were about perhaps
we could go about it better.

Abraham Lincoln

5

Management

Sybil E. Johnson

We have available today the knowledge and experience needed for the successful practice of management. But there is probably no field of human endeavour where the always tremendous gap between the knowledge and performance of the average is wider or more intractable.

(Peter F. Drucker)

INTRODUCTION

How many times has the plea, 'Why do I need to learn about management? I don't want to be a head occupational therapist, I want to treat patients' been heard, one wonders? Most of us, at one time or another, have had much of our educational and working life organised and managed for us; hence, there is a tendency to overlook the fact that management is an integral part of daily life. People need to organise themselves, to plan their working day, to communicate with others, to be in the right place at the appointed time and to prepare themselves for future tasks and activities. Therefore, whether the individual is a parent, an employee, a student or an employer, she requires management skills in order to achieve her goals.

It may be said that there are as many definitions of 'management' as there are managers. As Heller (1972) remarks: 'Any definition of management must be right, because almost any definition must fit something so amorphous and shifting'.

Moreover, people's descriptions are influenced by their background and personal viewpoint. However, any definition of management, whatever its origin, has common themes, e.g. that management is a *process* which involves achieving objectives through people, and thus cannot be carried out in isolation. A manager directs human resources and activities within the constraints of available finance, buildings, equipment and materials, with the purpose of achieving an organisation's overall aim.

Innumerable management texts debate the question of whether managers are born or made. Whichever belief is held, managers at all levels must have certain inherent qualities in addition to appropriate education and experience. This applies to occupational therapy as it does to any profession, workforce or organisation, and the intent of this chapter is to encourage the reader to formulate her own views and understanding of management and what it means.

All occupational therapy staff are involved in management to some extent. They all have to manage themselves and their daily allocated workload. For example, in certain settings a technical instructor may have day-to-day responsibility for a helper and will therefore need skills in supervising, directing, delegating and decision-making. A junior therapist will have to plan and organise her daily workload, communicate with colleagues and clients and, possibly, supervise a helper. A head occupational therapist will be involved in all management processes in order to ensure that departmental aims and objectives are met, that resources are used effectively and efficiently to meet specific needs, that staff morale and motivation are sustained. Figure 5.1 sets out the management skills required by occupational therapy staff.

This chapter is organised into six sections. Section 1 discusses the concept of management in broad terms, glancing at the most influential theories of management and outlining the basic components of the managerial process. Section 2 describes the framework within which occupational therapy management takes place by outlining the historical and legal context of present-day health and welfare services. This section also describes the regulatory framework for occupational therapy provided by professional bodies such as the Council for Professions Supplementary to Medicine. Section 3 looks more closely at the legal and ethical principles that bear upon the therapist's professional practice.

Section 4 is intended to assist the occupational therapist in entering professional practice and developing her career. This includes discussion of: time management and prioritising; coping with pressure and stress; core skills and professionalism; and strategies for seeking and taking up a new post in an occupational therapy service.

Section 5 discusses the interpersonal skills that are necessary to occupational therapy managers and staff, outlining the essential components of successful communication as well as various approaches that can be used to enhance communication within an occupational therapy service. Particular attention is given to the dynamics of meetings and committees.

The final section of the chapter examines in detail the various duties of the personnel and departmental manager. These include: staff recruitment, supervision and development; managing change; planning, developing and marketing the service; resource management (including data); quality control, finance and caseload management; and day-to-day administration.

It is hoped that the new as well as the more experienced therapist will be able to apply many of the management principles described in this chapter to her own practice, and that she will welcome the challenges and opportunities offered by managerial responsibilities at all stages of her career.

SECTION 1: MANAGEMENT

The meaning of management

Approaches to the theory of management are many and varied. Although there is no generally accepted definition of management, Fayol's statement in 1916 (Storrs 1949) that 'to manage is to forecast and plan, to organise, to command, to co-ordinate and to control' is still valid, despite

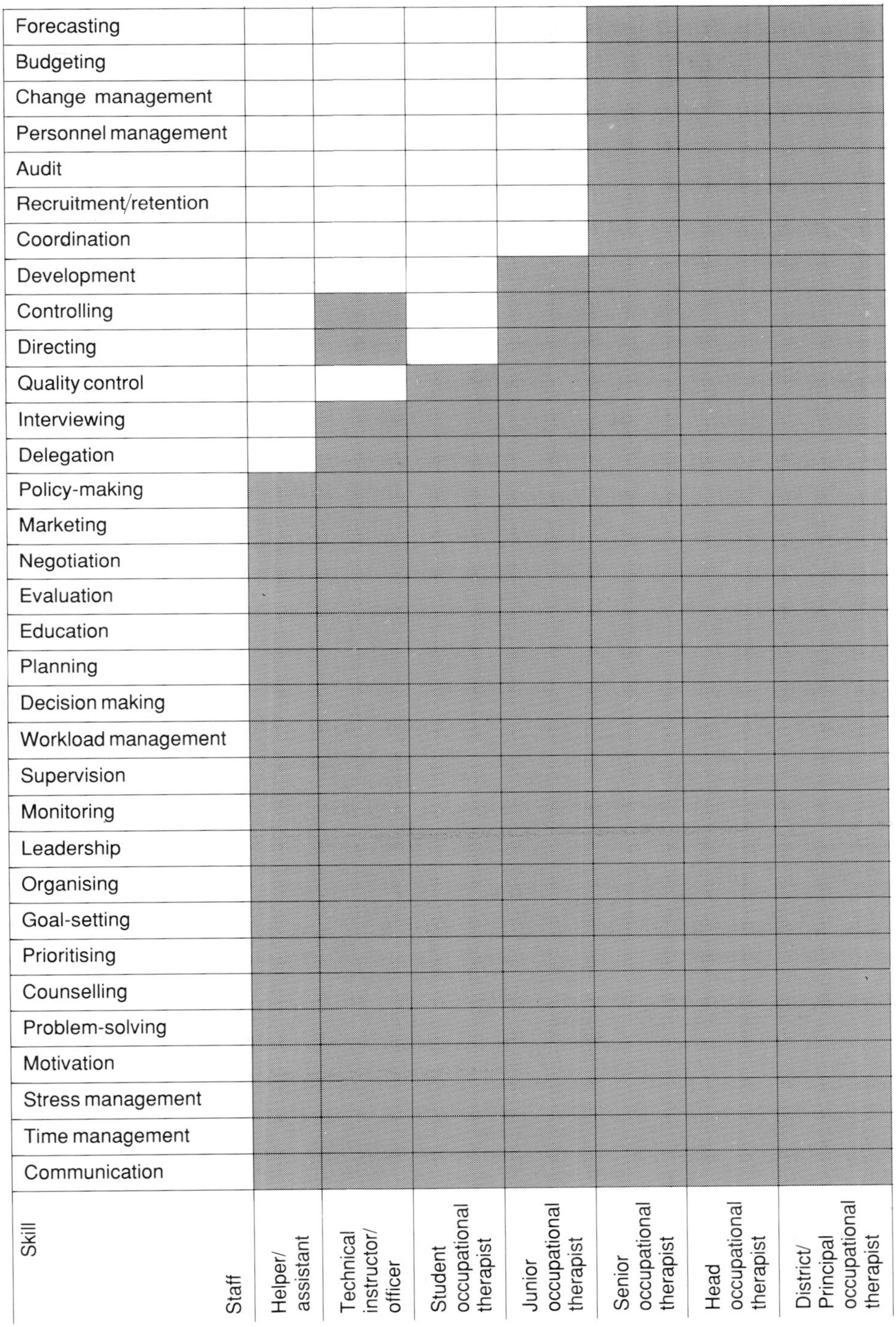

Skill	Helper/assistant	Technical instructor/officer	Student occupational therapist	Junior occupational therapist	Senior occupational therapist	Head occupational therapist	District/Principal occupational therapist
Forecasting					■	■	■
Budgeting					■	■	■
Change management					■	■	■
Personnel management					■	■	■
Audit					■	■	■
Recruitment/retention					■	■	■
Coordination					■	■	■
Development				■	■	■	■
Controlling		■		■	■	■	■
Directing		■		■	■	■	■
Quality control			■	■	■	■	■
Interviewing		■	■	■	■	■	■
Delegation		■	■	■	■	■	■
Policy-making	■	■	■	■	■	■	■
Marketing	■	■	■	■	■	■	■
Negotiation	■	■	■	■	■	■	■
Evaluation	■	■	■	■	■	■	■
Education	■	■	■	■	■	■	■
Planning	■	■	■	■	■	■	■
Decision making	■	■	■	■	■	■	■
Workload management	■	■	■	■	■	■	■
Supervision	■	■	■	■	■	■	■
Monitoring	■	■	■	■	■	■	■
Leadership	■	■	■	■	■	■	■
Organising	■	■	■	■	■	■	■
Goal-setting	■	■	■	■	■	■	■
Prioritising	■	■	■	■	■	■	■
Counselling	■	■	■	■	■	■	■
Problem-solving	■	■	■	■	■	■	■
Motivation	■	■	■	■	■	■	■
Stress management	■	■	■	■	■	■	■
Time management	■	■	■	■	■	■	■
Communication	■	■	■	■	■	■	■
Staff							

Fig. 5.1 Management skills and occupational therapy staff.

modifications by more recent writers. In 1980, for instance, Koontz et al changed the emphasis, describing 'the five essential management functions' as 'planning, organising, staffing, directing and leading, and controlling.'

These statements point to the understanding of management as a *process* that enables any organisation to achieve its objectives by planning, organising and controlling its resources, and offering staff leadership (Fig. 5.2).

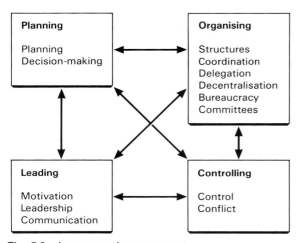

Fig. 5.2 A process of management.

Administration versus management

There are occasions when the words 'administration' and 'management' are confused or used interchangeably. However, there are differences which need to be understood:

- *Administration* is a relatively narrow activity, involving day-to-day maintenance of procedures such as stock control, record keeping and dealing with daily correspondence.
- *Management*, which will involve some administration, is on the other hand an activity which embraces the present and future of an organisation and its work. Hence, such elements as planning and forecasting, motivating staff, recruitment and retention, quality standards and controls assume importance.

Organisations

Management can only be considered realistically with reference to an organisation such as a family, a school, the local supermarket, a social service's office, a hospital or a particular department or service within a large organisation. An organisation in this instance is a social structure, rather than a process, and each one has certain essential features, i.e. people, a particular purpose and a structure or hierarchy.

One of the functions of an organisation is management, through which it furthers its own purpose whilst manipulating certain variables with given constraints. Handy (1976) describes these variables as people, work and structures, and systems and procedures, whilst the constraints in question are the organisation's goals, its culture (values, beliefs) and the technology available. All six of these interact such that change in one will probably result in change in one or more of the others. Successful management involves balancing the three variables with the three constraints in order to meet the organisation's needs at a particular time.

MANAGEMENT THEORIES

During the late 19th century, as large industrial organisations were established, systematic management thinking began to evolve. The theories that emerged during this period still influence the behaviour and attitudes of managers today.

Whilst a detailed knowledge of management theory is not essential in order to practice occupational therapy, some familiarity with theory facilitates understanding of present management approaches and is, as Mullins (1985) argues, important for aspiring managers because:

- They need 'to view the interrelationships between the development of theory, behaviour in organisations and management practice'
- They need to obtain an 'understanding of the development of management thinking', which will help them 'in understanding principles underlying the process of management'
- It is clear that 'many of the earlier ideas are

of continuing importance to the manager and later ideas on management tend to incorporate earlier ideas and conclusions'.

Management theories fall into three broad categories: 'classical', 'human relations' and 'systems'. These are described briefly below.

Classical

This school of management theory arose in the early 20th century; much of its early work is attributed to Henri Fayol. This theory considered the organisation in relation to its purpose and formal structure, with emphasis on work planning, technical requirements and the principles of management. It made assumptions about the 'rational and logical behaviour' of employees.

The business organisation was seen as a hierarchy with a very ordered structure, which contained bureaucracies related to specialisation. Emphasis was placed on authority, rules and impersonality.

Human relations

During the 1920s and the Depression greater attention began to be focused on social factors at work and on employee behaviour, particularly with reference to motivation. This theory was tested by Mayo's Hawthorne Experiments in the United States between 1924 and 1932 (described in detail in Cole 1984), in which the emphasis was on the worker rather than on the work. Major motivation theories were developed as a result of Mayo's conclusions, which stressed the need for managerial strategies which ensured that concern for people at work was afforded highest priority.

This approach was popular until approximately the mid-1950s, at which time people were beginning to work in more varied organisational environments and to express more complex needs.

Systems

This is a more comprehensive approach to the study of management in organisations and is based on General Systems Theory. It is an analysis of organisations as 'systems' with a number of inter-related 'sub-systems' (such as finance, personnel, marketing, research and development, production and services) which enable input to be converted into output.

The systems approach to organisation is generally 'open' (Fig. 5.3), as opposed to 'closed'; that is, the organisation interacts with its environment, relying upon it for input and for the distribution of output.

The organisation utilising this approach:

- specifies its objectives
- has defined sub-systems
- designs communication channels to optimise the flow of information
- groups activity areas to enhance communication.

Whilst, generally speaking, organisations still utilise a systems approach, development of management theory continues and more recent thinking considers that a management science approach is the next logical stage.

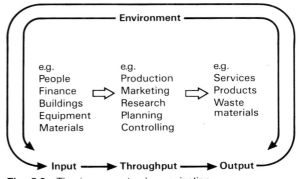

Fig. 5.3 The 'open system' organisation.

THE PRACTICE OF MANAGEMENT

The day-to-day practice of management has already been described as a process which involves a variety of activities. These activities may be divided into four groups: planning, organising, leading and controlling (Fig. 5.2).

Planning involves setting the objectives of the organisation and preparing strategies which will meet them. It also entails making decisions, plans and policies and anticipating results or outcomes. Planning must be carried out within an environmental framework, taking into account the organisation's strengths and weaknesses, its short- and long-term requirements, and the services and/or products it provides.

Organising is fundamentally concerned with putting plans into operation. It involves the coordination, delegation and decentralisation of tasks and resources, and, in order to achieve the required results, must take place within some form of structure.

Leading. Every manager is a leader who needs to motivate and gain the commitment of staff. The importance of effective communication cannot be underestimated and the individual's style of leadership/management will often have a major impact on the success (or otherwise) of the team.

Controlling involves establishing standards and measuring performance against those standards; taking corrective action when and where necessary and dealing with conflict if and when it arises. These types of tasks act as a feedback system for all management activity and are therefore vital to success.

SECTION 2: HEALTH, WELFARE AND OCCUPATIONAL THERAPY

HISTORICAL PERSPECTIVE

The management of occupational therapy has changed immeasurably since therapists first began practising in the United Kingdom. Change in public sector care provision, whether caused by internal or external influences, has been continuous. While the development of health and welfare services is explained in detail in other texts, the following summary should provide the reader with an historical context for current management practice in occupational therapy.

Prior to the existence of the 'welfare state', the voluntary sector initiated and provided a wide range of social services. Virtually all state provision is able to trace its origins to those early initiatives, primarily in the second half of the 19th century, when innumerable small charities, established by individual reformers and the churches, recognised that many people needed assistance of one kind or another and provided help in the form of education, charitable funds and workhouses (many of which later became hospitals).

Of equal influence during the 19th century was the Poor Law, the roots of which can be traced back to the Middle Ages. From the introduction of the Poor Law into the early years of the 20th century assistance included: cheap meals; health inspections for school children; health and unemployment insurance; old age pensions; probation for offenders; resettlement of the unemployed and care for 'mental defectives'. Many reforms instituted in the early 1900s were based on the methods developed by voluntary and charitable organisations in the 1800s. These measures enabled many people to receive assistance in time of need, avoiding the stigma of the Poor Law. However, there were still gaps in services exacerbated by two world wars, limited finance and industrial depression (Mays et al 1983).

The public sector services of today began with: the Education Act 1944, which was designed to provide equality of opportunity for children of all classes; the National Health Service Act 1946; legislation concerning family allowances and social security; the Town and Country Planning Act 1947, which enabled the government to control the physical environment in which people lived; and the National Assistance Act 1948.

The first NHS Act gave to the then Minister of Health the responsibility of promoting the establishment of a 'comprehensive health service designed to secure improvement in the physical and mental health of the people', with free care, advice and treatment. 1948 saw the birth of the NHS. Health care was divided into hospital services, teaching hospitals, community health (run by local authorities) and independent contractors. This cumbersome service remained in operation until 1974, when local authority health services were embraced by the NHS and a new management structure was established, consisting of the Department of Health and Social Security (DHSS), Regions, Areas and Districts. This top-heavy structure functioned for eight years. In 1982 the Area tier was abolished, Districts gained greater autonomy and Units were introduced, based on single hospitals, groups of hospitals, or services such as mental health or community health. In 1983, the Government and the then DHSS, still uncertain about management in the health service, commissioned Mr Roy Griffiths, now Sir Roy Griffiths, to consider management practices, and to report with recommendations. Griffiths was instrumental in introducing the idea of general management to the NHS — yet another significant change, which took effect in 1984/85. Devolution of responsibility, accountability and the resources to manage and provide services were introduced quickly, affecting all services and departments. In the late 1980s, government attention was still focused on health services. Consultative documents and a White Paper, subsequently to become part of the National Health Service and Community Care Act 1990 provided a framework for further internal change and gave new emphasis to community care for people living in their own homes.

Whilst one upheaval in the NHS followed another, local government was not without its share of change. The 1948 National Assistance Act established the welfare role of local authorities, for example, residential care for elderly people and services for those with long-term and permanent disabilities. In addition, the provisions made by housing departments, public and environmental health departments and education authorities had a far-reaching impact on personal social services. Housing departments in the 1950s, for example, were encouraged to provide purpose-built dwellings for people with disabilities, and environmental health grants were made available for certain people and/or properties in order to provide basic amenities. Education provision changed radically, from no education department arrangements for children with learning difficulties prior to 1970 to present-day opportunities for all children, including those with special educational needs.

The legislation affecting personal social services/departments is vast, covering responsibilities for children and families, adults with special needs, elderly and physically handicapped people, those with mental health problems and those with learning difficulties. Services provided are as diverse as those in health care and include: residential care; sheltered workshops; home care/help; social work; occupational therapy; adaptations to and equipment for people's homes; intermediate treatment for young offenders; specialist help for those with sensory impairments; and liaison with other agencies such as health, the police, courts, probation services, educational psychologists and the voluntary sector. Indeed, the responsibilities appear endless.

Whilst the public sector has been developing at a faster rate than its allocated resources have realistically permitted, voluntary organisations (non-statutory) have continued to make a substantial contribution to the care of people in need. Their involvement in care in the UK is of immeasurable value. They are not confined by legislation, accountability to the government or local electorates or by politics. Whilst the statutory bodies have major responsibilities governed by law, voluntary agencies now occupy a supplementary role, attempting to fill the gaps left by the inadequacies of state provision, yet working in partnership with health and social services. They provide:

- direct services to individuals or groups of people in the form of information, advice, support and care
- mutual aid and self-help centred on common interests or needs
- pressure group activity, coordinating information and debate related to specific causes or group interests and bringing these concerns to public attention through campaigning, advocacy and direct action
- resources, for example, services to other organisations both public and voluntary; research; expertise in specific areas such as disability and finance
- a coordinating function, i.e. representing the membership of other voluntary bodies, liaising and coordinating activities of common interest and lobbying the government, its ministers and departments, in order to influence local and national policies

The changes in both health and community care which will accelerate through the 1990s and into the next century have extensive implications for all organisations and professions involved in care services. Increasingly, both statutory and non-statutory service providers will work in partnership to enable the increasing numbers of less able and elderly people to remain in their own homes. The National Health Service and Community Care Act 1990, mentioned above, has introduced new structures and internal organisation to health care, local social service authorities and general practitioner services.*

Hospitals and community health services (excluding general practitioners) now contract to provide health care on behalf of health authorities, who act as purchasers of services for their resident population. Emphasis is placed on health promotion, quality, equity, effective and efficient resource management and offering people choice. These factors relate to all health authority providers of care, whether they are a self-governing or a directly managed unit.

Social service departments' provision for individuals and families emphasises assessment of need, care programmes, case management, the development of domiciliary, day and respite services, greater support for carers and the development of the independent care sector. The funding for certain social services has changed, particularly for people requiring residential care.

The reforms of recent years encompass general medical practices. Changes began with 'Promoting Better Health' (1987), which aimed to put the patient first. Today, Family Health Services Authorities (FHSA) are responsible for managing primary health care services, i.e. those provided by general practitioners, dentists, chemists and opticians.

Readers requiring in-depth information about recent changes are advised to refer to: 'Better Management, Better Health' (NHSTA 1985), 'Promoting Better Health' (HMSO 1987), 'Working for Patients' (HMSO 1989), 'Caring for People' (HMSO 1989) and the NHS and Community Care Act 1990.

LEGISLATION RELEVANT TO OCCUPATIONAL THERAPY PRACTICE

Law affecting the professional practice of health and welfare workers is extensive, sometimes complex and warrants some explanation. Many aspects of an occupational therapist's work have their roots in legislation and, depending upon her specialisation, the therapist must have a working knowledge of those statutes. If she works in mental health, for example, she must have a thorough working knowledge of the relevant acts in order to contribute appropriately to her clients' care. If she works with people with physical disability, familiarity with laws making provision for home care or home adaptations is important. Children receiving occupational therapy may need certain services within the auspices of educational legislation and the therapist must be *au fait* with such provisions.

Both local authorities and health services derive their powers and responsibilities from Acts of Parliament, certain sections of which 'require' them to undertake particular functions whilst others 'allow' them to do so. This legislation provides a framework within which occupational therapists and others function. The legislation described in Box 5.1 is that which is relevant to England and Wales. Readers in Scotland and Northern Ireland will need to refer to their own specific statutes, which differ from those listed.* In order to simplify reference, the relevant legislation is dealt with by subject i.e. Education, Employment, Health. For greater detail, reference should be made to the specific acts.

Legislation is supported directly and indirectly by Health Circulars, Executive Letters, Health Notices and Local Authority Circulars and No-

---

*Models of these revised structures and their organisation are not described in this text. It is envisaged that a variety of local models will emerge; these may include combining a district health authority with the local FHSA, and establishing trusts which would provide all community services for a particular client group in a particular area.

---

* The authors apologise to readers who work within a legislative framework which differs from that in England and Wales. Space precludes inclusion of every statute relevant to occupational therapy in the United Kingdom.

tices. These are issued by government departments for a wide variety of administrative, managerial and guidance purposes. They frequently explain recent legislation or case law as it is likely to apply to NHS local authority and FHSA activities. In addition, authorities receive government reports and White Papers regarding specific services; for example, 'Promoting Better Health' (1987) set out

Box 5.1 Legislation relevant to the practice of occupational therapy (Cont'd overleaf)

Act	Summary of relevant provisions	Act	Summary of relevant provisions
NHS			audit, provision of welfare services, planning, assessment of needs, taxation.
NHS 1946	Establishment of a comprehensive health service designed to secure improvement in the physical and mental health of the population; a free service of 'medical and ancillary care, advice and treatment for all'. Rehabilitation seen as an important element.	***Local Authority Social Services (LASS)***	
		National Assistance 1948	Local authorities given power to make arrangements for promoting the welfare of people with substantial and permanent handicaps, e.g. assistance in the home, residential accommodation.
NHS 1973	Reorganisation Act: all health services (community health previously with local authorities) to be provided by the NHS. Management arrangements very cumbersome. Between 1973 and 1989 there were numerous and substantial changes in the management structures and organisation of the NHS. These were initiated by the 1979 Royal Commission and documents such as 'Patients First' and health circulars.	*LASS 1970*	Preceded Local Government reorganisation in 1971. Described duties of new Social Services' departments and listed relevant legislation. United previously separate welfare services for elderly people, children, physically handicapped and mentally ill people into a service which was community based and family orientated. With the reorganisation of Local Government in 1974, LASS provided social work support to NHS, which had previously supplied own service.
NHS 1986 (Amendment)	NHS lost its Crown Immunity, becoming subject to all Health and Safety legislation, including food hygiene.		
NHS & Community Care 1990	Detailed in the White Papers 'Working for Patients' and 'Caring for People', this complementary combination provided a framework for health and community care for the 1990s and beyond. Includes: establishment of Hospital Trusts, further devolution of responsibility, management, family health services authorities, GP fund holding practices, funding,	*Chronically Sick & Disabled Persons 1970*	Extended provision of National Assistance Act 1948. Describes specific services for people in the community, e.g. practical help, information, register of disabled people, access to public buildings, accommodation for under-65s, disabled drivers/passengers car badges.

Box 5.1 Cont'd

Act	Summary of relevant provisions	Act	Summary of relevant provisions
Disabled Person's 1981	Amendments to CSDP Act 1970. Imposes duties on Highways and Planning authorities in particular, so that roads, new buildings and so on are planned and built to facilitate easy access for disabled people.	*Rating (Disabled Persons) 1978*	Amended the law re rates relief in premises occupied by disabled people, i.e. own home, residential care.
Disabled Persons (Services, Consultation & Representation 1986)	Resulted from concern over deficiencies in CSDP Act 1970, the inability to enforce its provisions, and disquiet concerning community care. Considered an addition to the legal rights and protection of disabled people. Being implemented in sections. Includes: needs assessment for individual and carer(s), provision of information, consultation with recipients of services, meeting the needs of those leaving special education, authorised representatives (advocates) for individual disabled people.	*Housing 1979*	Housing authorities responsible for adaptations in their own housing stock.
		Housing 1980	Criteria for grants (ref. Housing Act 1974) waived for disabled people.
		Housing 1985	Section 8 consolidated provisions of previous legislation requiring Housing Authorities to have regard for the special needs of disabled people (made explicit in CSDP Act 1970).
		Local Government & Housing 1989	Part VIII, 'House Adaptations for Disabled People', deals with new house renovation grant system, introducing Disabled Facilities Grant which replaced home improvement grant system. Seeks to build on established practice and reinforces community care philosophy by requiring housing and welfare services to cooperate. A summary of the Disabled Facilities Grant (Section 106) is offered in the Occupational Therapists Reference Book 1990 pp. 95–96.
NHS & Community Care 1990	Refer to NHS section.		
Local Government *(Housing, Rating, Grants)*			
Housing 1957	Introduced 'wheelchair' and 'mobility' housing.	**Mental Health**	
Local Government 1958	Introduced sheltered housing/warden schemes for elderly people.	*Mental Health 1983*	All previous mental health legislation repealed. Main changes include: establishing Mental Health Commission to protect interests of detained patients: new requirements regarding treatment of detained patients; changes in Mental Health Review Tribunal procedures; introduction of 'Approved Social Workers' in mental health; new powers for courts to remand people to hospital for reports or treatment; informal patients able to be included in electoral register.
Housing 1974	Availability of grants for home improvements and adaptations for disabled people. Criteria re property's rateable value and age had to be met.		

Box 5.1 Cont'd

Act	Summary of relevant provisions	Act	Summary of relevant provisions
Education			Education Authorities in reviewing their assessment and statementing procedures. Education for those with special educational needs up to 19 years.
1944	Schools for all children *except* those with a 'mental handicap'.		
1970	Special education provision for children with 'mental handicap'.	**Health and Safety**	
1976	Handicapped children categorised for educational purposes.	Health and Safety at Work 1974	Updated and clarified previous legislation. Responsibility of all to ensure the health and safety of themselves and others in their care or under their supervision. Now applies to all organisations, as NHS lost its Crown Immunity in 1986.
1981	Followed 1978 Warnock Report re special educational needs with change in law on special education. All previous categories abolished and replaced by more general terms, e.g. 'learning difficulty' and 'special educational needs'. Children to be educated in mainstream schools as far as possible. Parents to be more involved in assessment, placement and reviews of their child. Introduction of statementing.	**Employment**	
		Disabled Persons (Employment) 1944/1958	Introduced, and later reinforced, employment and training opportunities for disabled people of working age. Introduced quota scheme, Disablement Resettlement Officers, sheltered employment.
Education (Reform) 1988	In addition to introducing the National Curriculum and local management of schools, act offers advice to Local	Employment Training 1973	Services for disabled people of working age unchanged.

the government's plans for improving primary health care services.

Both the NHS and Local Authority Social Services (LASS) receive advisory visits from independent organisations. The Health Advisory Service (HAS), established in the early 1970s, undertakes regular visits to advise authorities regarding services for mentally ill and elderly people. In the mid-seventies the National Development Team (NDT) was established to advise authorities about services for people with learning difficulties. Both the HAS and the NDT are composed of people with experience of health and social service provision. Social service provision is usually represented by the Social Services Inspectorate (SSI). At the time of writing the fu-

ture of these two groups is unclear. What is certain is that the Audit Commission will develop a greater role within health care, to complement its long-standing functions within local government.

These frameworks are intended to be supportive, helpful and advisory and to assist authorities to monitor and audit the quality and quantity of their services, much as quality control might be managed in the private sector.

The plethora of statutes, reports, plans and so on are public documents. All are published and available to the general public through local libraries, community health councils and, for staff in particular, from medical, polytechnic and university libraries.

PROFESSIONAL FRAMEWORK FOR PRACTICE

Occupational therapy practice is affected not only by legislation relating to health, welfare and other public sector services but also by that concerning state registration, common and case law. As well as the law, there are ethical principles to which therapists are expected to adhere, such as maintaining confidentiality, updating clinical knowledge and skills, and managing resources appropriately.

A therapist's professional framework for practice commences with a recognised pre-registration course in occupational therapy. These courses must be approved by the Council for Professions Supplementary to Medicine (CPSM) and the College of Occupational Therapists (COT), the institution (polytechnic or university, for example) offering the course and, ultimately, by the Privy Council.

The CPSM

This body was established following the enactment of the Professions Supplementary to Medicine Act 1960. The Council is accountable to the Privy Council and its general function is to coordinate and supervise the activities of its seven Boards (Fig. 5.4). It includes representatives from the Privy Council, Northern Ireland, the Department of Health, several of the Royal Colleges (e.g. Physicians) and the General Medical Council. Box 5.2 summarises the functions of the Council and its Boards.

The Occupational Therapists' Board

This body is composed of nine registered occupational therapists (who have alternates) who are elected by state registered therapists, and eight other members representing the medical profession and education. The three statutory responsibilities of the Board are to:

- approve training courses and be satisfied that educational institutions maintain standards for educating students
- regulate and maintain proper standards of professional behaviour through its disciplinary powers
- consider applications, including those from overseas, for registration and publish a register annually of those approved for professional practice in the UK.

The Board is required to have both a Disciplinary and an Investigating Committee to regulate professional conduct issues. The Disciplinary Committee is independent of the Board and is responsible for preparing and circulating a statement of conduct to all registered occupational therapists. The Investigating Committee deals with allegations of professional misconduct made against registrants.

The COT

This body has a clearly defined role in pre-registration education and works closely with the CPSM. The COT is concerned with maintaining professional education standards in full- and part-

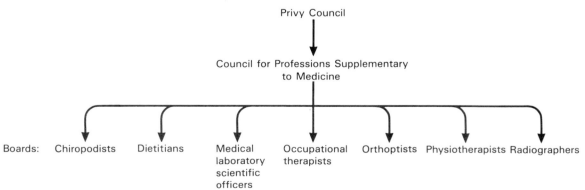

Fig. 5.4 Structure of the Council for Professions Supplementary to Medicine.

Box 5.2 Functions of the Council for Professions Supplementary to Medicine

Statutory role: PSM Act 1960
- *Aims*. To protect the public by regulating:
  —standards of pre-registration education
  —professional conduct
- *Functions*. Legal powers to:
  —register appropriately qualified individuals
  —approve standards of qualification, examination, education (i.e. the institution, course and final qualifying examination)
  —produce the Statement of Conduct and implement disciplinary procedures if necessary
- *Statutory visits*
  —a year following appointment of new head of course or as considered necessary
  —every five years with COT representation
  —joint revalidation with COT
  —tripartite validation in conjunction with COT and degree-awarding body
- *Visits include*:
  —tour of facilities
  —meeting with staff, students and managers
  —viewing the curriculum, coursework and assessments
  —visiting a selection of local and distant clinical and fieldwork placements
  —submission of report to relevant Board and the institution

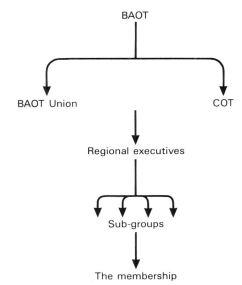

Fig. 5.5 Structure and organisation of the British Association of Occupational Therapists.

time courses to enable newly qualified therapists to state register — a statutory requirement for public sector employment — and to facilitate the continuing education and development of all occupational therapy staff.

The British Association of Occupational Therapists

It is probably useful at this point to summarise the structure and activities of the British Association of Occupational Therapists (BAOT), as they have a bearing on both professional practice and employment conditions of service. The Association functions both as a union and as a professional body; hence, the BAOT, the parent organisation, consists of the BAOT (Union) and the COT, which deals with issues of professional concern. An outline of the national structure of the Association is

given in Figure 5.5. BAOT business is dealt with at all levels but is led and coordinated by Council and its committees. This structure is shown in Figure 5.6.

The union provides a wide range of services to members nationally and locally, including: working with the Federation of Professional Organisations (a joint body which includes occupational therapists, physiotherapists, chiropodists, dietitians, radiologists, medical laboratory scientific officers and orthoptists) on matters relating to remuneration, conditions of service and grading structures; providing specific information, advice and support related to employment to regional and local stewards and to individual members. It seems likely that the Federation will become a 'local' organisation in the not-too-distant future, when issues regarding remuneration in particular might be negotiated regionally rather than nationally.

The Association produces and updates a variety of codes, guidelines and standards, for example the Code of Professional Conduct (1990), COT Advisory Service publications, the Good Management Handbook (1986), Research Advice Handbook, Stewards' Handbook, Health and Safety leaflets and an increasing range of standard guide-

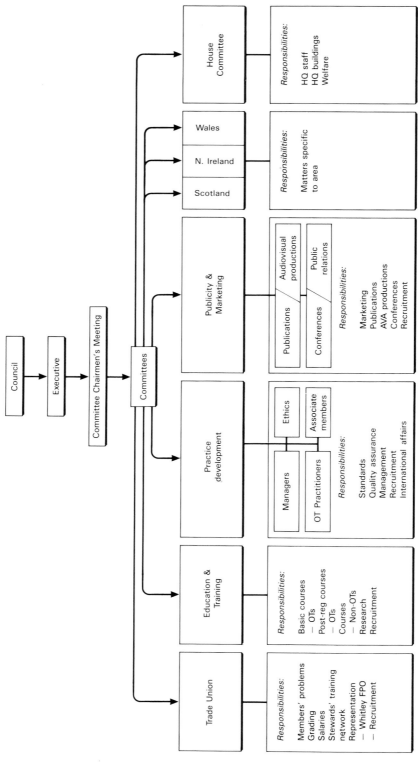

Fig. 5.6 British Association of Occupational Therapists: Committee Structure 1990.

lines such as the 'Statement on Professional Negligence and Litigation' and 'Occupational Therapy Services for Consumers with Physical Disabilities'. Whilst these documents do not impose any legal obligations on practitioners they do provide valuable sources of guidance and information. Further, more detailed, information about such publications and the work of the BAOT is described in the Occupational Therapists' Reference Books, issued regularly by the Association.

SECTION 3: PRACTICE AND THE LAW

The upsurge in litigation in health and social care in recent years has resulted in the need for occupational therapists to raise their awareness and knowledge concerning their practice and how it relates to the law. The following discussion summarises legal issues relevant to the practice of occupational therapy. The reader is advised to refer also to the Association's 'Statement of Professional Negligence and Litigation' and 'Code of Professional Conduct' and to other professional literature for more detailed information.

Practising within the law implies that occupational therapy staff carry out their duties in a manner which 'takes account of current acceptable practice and professional standards' and that they 'record their actions clearly and routinely'. Staff have a duty to be 'careful, considered, responsible and educated in carrying out professional responsibilities', i.e. they have a 'duty of care' to those people accepted for treatment (BAOT 1989).

Duty of care

The duty of care to be undertaken by a person has been defined in law in the following manner:

You must take reasonable care to avoid acts and omissions which you can reasonably foresee would be likely to injure your neighbour. Who then, in law, is my neighbour? The answer seems to be persons who are so closely and directly affected by my act that I ought reasonably to have them in contemplation as being so affected, when I am directing my mind to the act or omissions which are called in question.

(Donoghue v. Stevenson, House of Lords 1932; Wilsher v. Essex AHA)

This means that the occupational therapist's duty of care demands responsible behaviour which is in keeping with the education and training she has received, her professional skill and the post she holds.

Professional Judgement and Standards

The fundamental requirement for a therapist is to act 'in accordance with the practice accepted at the time as proper by a responsible body of opinion in the field of occupational therapy' (BAOT 1989). Therefore, the practitioner is expected to continually update her knowledge and skills in keeping with the ongoing development of professional practice.

Negligence

Negligence can only be implied in circumstances where harm has been caused. Legal action can arise in response to negligence caused by act or by omission:

- Negligence by act relates to an action which ought *not* to have been undertaken
- Negligence by omission relates to an action which was not undertaken, but *should* have been.

Negligence has two components: breach of the duty of care and any proven, resulting damage.

Breach of the duty of care

A duty of care is undertaken by the therapist once she accepts a referral. The therapist must ensure that her actions are accepted practice within the profession. If she acts contrary to such practice she may be liable to an action in negligence on the grounds that she has breached her duty of care. However, there are exceptions: the law accepts that people do make mistakes. Therefore, the therapist acting 'in good faith' who makes 'an error of judgement' may not be seen as in breach of her duty of care. It is vital, none the less, that staff are able to justify their choice and method of intervention according to current practices.

Vicarious Liability

An employer is usually liable for harm wrongfully caused by employees, and damages may be awarded against him or her if an employee is negligent. According to the concept of vicarious liability, 'provided you are acting within the agreed responsibilities of your job, then your employer accepts that damage caused during the course of your legitimate duties is his responsibility' (BAOT 1989).

However, if a staff member causes damage to a third party whilst acting *outside* her legitimate duties she will be said to be 'on a frolic of her own'. The employer can then refuse to accept vicarious liability and the individual could become personally liable. Therefore, it is wise for practitioners to have professional indemnity, such as that offered by the BAOT.

Referrals for treatment

The CPSM states that a therapist should treat an individual only if he has been referred by a registered medical practitioner *or* where there is direct access to that individual's doctor. In practice this means that a doctor's signature is *not* obligatory but that there must be communication concerning the treatment. Blanket referrals or other arrangements must be well established, accepted locally as 'custom and practice' and adopted with the 'knowledge and approval of a supervisor and/or management' (BAOT 1989).

Following acceptance of the referral a duty of care to that individual will have been initiated. Therefore, any intervention must be at least of an acceptable minimum level and standard. If for any reason these basic standards cannot be met, occupational therapy staff should not accept a referral or commence treatment.

Clientele's acceptance of treatment

An individual participates in treatment by consent, the only exception being for those detained under certain sections of the Mental Health Act 1983. The individual's participation in an activity is an implicit acceptance of any risk involved, provided that the activity has been explained and the risks are comprehended. An individual has the right under common law to give or withhold consent prior to examination or treatment. (Exceptions include urgent or life-saving treatment, statutory requirements to examine individuals under Public Health legislation, and detention under certain sections of the Mental Health Act 1983.) People are entitled to receive sufficient information, in a manner they understand, about the proposed treatments, any alternatives, and any substantial risks, in order that they can make a balanced judgement, and care should be taken to respect an individual's wishes.

Consent to treatment may be 'implied' or 'express'. It is implied by compliant actions, for instance attending for assessment and treatment and offering an affected hand for the fitting of an orthosis. In express consent the individual confirms his agreement in explicit terms, orally or in writing. Oral consent may be sufficient for the vast majority of contacts with clients by a profession such as occupational therapy. Written consent should be obtained for any procedure or treatment that carries any substantial risk or has a significant side effect. Both types of consent should be recorded in clients' notes.

More detailed information should be sought from 'A guide to consent for examination or treatment', issued by the NHS Management Executive in 1990 (HC (90) 22).

Levels of competence

Staff are required to act within their capabilities and job specification. Demands which exceed these limits must be met by appropriate training. This is particularly important as occupational therapy services change in emphasis and as therapists and their support staff change their working practices and environments. Such change must be accompanied by agreement from service managers.

Supervision

Supervision ensures that professional practices and standards are maintained and developed. All staff need such support but the amount and type they require will vary and this should be negotiated between supervisor and staff member. Staff with supervisory responsibilities must delegate and supervise at an appropriate level; that is, they must delegate within the skill and competence of the junior staff member, supervise adequately in terms of quality and quantity (time) and retain overall responsibility for the delegated task.

Record keeping

Written records of intervention, advice and outcomes are a requirement of good practice, as the primary purpose of records is to facilitate the care, treatment and support of an individual. Records are legal documents in that they are a record of the services provided by the employer. Any record must contain fact and represent an objective opinion of the intervention and outcomes. Records may be used in evidence long after an episode of treatment has ceased and each employer will have arrangements for their retention and disposal based on guidelines issued by the Department of Health. Box 5.3 offers guidance on record keeping and report writing.

Products used by occupational therapy staff

The Health and Safety at Work Act 1974 (Section 6) requires any person who designs, makes, imports or supplies any article for use at work to ensure that the 'article is so designed and constructed as to be safe and without risks to health when properly used'. Additionally, the Consumer Protection Act 1987 'creates a regime of strict civil liability for damage caused by defective products'.

Box 5.3 Record keeping and report writing. (Reproduced by kind permission from BAOT Statement on Professional Negligence and Litigation, Appendix 1 1989)

1.1 Reports should contain:	other written or verbal communications or exchanges of information pertaining to the individual, duly dated and signed
1.1.1 accurate, concise and relevant information recorded at the time of, or immediately after, any action or intervention	
	1.2 General points to be noted:
1.1.2 facts, not opinion	1.2.1 written information must be legible
1.1.3 patient's name, address, date of birth, name and address of personal doctor and any other relevant personal details	1.2.2 entries must not be obliterated or altered by the use of correction fluid such as Tipp-Ex or other proprietary product
1.1.4 where possible, written confirmation by a medical practitioner of diagnosis and any contraindications	1.2.3 written records are subject to scrutiny and are the property of the employer, not the employee
1.1.5 a statement to that effect if the patient is unaware of the diagnosis	1.2.4 information about a patient is confidential to the employer, not the employee
1.1.6 date of receipt and method of referral	1.2.5 legal action must be initiated within 3 years of an incident occurring
1.1.7 assessments; type and method undertaken; outcome	1.2.6 a legal case must be settled within 7 years of its initiation
1.1.8 treatment objectives	
1.1.9 intervention to meet objectives; outcome	1.3 Information to be excluded from any record:
1.1.10 the date of each assessment and intervention and the signature of the person making it, and on whose instruction it was made if applicable	1.3.1 unconfirmed diagnosis
	1.3.2 anecdotal comment
1.1.11 any documentation, correspondence and	1.3.3 discursive description

From 1990, public sector authorities have had to adhere to the Control of Substances Hazardous to Health (COSHH) Regulations. These require employers to evaluate and control the risks to health for all their employees and visitors to the work premises from exposure to hazardous substances such as various types of dust, paint strippers, disinfectants, paints and printing ink.

Occupational therapy staff are suppliers, keepers and producers of a wide range of products; therefore, they must keep accurate and up-to-date records as an essential safeguard in the event of any claim.

Educational and professional development

Therapy staff have a duty to ensure that their knowledge and skills are kept up to date; therefore, time off for study is vital. Employers who refuse such study time can be liable, should harm be caused to an individual because a staff member was not conversant with current practices.

Student education

The general principles of care applicable to occupational therapy staff also apply to students and those involved in their pre-registration education. For example, a clinical supervisor is responsible for a student's practice, ensuring that delegated tasks are within the latter's sphere of competence.

Confidentiality

Staff have a duty not to divulge information concerning an individual to an unauthorised third party without his consent. However, all notes which relate to that individual's treatment can be made available to a court of law in certain circumstances. Information is given to colleagues who are taking over the individual's care or to other team members involved in his care only on a 'need to know' basis; here, it is considered that the individual's consent is implied, as the transfer of information will facilitate the continuation of his treatment. In practice, the therapist will inform the person about the release of information. Doubt is frequently expressed when essential information is needed by colleagues in another authority, for example if a home visit report prepared by a hospital-based therapist needs to be passed to home care, nursing and occupational therapy colleagues in the community. This is legitimate on a 'need to know' basis, but the report initiator may need to mark the report 'confidential' or 'not to be copied' in order to safeguard confidentiality. Additional information regarding data protection is included in Section 6 on p. 138.

Discharge home visits

During the course of her duties an occupational therapist will undertake many home visits with hospital-based clients. Most of these are an integral element of the individual's treatment programme and aim to establish his abilities and difficulties within his home environment.

If, during the course of a routine home visit, the individual refuses to return to hospital, the therapist in charge of the visit must ensure that he signs a disclaimer or a self-discharge form after she has discussed the matter with the individual and his carers and made contact with the ward to explain the circumstances.

Health authorities may require staff to undertake discharge home visits. These should only take place with the consent of the consultant in charge of the case, who retains the overall responsibility for that individual until he is discharged to the care of his general practitioner.

The occupational therapist's legal responsibilities (Fig. 5.7) also include requirements related to health and safety, employment, data protection and specific mental health and disability statutes. Where appropriate, these are referred to in other sections of this chapter.

SECTION 4: SELF-MANAGEMENT AND PREPARATION FOR PRACTICE

Managing oneself well and being prepared for practice and a particular post offers a professional and managerial baseline upon which the therapist

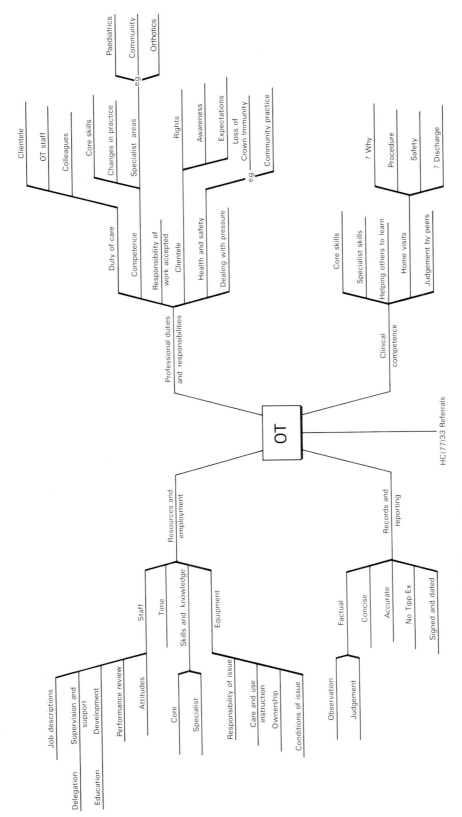

Fig. 5.7 The legal responsibilities of occupational therapy staff.

can build. She needs to understand how the organisation and systems (services) in which she is employed work and to comprehend her own role and its parameters within this framework. Additionally, the therapist needs to know what motivates her and encourages her to perform well. She should also understand the meaning of professional standards and competence to practice, how these are interpreted locally, and how they influence daily practice. A responsible therapist will also be concerned with her own development. By examining her own work and her strengths and weaknesses, she should be able to define personal objectives and further education and training needs.

Time management and prioritising

Time is an extremely valuable resource; therefore, using it effectively and efficiently is one of the most significant contributions that a therapist can make to a service's work. When asked to undertake an additional task one therapist's response may be 'I haven't the time', or 'I can't do it today, will next week do?' or 'Have you asked Jim?'. Another therapist, perhaps even someone who always appears exceptionally busy, might accept with alacrity. Why? Probably because she is well organised — she plans and uses her time to the optimum, works to priorities and is prepared to negotiate deadlines.

The following paragraphs attempt to identify the problems which beset time management and to offer a number of solutions.

Problems with time management

- An out-of-date (or non-existent) job description or job specification
- unclear personal or service objectives (or a lack thereof)
- inadequate use of planning diaries
- no day-to-day, weekly, monthly or longer-term planning schedule for individuals or the service
- other people organising one's time
- a variety of interruptions, e.g. colleagues, telephone calls, impromptu meetings

- crises of one sort or another of varying severity
- poor leadership, line management and example
- poor information systems
- the environment generally
- an excessively heavy caseload.

The potential solutions

- *Job description/specification.* Ensure that this is up to date. Ideally, it should be reviewed formally on an annual basis during the therapist's individual performance review with her line manager. It offers a profile of her job and defines her key tasks, often in priority order; for example, activities related to clientele and their treatment will be listed before more general departmental activity such as health and safety or statistical returns.
- *Objectives.* In addition to understanding her own role, the therapist should be aware of the service's objectives for the current year in order that she sees the significance of the personal objectives she sets with her line manager. She requires these in order to help her to prioritise tasks and organise her time accordingly.
- *Use of a diary.* Most people are accustomed to using a personal or pocket diary in which they record appointments, addresses and telephone numbers. In a simple way they are using the diary as a planning and organising tool. A diary used at work, or elsewhere for that matter, is a primary instrument of management, and without it the owner may, almost literally, be lost.

Using a diary effectively is a skill which is easy to develop and each therapist will find that she uses it for an increasing number of tasks, such as:

1. Scheduling regular commitments, including appointments with specific clientele/families, multidisciplinary team meetings, case conferences, ward-based sessions, therapy staff meetings, weekly ward rounds, monthly staff training.

These are relatively straightforward to incorporate into the weekly or monthly schedule. The three uses listed below are slightly more difficult to incorporate, but with practice the therapist will begin to automatically use her diary to timetable them.

2. Scheduling time for certain tasks, for example 4.00 p.m. daily for report writing and updating treatment notes; 9.00–9.30 a.m. for local telephone calls; every third Thursday (afternoon) for reading and study in the medical library.
3. Scheduling 'breathing space' between regular commitments in order to deal with: urgent telephone calls, a colleague's query, 'catching up' with notes, seeking advice from one's team manager.
4. Implementing a 'bring forward' system which will prompt preparation for future activities, e.g. contributing to the service's policy concerning study time, preparing for an annual performance review, or undertaking pre-course research and reading.

Utilising her diary in this way will enable the therapist to see, at a glance, how much time is committed each day and what hours/sessions are available. In this way she can retain a certain degree of flexibility which will assist the effective use of her own time.

- *Visual planners* based on calendar and/or financial years are frequently used by departmental and team managers in order to plan and record events such as staff's annual, study and sick leave, student placements, and particular deadlines. They offer an 'at-a-glance' picture of selected events.
- *Time analysis.* A periodic, accurate and realistic analysis of exactly how working hours are spent is often salutary. Some departments/services include this type of analysis in annual staff performance reviews and utilise it to monitor and review tasks and activities and the time allotted to them.

Figure 5.8 shows a sample work diary and time analysis form, which would be completed over a period of at least five consecutive working days. The variety of tasks undertaken and the time they consumed would be analysed, including any activity involving colleagues. Evaluation of the analysis would determine whether the right proportion of time has been allocated to the highest priority tasks and what adjustments might be required in the future.

- *Planning one's time.* This must take place within the framework of the purpose of one's job and the scope of authority it entails, one's lines of accountability, current objectives, and the required standards of performance. The therapist has to decide:

1. How long she wishes to spend on a particular task (this is generally determined by its importance) and
2. How quickly she has to complete it (i.e. its urgency).

Importance and urgency are not the same. An urgent activity is not necessarily important but needs to be dealt with immediately; an important activity will generally require more thought and, hence, more time to complete.

Planning and controlling the use of time must be done on a short- and long-term basis and take account of absences from work. Planning time relates to effective use of the diary. Controlling time is more difficult. The therapist needs to be able to identify what comprises 'lost' time and whether this is her fault or that of others. A degree of assertiveness is essential in order to:

— concentrate on one task at a time
— restrict interruptions by setting aside periods of time for specific tasks and informing colleagues of this arrangement
— influence the environment in which one works and work around its constraints, for example by using the library or the line manager's office in order to write an important report because one's own desk is in an open-plan office
— ensure that any information required is readily available to enable the completion of the task in hand, i.e. extracting all the required case notes during a single visit to central records.

Prioritising

Establishing priorities is an integral part of plan-

DAY _MONDAY : PM_   _1·30 PM_ to _5·30 PM_   TIME

ACTIVITY	1.3	1.4	1.5	2.0	2.1	2.2	2.3	2.4	2.5	3.0	3.1	3.2	3.3	3.4	3.5	4.0	4.1	4.2	4.3	4.4	4.5	5.0	5.1	5.2	5.3
A. CLINICAL — Face-to-face	▨	▨	▨	▨	▨	▨	▨	▨	▨	▨						▨	▨	▨							
— Patient related											▨	▨	▨												
— Patient related and involving Social Services																									
B. ADMINISTRATION — Records																									
— Reports																			▨	▨	▨				
— Letters																						▨	▨	▨	▨
— Other																									
C. COMMUNICATIONS — Telephone in																									
— Telephone out														▨											
— Informal meetings: — one-to-one																									
— group																									
— Formal meetings: — staff																									
— committees																									
— other																									
D. TRAVEL — Between rooms																									
— Units																									
— Sites																									
E. PERSONAL TIME — Coffee, loo, etc.															▨										
F. PERSONNEL MANAGEMENT — Staff Supervision																									
— Counselling/grievances																									
— Recruitment																									
— Induction																									
G. FINANCE — Day-to-day																									
— Printouts																									
— Other																									
H. PUBLIC RELATONS — Talks																									
— Presentations																									
— Other																									
I. OTHER — Please specify																									

Fig. 5.8 Tools for analysis. (A) A sample 'work diary'.

Activity	Total time spent	% of working day (p.m. only in this sample)	Difference between predicted and actual time
A. CLINICAL	160 minutes	64%	+30 minutes
B. ADMINISTRATION	70 minutes	28%	
C. COMMUNICATIONS	10 minutes	4%	-20 minutes
D. TRAVEL			
E. PERSONAL TIME	10 minutes	4%	
F. PERSONNEL MANAGEMENT			-10 minutes
G. FINANCE			
H. PUBLIC RELATIONS			
I. OTHER			

Fig. 5.8 Cont'd. (B) A sample 'analysis of time'.

ning. The framework for prioritising is identical to that of planning one's time. Something which is of top priority takes precedence over all other activities in relation to one's time, i.e. it is *first* in time, place or rank. Priorities are frequently stated for an employee. They may be set by the therapist's line manager or employing authority, and even by the government. The individual often has to set her own priorities within these parameters.

Priority setting commences with questions. What is my job? What is its prime purpose? What tasks are of secondary importance? How much time do I have to complete certain activities and achieve certain goals? Having answered these questions the therapist has to balance the needs and demands of her job with the time and other resources at her disposal.

The following suggestions may assist the occupational therapist in identifying and setting priorities:

- Write down the tasks requiring attention, including both regular and one-off commitments
- Decide whether these are urgent or can wait, whether they are small or large, short term or long term, and whether they are interesting or dull
- Identify a time-scale and whether this is set by the line manager or the individual
- Identify which of the tasks are a regular element of the work schedule

- Establish whether any of the tasks can be delegated and to whom
- Establish which tasks, if any, can be simplified or eliminated
- Organise the remaining tasks into related areas in order to deal with those which are similar consecutively
- Set aside specific time to deal with priority activities, for example caseload management and the prioritising of client's needs
- Use a diary, visual planner or bring-forward system to maximum effect
- Set deadlines and adhere to them even if this requires negotiation with the line manager
- Be proactive.

MANAGING STRESS

Occupational therapists, like other people, are subject to varying degrees of stress in the course of their work. Stress is a common experience. Many people thrive on it, while others find it intolerable. Wilson (1984) describes stress as, on the one hand, 'a positive force' which produces 'drive to achieve full potential'; conversely, it may be 'an unpleasant experience', upon which both internal and external factors — for example, an illness or a hostile environment — have an influence.

In order to manage stress one must understand it; i.e., one must recognise stressful circumstances and their symptoms or warning signs.

Feelings of stress may arise in response to:

- working in isolation from professional colleagues
- poor definition of roles in a multidisciplinary team
- rapid throughput in an acute ward
- the seemingly unmanageable proportions of a caseload
- a growing waiting list
- resource shortages
- impending closure of a hospital
- relocation of the service and/or individuals
- staff turnover
- change in the organisation.

The symptoms or warning signs of stress can be divided into four distinct categories, which the reader should recognise from her clinical theory and practice:

- *physical*: headaches, disturbed sleep patterns, exhaustion, gastrointestinal upsets
- *emotional*: lack of enthusiasm, negative attitudes towards clientele, irritability, anxiety, anger, mood swings, depression, feelings of hopelessness
- *behavioural*: poor work, taking longer over tasks, double-checking work, making more errors, absenteeism, resistance to change, rigid views, withdrawal
- *cognitive*: impaired memory function, difficulty concentrating and making decisions, problems with 'switching off', decreased ability to problem-solve.

Strategies for coping may be sub-divided under the headings 'personal' and 'organisational', as follows:

- personal:
  — being able to ask for help
  — knowing and understanding oneself at home and work and the relationships within those environments
  —knowing and understanding one's own work requirements, i.e. priorities, the knowledge and skill levels needed, the volume to be dealt with and the time available and required to complete tasks

  — recognising the symptoms in oneself and being able to take corrective action
  — leading a balanced life-style in which work assumes its correct proportion
  — keeping healthy and fit
  — relaxing
  — developing one's assertion skills
  — fostering one's self-confidence
  — encouraging individuals to gain control over their work pattern
  — specific counselling with supervisor
  — career evaluation
  — recognising and analysing personal feelings
  — withdrawing temporarily and writing down and prioritising tasks awaiting attention
- organisational:
  — reviewing individual performance
  — forming staff support groups
  — providing stress awareness training
  — providing stress counselling
  — encouraging awareness of others at work
  — modifying, where possible, the working environment
  — clarifying policies and procedures within the service, for example study leave, selection and promotion criteria, grievance procedures
  — encouraging participation in service planning
  — clarifying delegation authority
  — defining service/departmental priorities
  — understanding individuals' personal circumstances
  — modifying the volume of work an individual is expected to manage.

Coping with stress is never easy. However, a supportive environment in which activity is planned and prioritised and delegation and supervision are handled realistically, and where people share, care and communicate and have permission to acknowledge stress will help to make stress manageable even though many of the factors contributing to it remain.

CORE SKILLS AND PROFESSIONALISM

All professionals possess core skills which translate

their philosophy and essential role into daily practice. The philosophy of occupational therapy focuses on human occupation and occupational behaviour and on how these are affected by health and ill health. Each therapist must base her practice on knowledge (i.e. theory), to which must be added certain skills and attitudes.

Pre-registration education provides occupational therapists with a knowledge base which is enhanced, with the passage of time, by experience and post-registration education. Likewise, the core skills of the profession are established prior to state registration and continue to develop, particularly in specialist areas, following qualification. Students may well base their attitudes on the role models they meet during their education, but as they develop as therapists they will be able to modify their own attitudes to a variety of circumstances.

Core skills

These could be described as the 'bread and butter' of practice. In occupational therapy they focus on activity and the needs of clients to function in their own particular environments. In terms of the occupational therapy process, discussed extensively in Chapter 4, core skills may be described as:

- the effective seeking and gathering of relevant information
- undertaking appropriate assessments
- setting objectives
- planning and implementing intervention
- selecting activity to meet objectives
- modifying activity to meet needs
- modifying the treatment environment
- monitoring and evaluating intervention outcomes
- motivating people.

In order to fulfil the requirements of the above process and thus meet individuals' needs, the therapist must possess certain other core skills. These are the ability to:

- analyse activity for therapeutic use
- problem-solve and enable others to develop their own strategies

- communicate, verbally and non-verbally, factually, succinctly and accurately
- make decisions, initially at a clinical level
- understand professional standards and implement them
- lead others and model a number of roles
- counsel others; this entails being an effective listener and understanding human behaviour
- interview people in a manner which encourages their cooperation
- provide an optimum learning environment and impart knowledge, skills and attitudes to others.

Each of these skills is dealt with extensively in other chapters and in other sections of this chapter. Here, we need only say that each student occupational therapist needs to develop these skills so that she is adequately prepared to assume responsibility for her own caseload in her first post as a state-registered therapist.

Professionalism

According to Chambers Twentieth Century Dictionary, 'profession' means 'an employment not mechanical and requiring some degree of learning: the collective body of persons engaged in any profession'. 'Professionalism' refers to 'the status of a professional: the outlook, aim, or restriction of the mere professional'. Professionalism may also be defined as acting in pursuit or protection of the interests of one's profession.

In past decades, 'professionalism' was perceived largely as a matter of a therapist's behaviour and appearance — whether she was punctual, wore a clean uniform, had tidy hair, and so on. Whilst these behaviours are still relevant, being professional is now interpreted rather more extensively and includes such considerations as the occupational therapist's clientele, education, behaviour and autonomy:

- *Clientele*:
  — the profession aims to provide a service for its clients
  — that service should be in the clients' best interests

— interaction between client and therapist should be based on mutual trust and confidence
— intervention should be conducted confidentially
— the profession may be expected to make objective decisions about clients and to make decisions on their behalf

- *Education.* At an educational level, professionalism involves:
  — acquiring a systematic and scientific body of knowledge
  — undergoing a lengthy period of education
  — continuing to update knowledge and skills
  — setting one's own standards of competence to practise and auditing oneself
  — participating in the training of students and junior colleagues

- *Behaviour.* Behavioural standards are stated in the profession's Code of Professional Conduct, a set of rules which guide professional practice. The standards are described under the following headings:
  — relationships with, and responsibilities to, clients
  — professional integrity
  — professional relationships and responsibilities
  — professional standards

- *Autonomy*:
  — a profession forms a professional association and writes self-governing rules
  — it draws up a code of ethics to regulate members' standards of behaviour
  — it defines its own sanctions for members
  — it negotiates and collaborates with the state and other groups to maintain and extend its status
  — it may form pressure groups to initiate changes in social policy
  — it may monitor and evaluate the effects of changed policies.

Translating professionalism presents occupational therapists with a constant and worthwhile challenge, supported by their association's guidelines, statements and standards, which enables them to continually 'advance their expertise to the benefit not only of their clients but also of their field' (Wallis 1987).

PREPARATION FOR PRACTICE

The guidance offered in this section is intended to assist the individual to make the transition from student to therapist and to remind those returning to work following a break in service of a number of the procedures involved in identifying, applying for and accepting the ideal post.

Career opportunities in occupational therapy are extremely varied and numerous. Therefore, selecting the ideal job requires forethought, investigation and making choices. During the final year of a pre-registration course, most students will have formed an idea or plan for their first step on the career ladder. The choices available are considerable and may include:

- a post in a particular speciality, such as paediatrics or mental health
- a fixed rotation, for example two years divided into four six-month blocks, offering care of the elderly, orthopaedics, acute psychiatry and a younger disabled people's unit
- a negotiable rotation in which the first block may be allocated but where subsequent blocks may be negotiated according to individual preference.

In the latter instance in particular, personal choice will have to be weighed against client and service needs, hence the need for the newly appointed therapist and her manager to negotiate the rotation. In addition to the *type* of post being sought, an individual will often have other criteria to consider, such as geographical area, reputation of the service, and further education opportunities in local higher education facilities. Whatever the individual circumstances, it is important that the therapist seek a position which will offer continuing development and support; this will enable her to make a valued and satisfying contribution to the profession. Lansdowne (1989) investigated rotations for basic grade therapists and identified ten points pertinent to the selection of a first post. These are listed in Box 5.4.

Box 5.4 Priorities: Preparation for practice. (After Lansdowne 1989)

```
 1. Commitment of authority to provide
    continuing education, especially in
    developing specific skills
 2. Commitment of occupational therapy service
    to the provision of planned rotations
 3. Frequent supervision and support from senior
    staff; peer group support opportunities
 4. Temporary accommodation
 5. A pleasant location
 6. Easy access/transport system to home area
 7. Personal ties dictating location of first post
 8. Prior knowledge of the service/department
    from clinical education block or peer group
 9. An informal atmosphere in occupational
    therapy
10. Staffing structures within the authority for
    future career development.
```

The next stage involves examination of advertisements for posts and/or following up offers made during clinical education placements. Advertisements in the profession's journal and other publications should be read carefully, as they may offer comparatively limited information (health authorities have to adhere to advertising restrictions) and will raise a number of questions. They will describe the service and/or rotation, as well as specialities and the support and education available. Opportunities for obtaining further information and for making an informal visit are usually offered and it is advisable to pursue these offers prior to or in conjunction with requesting job descriptions and application forms.

Informal visits provide an opportunity to meet one's potential future colleagues, to view the facilities and resources available, to talk to junior staff, to ask questions and to obtain a 'feel' for the department and its philosophy. Such visits also benefit the potential employer, who can meet and talk with individuals informally and ascertain their possible suitability.

Job descriptions vary in format but the description of the function and main tasks of a particular grade of post will be broadly similar. One would expect to see the following tasks enumerated in a basic grade job description: assessment, treatment and resettlement of clients; administration associated with clinical work; liaison with colleagues; continuing education; contribution to departmental tasks; health and safety. Figure 5.9, a sample job description, also includes information regarding the post title and grade, its location, and to whom the individual is responsible. One should also expect to see a date indicating when it was last revised.

Applying for most junior posts will require the completion of application forms. These also vary in format but request similar information e.g. personal details, a summary of education completed or nearing completion, relevant experience to date, the skills and qualities the applicant has to offer and the names of at least two referees.

An application form should be treated as an opportunity to market oneself on paper. It should be filled out neatly by hand or typed, offer information in a logical sequence and help the recipient to form a picture of the writer. Two of the most important sections will be 'relevant experience' and 'skills and qualities'. The former may include experience obtained prior to, as well as during, pre-registration education, for example a year's work as a volunteer in a residential home. The 'skills and qualities' section might include, for instance, information about a research study, the satisfaction gained when working with a particular age group or the additional knowledge and skills obtained during an elective placement.

Any information which is pertinent to the post ought to be included and may be added on additional sheets if the form offers limited space.

Many people maintain a curriculum vitae (CV) containing personal and professional information. Box 5.5 suggests one format which could be utilised. A CV can be attached to an application form, providing appropriate reference is made to it on the form or in the accompanying letter.

Applications for jobs usually require the provision of two referees. In applications for a first job one of these must be the principal or head of the course attended. The other may be a clinical supervisor or a previous employer, for example a head occupational therapist for whom the individual worked in a voluntary capacity. It is essential, as well as courteous, to ask permission to use people as referees *before* completing an application

MIDSHIRE HEALTH AUTHORITY: SOUTHERN GENERAL HOSPITAL

JOB DESCRIPTION

POST: Occupational Therapist

GRADE: Junior/Basic

LOCATION: Southern General Hospital's 3 departments, including the
                   Psychiatric Unit

RESPONSIBLE TO: Head Occupational Therapist, and on a daily basis the
                   Senior Therapist in charge of the section/speciality

FUNCTION: On rotation, clinical duties with in, out, day
                   patients

MAIN TASKS:

1.   To undertake clinical duties within allocated work areas and
     participate in all tasks allied to the assessment, treatment and
     resettlement of patients.

2.   To liaise with colleagues within and outside the hospital regarding
     the treatment, care and resettlement of patients and their carers.

3.   To assist Senior Therapists in the support of occupational therapy
     helpers.

4.   To participate in the development and education programmes for
     occupational therapy staff, including the authority's Junior
     Therapist programme.

5.   To assist Senior Therapists with administrative duties as required.

6.   To comply with Health and Safety at Work regulations, ensuring that
     health, safety and security standards are maintained within work
     areas.

7.   To undertake other tasks related to occupational therapy as required.

April 1991
AMS/TFJ

Ref. J.D.S.

Fig. 5.9 Example of a junior therapist's job description.

form. This offers them an opportunity to discuss the matter with the individual.

A letter to the personnel officer or head occupational therapist should accompany the application form and/or CV. It need only be brief, explaining the purpose of the correspondence and referring to the enclosures.

If one is short-listed for an interview the next stage of preparation commences. The authority will provide details of the date, time and venue of the interview and may ask interviewees to take certain information with them, for example their diploma and state registration certificate if available. It is always advisable to prepare carefully for

Box 5.5 Sample format for a curriculum vitae

Title page

- Name, address, date

Subsequent page(s)

- Personal details:
  — date of birth
  — marital status
  — dependents
  — health
  — car owner/driver
  — interests
- Education and qualifications
  — schools attended
  — college(s)/course(s) attended (dates, qualifications)
- Previous employment/clinical education placements
  — commencing with most recent
  — dates of employment/placement
  — summary of duties/experience for each
- Qualities/other experience relevant, e.g.
  — committee membership
  — relevant professional interests
  — voluntary work

Box 5.6 Checklist: preparing for an interview

The job

- Research the organisation/service
- Familiarise self with information attached to job description
- Analyse and evaluate the job description
- Try to anticipate questions you may be asked and decide how to answer them
- Visit the service
- Be clear about your qualities, personal and professional, and your abilities related to the job
- Be clear about relevant experience
- Consider questions you may wish to ask

Other preparation

- Allow time on/before the day of the interview to travel and locate the venue
- Know for whom you have to ask
- Consider your appearance, i.e. are you neat, tidy, comfortable
- Practice, if necessary, how to sit, to appear relatively relaxed (but not 'laid back')
- Consider where you might place any papers you take with you

any interview and to think about questions and answers from a dual perspective, i.e. the panel's and one's own.

The panel will probably be comprised of the head occupational therapist, the post's line manager and a personnel officer. They will be interested in the interviewee as a person and as a therapist, and will focus many of their questions on the application form contents. In addition, they may wish to know how the applicant copes with particular circumstances, with anger, and with stress. They may ask about ambitions and professional and personal interests. The applicant should always be offered the chance to ask questions of the panel members. It is wise to consider these beforehand and to note them down — interviews can cause memory lapses. In order to prepare well for an interview, whether it be formal or informal, the suggestions in Box 5.6 may help. Further guidance is offered by Fletcher (1983).

On completion of interviews the panel will need to decide which applicant is best suited to the service and the post. This frequently requires much discussion but interviewees will be informed of the

outcome as soon as possible. Therefore, applicants should be prepared to wait or to let the panel know when and where they may be contacted later that day or the following day. Interviews are sometimes exhilarating experiences but they can be quite the opposite. Be prepared for pleasure or disappointment, and be certain whether the post is the right one or not. One is not obliged to accept a job if it is offered. If an individual is not offered a particular post, disappointment and a feeling of failure will ensue. However, this soon abates as one becomes philosophical about it, puts it down to experience and tries again.

Once a post is accepted a medical will be required and a contract will be prepared. The medical element may comprise the completion of a form which asks both general and specific questions about one's health and medical history. An individual may or may not be called for a medical examination, depending on the authority's policy. The contract of employment is usually signed on the day duty commences. This is an agreement between the individual and the employer regarding the conditions of employment and will include the date duty commenced, the hours to be worked, salary scale, intervals at which one is to be paid, holiday entitlement and notice of resignation required. Authorities may also provide at this stage information about their health and safety policies and procedures, grievance and disciplinary procedures and pension schemes.

Issues surrounding employment can seem rather complex at times and an individual may wish to seek advice from her prospective employer or from an independent source. If queries relate to the authority and its employment policies these are best asked of the personnel department. If they concern employment as an occupational therapist generally, the BAOT's Industrial Relations department is often an ideal starting point, in conjunction with their leaflet 'Starting Work', which is available to all third-year student contributors.

SECTION 5: INTERPERSONAL SKILLS

Occupational therapists require a wide range of interpersonal skills if they are to function effectively as individual clinicians and team members and to provide quality services to an authority's clientele. The individual therapist must remember that her interpersonal skills, which readily appear during face-to-face contact with clients and their carers, are equally important during dealings with colleagues in both clinical and managerial settings. Interpersonal skills are concerned with communication and relationships; therefore, this section will deal with such skills under those two subheadings.

COMMUNICATION

Imparting or sharing information of one sort or another is the essence of communication; as the word 'sharing' implies, it is a two-way process. The process of communication is frequently described as the 'life-blood' of an organisation and an activity to which managers devote an overwhelming proportion of their time. However, if communication is to further an organisation's goals it must be used effectively by everyone in the organisation's employ. It is essential, therefore, that communication:

- is effective, in order to utilise all resources, particularly time, efficiently and successfully
- has an objective or purpose which has to be heard, understood and accepted by others
- occurs in an environment which is conducive to the interchange
- facilitates required actions
- is offered at an appropriate level, i.e. in terms of vocabulary, language and level of understanding
- considers the dynamics of a particular situation, for example the newly established vis-à-vis the long-standing team.

Networks

The level and success of any interaction will be influenced by the networks utilised in the service and organisation. Figure 5.10 illustrates four of the most well known of these, which are as follows:

- Wheel or Star: the most centralised and the most efficient for simple tasks. The central person acts as a focus for the network's activities and is perceived as the leader. This is the least satisfying network for people on the periphery.
- Circle: more decentralised and, overall, less efficient. The group will tend to be disorganised and performance will be erratic and slow. It will, however, solve complex problems and cope with change and new tasks more quickly and efficiently than the wheel/star. It is the most satisfying network for all members.
- All channel: involves full discussion and participation and works most effectively where a high level of interaction between members is needed in order to solve complex problems. It provides a fairly high level of satisfaction for its members.
- Chain: this may be appropriate for dealing with simple tasks which need little interaction, as information travels along

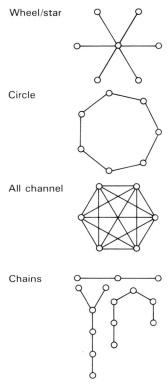

Fig. 5.10 Communication networks.

pre-determined channels. However, it provides a relatively low level of satisfaction for its members.

In summarising the above one might state that: centralised networks are satisfactory for solving simple problems; a network determines to an extent who will be its leader; and a network can affect members' motivation levels in that the more decentralised it is the greater the satisfaction for all members.

Vertical and lateral communication

Whilst an organisation will contain innumerable networks it should, ideally, possess both vertical and lateral means of communication to assist it to meet its overall purpose.

Vertical communication tends to be formal. In an upward direction it provides the organisation's senior managers with information about activities at every level; this may take the form of progress reports, suggestions, explanations, and requests for help and/or decisions. The downward flow of information is intended to advise, inform, direct, instruct, and evaluate, and to provide staff with information about the organisation's goals and policies. This may be done through in-house journals, codes of practice, memoranda, short-term programmes and so on.

Lateral communication usually follows the line of workflow and occurs between different team members, teams and departments. Its purpose is to provide a direct channel for problem-solving and coordination and it should foster the development of sound working relationships among peers.

Types of communication

There are three types of communication: verbal, non-verbal and a combination of these two, i.e. paralinguistic.

Verbal communication includes:

- talking face to face, as in meetings (committees, case conferences, working parties), workshops and seminars, public speaking, the grapevine
- written information in the form of letters, reports, service business plans and objectives, circulars, memoranda, overhead transparencies
- communication by telephone.

Non-verbal communication relates to the behaviours people display, such as gesture, facial expression, body language, posture or silence which, when used with or without language, communicate a great deal to the observant recipient.

Paralinguistic communication could be described as a combination of verbal and non-verbal communication in which the giver of information displays, for example, a particular posture or expression and accompanies it with some form of verbal communication such as a grunt or laugh.

Facilitating effective communication

If communication is to be effective, i.e. to achieve its objective, both the sender and receiver must ensure that the interchange takes place in a man-

Box 5.7 Facilitating effective communication

People

- Clarify ideas before communicating
- Communicate face-to-face
- Use feedback
- Be sensitive to receiver's mood, attitude, personality, interest, memory, difficulties
- Use direct, simple language or language common to sender and receiver
- Reinforce, i.e. provide information more than once in different ways
- Select ideal means of communicating particular message
- Grasp opportunities to convey information of help/value
- Examine the reason for each communication
- Be clear
- Beware of overtones
- Use silence to enable people to think
- Know level of pre-communication understanding in order to avoid assumptions/misunderstandings
- Use appropriate communication networks and cascade systems
- Use ideal volume
- Try to understand as well as being understood
- Support words with actions
- Communicate for the future as well as the present
- Follow up communications

Environment

- Select an environment, wherever and whenever possible, which is conducive to sending and receiving accurate information which is clearly comprehended
- Environment should be appropriate, e.g. formal for a formal meeting, comfortably informal for supervision
- Consider lighting levels, position of windows
- Avoid very noisy environments
- Select a telephone-free environment where appropriate
- Place notices on doors to notify others of communication in progress, e.g. to signify confidential nature

---

ner which is conducive to success, that is, which overcomes any barriers. Box 5.7 lists the elements required for effective communication.

RELATIONSHIPS

The second major aspect of interpersonal skills concerns the therapist's relationships with others, the behaviour she displays, the roles she enacts and the settings in which this takes place. People will behave in different ways depending on the circumstances and/or the environment, the others involved and the purpose of the interaction; additional ingredients are personality, character and professional traits.

Relationships in the context of interpersonal skills can be considered in relation to the roles (see also Ch. 13) an individual adopts with staff, the organisation and within meetings.

Staff

Staff roles relate to each individual's status and authority within a service. The departmental manager, for example, will be:

- a leader, the figurehead responsible for her staff, their support, guidance and motivation
- an educator, of her own staff and others in the organisation
- a liaison officer, linking her service to those of others both within the organisation and in the external environment
- a counsellor, identifying needs and solving problems, handling conflict and managing change
- a motivator, facilitating her staff's participation in all appropriate service activity.

The organisation

An individual's roles and functions, in relation to her position in an organisation, may include:

- facilitation: enabling necessary tasks to be accomplished easily and without disruption
- coordination: integrating the various activities within a department, thereby ensuring that all the aspects of a service form a 'whole'
- monitoring: receiving information which will enable her to understand the working of the organisation and relevant departments and their relationships with their environments, enabling her to advise, check, and audit
- controlling: in relation to her responsibility

for resources and service provision, she maintains control by checking, restraining or regulating, and by authorising decisions to be implemented
- negotiation: conferring for the purpose of mutual agreement, both within and outwith her service
- resource allocation: the authority to deploy resources according to a service's objectives and needs.

Occupational therapists always work with other people. These may be colleagues within their own department or those in other disciplines; thus, therapists work in one or more teams and a number of environments. Working in teams requires effective communication, cooperative planning and harmonious working relationships. The informal manner in which individuals may work together is described under Communication, above, but groups of people periodically need to communicate on a more formal basis, for example at a case conference or planning meeting.

The advantages of groups of people working together are that:

- the group has greater knowledge, information and expertise available
- more ideas are forthcoming, offering more approaches to problem-solving and potential solutions
- there is increased acceptance of solutions and their implementation
- better quality decisions are made.

However, there is a key disadvantage, namely the lack of responsibility of individual members for decision implementation, with the exception of the group leader.

Meetings

It is valuable, at this point, to consider meetings and the formal and informal relationships which occur within their framework in some detail. A meeting is an organised group of people of one or more disciplines who assemble for a specific purpose. The sub-sections below describe: the types and purposes of meetings; their organisation, structure and content; the roles of key personnel; dynamics and interactions.

Types

Meetings may be:

- ad hoc, the chance meeting with a colleague with whom one wished to discuss an item of mutual interest
- unplanned informal: casual conversation among colleagues during a break which includes some item of business
- planned informal: an arranged meeting in an informal setting for a general discussion concerning an agreed subject of mutual interest
- formal: planned meetings for which there will be an agenda, minutes, a chairperson and secretary. These may be regular or one-off assemblies. Specific meetings could be included in this type, for example an annual general meeting, a working party, a briefing for a future meeting, or a project team's regular development and planning forum.

Purposes

The purpose of meetings, particularly those of committees which meet regularly, need very clear terms of reference (an example is given in Fig. 5.11) to enable every member to contribute effectively to the task at hand. Reasons for meeting may include one or several of the following:

- coordination, i.e. liaison; dealing with service-wide issues, policies and procedures; working towards a common goal
- consultation and advice, which may involve helping colleagues to make decisions
- development, to provide opportunities for free thinking or brain-storming on a particular topic, for example marketing the service
- state of play: regular gatherings to discuss specific projects or targets, such as staff education
- solving problems and making decisions involving commitment by all members

RESOURCE MANAGEMENT SUB-COMMITTEE: TERMS OF REFERENCE

Aim: To provide a professional forum for the monitoring and evaluation of all elements of Resource Management, i.e. clinical and managerial information, patient administration system, clinical audit, performance indicators, quality assurance, performance review and budgeting/financial information.

Key tasks

1. Identify R.M. information needs in the short, medium and long term, including Korner data over and above M.D.S.

2. Evaluate potential information systems and their appropriateness for Unit and District-wide information, including integration with P.A.S. district-wide

3. Consider clinical audit processes/systems appropriate to occupational therapy

4. Monitor and evaluate performance indicators

5. Establish minimum quality standards for district-wide use which facilitate the formation of minimum standards in all specialities/sub-specialities and consider means of monitoring, evaluating and developing those standards

6. Encourage every Unit's service to undertake performance review which embraces all elements of Resource Management

7. Facilitate the provision of financial information, initially from Korner M.D.S.

8. Support all occupational therapy managers in the development of Resource Management

9. Liaise with colleagues of other disciplines as appropriate to the group's and profession's needs

10. Encourage/facilitate evaluative work

Membership/meetings

1. The sub-committee will be accountable to the District/Head Occupational Therapists' Committee

2. Membership will comprise: District O.T., Head O.T.s: SCH, RHH, NEH, NGH, M.I.U. (1), M.H.S. (1), F. & C.S.

3. The sub-committee will meet a minimum of six times per annum

4. Chairman and secretary to be elected by committee

5. Others may be co-opted at the committee's discretion

SEJ/EB/2.4
April 1990

Fig. 5.11 Terms of reference: an example. (Reproduced by kind permission of Sheffield Occupational Therapy Services.)

- making recommendations to higher or lower levels in the organisation
- giving and receiving information
- giving permission for action.

A group of people will be enabled to achieve the above purposes because they will be able or encouraged to:

- pool their knowledge, skills and resources
- share ideas with one another
- listen, in order to understand
- divide tasks to be achieved
- be flexible, demonstrating a willingness to be persuaded to change one's viewpoint
- participate fully
- find challenge and stimulation in disagreement
- reach a genuine consensus.

Organisation, structure and content

Formal meetings will require a prepared agenda and an agreed order of business.

An agenda, or programme of business for a meeting, should itemise specific topics for discussion in order of priority. It should indicate which member is to introduce the item and refer to any supporting information attached to the agenda or circulated previously (Fig. 5.12). The agenda should be circulated to members well in advance of the meeting date, thereby enabling them to be well prepared for their presentation and/or discussion.

The order of business at a meeting will probably be as follows:

- it will start on time
- the agenda will be adhered to
- discussion should be structured and debate encouraged
- a record of the proceedings will be taken, i.e.
  —date
  —time
  —venue
  —those present/absent
  —the chairperson
  —acceptance of minutes of the last meeting
  —matters arising from those minutes
  —major agenda items: a summary of discussion, decisions made, action to be

taken, by whom, by a set date
  —any other business may or may not be included, depending on the committee's custom and practice
  —confirmation of the date of the next meeting
- it will finish on time.

Committees

People who are members of a committee will all have particular roles within that forum. These roles may entail specific duties such as those of a chairperson or they may be more general. Specific roles are described below:

- Chairperson:
  —acts as the group's facilitator (not master)
  —assists the team to make the best decision in the most efficient manner possible
  —guides, mediates, probes, stimulates, interprets, clarifies and summarises
  —steers the debate/discussion forward, aiming to arrive at a resolution acceptable and understood by everyone
  —ensures fair play by controlling the garrulous and the interrupters, encouraging the reticent and protecting the weaker members.

It is worth remembering that the perfect chairperson does not exist, but that an individual's performance in this role will be enhanced with experience.

- Secretary
  —prepares the agenda in consultation with the chairperson
  —takes the minutes
  —deals with correspondence which is sent to or from the meeting
  —circulates all relevant information to committee members
  —deals with the administrative arrangements for each meeting, i.e. books the venue, orders refreshments, issues travel directions
  —may or may not participate in the discussion, depending on the purpose and

membership of the committee; for example, the secretary of a BAOT sub-group will contribute to discussion but the secretary who is also the chairperson's secretary will not generally participate unless asked to do so.
- Treasurer

—monitors and controls income and expenditure
—deals with all financial transactions
—has the accounts audited annually.
- Committee members:
  —attend and participate in all meetings, addressing all discussion through the chair

MIDSHIRE OCCUPATIONAL THERAPY SERVICE

HEAD OCCUPATIONAL THERAPISTS' COMMITTEE

The next meeting of the committee will take place on Wednesday, 25 September 1991 in the Board Room at Southern General Hospital, commencing at 9.00am.

AGENDA

1. Apologies for absence: Y.B., F.C.

2. Minutes of the last meeting: to approve as a correct record

3. Matters arising:

    45/91: Clinical education placement review (to report action — D.O.T.)

    59/91: Food Hygiene training (to confirm dates/venues — M.H.)

    61/91: N.V.Q. and support worker training (to report outcome of 28.8.91 meeting — E.L.).

4. Community Care Plans: to receive Units' comments and observations re plan for care of elderly people (All)

5. Quality Standards Guidelines: to review 1990 document. Discussion to be led by R.B.

6. Clinical Audit: to receive report from M.H. of evaluation of pilot at S.G.H. (Report attached)

7. Sub-Committee Reports:

    (i) Staff Development (D.O.T.)

    (ii) Resource Management (S.M.)

8. Any other business

9. Confirm date, time, venue of the next meeting

DOT/PS

Ref. O.T.4

11.9.91

Fig. 5.12 A sample agenda.

—should prepare for the meeting in advance, for example by reading appropriate papers, considering the options for an item requiring a decision

—should be clear and logical in discussion

—should seek the most acceptable solution and accept only those which are logically sound

—should be prepared to participate in the group's work, some of which may take place in sub-committees.

Dynamics and interaction

If a committee is to fulfil its purpose, positive dynamics and interaction are essential, and require at least as much attention as preparing an agenda or selecting a chairperson. Group dynamics concerns the behaviours (interaction) and forces within a group of people; understanding group dynamics involves understanding one's own behaviour and perceiving oneself as others do.

Group cohesion is vital. The members of the group need to develop in order to offer one another and the team loyalty and to be able to adhere to agreed and established standards. Factors which aid cohesiveness include:

- similarity of work, i.e. occupational therapy
- physical proximity to one's workplace — the security of being on one's own territory
- the environment in which the group meet and work — the venue and seating arrangements should be conducive to interaction
- group size — too large a group may hinder debate and interaction; too small a group may limit the group's ability to fulfil its task
- knowing what motivates members individually and collectively
- respecting one another's roles, opinions
- a leadership style that facilitates the group's function by offering support and clarification, enabling facts to be analysed critically, controlling confrontation, and arbitrating
- common social factors and group norms — a team will develop its own norms or common standards of behaviour, which may be influenced by management styles, policies and procedures
- the prospect of rewards, for example the publication of practice standards for the service or the chairman's seasonal treat
- threats from outside the team — questioning the group's purpose or effectiveness, for example.

If a team is to become sufficiently cohesive to be able to work together effectively it has to develop through four clearly identifiable stages:

1. Forming: members learn about the task to be completed; identify and learn the group rules and methods of operation; acquire information and other resources. There is great reliance upon the leader at this stage.
2. Storming: internal conflict develops and members resist the task at an emotional level.
3. Norming: the conflict has settled and cooperation develops. Views are exchanged and new standards (norms) developed.
4. Performing: teamwork is achieved, roles become flexible. Solutions are found and implemented.

Working through these stages whilst endeavouring to conduct the group's business may take a considerable time. The process of developing into a cohesive unit can be encouraged by taking specific time out for team building, enabling individuals to begin to identify with the group. The content of team building events will vary but will include opportunities for individuals to describe and discuss their particular roles and functions, the constraints they work with and the pleasures of their jobs. An event may also involve a series of exercises in which small groups work on a given task requiring discussion and debate, problem-solving, decision-making and cooperation. Beginning to understand colleagues and how they think and work provides an invaluable baseline from which the whole group can assess its development.

Interaction among group members will depend upon leadership, motivation and setting and upon adherence to agreed rules and procedures. Successful interaction involves achieving a balance between attention to the task in hand and attention to the people concerned. It also requires commitment to the group and a high degree of collaboration (team spirit) to enable members to be more open and more comfortable with their pursuit of the team's objectives.

A therapist's interpersonal skills underpin all her roles and functions. Successful intervention programmes, planning meetings, multidisciplinary team work and the many other settings in which she works require her to understand herself and others with whom she has contact, whether on a one-to-one basis or within a group setting. Effective communication and sound working relationships can only enhance the effectiveness of a service and the organisation within which it operates.

SECTION 6: PERSONNEL AND DEPARTMENTAL MANAGEMENT

We trained hard but it seemed that every time we were beginning to form up into teams we would be reorganised. I was to learn later in life that we tend to meet any new situation by reorganisation, and a wonderful method it can be for creating the illusion of progress while producing confusion, inefficiency and demoralisation.

(Caius Petronius AD 62)

Today's manager lives in a world of rapid change, and yet the rate of change is likely to increase in the years ahead. Unless he can keep up with this change he's likely to find himself obsolete.

(Dale & Michelon 1966)

These two remarks made in very different times, perhaps serve to articulate many people's feelings about the constant changes in public sector health and social care since the late 1940s. Many excellent managers, in occupational therapy and other disciplines, continue to struggle with elements of their managerial and other tasks because they are operating in times of continual change and with resources which need to be increasingly elastic. However, the reader who feels somewhat daunted by the sheer size of the management function is urged to take heart and look for the opportunities, challenges and satisfaction to be gained in any sphere and at any level of management.

Section 1 discussed management, organisations, management theories and practice in relation to planning, organising, leading and controlling. This section deals with the practicalities of managing on a day-to-day basis. It will become evident to the reader that managers undertake some activities which are clearly managerial and others which may be described as administrative or clinical.

The managerial element is a matter of making decisions about the section of a service or organisation for which the individual is responsible. The non-managerial element may include tasks in which her staff will be participating daily, i.e. the treatment of clients and its accompanying paperwork. In many instances the latter element is important because it helps the manager to maintain her practical knowledge and skills. However, she must not allow her clinical work to deprive staff of their responsibilities and interest, nor should she allow it to prevent her from managing effectively. Occupational therapists have to learn to manage themselves and their time appropriately, regardless of their grade. Promotion entails greater management responsibility; the higher the position the more one manages and the less one participates in the service's practical work.

The daily activities undertaken by a manager will take many shapes and forms, but they will fall into broad categories which, when drawn together, integrate the resources and functions of a service. The sub-sections which follow deal with departmental and personnel management within practical headings, i.e. personnel, planning and development, managing change, resource management and administration.

PERSONNEL

The therapy staff who provide services to clients are the most important resource a manager possesses. They have skills, knowledge and expertise which are supported by the service's other resources (its facilities, procedures, systems and so on). Staff are individuals as well as team members; in addition to common basic needs they have individual requirements which are reflected in creative, exploratory and self-fulfilling activities. The manager should remember that all human behaviour must be goal-directed in order to satisfy needs and that this has substantial implications for managing a service's most expensive resource.

A manager has a number of personnel functions which she fulfils with the support of the organisation's personnel department. These functions are:

- obtaining, developing and motivating the staff needed to achieve the service's objectives
- developing a service philosophy and structure and evolving a management style which promotes commitment and cooperation
- utilising staff's skills and capacities to optimum effect
- ensuring that the organisation meets its social and legal obligations towards its employees.

Much of the personnel department's support and advice will concern the authority's policies, procedures and services for employees:

- practical assistance with recruitment, such as placing advertisements, arranging interviews, sending for references
- employee relations — consultative committees (management and union)
- employee services — health and safety, occupational health, welfare, personnel records and information systems
- social responsibility — equity of attitude, consideration, quality of working life and environment
- employment policies — the people the organisation wishes to employ, the qualifications, experience and personal qualities required
- remuneration — level of pay and other benefits, such as flexible working hours
- promotion — from within the organisation and through the introduction of new employees; reconciliation in potential conflict
- education — schemes, levels, type (i.e. clinical or managerial)
- employee relations — union recognition, representation and participation.

Employment law

Most of the framework for the above is provided by legislation, current national management and staff-side agreements and a wide range of health and local authority circulars. A number of the key acts are summarised in Box 5.8. NHS staff are currently employed on remuneration scales and conditions of work agreed nationally. However, at the time of writing it seems likely that this arrangement may change so that NHS staff work to locally agreed pay scales and conditions. Those staff employed by local authorities are also subject to scales and conditions set nationally, although currently there is no nationally agreed range of salary points for occupational therapy staff. In addition to present national agreements for public sector employees, there will also be existing local agreements, that is, policies and procedures, which an employing authority has set within national guidelines; these concern, for example, accident reporting, fire policy, grievance and disciplinary procedures, and health and safety.

Grievance and disciplinary procedures

These procedures, which form part of the contract of employment, exist to ensure fairness, consistency and equity and to facilitate the management process. They aim to establish particular standards of performance and to assist in the management of difficult situations. Public sector employers issue all employees with a copy of the authority's procedures.

In the event of a *grievance*, an employee formally takes up an issue of concern with her line manager, e.g. grading, behaviour towards employee.

A *disciplinary procedure* is a formal process for improving performance and/or behaviour which is judged inadequate for the job by the manager. This procedure includes verbal and written warnings to ensure employee compliance with the organisation's rules. There will be penalties for misconduct and poor performance, including summary dismissal for certain offences such as theft.

Box 5.8 Employment law relevant to personnel management in occupational therapy

Act	Key provision		
Professions Supplementary to Medicine 1960 and NHS (PSM) Regulations 1974	State registration of therapists employed in the public sector.		Maternity Pay Fund. Extends jurisdiction of industrial tribunals. Employees have right not to be unfairly dismissed.
Health & Safety at Work 1974	Safe working conditions and safer systems of work. *Employer*: duty to appoint competent and properly qualified staff; provide and maintain safe equipment; provide and maintain safe workplace; provide and maintain a safe system of work. *Employee*: duties relate to same four areas as above, i.e. to be competent at level employed, to use equipment safely and for intended purpose, to maintain safe workplace, to utilise safe working systems based on cooperative practice and safety precautions. Occupier liability and employers' liability for conditions in which employees are instructed to work. Employees have general duty to take 'reasonable care' and to report dangers.	*Sex Discrimination 1975 and Race Discrimination 1976*	These two acts apply generally to all employment issues and make it unlawful to discriminate, directly or indirectly, against men or women on grounds of race, sex or marital status, regarding recruitment, terms and conditions of employment, opportunities for development, dismissal. There are exceptions permitted within the law, e.g. if the essential nature of job requires particular sex or racial characteristics; if the organisation is a single-sex establishment and it is unreasonable for post to be held by a person of the other sex; if the job requires a married couple. The *Equal Opportunities Commission* was established to oversee these two acts (and Equal Pay Act 1970).
Employment Protection 1975	Promotes improvement in industrial relations. Amends law relating to rights of employees. Amends law relating to employees, employers, trade unions and employers' associations. Provides for establishment of	*Employment Protection (Consolidation) 1978*	Set minimum standards re contracts and in nationally negotiated conditions, e.g. antenatal care, maternity/paternity leave and pay, rights to return to work; trade union membership with entitlement to time off work in certain specified circumstances.

In order to ensure consistency, equity and fairness these procedures must:

- be agreed between management and staff side, i.e. legitimate and written down
- promote consistency in similar situations
- define the authority of the individuals operating them

- structure and therefore clarify the relationship between managers as delegated power-holders of the authority and the authority's appeals system
- be logical, i.e. follow proper procedural stages
- enshrine and legitimise employees' rights to representation and eliminate victim isolation.

Staffing a service

In the past, an occupational therapy service was staffed according to its establishment, i.e. a specified number of employees by grade for which the service was provided with a pay budget. Increasingly, the trend is to staff a service within a cash limited agreed budget, which must allow for staff salaries, travelling and subsistence, study leave, uniform or mufti allowance (NHS), equipment, materials and publications. Within this framework the manager has to provide a staffing structure, i.e. the ideal skill mix to accomplish the service's objectives and undertake the daily workload. The manager will thus utilise her resources flexibly, continually weighing service demands against both staff and non-staff resources at her disposal.

Manpower planning

In order to provide the most cost-effective, high-quality service, a manager must plan and develop her staffing requirements. This will involve assessing the skill mix needed, i.e. identifying by grade how many staff will be needed to meet the needs of future clients. Information from business plans and planned future developments will enable the manager to submit requests for further resources. Manpower planning relies upon the manager's past experience, professional judgement and knowledge of the number of staff required per client group already served. Additionally, she may consider the following:

- the needs of the local population, taking into account any special characteristics such as the proportion of elderly people or the presence of a particular industry
- current and potential future activity levels
- imminent retirements, the mobility of junior staff, incidence of maternity leave, turnover in past years
- productivity and throughput of the service (see p. 143) and whether these can be improved.

A major part of manpower planning involves examining skill mix, i.e. the grades of staff needed and in what proportions. In order to do this the manager needs to identify the various roles of the different grades in each speciality and attempt to match existing staff to client need in the most cost-effective way. As well as helping to create a service that is responsive to clients' needs, this will enhance the job satisfaction of staff members, whose skills will be used optimally. Managers should review skill mix continuously as client needs and service delivery change with time. Additionally, changes in employment training, such as National Vocational Qualifications, will continue to have an impact on the staff skills available.

Recruitment and selection

Authorities have recruitment and selection policies and procedures which enable them to obtain the number and quality of employees they require to satisfy their objectives and needs. There are three key stages in the recruitment and selection process:

1. defining requirements: job description and specification, terms and conditions of service
2. attracting candidates: reviewing and evaluating sources of applicants from within and outwith the organisation; advertising
3. selection: short-listing, interviewing, assessing, obtaining references, offering employment, drawing up contracts

Section 4 (p. 102) referred to a number of the points above from the applicant's perspective. This section will consider them from the employer's viewpoint.

Defining one's requirements will include:

- evaluating the job description and updating it if necessary
- drawing up a job specification — identifying what is essential and desirable in relation to skills, knowledge, attitudes, experience
- deciding how to assess and evaluate applicants against essential and desirable skills and qualities. Some people use a numerical point plan in which a score of 1 to 5 is allocated to seven requirements; this is illustrated in Table 5.1.

Table 5.1   Interviewing: the seven point plan of specifications

Specifications	Examples of essential/desirable requirements
1. Health and appearance	Physical and mental fitness, broadly acceptable appearance
2. Attainments	Appropriate knowledge, skills, abilities, qualifications; positive attitude to job
3. General intelligence	Flexibility, ability to adapt, ability to learn
4. Special aptitudes	Skills, techniques, computer literacy
5. Interests	Motivation, creativity, problem-solving skills, potential for positive contribution and development
6. Disposition	Active, pioneering and persevering temperament; maturity in outlook; discretion; reliability
7. Circumstances	Willingness to move house; ability to drive; flexibility re working hours, on-call rotas

Attracting candidates may involve:

- examining the factors likely to attract or repel potential applicants, for example:
  - reputation of the authority as an employer, including its equal opportunities policy
  - occupational therapy's reputation
  - security of employment
  - flexibility for employees of varying cultures, for example, re uniform, feast days, prayer times
  - working conditions
  - opportunities for continuing education
  - location
  - career prospects
  - structured support and supervision
  - team work
- selecting selling points and preparing written and visual information
- considering internal and external sources, including professional journals, agencies, educational establishments and 'job shops'.

Advertising must meet legal requirements. It should also be justifiable, create and maintain interest, and stimulate action.

Selecting staff involves:

- short-listing candidates into categories —

'possible', 'marginal', 'unsuitable' — using the job specification mentioned above
- interviewing in order to obtain and assess information about each candidate for comparison after the interview
- using assessment criteria such as those described in Table 5.1. Selection 'tests' are rarely used for clinical occupational therapy posts; for more senior grades they may include presentations, psychometric testing, aptitude and attainments tests
- offering the most suitable candidate the post; assuming she accepts, the formalities of references, written confirmation of the offer, contract and starting date are then dealt with.

Retention

Retaining staff is a challenge which stretches the imagination of most managers at some time or another, and occupational therapy managers are no exception. The profession's workforce is relatively young, predominantly female, highly mobile and a much sought-after 'commodity'. The discussion of motivation, in the following sub-section (p. 119) is relevant to the issue of staff retention, but first we might consider conditions which will encourage staff to remain in their jobs. These may include:

- a wide range of development and educational opportunities such as post-graduate courses, in-service development, regular study days, in-department seminars and secondment to local polytechnics or universities for multidisciplinary degree or research courses
- management practices that foster job satisfaction, e.g. utilising caseload management, maintaining appropriate levels of support and supervision within the team, operating an 'open door' policy in which the manager is always available at specified times of the week, valuing staff and enabling them to have time out to read and study, offering them an interesting workload within the service's parameters
- creche or other child-minding facilities, particularly if these are on-site, for staff with young families

- flexible employment scheme whereby staff can negotiate working hours and/or holidays to fit with departmental and family requirements; job sharing; career breaks with retraining schemes and regular contact built in
- high profile and status of the service
- appropriate promotion policy within the department or service.

Motivation

'Motivation is inferred from or defined by goal directed behaviour' (Armstrong 1988). The ability to continually motivate staff is an essential management skill and is of vital importance in times of change, pressure and stress. The following is a summary of methods which may be used for motivating staff. The reader is advised to refer to specific texts for theories of motivation.

- implementing an external reward system; this might include performance related pay (PRP, applies primarily to senior managers at present), fringe benefits such as regular time out, security, promotion, recognition and pleasant working conditions
- creating inherent conditions, i.e. those contained within the job, which provide satisfaction and feelings of accomplishment, enable staff to express and use their abilities and give them decision-making authority
- improving individuals' skill levels through ongoing education
- encouraging understanding and acceptance of the individual's and other people's roles, ensuring clear role definition
- setting clear targets
- providing adequate supervision
- encouraging staff's sense of commitment to and identification with the service and its objectives, using development activities which improve integration (e.g. team building) and adopting a more participative and democratic style of management
- fostering understanding of service/ organisational rules so that staff are aware of expected standards of performance and behaviour.

There are occasions when staff will adopt a variety of defence mechanisms in response to frustration at some element of their work or the service. They may display aggression, apathy, withdrawal, projection, regression or repression. A manager must be alert to these behaviours, endeavour to uncover the cause and work with staff to provide solutions and to raise motivation levels and avoid burn out in a mutually agreed manner.

Interviewing

Interviewing is described in Section 4 (p. 105) from the point of view of the interviewee. This section considers the types, purposes and principles of interviews from the interviewer's perspective.

An interview may be of one of the following types:

- selection: to obtain the best available candidate for the job and the service
- induction: generally a discussion on first day of employment, followed by induction programme and a follow-up after a specified period of time
- disciplinary: to inform the interviewee of her unacceptable behaviour or errors, to correct and prevent recurrence. A union representative and/or a 'friend' of the interviewee may be involved. Future checks will be made of behaviour and performance
- grievance: enables individual to air complaint and to discover and remove causes of dissatisfaction if possible. Requires follow-up to ensure agreed action is implemented
- review/appraisal: to review employee's performance over set period of time against agreed objectives; to build on strengths; identify weaknesses; identify areas of improvement; decide how to overcome weaknesses; identify subsequent development needs and discuss future potential prospects. Widely used as a stage in staff development programmes
- exit: to discover an individual's true reason(s) for leaving with a view to taking any

required action to prevent others leaving for the same reason(s). To secure the employee's goodwill and the service or organisation's reputation

- consultation/fact finding: to gather facts and other relevant information from specific people in order to complete a particular task
- counselling: to listen to an individual and help her to consider options to solve or come to terms with a problem.

Interviews may be conducted with one or more of the following purposes in mind:

- to exchange information
- to seek behavioural change
- to solve problems
- to make decisions
- to gather new information.

Interviews may be described as a four-step process:

1. defining the purpose of the interview
2. preparing: selecting interviewees, choosing an appropriate environment, ensuring privacy, setting time, establishing any policies, procedures or rules needed
3. conducting the interview: stating its purpose, establishing rapport, listening, probing, measuring feelings/facts, using open questions, being impartial, deciding course of action
4. following up, to check that proposed action has been taken.

Interviewing, like any other skill, has to be learned and should improve with practice and experience. The checklist in Box 5.9 and the do's and don'ts of interviewing in Table 5.2 provide various rules of thumb for the objective and successful interviewing of clients, carers and staff (as well as advice for the interviewee).

Induction

Induction, or orientation, is usually a relatively formal programme designed and implemented by a manager to introduce a new employee to her job. The hours spent in induction are invaluable, as

Box 5.9 Interviews: the key elements

I	Information
N	Naturalness
T	Technique
E	Eye contact
R	References
V	Verbal skills and fluency
I	Interaction
E	Experience
W	Weaknesses
I	Interests
N	Non-verbal communication
G	Getting to the interview
G	General impression
E	Effectiveness
N	Nervousness
E	Encouragement. Enquiries
R	Relaxation. Reception
A	Application. Attitudes. Attributes. Alertness
L	Listening
C	Communication
H	Humour. 'Homework'. Hypothetical questions
E	Environment
C	Control
K	Knowledge
L	Leading questions
I	Initiative
S	Skills. Selection/suitability. Selling. Smiling
T	Type

they offer new staff a starting-point for full participation in the service. During the induction period new staff should be given time to:

- familiarise themselves with the geography/layout of their work area
- read and understand information concerning the authority and service
- meet relevant colleagues, particularly those within their allocated team
- observe the service and the individuals and teams working within it
- understand the service's objectives
- discuss policies, procedures, paperwork, caseload management practices, support and supervision.

Induction programmes will vary according to local circumstances and individual needs. A sample induction programme is offered in Box 5.10.

Table 5.2 The do's and don'ts of interviewing: tips for the interviewee and interviewer (cont'd overleaf)

Checklist	Do	Do not	Checklist	Do	Do not
Information	Keep to the point Listen and absorb Ask for clarification	Waffle Try to bluff if you have misunderstood or were not listening	Interaction	Try to relate to interviewer by listening and making appropriate non-verbal signs	Try to 'take over' Overdo the 'listening' so that you give nothing
Naturalness	Aim to be yourself in your professional capacity	Overdo your intro/extrovert tendencies	Experience	Ensure that interviewer is aware of relevant past experience: pre-training, during and since	Waste time or effort on what you consider inappropriate information, *unless* you are asked
Technique	Practise — it helps if you appear relaxed, knowledgeable, interested Remember that interviewing and being interviewed should improve with experience	Ignore preparation — to do so is to fail Think that 'it'll be alright on the day' — nervousness will probably get the better of you	Weaknesses	Remember that everyone has them Know your own, and be able to admit them	Pretend that you are perfect Be afraid to admit a weakness, but follow it with an explanation of what you are doing/going to do about it
Eye Contact	Maintain it appropriately Remember non-verbal communication	Try to outstare interviewer Avoid eye contact by looking around room or at a point behind interviewer	Interests	Include these in your CV/Application. Both personal and professional interests provide information about you	Underestimate the value of personal interests — they show signs of the 'real you' Admit to having no professional interests
References	Choose your referees carefully Select those whom you know professionally, unless a 'personal' one is also requested Always ask if someone is prepared to give a reference	Ask friends to act as referees — they don't always say what the panel wishes to hear Assume, ever, that someone will act as referee. It may be inappropriate or they may not wish to act on your behalf	Non-verbal communication	Be aware of it — in yourself and others — and what it tells you, or the panel	Ignore your less endearing traits — do something positive to overcome them
			Getting to an interview	Allow ample time for travel, finding the right building/office/department, and for freshening up	*Ever* arrive for an interview at a run, dishevelled, or late
Verbal skills and fluency	Be sure of your facts/reasons for application Practise your skills Try to predict what you may be asked so that you have an answer Prepare your questions if you are interviewing Pause before answering/asking a question — it gives you valuable seconds of 'thinking' time	Try to bluff; your fluency and skills will be lost Go unprepared (see Technique above) Overdo the 'chatter' 'Dry up'; if you do, ask interviewer to clarify/repeat question	General impression	Remember, first impressions can be lasting ones — what sort do you create?	Try to be clever and over-impress on first meeting, or withdraw and create no impression at all
			Effectiveness	Know yourself, both as an individual and as a therapist Convey this to your interviewer calmly, thoughtfully, objectively	Attempt to prove how effective you are by giving examples which indicate something else!

Table 5.2 Cont'd

Checklist	Do	Do not	Checklist	Do	Do not
Nervousness	Remember everyone is nervous sometimes Learn to cope with the visible signs Remember that an interviewer will encourage you to talk and to relax	Admit that you are nervous to an interviewer Forget that the nervousness keeps the adrenalin flowing, which is good — so don't try to rid yourself of nervousness altogether		professional attitude throughout the interview	attitude to any topic other than professional issues
			Attributes	Remember that personal and professional characteristics may have a bearing on the job for which you have applied Remember that your general health will be important too	Be sexist Be over-familiar
Encouragement	Encourage someone if you are interviewing them, i.e. help them where appropriate, give the right non-verbal signals	Discourage someone by being over-assertive, doing all the talking, giving no non-verbal response			
			Ambition	Admit to being ambitious, within reason. It shows that you are well motivated	Overdo it. You may need to tone down your true professional ambition(s) for the sake of the interview, i.e. don't tell the chairman (Head OT) that you are aiming for her job in a year or two!
Enquiries (questions)	Use questions in a positive/specific way, even if some are hypothetical or reflective Remember that questions which could be construed as discriminative are unacceptable Prepare your questions beforehand, ensuring that they are sensible and relevant	Ask leading questions, or those which only require a 'yes/no' answer Be afraid to ask questions about the job, structure of department and so on Ask questions about salary, holidays. You should be told the answers to these			
			Alertness	Be alert throughout the interview, especially mentally	Look bored Yawn Fidget
			Listening	Really listen and understand what is being asked/said Learn to listen if it's not one of your strong points	'Switch off' — this can be fatal to your chances of a job
Relaxation	Do give the appearance of being relaxed in manner and speech Practise the techniques which help you to relax *before* interviews/trying situations	Relax, literally, by sprawling or sounding lackadaisical			
			Communication (Written and Verbal)	Be clear and concise Keep to the point Demonstrate that you are an efficient and effective communicator	'Waffle, talk of irrelevant issues Distract others with non-verbal signals
Application	Ensure it's legible and to the point Apply yourself wholeheartedly to the interview Remember that short-listing is carried out on the basis of your written application	Ignore the importance of the first impression of a telephone enquiry or application form	Humour	Ensure that you have your sense of humour with you 'on the day'	Be flippant Tell jokes Appear miserable
			'Homework'	Prepare yourself thoroughly for interviewing and being interviewed. This preparation shows interest, foresight and good sense	Try to get away with lack of preparation. It leads to failure because it creates a bad impression
Attitudes	Be positive Display a	Try to impress with your personal			

Table 5.2 Cont'd

Checklist	Do	Do not	Checklist	Do	Do not
Hypothetical questions (see Enquiries)	Be prepared for these. Interviews for OTs do not always include a practical assessment; therefore, the interviewer needs to ask you what you would do in a specific case	Rush your response or try to over-impress. Use phrases such as 'in my experience . . .' Insist on telling of your experiences in 'X' hospital ad nauseam			accordingly, or seek the answer outside the interview
			Initiative	Demonstrate that you possess it, in your application, in your replies to questions Remember that interviewers are seeking someone who has the initiative to 'get on with the job' and to continue their professional development	Over or underdo it Give the impression that you could undertake the Head OT's job tomorrow Be so reticent that you display no initiative at all
Environment (see Reception)	Prepare the room for interview carefully. It must: be reasonably comfortable, have a pleasant atmosphere, afford absolute privacy and enable panel and candidate to observe behaviour and to see and hear Help the interviewee to be at ease	Accept any interruptions Blind the candidate with bright light Give her a creaky, uncomfortable chair Fill the room with distracting items			
			Skills	Elaborate upon skills you possess (personal and professional) which are applicable, as asked Explain your particular interest in specific skill(s)	Undersell the skills you have Overstate. You may well be able to improve the level of skills in this post
Control	Be in control of yourself and the interview (as panel member) Be in control of yourself (as interviewee) physically and mentally	Ask questions which enable the interviewee to ramble at length; if this happens interrupt at a pause and say 'thank you' and ask your next question Take over the interview if you are being interviewed!	Selection/ suitability	Remember that the interviewer is trying to ascertain whether you are suitable for this job and this department. It is up to you to prove yourself Think carefully before applying — is the job right for you? Remember that there are always other chances and you will be successful	Expect success every time Be disappointed by failure — think of it in terms of experience and your own learning
Knowledge	Show that you are knowledgeable about OT Show that you have some knowledge re the job applied for, i.e. you have done your 'homework' Be modest, but sell yourself objectively	Blind everyone with science, e.g. by talking about a technique you've just learnt			
			Selling	Remember that you have to sell yourself at an interview. It is not just your qualifications, knowledge and skills which are being tested, it's also you as a person Remember that your 'performance'	Be too modest or too outgoing so that you under- or oversell yourself 'Get on your soapbox' — it will not be appreciated!
Leading questions (see Enquiries)	Answer objectively if asked a leading question, e.g. how long would you stay if offered the job	Ask leading questions yourself. If you need an answer to a delicate subject, then phrase it			

Table 5.2 Cont'd

Checklist	Do	Do not
	and your references 'sell' you	
Smiling	Try to smile in a natural and relaxed way, and to appear at ease Remember to smile with your face and eyes not just with your mouth	Grin or pretend you are advertising toothpaste! It is highly suspect and and your face will ache!
Type (of interview)	Remember the purpose of the interview you are attending/holding Be prepared	Underestimate the importance of interviews, be they formal or informal

Staff development and education

Staff development is an essential component of personnel management, offering many benefits to the authority, the service and the individual.

To the organisation it offers:

- staff versatility, which will help the service to provide continuity in times of staff shortages
- increased quality of skills
- greater efficiency in meeting objectives
- the opportunity to produce senior staff
- enhanced competition and recruitment, particularly if the authority has a good reputation
- reduced turnover
- a continual flow of ideas
- cost effectiveness in the short and long term.

Services benefit from developing their staff in an environment which:

- enhances the delegation process
- enables more effective decisions to be made at all levels
- offers opportunities to develop individual's potential
- promotes confidence in additional responsibilities when deputising.

Individuals benefit in a number of ways:

- Their skills, self-esteem and job satisfaction are enhanced

Box 5.10 Example of an induction programme

Day 1

- Ensure contract has been signed
- Point out to new staff member location of: her desk, office and department facilities such as toilets, changing room, fire exits, refreshment areas
- Introduce her to immediate/team colleagues
- Conduct induction interview, discussing first two weeks of programme, establishing immediate needs
- Give tour of relevant facilities
- Describe structure of department and where new employee fits in
- Ensure that she has something positive to do if her line manager is called away
- Provide concise, clear, written information to support verbal input

Weeks 1–2

- Ensure programme is flexible so new staff member can contribute and gaps in knowledge/skills can begin to be addressed
- Encourage her to shadow appropriate colleagues in department and to meet and talk with other relevant colleagues e.g. team physiotherapist, social worker
- Clarify service objectives, priorities, expected standards
- Deal with departmental policies and procedures
- Clarify lines of accountability
- Establish ground rules, e.g. behaviour, dress, time
- Introduce employee to work schedules and own caseload
- Ensure that she attends authority's induction course as soon as possible
- Begin to identify support network(s)
- Have line manager review induction with employee

Weeks 3–4

- Review induction to date
- Increase employee's contribution to caseload
- Plan to meet needs

- Their confidence, security and interest are increased
- They develop specialist knowledge and skills
- Their career prospects are enhanced
- They feel valued.

After an induction programme and education to meet immediate needs, each employee should participate in a system of performance review (appraisal) which will form the basis of her continuing development.

Individual performance review (IPR)

In its present format, IPR was initiated by Personnel Memorandum (86)10, which explained the process of IPR for NHS managers. IPR is now widespread in the NHS and is a *formal* means of reviewing and evaluating an individual's ongoing performance with the intention of discussing progress, locating strengths and weaknesses and setting goals to meet identified needs. IPR enables the manager to formally record staff performance on a regular (usually annual) basis and assists the individual to take a considerable degree of responsibility for her own career development.

The techniques used may vary but the process, essentially, is carried out in three stages — pre-interview, interview and post-interview — and is accompanied by documentation.

• *Pre-interview stage*: both manager and staff member will undertake preparation for the interview. This may entail the manager considering the individual's performance vis-à-vis the previous year's objectives or her job description if it is a first IPR. The individual may complete a time and task analysis (Fig. 5.8) as well as a review of her past twelve months' performance, explaining which tasks have given her the greatest or least satisfaction and why, and which have caused her most anxiety and why (Fig. 5.13A). She will also identify her objectives for the forthcoming year. Her analysis and comments are forwarded to her manager, who will consider them prior to the interview.

• *Interview stage*. The interview is a continuation of the two-way dialogue. It should be conducted in privacy and relatively formally, offering both parties opportunities to review, discuss and plan ahead objectively, to consider the performance standards achieved, review accomplishments against objectives and agree on objectives and an action plan for them both.

• *Post-interview stage*: the agreed action should then be implemented by the manager and/or individual according to the actions and time-scales agreed. Interim reviews will enable both parties to modify objectives in response to changing circumstances. This may occur during supervision sessions (see p. 127).

Education

Once a service has established an IPR system it is able to plan, systematically and objectively, a strategy for formal or informal staff education to meet identified needs. Ongoing education equips employees with the necessary knowledge, skills, behaviours and attitudes to meet standards, improve performance, and, if appropriate, prepare for the next grade. By applying a professional development framework, incorporating all staff grades, a manager can identify, very broadly, the key tasks required by grade, the competencies expected after, for example, six months, the knowledge and skills required to develop within a grade or to progress to the next level and how these needs might be met. This system can be utilised for individuals or for groups.

How do managers and staff meet these identified needs? Traditionally, courses have been considered the mainstay of continuing education, but experience demonstrates that there are other, more effective, means by which staff can develop skills. Examples include: being coached on the job by mentoring staff; job rotation (particularly in the case of junior therapists and helpers); undertaking research; working alongside a more experienced colleague; utilising opportunities offered by the Open University and other organisations; using self-development or learning packages developed in the service; and experiential learning, which provides new experiences in a practical setting.

Two particular areas of continuing education for therapists should be mentioned at this juncture: training staff to be trainers of others and clinical supervision training.

1. *Training the trainers*. All occupational therapy staff adopt the role of teacher because they

(A)

1. What is the main purpose of the job I do?

2. What do I think is the main purpose of my boss's job?

3. What have I achieved over the last few months or particularly enjoyed doing?

4. What has been difficult to do?

5. Have I had opportunities to improve myself and the way I do the job?

(B)

1. What areas of work would I like to improve my performance in over the coming months?

2. What opportunities and help am I looking for?

3. What aspects of my work do I want to concentrate on?

4. What objectives would I set myself for the next few months?

Fig. 5.13 Pre-interview questionnaires. (A) Reviewing the past year. (B) Considering the forthcoming year.

facilitate the learning of clients, carers and themselves. However, most staff will require specific, additional knowledge and skills to enable them to supervise and develop colleagues, particularly junior and support staff and students. Helping others to learn is a responsibility which should be taken seriously. The trainer will need:

- an understanding of the knowledge and skill competencies demanded by the area of work in question
- an understanding of the objectives of the development programme
- effective presentation skills and an understanding of the learning process
- sound evaluative techniques.

2. Clinical supervision training for occupational therapists who supervise the clinical education of students is undertaken sequentially, working from level 1 to 6. Levels 1 to 4 are organised locally by pre-registration course staff and/or authorities. Levels 5 and 6 cover topics offered in institutions of higher education. A summary of the content of each level is described in Box 5.11. The object of this approach is to offer course organisers a certain degree of flexibility to accommodate local developments and variations whilst maintaining national standards. Levels 1 and 2 may be attained after a therapist has consolidated her pre-registration education, i.e. during, at the earliest, the second year after qualification. Levels 3 and 4 are aimed at senior therapists, as are levels 5 and 6, which also include departmental managers.

Supervision

Supervision may be defined as regular, informal discussion between an individual and her manager. It is non-directive in that it encourages the therapist to take responsibility for her own practice, standards and development. It may be useful to consider the elements of supervision as follows:

- What is it? Supervision takes the form of free, unstructured discussion between two people. It is used at all grade levels to facilitate learning, offer guidance, promote the sharing of information, air concerns and problems and foster the maintenance

Box 5.11 Sequential approach to clinical education supervisor training: a summary

Level	Content summary
1	Role of clinical education; appreciation of basic learning theory; sources of information available to students, including self as a model; understanding the learning objectives for each stage of education and the need to identify specific needs of individual students
2	Planning and implementing clinical education; planning and organising placements within own work setting; recognising and responding to needs/changes; teaching and assessment techniques; evaluation and non-performance
3	Management of learning, recognising the variety of ways in which attitudes, cognitive and practical skills can be acquired; applying selected techniques to improving this understanding and performance of students and staff; assessment of students' performance
4	Professional development; developing and evaluating opportunities for learning; observing own and others' progress and relating strategies and outcomes to learning/education theories; planning programmes for individual students using a variety of settings and resources
5	Curriculum design; design of curricula for professional education at different levels based on own knowledge, skill and experience, familiarity with education theory and needs of students
6	Research and evaluation; skilled continuing observation of learning in various settings; analysis of strategies and outcome leading to structures of controlled innovation

of standards. It gives support and encouragement to staff as they develop skills and confidence. This particular management tool should not be confused with IPR.

- Who is involved? The individual therapist and her line manager.

● Why is it needed? Supervision is a valuable means of overseeing a therapist's caseload, enabling her to take responsibility for managing her current work and to measure her performance against established standards. It assists both people concerned to monitor the therapist's practices and procedures and to deal proactively with any potential difficulties with individual cases and with broader issues related to her daily work.

● Where does it occur? In the work place, in a private, quiet environment.

● When does it occur? Supervision discussions should take place for an hour or so at regular intervals, such as every week or month. The exact timing depends on the therapist's needs, grade and objectives.

● How does it take place? Supervision often commences on a case review basis. This offers security to both parties by focusing on the daily workload. For example, it may take the form of discussion of a particular case, in which the outcome of an initial interview, the aims established and the therapist's short-term plan for intervention are analysed and evaluated.

As both parties become more confident and comfortable with the supervision process the informal agenda may include discussion of more general issues such as working with carers of people with a certain disability, report writing, or standards for a given element of practice.

The object of supervision is to help staff to retain existing and develop further competencies, to facilitate their understanding of themselves and others, to monitor their progress and to encourage them to make the most of their strengths and consider their weaknesses. Although the two must not be confused, regular, positive supervision can complement and aid the IPR process.

Counselling

There are occasions when staff may need assistance with a particular problem which they are unable to resolve alone. One type of help offered by their manager or someone outside the service may be counselling.

Counselling should be a voluntary process by which the therapist can identify, explore and resolve problems and more clearly define her needs. It should enable her, in a supportive, non-authoritative and confidential environment, to seek reassurance, handle conflict, manage change, interpret her behaviour in particular circumstances, and cope with authority or power. It should give her the opportunity to express herself freely without fear of prejudice or repercussions. The manager should be as non-directive as possible; she should listen carefully, and endeavour to help the individual to seek a resolution for her difficulty and to set herself goals.

Having counselled a staff member, the manager should communicate regularly with the individual, helping her to revise her plans if necessary and to consider any additional needs or problems which may have arisen.

Leadership

The most vital element of any management job is leadership. A manager must obtain the commitment of her staff to the service and the tasks to be achieved. In doing so, she must consider her staff's need for cohesion as they work toward a common purpose, as well as the individual needs of staff members.

Managers' styles of leadership will relate to the task and to the group, but will also depend upon the environment and the leader's qualities. Management styles tend to be described in terms of extremes, i.e.

authoritarian v. democratic
autocratic   v. participative
job centred   v. people centred
directive   v. permissive.

In practice, an effective manager will develop an approach on the continuum between, say, authoritarianism and democracy which meets the demands of particular circumstances. She may need to be more authoritarian when a specific deadline is imminent; conversely, she will be more democratic when involving staff in standard-setting. Whatever the approach utilised, she needs to ensure that it facilitates team cohesion, loyalty, trust, confidence, respect and motivation.

In order to achieve results with the staff and

other resources at her disposal, a leader must be capable of:

- setting certain standards and demonstrating them by example
- effective delegation
- accepting responsibility
- effective communication at all levels
- setting clear objectives
- praising, motivating and disciplining staff
- supervising and counselling
- selling ideas
- consulting others
- maintaining credibility, so that staff trust and respect her
- making the right decisions

Many of the qualities expected in a good leader are summarised in Box 5.12.

Box 5.12 The qualities of a good leader

Personal	*Professional*
Approachability	Ability to delegate
Ability to accept criticism	Ability to facilitate learning
	Availability
Decisiveness	Conciliation/negotiation
Dependability	skills
Empathy	Confidence
Emotional stability	Dedication
Energy and drive	Democracy
Fairness	Effectiveness
Foresight	Innovation
Initiative	Judgement
Integrity	Loyalty
Interest in people	Objectivity
Interpersonal skills	Political acumen
Judgement	Recognition of others'
Loyalty	abilities and limitations
Recognition of own	Reliability
abilities and limitations	Skill as chairperson
Reliability	Skill as organiser
Sense of humour	Supportiveness
Sincerity	
Tolerance	
Trustworthiness	

Delegation

Delegation is the art and practice of giving a subordinate/delegate the necessary authority to make decisions in a specified area of her work whilst the delegator retains overall responsibility. Delegation is an essential component of successful leadership and, like other elements of management, may be described as a process. The steps in this process are as follows:

- goal setting: identifying the task and its parameters
- programme planning: deciding how, when and where the task is to be implemented and completed
- the actual delegation to the staff member, ensuring that she is conversant with the task and how she is to fulfil her responsibility
- dealing with any issues which arise with the delegate
- monitoring and supporting the delegate, assisting her to reach a successful outcome.

Effective delegation has various benefits. It allows the manager to concentrate on major tasks without being distracted by lesser ones. It allows her to spend her time more creatively and to develop a more effective and motivated team.

Delegation offers team members rewarding challenges and a feeling of worth. It fosters the development of group decision-making skills and combined effort. It also accords to individuals appropriate recognition of their particular skills.

The involvement of groups and individual staff in delegation enhances job satisfaction, raises morale and ensures commitment to decisions which are made by those involved in the service's daily clinical work. Delegation fosters mutual trust and confidence, enchances the rate at which tasks are completed satisfactorily, and makes the service more effective overall.

However, delegating authority does carry a degree of risk; the manager should be fully aware of what is involved in tasks she is delegating and anticipate what might go wrong, bearing in mind that she retains overall responsibility.

The manager's role as delegator includes setting guidelines, providing parameters or limits, supporting staff and acknowledging their involvement. In order to delegate successfully and to accord an appropriate degree of authority to junior staff, the manager must know the members of her team in terms of:

- what motivates them
- their willingness to respond to challenge and opportunity
- their individual characteristics, knowledge, skills and competencies
- their creative abilities.

The following are essential elements in the manager's effective use of delegation:

- awareness that she retains overall accountability
- willingness to give staff freedom of action, usually within defined limits

- understanding of the responsibilities of her own job and that of the delegate's post
- realistic confidence that the delegate has the competence and potential to complete the task
- understanding of whether the task is of interest and whether it further develops the delegate's skills and knowledge
- effective communication
- realistic time-scales for task completion
- clear standards and targets set with the delegate
- programming review dates
- recognition of the abilities of the delegate and trust in her to complete the task, with support and review as required.

There are positive and negative aspects to delegation, as there are with any management tool; these are summarised in Box 5.13.

Box 5.13 Delegation: positive and potential negative apsects

Positive aspects
- Can relieve pressure on leader
- Job enrichment for leader and delegate
- Utilises others' skills
- Enhances relationships
- Encourages maximum involvement
- Develops people
- Offers leader time for other tasks
- Decisions made closer to daily work of service
- Encourages group cohesion
- Enhances communication
- Can enhance quality of work and of decisions made
- Enables delegates to take on additional responsibility in a supportive environment
- Can reduce time taken to complete tasks

Potentially negative aspects
- Time leader spends training staff to cope with added responsibility
- Risk of losing control
- Over-delegation, i.e. staff over-loaded, leader underworked
- Anxiety/stress in delegate
- Time spent monitoring, supporting
- Sub-standard work
- Fragmentation of work or group if one person overloaded
- Poor briefing
- Lack of clarity re targets, standards, time-scale
- Slow (democracy is slower than autocracy)
- 'Buck-passing'

Managing change

We live in times which are constantly changing in one way or another. As individuals and as therapists we need to be able to manage change in order to retain our sanity and effectiveness. Any change — be it a client's terminal diagnosis or increased disability, a new manager, a new type of support worker, a revised grading structure, or an organisational modification — will result in a number of reactions or stages through which one has to progress. These stages might be described as:

1. shock and disbelief
2. an emotional reaction: euphoria, anger, depression, denial
3. questioning: bitterness, anger, frustration
4. gradual acceptance
5. action to cope with the change.

Managing change can be likened to handling stress (see Section 4, p. 99). It entails being creative in finding ways to cope. It is helpful to understand the levels at which change can occur, and that there are different types of change, namely:

- that which is thrust upon people — the most difficult to manage
- that which is foreseen, and about which one

is consulted, although decision-making power is held by someone else
- that which one desires and about which one makes the decision.

Individuals are often able to contribute to debate and influence decisions concerning proposed change at a local level. They may be consulted about change at higher levels but are less likely to be able to influence the outcome.

Prior to considering managing change stages and strategies it is necessary to discuss the elements of creative management. First, one has to understand organisations (refer to Section 1.1) and individuals within them including their needs, drives and ambitions, and how the work is completed including planning, leadership and coordination. Second, one needs to comprehend the creative process, that is the development of insight into problems, recognising barriers and pre-conceptions, understanding entrepreneurship and the use of mentors. Thirdly, there is the need to develop creative problem solving techniques: lateral thinking, brain storming, experimenting with ideas, enabling through sensitivity, patience and the addressing of failure. Once these elements have been grasped, a manager should be able to initiate the 'change management' stages.

The successful management of change demands an understanding of: the need for and processes of change; the underlying conflicts and problems implied or created by change; methods of developing relevant responses and coping mechanisms. The individual will need to identify her own roles, needs and feelings within the change process:

- is change based on unmet/met needs, indicated by staff or clients?
- the skills required i.e. problem solving, communication, decision making
- motivational factors such as leadership, support networks
- personal responses to fear, anger, aggression, uncertainty.

Managing one's own and others' responses to change entails:

- effective leadership and assertion
- very thorough and open communication
- support systems/networks for all staff

- making counselling available for those who request it
- analysing problems, options and decisions.

Change demands the development of coping mechanisms within the team. Initially, the leader of the team should never assume that others understand or interpret change in the same way. Change management must start with discussion and clarification of individual conceptions about the change. This will form the basis of a common understanding. Thereafter, coping mechanisms such as counselling, support and advice networks, or training can be agreed and established.

Managing change within a particular service such as occupational therapy is a task to which all staff can contribute. Small teams can research and evaluate ideas, review specific areas of the service, evaluate techniques utilised, review policies and procedures, monitor actual outcomes against agreed measures of quality and utilise their knowledge of human behaviour to understand how change will influence and affect groups and individuals. The service manager will facilitate and coordinate these efforts whilst undertaking her own analyses, review and evaluations of public sector legislation and policy and its influence on her department.

A service can prepare for change by establishing the nature and extent of existing services and their strengths and weaknesses. Visiting work areas, listening to staff and clients, reading relevant documents and undertaking surveys will enhance this preparation, which should be followed by a needs assessment and analysis based on client demand, market research and information analysis.

Planning for change

Strategies that might be used in planning for change include:

- examining current policy. This involves considering the implications of current national trends in care, local demography and epidemiological patterns and trends, local planning proposals, consumer wants and needs and any issues regarding general service provision

- clarifying the service's vision of the future and agreeing on the steps required to turn this vision into reality. This may involve:
  — sharing aspirations, dreams, ideals
  — putting these ideals in a realistic perspective
  — agreeing on a common purpose
- identifying agents of change; these may include group discussion, planning, consumer and/or staff forums, partnerships with other services whose objectives are similar to one's own, networks, the political climate, local and national policy changes and pressure groups. Whichever change agents are used, they must be coordinated by an identified leader who can ensure that the object of the exercise remains clear and that change proceeds according to the agreed strategy
- designing a strategy (including time-scales, people involved) and, if the change is major, piloting the strategy
- implementing the strategy and following this with consultation with and participation of all staff on a continuous basis
- preparing to meet the resulting challenges and opportunities with the networks for support and counselling described above
- building in evaluation.

Managing change successfully presents many challenges and opportunities and requires managers and staff to utilise all of their personal and professional knowledge and skills. If change is planned, those concerned should agree its purpose and monitor changes in need and demand through consultation and review. They will also need to market their vision of the future, persuading consumers of the benefits of change and creating an environment conducive to creativity and innovation (see Marketing, p. 134).

PLANNING AND DEVELOPMENT

Planning is one of the four major elements of management. In health and social care it occurs within a national framework of legislation, government priorities and policies, circulars and economic constraints. It takes place within varying parameters i.e. long-term, short-term and on a daily basis, utilising the same principles for each. In practical terms it involves: business planning, i.e. forecasting needs; defining objectives to meet those needs; making decisions, including how one deploys staff and other resources; negotiating change; and marketing the service.

The process of planning entails:

- reviewing existing services
- identifying gaps in services, the needs of the population and any particular characteristics affecting health and social care, such as the increase in people aged 85 and over
- participating in the development of draft plans or service agreements outlining care services
- identifying the resources to meet specific needs
- consulting with key health and/or local authority teams, other statutory and non-statutory organisations, unions and the public about the proposed plans
- developing aims and stages, including a timetable of implementation, the implementation itself and monitoring and evaluation.

It is also vital to consider the above within the context of the management of change (see p. 130). In order to review existing services and to identify needs, gaps and problems, the information and Information Technology (IT) available to planners must be carefully analysed and evaluated. All authorities collect information about their services based on Körner sets; to this may be added:

- needs assessment surveys conducted with the assistance of health and social care consumers, the general public, service providers, referral agents
- demographic studies
- epidemiological studies and reports
- health and local authority revised structure plans which have implications for how and where services may be delivered
- performance indicators (see p. 140)
- the result of work undertaken by specific task groups, which include a user/consumer contribution.

Planning for health and social care now operates within the framework described in the NHS and Community Care Act 1990. Fundamentally, this means that health and local authorities, with FHSA's and local users, plan together to meet the needs of their resident population. For example, the planning of acute health services should consider the after-care and support required by people on discharge from hospital, including collaborative care arrangements among all agencies. This process applies to any client group and will occur within local purchaser/provider roles and frameworks; its outcome will often depend on the coterminosity of authority boundaries, local pressure groups and the pattern of existing services.

Planning a service

Planning, developing and coordinating an occupational therapy service take place within the frameworks described above and in Section 2. Occupational therapy managers examine the relevant statutes, priorities, policies, business and care plans and establish the implications of these for their particular service. For instance, if the authority states that health care for elderly people or treatment at home for young people with physical handicaps are priority areas, occupational therapy plans must reflect this.

When planning her service a manager must consider the following elements:

- definition of the service's aims and how action can be unified in order to achieve those set goals. For instance, occupational therapy's aims for neurological services may include the formation of an informal yet effective cross-Unit team of therapists, whose expertise will ensure that individuals transfer from acute care to the rehabilitation unit and subseqently to community care with minimum disruption to their intervention programme
- planning within the service's aims, which includes review, integrating relevant information and communicating with those concerned. For example, therapists working

with children with multiple handicaps should contribute to the planning of future services for this group.

- organising services, including the effective deployment of existing and any new resources, ensuring that leadership, supervision and monitoring are included in each team
- issues related to staff, such as communication, development and education on a unidisciplinary or multidisciplinary basis, as appropriate issues which may cause difficulties if not adequately addressed, for example:
  - distances, if the service covers a large geographical area or a large hospital site
  - staff's physical working environment
  - the size of the service, whether large or small. (Each presents its own problems of organisation and coordination)
  - status, attitudes, preconceived ideas, personal dislikes, personality conflicts, traditional accountability structures and lack of awareness of other team members' roles. Organisational weaknesses must be borne in mind and may include poor leadership, ineffective communication, lack of planning at all levels or narrow (specialist) interests.

The development of any service occurs within its host Unit's or section's business plan, a document which describes in general terms the services offered to users, i.e. the general public, doctors and other colleagues. Within this framework, services such as occupational therapy will prepare a service agreement which describes in a little more detail the types and numbers of people accepted for treatment, location and timing of treatment, the interventions to be used, and the standards, including monitoring and evaluation strategies, to be applied in the forthcoming year.

Service development does not necessarily mean an increase in resources. It *may*, if new specialities are planned and implemented, but more often than not services must develop within their *existing* resources, to which may be added income generated such as by marketing therapy to a speciality not previously included in the service or 'selling' staff education programmes. Generally, the manager will have to consider whether the status quo is viable or whether she needs to rationalise present provision and resource deployment. In doing so she will ask:

- What does occupational therapy provide now, to whom, why, where, when, how?
- What is needed, according to the authority's predictions, to meet the needs of the population?
- What implications does this have for occupational therapy?
- What needs to be provided?

Frequently, the only means of providing a revised or new service is to eliminate or reduce an existing one and to redirect resources to the priority area. Alternatively, a health and local authority may consider the provision of a joint occupational therapy service which facilitates joint planning and coordination and deploys resources more effectively and efficiently.

Achieving effective coordination of and within a service requires high-quality leadership, effective communication, the development of efficient and effective teams and realistic management practices.

Marketing

Marketing entails creating and developing a demand and ensuring that this demand is matched by supply. Occupational therapy staff need to explain and promote their service both informally and formally, and the profession could benefit by applying certain techniques to its marketing strategies.

Marketing is not merely a process. Penn and Penn (1990) describe it as 'a philosophy, an attitude of mind that accepts the idea that customers should be the focus of everything that is done by the organisation'. This attitude should direct the organisation's activities towards a common goal, i.e. 'to discover and satisfy the present and potential needs of consumers using all the skills and resources of the organisation'.

The marketing process applies a number of techniques which, when combined, are described as the 'marketing mix'. This 'mix' comprises ten elements, described below:

1. *Marketing research*: gathering information systematically and objectively. Occupational therapy's marketing research might commence by identifying current and potential clients and their needs and the key referring agencies.

2. *Product policy*. The product or, in the case of occupational therapy, service is the means by which clients may be satisfied. If the profession's aim is to enable people to be as independent as possible it needs to develop policies regarding: the types of intervention best suited to particular client groups; being proactive in times of change, i.e. modifying services to meet needs; the evaluation and audit of outcomes; and the development of staff.

3. *Packaging* is not a concept commonly associated with occupational therapy but it is one worth considering, as packaging includes such things as staff attitudes, behaviour and appearance, a department's atmosphere, a welcoming environment, and logos on stationery and leaflets. Effective packaging facilitates the development of an easily recognised organisational or professional identity.

4. *Pricing policy*. Pricing is a complex process which must take into account the amount purchasers are prepared to pay for a service. Costs must also be considered in relation to the convenience to clients of treatment times and locations, and the success of interventions.

5. *Distribution policy* includes: (a) physical distribution, which entails getting the service to the consumer, i.e. is the service available locally, within travelling distance or not at all? and (b) choice and use of intermediaries, i.e. the type of referrals received and from whom, and how the client accesses the service.

6. *Public relations* includes improving public awareness, projecting credibility, evaluating new markets and motivating staff. Within occupational therapy it is the function of all staff, supported by their managers and the BAOT's Public Relations Officers' network, to raise the profession's profile and to help people to understand the purpose of occupational therapy.

7. *Advertising* in occupational therapy might entail marketing the service to purchasers, e.g. a health authority, a Unit's clinical directorates, or a community team. The service will need to consider why it needs to market itself; whether to deal with advertising in-house or through an agency; the target audience; the media to be used; how to measure the marketing campaign's effectiveness; and how it is to be financed.

8. *Sales promotion* in occupational therapy could be likened to (7) above. It tends, however, to be utilised for different purposes, such as recruiting potential people for training or staff for a particular speciality. Media used may include displays, exhibitions, open days and careers conventions.

9. *Personal selling* involves individual members of the profession promoting the value of occupational therapy for a particular client or group of clients to colleagues and others, for example to a doctor during a ward round, to a local councillor or to a voluntary organisation.

10. *Customer service.* The whole process of providing a service to clients and referral agents needs continuous monitoring to ensure that the right level and type of service is offered to people who need it, at a time when it is most effective and at the right 'price'.

Occupational therapy may not use all ten elements of the 'marketing mix' at once, but individuals and services need to consider them all in order to select the appropriate ones for the circumstances. It should be remembered that, essentially, marketing is a matter of providing the right service at the right time, in the right place, at an acceptable price and to an agreed standard.

Decision-making

Making decisions is part of everyday life and most people develop considerable personal skill in clarifying issues, weighing options and deciding upon actions in the private sphere. In relation to the management of oneself at work, a more structured approach can often ensure that all relevant issues are considered thoroughly. One decision-making process, described as the five 'C's —

i.e., Consider, Consult, Crunch, Communicate and Check — may provide a useful guide:

1. Consider
   — First clarify the issue or problem. Is it genuinely a problem? Does it need specific action?
   — If it requires action, define the objective(s) to be achieved.
   — Decide who should make the ultimate decision.
   — Clarify a time-scale, including a date by which a decision must be made.

2. Consult
   — Collect all relevant information in the time available. This may include local, regional or national information gleaned from colleagues.
   — Organise and analyse the information.
   — Call a meeting of those involved, if appropriate, to identify causes, to consult and to seek options and ideas.
   — Determine when any discussion about the issue has to cease due to time constraints.

3. Crunch
   — Weigh up the options and, if time permits, think about them for a day or so.
   — Select an option, i.e. make the decision.
   — If the arguments of those involved are balanced the decision maker must take her own reasoned course to the decision, having listed the pros and cons, examined the consequences, and measured them against the objective(s).

4. Communicate
   — Write an implementation plan, if applicable.
   — Brief all those involved or affected on the action and subsequent outcomes.
   — Aim to obtain acceptance of the decision. Agreement will not always be forthcoming or vital.

5. Check
   — The decision maker must check that the decision has been implemented.
   — This will be followed by monitoring and review and, if necessary, by further corrective action.

— The decision maker should bear in mind that it is not possible to please everyone involved all the time.

Negotiation

Negotiation forms a part of the decision-making process and is another personal skill which is learned and used by people in their daily lives. Fundamentally, it concerns influencing other people through the exchange of ideas or something of material value, such as salaries. It is used to satisfy one team's or individual's needs when someone else controls what they want or need. 'Bargaining' and 'persuading' are other words used to describe negotiation. The term used may be influenced by particular circumstances; for instance, one may 'bargain' with an employer for a pay rise in return for increased productivity, 'persuade' a colleague to undertake a particular task for the status it offers or 'negotiate' a treatment contract with a client. Regardless of the term used or the circumstances, negotiation will usually follow a particular pattern. Brewster (1984) describes negotiation succinctly and offers practical suggestions which are summarised in Box 5.14. In addition, therapists should utilise their knowledge of motivation theory to enhance their negotiation skills.

Box 5.14 The four stages of negotiation

Before	During
• Aim for a positive atmosphere	• Listen carefully
• Collect relevant information	• Take your time
• Assess strengths and weaknesses of both parties	• Ask questions
• Identify own objectives	• Keep calm
• Consider possible tactics	• Use summaries
• Select your negotiating team	• Clarify stage of negotiation reached periodically
• Allocate roles to team members	• Use adjournments if necessary
• Ensure everyone is clear about both objectives and tactics	• Make concessions and obtain concessions in return

At the end	After
• Proceed with caution on 'final' offers	• Ensure agreement is communicated
• Ensure both parties can claim success	• Implement the agreement
• Summarise	• Monitor its results
• Put agreement in writing	• Review with your team
• Congratulate both parties	

RESOURCE MANAGEMENT

Resources in any setting include staff, their skills and expertise, accommodation, equipment, materials, information and finance. Effective and efficient management of these resources should facilitate the provision of a quality service or product to an organisation's clients. Resource management (the Resource Management Initiative in the NHS) enables a manager to make more informed decisions about how the resources she controls can be used to maximum effect, whilst relating service activity to running costs. This section describes the key areas of resource management within occupational therapy; these are summarised in Figure 5.14.

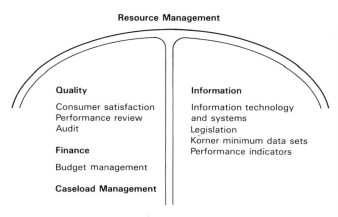

Resource Management

Quality
Consumer satisfaction
Performance review
Audit

Finance
Budget management

Caseload Management

Information
Information technology and systems
Legislation
Körner minimum data sets
Performance indicators

Fig. 5.14 Components of resource management.

Information

Data concerning local populations, their health and ill health, welfare needs, birth and death rates and predominant illnesses have been collected by health and local authorities for many years. This information has enabled the DoH, the Regions and local providers of services to plan services in a very general way, but it has never provided an adequate basis upon which therapists, nurses, doctors, home care or social work services could monitor, evaluate, plan and develop services to meet identified needs. This state of affairs has hindered the management of static or decreasing resources, which are now unable to match increasing and/or changing demands.

During the late 1980s the collection, collation and storage of health care information changed radically, primarily with the advent of Körner minimum data sets (basic information required by the DoH) and the need to provide evidence of cost effectiveness, efficiency, quality, effective resource deployment and the changing needs of the population.

If information is to form the basis for all planning, development and service coordination, managers will need to make use of various kinds of data. Information may be needed with reference to:

- diagnostically related groups (a system initiated in the United States for coding people by diagnosis and identifying a cost for examination and treatment for a particular condition)
- other groups, classified by, for instance, history, diagnostic procedures, drugs, appliances, preventive procedures and health status
- performance indicators such as cost of occupational therapy by client type, outcomes of intervention
- priorities at all levels
- Regional and District plans
- local epidemiological and demographic trends
- financial position of the health or local authority
- alternative funding sources such as Joint Finance

- modern treatment methods and future trends
- educational needs and methods at pre- and post-registration levels
- the effectiveness of existing services
- future staff recruitment and retention
- staff, i.e. motivation, job satisfaction, attendance, special skills/qualifications, preferred areas of work, past experience, clinical teaching experience
- implications of change, such as the shift from hospital to community care, for staff education and development
- plans of other professions
- other authorities' plans and their implications.

Access to information which is accurate, up-to-date and easily retrievable enables a manager to:

- deploy staff effectively and efficiently
- ensure all staff use their time effectively and efficiently
- make economic use of buildings and equipment
- delegate
- monitor performance of service and staff
- concentrate on treatments with proven, effective outcomes
- use staff grades correctly
- accept and respond positively to change.

Information systems and technology

Until comparatively recently, most information was collected and stored in manual systems from which it was difficult to retrieve essential information for detailed and meaningful analysis. At the time of writing, information technology systems within health and social care are developing rapidly and are changing the face of data collection, collation and analysis, enabling individuals and managers to obtain relevant information about staff, clients, treatments, outcomes, and finance, thus facilitating decision-making and planning.

Information technology is developing continually, as are people's abilities to use this technology effectively despite time limitations and financial restraints. Technical systems have increased the availability of information to such an extent that public sector managers can make more realistic forecasts and plans, coordinate and deploy resources in an informed manner and relate costs to activity.

Legislation and data protection

During the 1980s, the proliferation of computer-based systems for the storage of personal information gave rise to new legislation regarding data protection. Occupational therapists need a working knowledge of this legislation, which is summarised in Box 5.15.

Client information

All authorities have a manual or computerised central client record system — Patient Administration System (PAS) in health authorities — which contains health and/or social care information concerning individuals and/or families. This information includes personal details such as full name, age, sex, address, status; social, medical and other relevant histories; previous referrals or admissions; treatment given and its outcome. It is anticipated that these systems will provide most of the data necessary for analysis and subsequent planning of services.

Occupational therapy services have always collected information about clients and their treatment, and since April 1988 the Körner minimum data sets have shaped the collection of client-related activity. Figure 5.15 illustrates the minimum data required in 1990 for six professions, collated from information about individual clients, by speciality, referral source, type (i.e. in, out, day or community patient/client) and by treatment location. This data facilitates analysis of the contacts by staff according to the above criteria and enables costs to be apportioned to specific service areas. Currently it provides rather crude measures of activity, and is due to be changed.

Staff activity data

The 'sample enquiry' shown in Figure 5.15 is designed to provide information about the per-

Box 5.15 Data and information protection legislation

Act	Key points
Data Protection 1984 Further references: 1. Modified Access to Personal Health Information: HC(87)14	Purpose is to control all personal information which is processed by computers. Requires all users of personal data to register their system and its purposes. Allows individuals to: consult a public register containing all organisations using computerised data; obtain a copy of personal data stored on payment of a fee; have inaccuracies erased or corrected; obtain compensation for any damage or distress caused by lost, inaccurate or misused data. Some categories of information are exempt from the act, e.g. that which safeguards national security.
2. Personal Social Services — disclosure of information to clients LAC(83) 14	
Access to Personal Files 1987	Applies to local authority social service and housing authorities and covers information recorded *after* 1 April 1989. Provides clients with right of access to personal information held by local authorities and allows them to obtain copies.
Consumer Protection 1987	Rationalises consumer protection legislation and outlines new responsibilities for producers and suppliers. Requires that records of products, suppliers and receivers, including clients, are kept.
Access to Medical Reports 1988	Establishes right of access by individuals to reports relating to themselves provided by a doctor for employment or insurance purposes. This may include information supplied by other health professionals.

DATA BASE INDEX

Entity name	Attribute name	Ch	CP	O	OT	Pt	Sp
● Face-to-face contact	Age	●	●	●	●	●	●
	Community based	●					
	Date of contact	●	●	●	●	●	●
	Duration of contact				●		
	First contact in financial year	●	●	●	●	●	●
	Initial contact	●	●	●	●	●	●
	Last contact in episode						●
	Sex	●	●	●	●	●	●
	Source of referral	●	●	●	●	●	●
● Location	Type of location	●	●	●	●	●	●
● Sample enquiry (staff)	Proportion of time (face-to-face)	●	●	●	●	●	●
	Proportion of time (telephone contacts)	●	●	●	●	●	●
	Proportion of time (home assessment)				●	●	
	Proportion of time (other professional activities)	●	●	●	●	●	●
● Home assessment visit	Date of contact				●	●	
● Patient episode of care	Duration of episode						●

Fig. 5.15 Körner implementation: paramedical services.

centage of time staff spend in face-to-face contacts with clients or their proxy, telephone contacts, other professional activities and home assessment visits. These, too, are relatively broad measures to which services have added categories related to their own activity areas, such as education received and given, treatment media and techniques used, and intervention outcomes. As computer-based systems are incorporated in the management of occupational therapy, managers are becoming better equipped to monitor, review and evaluate service quality measures and outcomes in relation to set standards.

Manpower information

Every authority has a manpower or personnel information system which contains details on all staff. In addition to personal information, it may include such data as qualifications, state registration, post-registration education, absence leave, employment commencement date, salary, annual increment date, holiday entitlement and allowances. As these systems become more sophisticated they aid manpower planning, recruitment and retention.

Performance indicators

These indicators are produced annually in the NHS and offer rough comparisons of the activity and resources of specific services between districts and against national standards. Their usefulness is limited, as like is not compared with like and they do not measure particular practices or quality. They present a distorted picture, as they do not take account of, for example, the number of beds or day hospital places, or the regional specialities in one district.

Three performance indicators are produced for occupational therapy; for the reasons given above, they are of limited value.

1. total occupational therapy costs related to the authority's resident population
2. the number of qualified occupational therapists (full-time equivalent) to the population
3. the ratio of qualified to 'unqualified' occupational therapy staff in the authority.

It seems likely that these types of indicator will be replaced or merged with other resource management data.

Quality

Quality became an increasingly important issue in the public sector during the 1980s and continues to feature very prominently in all service provision, resource allocation, evaluation and out-

Box 5.16 Quality assurance: glossary of terms

Audit: a methodical clinical and managerial review or investigation of resources and activities

Concurrent review: a method of reviewing process and outcome of client care during an episode of care

Criteria: predetermined elements of care against which quality and appropriateness are measured

Effectiveness: performance and level of benefit under normal conditions by average practitioner for typical client

Efficiency: the probable benefit expected/intended in ideal circumstances for a defined population

Frame of reference: theoretical and moral basis upon which a particular intervention is founded

Indicator: professionally developed, clinically valid and reliable dimension of the quality and appropriateness of intervention

Input: see Structure

Monitoring: planned, systematic and ongoing collection and organisation of information and comparison with pre-determined performance levels

Outcome: results of structure and process related to improved health, restored or improved function and client satisfaction

Process: intervention/management activities, e.g. assessment, treatment, preventative input, documentation

Quality: the degree or standard of excellence

Quality assurance: a process in which desirable and achievable quality levels are described along with the extent to which they are achieved and the action taken to enable them to be reached

Reliability: reproducibility of findings

Retrospective review: review which focuses on data collection and analysis from clients' records and after discharge

Standard: an accepted/approved statement of something against which measurement and/or judgement take place

Structure (input): resources used to provide a service and the manner in which they are organised

Validity: the ability of a test to measure what it purports to measure

come analysis. It is often described as a degree of excellence which is measurable against set requirements. Quality assurance is regarded as an ongoing process. Some of the terms used in this area are defined in Box 5.16.

Three basic components of quality assurance are applicable to occupational therapy:

1. technical quality, which can be equated with professional performance
2. efficiency of resource use
3. consumer satisfaction vis-à-vis stated and unstated needs.

Quality must be viewed in its totality, taking account of available resources, the environment, staff needs, professional opinion, local and national health care targets, public opinion and the needs of the individual. This approach is called Total Quality Management (TQM). Authorities throughout the United Kingdom have produced TQM documentation to assist their staff to provide, monitor, review and evaluate quality. This approach also gives one discipline the opportunity to learn from another.

Professional performance and standards

Quality assurance comprises a range of procedures undertaken in order to promote better quality services. It requires an analytical and evaluative approach within which a manager and staff can analyse, appraise, review, evaluate, modify, observe, ensure equity of provision, consider client and staff needs, question, audit and identify satisfaction levels. It is a process which begins with general principles or the setting of standards. Its purpose is to:

- define acceptable minimum levels of performance and service delivery
- develop policies, procedures and administrative systems
- define goals for service delivery and set realistic objectives
- define goals for personal development and set realistic targets
- review performance and achievements
- consult with those involved.

In practice, the following procedure may be followed (after Crawford 1989):

1. Staff select a topic, for instance assessment of the person with hand dysfunction.
2. A care group is defined, i.e. outpatients.
3. Staff decide on their objective and justify it, for example the standardisation of hand assessment in the authority's outpatient occupational therapy units, which will aid evaluation and research.
4. They identify the process structure required in terms of input (the resources needed), the process (how intervention is to be conducted) and the outcomes (measurable and observable treatment results).
5. They prepare a standard statement about their agreed quality measure.
6. They agree a date by which the standard is to be achieved, using a realistic time scale.
7. They agree a review date, e.g. three months following acceptance of the standard.
8. Staff commit themselves to the standard, e.g. by signing it.
9. They begin to index standards in order to code them and to avoid duplication.
10. As they commence measurement of outcomes they identify the need for changes, if any.

Both staff and their managers have to assess the quality of the service provided and should select a method which best meets their needs, remembering that no one method is ideal. Broadly, assessment will entail asking questions about input, process, outcome (Box 5.17) and satisfaction and may include random sampling, measuring against agreed criteria and standards, and monitoring information about client and staff activity. Preliminary questions include (Graham 1990):

- What do we mean by 'quality'?
- What are the evaluation objectives?
- What sources of information are available and reliable?
- What resources are available and justified for inclusion in an assessment?
- Is a particular time-scale being used, i.e. retrospective, concurrent or prospective?
- What kind of treatment problems are envisaged?

Box 5.17 Example of a general quality standard

Input	Process	Outcome
Staff grade, time, facilities and equipment to undertake a specific assessment	Therapist will administer assessment(s) as appropriate to client group/ individual, e.g. — personal daily living — life roles — community living skills — cognitive function	Time and ease of completion during and after assessment Ease of analysis Relevance of information obtained from analysis Value of assessments in current use

In addition, the manager will consider:

- practitioner performance, i.e. knowledge, skills, qualifications, judgement, interpersonal skills
- the appropriateness of the service to the client group
- client participation (which is difficult to measure but is none the less important)
- accessibility of the service i.e. time, location
- continuity of care between home and hospital and vice versa
- the record system
- costs
- client satisfaction.

A manager should influence and implement change in order to provide better quality services. She can facilitate this change by developing her staff using some of the following methods (see also p. 130):

- actively encouraging support systems, staff advocacy and consumer forums
- improving organisation and communication skills
- developing caring approaches in her team
- improving the environment when and wherever practicable
- encouraging staff to set up quality circles

- helping them to learn how to monitor and audit their own performance.

Efficiency and effectiveness

An efficient and effective service is one that provides value for money, using measures that ensure that the service offered is the best within current available resources. It is also one with sufficient flexibility to cope with social, environmental and political change. Ensuring that a service is efficient and effective is an ongoing managerial task which can be divided into three elements, each of which includes aspects of quality and service provision mentioned in the preceding section:

- reviewing existing services by monitoring plans and time scales, budgets and staffing levels, and cost fluctuations
- considering the organisation's systems, including its plans, accountability structures, performance review, staff development, communication, flexibility and creativity
- adopting fail-safe systems by including health promotion and education in staff development programmes, caring for and motivating staff, setting and maintaining standards, encouraging self-review and career development, offering opportunities for creativity and innovation and allowing staff to be individuals.

By undertaking the above, the manager will help to ensure that her team is sufficiently motivated to provide the highest quality service they can in the given circumstances. She cannot measure efficiency and effectiveness merely by monitoring statistics such as client throughput; she must also take into account the criteria of quality, discussed above (p. 141).

Consumer satisfaction

Clients are all services' raison d'être and they have certain rights. Within health and social care they have rights to self-expression, independent decision, dignity, respect, privacy, information given in a form they can understand, as well as the right to consent to or refuse intervention. With the current upsurge in consumerism, services are continuously developing means of encouraging clients to participate in services and to obtain their help in improving satisfaction levels, whether these are related to waiting times, the environment or to actual care and treatment.

De Gilio et al (1989) describe consumer satisfaction in the following terms:

- being more accessible to clients in terms of: the location of services and their proximity to transport networks; the design of buildings and departments; social accessibility for people of varying cultures; availability in relation to speed of response, personalising services; informing clients about services using a variety of media
- enabling users to participate in the design, planning and delivery of services, equipment and systems; asking them to provide feedback through user groups, interviews or surveys; encouraging advocacy
- providing a service which is user friendly, i.e. one in which staff are courteous and respectful, handle any complaints with diplomacy, provide information which is readily understood.

Consumer satisfaction is often subjective, but, over time, interviews or surveys can provide much valuable information about a service and the environment in which it is provided and point the way toward beneficial change.

Service performance review

Unit and Service Performance Review have been operational in the NHS for a number of years. Performance is reviewed annually against previously agreed objectives. This is a formal process, much like IPR, in which Regions review Districts, Districts review Units and Units review their services. In the case of a service such as occupational therapy, the manager may compile a report of the past year's activities and achievements, describing how objectives have been met, what shortfalls there have been and why. Alternatively, her line manager may conduct the review according to the more structured format used for senior managers in the NHS in which objectives, actions to be taken (and by whom), time-scales, success criteria, and anticipated problems are identified. Senior managers' annual salaries are linked to this process in the form of performance-related pay. Few occupational therapy managers participate in this system as yet, but may well do so in future, particularly in NHS Trusts.

Clinical audit

An audit is a method of competence assessment which has been practised informally for many years. It operates within the quality framework of input, process and outcomes (see p. 141), measuring performance or standards qualitatively and quantitatively. Within the NHS, audit concerns all staff who may influence health care outcomes. In social service departments, audit is less formal than in the NHS, although the principles are identical and relate to Social Service Inspectorate (SSI) guidelines.

Audit is a method of quality promotion and review in which cases are analysed by an individual's peer group. There are five objectives:

- to identify common patterns and changes in health and social care needs
- to monitor the delivery of occupational therapy
- to monitor intervention, programme and technique outcomes
- to develop intervention models and strategies which ensure that resources are used to maximum effect and meet clients' needs
- to further research.

Successful and effective audit depends on accurate and up-to-date records and on staff being prepared to allow policies and procedures affecting practice to be modified as the result of audit.

A number of steps are necessary for successful audit:

- identifying the areas of intervention to be audited
- deciding what objectives and criteria are important. This may involve, for example, making four or five statements which

describe practice standards and how the performance of each standard will be recorded. The staff involved discuss these standards and decide how they should be measured.

- being aware of the latest research results in the area being audited
- deciding which formal and informal standards and time-scales are to be used and what records should be kept for audit purposes
- extracting relevant information from clients' occupational therapy or other records
- reviewing the results of intervention, e.g. by comparing the effects of two techniques used in the treatment of a specific condition
- identifying any strengths or weaknesses in interventions
- deciding how any future treatments could be modified and incorporating such modifications into standard procedures.

Audit may be approached in several ways — for instance, by problem (such as depression in CVA), by diagnosis, by age group or by a particular element of a service, (e.g. an upper limb clinic for children).

Audit can be undertaken within a single discipline or within a multidisciplinary team; the principles and the process are identical whichever approach is used. Both favourable and unfavourable outcomes should be identified so that good practice methods may be promoted locally and nationally.

Finance

Money may be described as the major resource in any organisation as it pays for staff, expertise, accommodation, education, research, public relations, and so on. The main component of NHS funding is the government's allocation issued via Regional Health Authorities. Additionally, Health Authorities generate income and supplement their financial resources from trust funds, joint finance and grants. Local Authorities obtain their finance primarily from government grants and the local community charge, and supplement it with income generation and joint finance.

Every manager has a budget with which to operate her service, allocated for staff and for non-pay expenditure. Budgets may be discipline-based, e.g. occupational therapy, or clinical or social service based, e.g. neurosciences or child care. Whichever system is used, the principles of budget management are identical.

Budget management and control is undertaken with assistance from an authority's finance staff. First, a manager must understand all the factors which contribute to her budget, i.e. staff and non-pay components. Second, she must have a working knowledge of the authority's standing financial instructions. (The Glossary of Terms given in Box 5.18 may be of assistance here.) Financial issues are best explained in terms of the budgetary cycle, described below.

1. Midway through a financial year a manager will discuss her present budget with the finance officer (and general manager on occasions). They will consider the adequacy of the current year's budget, any under- or overspending, changes in workload affecting the budget and the financial implications of any forthcoming developments. In addition, they will discuss the following financial year's allocation.

2. Before the financial year-end (31 March) the manager will receive information about her next year's budget.

3. She must study the contents of her budget under the pay and non-pay headings, ensuring that all ongoing needs are accounted for.

4. Budget statements like the one illustrated in Figure 5.16 reflect past activity under broad headings. The manager will monitor these as described in (6), below.

5. Budget adjustments are required periodically to take account of service changes or monetary factors such as pay awards, on costs and inflation. The two former categories are generally added to a budget automatically. However, inflation and price rises affecting non-pay items may be adjusted in accordance with the Hospital Services Price Index (HSPI) or with the percentage calculated for authorities for a particular year (i.e. local authorities work on a base percentage rate for supplementing budgets which operates in a similar

Box 5.18 Finance: glossary of terms

Accounting code: set of digits giving information about where expenditure is incurred, budget it is costed to and type of items purchased/produced

Budget: total amount of finance allocated to a budget holder/manager to run a service for one year

Budget holder: person delegated overall management responsibility for a service's budget. Has overall control of service

Budget manager: day-to-day spender of budget

Budget statement: a paper issued monthly and annually detailing the elements of spending and funding

Capital expenditure: annual sum allocated to RHA by DoH for minor capital works, larger capital schemes (e.g. a new health centre) major capital (e.g. a new hospital)

Cash limit: finite sum given to each authority annually which includes estimated sums for pay awards and inflation

Cost centre: a hospital or centre

Cost code: accounting centre to which costs are attributed and identified, e.g. ward, occupational therapy

Development: scheme to change the level or type of service provided

Establishment: total number and grades of staff in a particular service

Expense code/number: usually last two digits of accounting code, relate to type of item to which expenditure is allocated

Expenditure:
Non-recurring: one-off allocation/expense, e.g. piece of equipment
Recurring: continuous expenditure recurring each year and throughout the year, e.g. salaries

Flexibility: ability to move money within budget headings

Funding: allocation of money to budget holders

Hidden costs: expenditure incurred outside one budget chargeable to another function, e.g. taxis for home visits

HSPI: Hospital Services Price Index — an index of relative prices

Incremental drift: cost associated with staff in post receiving annual salary increments, causing manpower costs to rise year by year

Index linking: automatic baseline adjustment to take account of inflation

Non-pay budget: all expenses of a service, except staff salaries

On costs: additional costs of staff over and above salaries, i.e. employers contribution to employee national insurance and superannuation

Pay budget: budget to cover staff salaries only

Revenue: day-to-day running expenses of service

SFI: Standing Financial Instructions — outline of rules regarding all financial matters

Top slicing: taking first call on allocation prior to distributing to budgets

Virement: ability to switch funds within and/or between budget headings dependent upon local policy

way to the HSPI). There will be instances in which adjustments are not made, usually due to an authority's or unit's financial status, which leads to a devaluing of a budget over time.

6. The manager must monitor expenditure against income. Although pay is automatically charged to the appropriate service's budget, a manager also needs to monitor expenditure in relation to recruitment, resignations, maternity leave, vacancies and frozen posts.

Under the non-pay heading the manager needs to monitor orders and requisitions for goods and services. Additionally, she will consider income generated by the service, such as sale of any items produced (a continually decreasing element of most occupational therapy budgets) or income from courses, and ensure that this is credited against planned expenditure.

7. Overall, budget management relies on the regular receipt of information about the state of a budget, issued on the statements mentioned in (4), above. The manager will check the staffing position against the agreed pay allocation, bearing in mind any vacancies or maternity leave. Non-pay

MIDSHIRE HEALTH AUTHORITY
30 SEP 90

COMPARISON OF BUDGET WITH EXPENDITURE FOR THE PERIOD 1ST APRIL 1990 TO 31ST AUGUST 1990

UNIT — OUTPATIENTS, GENERAL HOSPITAL

BUDGET REPORT — OCCUPATIONAL THERAPY

BUDGET MANAGER — A. B. BROWN
HEAD OCCUPATIONAL THERAPIST

MANPOWER CONTROL		SUBJECTIVE ANALYSIS	BUDGET FOR YEAR	BUDGET TO DATE	EXPENDITURE TO DATE	OVER-SPENDING	UNDER-SPENDING	BUDGETARY CONTROL	
ESTAB. CONT. HRS. W.T.E.	EMPLOYED MONTH-END W.T.E.							A.F.E. W.T.E.	CUM AV IN POST W.T.E.
			£	£	£	£	£		
		PAY							
1.0	1.0	OCC THERAPIST — SENIOR I	17100	7125	7140	15		1.0	1.0
0.4	0.4	OCC THERAPY HELPER	3700	1540	1475		65	0.4	0.4
1.4	1.4	TOTAL PAY	20800	8665	8615		50	1.4	1.4
		NON-PAY							
		OCC THER EQUIP-PURCHASE	200	80			80		
		OCCUPATIONAL THERAPY MATERIALS	100	40	55	15			
		AIDS TO DAILY LIVING	100	40			40		
		INSTRUCTIONAL PUBLICATIONS	200	80			80		
		SUB TOTAL	600	240	55		185		
		UNIFORM ALLOWANCE			28	28			
		SUB TOTAL			28	28			
		OT SALES — MANUFACTURED ITEMS	−100	−40	−44		4		
		SUB TOTAL	−100	−40	−44		4		
		TOTAL NON-PAY	500	200	39		161		
1.4	1.4	TOTAL	21300	8865	8654	28	211	1.4	1.4

Fig. 5.16 Example of a budget statement.

expenditure will be monitored by comparing expenditure-to-date against the allocation-to-date, allowing for any orders and requisitions as yet unpaid. Each manager will develop a system of ensuring that the non-pay budget is expended in such a way as to avoid underspending or year-end panic purchasing. Overspendings in any part of the budget need to be corrected; this may be done through virement from underspent areas, providing the authority or unit does not recover such surpluses to balance overspendings elsewhere.

Occupational therapists are well able to monitor, review and control their budgets providing they receive accurate and regularly updated budget statements and seek advice and support from their finance colleagues who appreciate the finer nuances of health and social care funding and budgets.

Caseload management

Pressure on services in which demand outstrips available resources frequently means that work has to be prioritised. Case management is a system or tool for facilitating prioritisation. It helps an individual to manage her time in relation to her caseload and a manager to monitor and manage the service, thus ensuring that agreed quality standards are maintained and that staff do not suffer from overload.

Before describing the process of caseload management it is necessary to define certain terminology:

- referral: any request for assistance or a service which requires face-to-face contact and interaction of some sort
- case: a client *accepted* for assessment and/or intervention. The client remains a case until discharge from the service
- waiting list: people who have been referred who are awaiting allocation to a therapist
- caseload:
  — annual: total cases dealt with in a particular year
  — current: cases for which the service has ongoing responsibility
  — potential (contained): in a particular work

area such as a ward all people could be potential but not actual cases
  — potential (very large): e.g. people living in a particular geographical area
- workload: daily work with current caseload, plus related administration, liaison, teaching and managerial tasks
- case mix: the type and complexity of cases on a therapist's caseload
- priority: a person who comes before other clients when his needs are analysed against set criteria
- weighting: the weighting allocated to a client will depend on the complexity of his needs, the input required at the caseload review date and the resources needed to meet his current needs. Haylock (1989) weights acute health care in terms of minimal input, short-term rehabilitation without complications and more complex rehabilitation needs. Weighting of individual clients will depend on professional judgement and the allocation of time to a particular type of case over a weekly or monthly time-scale.

The system or process of caseload management employed by a service needs to be simple to use, take as little time as possible to operate and be sufficiently refined to identify the optimum number of clients each therapist can manage in view of her grade, experience and need for supervision.

Caseload management is becoming increasingly important with the advent of new legislation, quality standards, audit and costings. Service agreements need to identify the available resources which can be used to assess and treat a certain number of people with varying needs at an agreed standard at a particular time. Managers can then also identify and justify the difference between actual and estimated shortfalls in service provision in relation to their existing resources.

The ultimate outcome of improved resource management systems is to enable government departments, the Social Services Inspectorate (SSI), Regions, and local health and social service authorities to monitor, review, evaluate and analyse data with a view to obtaining the highest quality of service for the greatest number of people within available resources. Health care social services will see a good deal of change in the forthcoming decade and beyond; as resource management becomes more sophisticated, managers will be better informed and will be able to make more informed judgements.

ADMINISTRATION

In contrast to the proactive nature of management, administration is a reactive activity which deals with the day-to-day tasks which support the overall function of a service or department. Administrative activities are dealt with by managers, therapy staff and any clerical support allocated to the service. These activities include record keeping and report writing, stock and equipment control, monitoring staff absences, collecting and collating information, coordinating staff rotas for particular duties and organising clerical support for typing, filing and telephone reception.

Record keeping

Records are administration's memory bank. They contain information about a service, its clients and staff, supplies, equipment and so on. They take a number of forms, for instance files, written reports, charts, tapes and discs, and are important in the control and assessment of work. They assist a manager, and others, to monitor what is happening or has happened, to make effective decisions and to assess progress towards goals. They must be accurate, accessible and informative and each manager needs to consider the following questions when deciding whether or not to keep records:

- Will the information be useful? How? When? To whom?
- What part will it play in decision-making and evaluation?
- Can it be collected accurately enough to serve its purpose?
- Will it be accessible?
- Will it be available when and where it is required?
- Can it be stored at a reasonable cost?

Rather than describing types of records in detail in this text we refer the reader to Creek 1990 (Ch. 28), which provides a thorough overview of record keeping generally, occupational therapy records in particular and the systems which are commonly used.

Report writing

Reports contain information which has to be communicated to clinical colleagues, others in the organisation and those in other agencies. Information concerning report writing is contained in Section 2 (p. 93), Box 5.3 and in Creek 1990 (Ch. 28). In preparing to write a clinical or managerial report, it is useful to formulate a clear picture of its purpose and intended audience; the report writer may find that posing the following questions will help her to define an appropriate strategy:

- What is the purpose of the report? e.g.
  — to impart information
  — to fulfil a legal requirement
  — to present an annual review
  — to propose a development
- To whom is it addressed? e.g.
  — a colleague
  — one's manager
  — the management team
  — another committee
  — another service
- What is its subject matter? e.g.
  — a client's progress
  — results of a particular clinical study
- What type of language should be used? e.g.
  — lay terminology
  — technical
  — a mixture
- Is consultation required?

The following aspects of presentation and layout should also be considered:

- Structure
  — How much detail is required?
  — Are appendices needed?
  — Is there a maximum length?

- Layout
  - Should it be formal, with summary and recommendations?
  - Can it be informal, as in a memorandum?
  - Should it take the form of a letter?
- Organisation of information
  - Is the material presented in a logical sequence?
  - Are there sufficient headings to guide the reader?
  - Are appendices given in the relevant order and referred to clearly in the text?
- Presentation
  - Is presentation appropriate to the report's purpose, audience and level of formality?
  - Have all necessary supporting materials (e.g. tables, figures, references) been provided?
  - Is there a title page clearly identifying the originator and subject of the report?

Stock and equipment control

A range of materials (stock) and equipment is needed to provide treatment. These items have to be budgeted for, controlled and maintained and all staff can contribute to their economical use and proper care. Records of all transactions regarding stock and equipment must be retained, whether these relate to orders and requisitions or to maintenance and repair. Every service also needs an audit system for interim and annual stock and equipment checks, not only for its own information but also for authority audit purposes. The following is an outline of the principles of selection, purchasing, storage and distribution of stock and equipment.

Selection

- Careful selection of both materials and equipment is necessary in order to provide satisfactory, current intervention techniques and to avoid wastage of staff and client time and materials.
- Those responsible for or contributing to the selection process should consult catalogues, obtain samples or arrange a demonstration in order to inspect any unfamiliar item prior to purchase.

- Colleagues and technical staff who may be more knowledgeable about a particular item should be consulted prior to its purchase.
- It should be remembered that the cheapest is not always the best or most economical in the long term.
- Equipment must be well made, safe and durable.

Purchasing

- Consider quality and value for money.
- Relate items purchased to types of client and their intervention needs.
- Consider whether materials and equipment will be used continually or occasionally.
- Relate quantities purchased to need and to storage space available; overstocking may lead to spoiling and services now have to keep stocks within an annually agreed value.
- Consider the rate at which materials will be used.
- Remember that costs *may* be reduced by ordering large enough quantities to avoid delivery charges.
- Ensure that purchasing takes place through the organisation's standard system, for both internally and externally supplied items.
- Needs and costs must be estimated per annum.
- Spending must be monitored against stock held.
- Replacements for obsolete or unrepairable equipment have to be planned for and costed.
- Maintenance of equipment has to be 'purchased'.
- Each manager needs a system which will enable her to monitor and control the purchasing function of the service.

Storage

Appropriate storage and care of both materials and equipment are essential if a service is to operate smoothly and offer effective intervention to its clients. The control of stock and equipment should be simple and systematic, so that it becomes automatic.

Distribution

- The sale of items made in occupational therapy, though still decreasing, requires that the manager adhere to the organisation's financial regulations and procedures for receipt of money from purchasers.
- Prices should cover the cost of the materials plus a percentage for wastage. Profits should not be made on items produced as part of a client's therapy.
- The short- or long-term loan of equipment such as daily living aids must adhere to the issue procedure agreed with the organisation.
- If the authority sells daily living aids to clients it must also follow financial regulations and procedures, including the issue of receipts.

Monitoring staff absences

Staff may be absent from work for a number of reasons, such as sickness, holidays, compassionate, study and maternity leave. Leave of absence should usually be requested or notified and agreed in accordance with established national and local policies and procedures. The salaries and wages department must monitor such absences in case remuneration has to be amended, as in cases of prolonged sick leave, maternity or unpaid leave. Additionally, a manager needs to monitor absences for the following reasons:

- to identify any patterns in sick leave which it may be possible to rectify, such as repeated one-day absences which may signify stress
- to support and counsel any staff member who has prolonged absence through illness
- to facilitate flexibility in the planning of services at particular times of year, for instance during the summer when many staff wish to take their main holiday
- to monitor leave taken and compare this with actual and potential departmental outputs
- to plan cover for staff whose prolonged absence is foreseen, e.g. in the case of maternity leave or a lengthy study course
- to monitor any industrial injuries, for example back injury or personal injury caused by equipment or clients

- to monitor the volume of annual leave carried over from one year to another and to implement limitations if appropriate
- to monitor time taken in lieu of extra hours worked and, if this is excessive and/or follows a particular pattern, to negotiate changes in daily or weekly duty hours with an individual
- last, but not least, to operate a monitoring system which cares for staff, which may involve the occupational/staff health department's assistance and advice and assistance from medical and other colleagues in cases of sickness or injury.

Staff rotas

Rotas are time plans by which certain activities are distributed among staff members such that each takes responsibility for a specific task for a particular period. Rotas in occupational therapy departments may be drawn up for tasks such as end-of-day security; printing press preparation and cleaning; general tidying/storage; refrigerator checking, cleaning and defrosting; collection of in-service training programme contributions; selected maintenance of equipment. They are common in most if not all organisations and are needed for the following reasons:

- to distribute work fairly and evenly during normal working hours
- to distribute uninteresting and interesting work equally among staff
- to provide staff with the opportunity to contribute to the overall function of the service, including daily housekeeping.

There are two clear rules for drawing up rotas. First, the period of time for each allocated duty must be the same for all staff. Second, if groups of staff are allocated a task, that task must be subdivided equitably.

Clerical duties

All occupational therapy staff have to undertake clerical tasks during the course of their work, whether or not clerical staff are available to support the service. If clerical support is available, tasks may be allocated specifically or be performed by a pool of clerical staff. Where support is provided, therapy staff will obtain assistance with typing, filing and telephone duties. However, there are still services which have to function with little or no support; therefore, therapists need to be able to devise clerical systems which facilitate rather than hinder their clinical duties.

Written communications

Most services will have assistance, however limited, for the typing of letters, reports and the like. However, staff may have to hand-write clients' treatment notes, memoranda and so on.

Filing

It is essential that all services and their work areas have an efficient filing system for clinical and managerial records. A filing system must be simple so that it is easily maintained and facilitates easy retrieval of papers. It should include a place for every type of record normally found within the service and organisation. Three key methods are commonly used in filing systems:

- alphabetical: files are arranged in alphabetical order regardless of subject. This is probably the most straightforward system in use.
- numerical: this requires each file to be allocated a number. This requires a master index which can be cross-referenced, if necessary, to a subject index.
- by subject: this is useful for general purposes and for small filing systems, but requires some type of indexing for easy reference and retrieval.

Whichever method is selected, all staff with access to it must learn how to use it correctly so that it maintains its effectiveness.

Telephone duties

Therapists may spend many hours each week on the telephone dealing with matters regarding particular clients. However, they may also find that they take calls and messages for colleagues, and

that this works satisfactorily providing those colleagues reciprocate. Calls can be screened by reception or clerical staff if this support is available; otherwise, each service or work area will need an appropriate and foolproof message relaying system which will enable staff to continue their clinical work with as few interruptions as possible.

Administration is not a popular task with occupational therapy staff, but if a service and its resources are to function at an optimum level of efficiency and effectiveness simple and reliable administrative procedures, practices and systems are indispensable.

RESEARCH

Research involves planned observation or experimentation using particular methods of recording and measurement. It is an essential component of clinical and managerial work. Informally, it may entail discussing cases with colleagues, thus stimulating discussion and speculation. Formally, it is undertaken to answer clearly defined questions, for example whether a particular technique is effective or an information system meets current and future needs.

The process of research includes:

- identifying a broad area of study
- undertaking a literature search and review
- specifying the question to be answered
- designing the appropriate methodology
- collecting appropriate data
- analysing the data
- disseminating the findings to colleagues.

Its overall purpose is to further the individual's and the profession's knowledge in a particular area.

Whilst all pre-registration occupational therapy courses include an element of research, therapists at all levels find that research courses organised by polytechnics and other establishments offer additional learning opportunities, advice and support. The reader is also referred to Creek 1990 (Ch. 30), the BAOT's Reference Books and its Research Interest Group, and to DoH and Regional documents on research and funding.

CONCLUSION

Management in all areas of public service has changed and continues to develop apace, not only as a result of legislation and government policies but as a direct result of the developments and trends in health and social care and the increasing need to use resources in a way which provides high-quality, cost-effective services.

This chapter has, it is hoped, placed management in a realistic and practical perspective, offering background information about the history, theory, legislation and practice of management and describing many of the day-to-day tasks which face staff at all levels. People's management skills, like their clinical abilities,

develop over time and with experience. Most skills are learned 'on the job', with occasional injections of theory from specific courses. Few, if any, managers are born. Most are *made*, and are shaped by their own personalities, knowledge, skills and attitudes, whatever their level of responsibility. Occupational therapists have an advantage over some other professionals in that the intervention processes they use give them the opportunity to develop many management skills (Fig. 5.2). Therapists should remember that 'management is not an activity that exists in its own right. It is rather a description of a variety of activities carried out by those members of organisations whose role is that of a manager' (Cole 1984). All occupational therapy staff are managers of something or someone, and most especially of themselves.

USEFUL ADDRESS

British Association of Occupational Therapists
6-8 Marshalsea Road
Southwark
London SE1 1HL

REFERENCES

Brewster C 1984 Understanding industrial relations. Pan Books, London
British Association of Occupational Therapists 1989 Statement on professional negligence and litigation (SPP 135). BAOT, London
British Association of Occupational Therapists 1990 Code of professional conduct. BAOT, London
Cole G A 1984 Management theory and practice. D.P. Publications, London
Council for Professions Supplementary to Medicine 1990 Statement of conduct. CPSM, London
Crawford M 1989 Setting standards in occupational therapy. British Journal of Occupational Therapy 52(8): 294–297
Creek J (ed) 1990 Occupational therapy and mental health: principles, skills and practice. Churchill Livingstone, Edinburgh
Dale E, Michelon L C 1966 Modern management methods. Penguin, Harmondsworth
De Gilio S, Bowden R, Burrows H 1989 The management manual for health care professionals. Winslow Press, Bicester, Oxon
Drucker P F 1968 The practice of managment Pan Books, London

Graham N O 1990 Quality assurance in hospitals: strategies for assessment and implementation. Aspen, Rockville, MD
Handy C B 1976 Understanding organisations. Penguin, Harmondsworth
Haylock S 1989 A method of caseload management. British Journal of Occupational Therapy 52(10): 380–382
Heller R 1972 The naked manager. Barrie & Jenkins, London
HMSO 1944 Education act. HMSO, London
HMSO 1944/58 Disabled persons (employment) acts. HMSO, London
HMSO 1946 National Health Service act. HMSO, London
HMSO 1948 National assistance act. HMSO, London
HMSO 1957 Housing act. HMSO, London
HMSO 1958 Local Government Act. HMSO, London
HMSO 1960 Professions supplementary to medicine act. HMSO, London
HMSO 1970 Chronically sick and disabled persons act. HMSO, London
HMSO 1970 Education act. HMSO, London
HMSO 1970 Equal pay act. HMSO, London
HMSO 1970 Local authority social services act. HMSO, London

HMSO 1973 Employment and training act. HMSO, London
HMSO 1973 National Health Service act. HMSO, London
HMSO 1974 Health and safety at work act. HMSO, London
HMSO 1974 Housing act. HMSO, London
HMSO 1974 National Health Service (PSM) regulation act. HMSO, London
HMSO 1975 Employment act. HMSO, London
HMSO 1975 Sex discrimination act. HMSO, London
HMSO 1976 Education act. HMSO, London
HMSO 1976 Race discrimination act. HMSO, London
HMSO 1978 Employment protection (consolidation) act. HMSO, London
HMSO 1978 Rating (disabled persons) act. HMSO, London
HMSO 1979 Housing act. HMSO, London
HMSO 1980 Housing act. HMSO, London
HMSO 1981 Disabled persons act. HMSO, London
HMSO 1981 Education act. HMSO, London
HMSO 1983 Mental health act. HMSO, London
HMSO 1984 Data protection act. HMSO, London
HMSO 1985 Housing act. HMSO, London
HMSO 1986 Disabled persons (services, consultation and representation) act. HMSO, London
HMSO 1986 National Health Service (amendment) act. HMSO, London
HMSO 1987 Access to personal files act. HMSO, London
HMSO 1987 Consumer protection act. HMSO, London
HMSO 1987 Promoting better health. White paper. HMSO, London
HMSO 1988 Access to medical reports act. HMSO, London
HMSO 1989 Caring for people. White Paper. HMSO, London

HMSO 1989 Local government and housing act. HMSO, London
HMSO 1989 Working for patients. White Paper. HMSO, London
HMSO 1990 National Health Service and community care act. HMSO, London
Koontz H, O'Donnell C, Weihrich H 1980 Management. McGraw-Hill, Japan
Lansdowne J 1989 To rotate or not to rotate. British Journal of Occupational Therapy 52(1): 4–7
Mayo E 1933 The human problems of an industrial civilisation. Macmillan, New York
Mays J, Forder A, Keidan O 1983 Penelope Hall's Social Service of England and Wales. Routledge & Kegan Paul, London
Mullins L J 1985 Management and organisational behaviour. Pitman, London
NHSTA 1985 Better management, better health. NHSTA, London
Penn B, Penn J 1990 Marketing occupational therapy: imperative for the future? British Journal of Occupational Therapy 53(2): 64–66
Storrs C 1949 General and industrial management. Pitman, London (Translation of Fayol H 1916 Administration industrielle et generale)
Wallis M A 1987 'Profession' and 'professionalism' and the emerging profession of occupational therapy. British Journal of Occupational Therapy 50(8): 264–65; 50(9): 300–302
Wilson M 1984 Occupational therapy in short term psychiatry. Churchill Livingstone, Edinburgh.

FURTHER READING

Adair J 1985 Effective decision making. Pan, London
Armstrong M 1988 A handbook of personnel management practice. Kogan Page, London
College of Occupational Therapists 1991 Research advice handbook. COT, London
College of Occupational Therapists 1986 Good management handbook. COT, London
College of Occupational Therapists 1989 Standards, policies and proceedings: standards of practice for occupational therapy services. SPP 120, SPP 105, SPP 100, SPP 125, SPP 130. COT, London
Cox C 1988 Practical aspects of stress management. British Journal of Occupational Therapy 51(2): 44–47
Craik C 1988 Stress in occupational therapy: how to cope. British Journal of Occupational Therapy 51(2): 40–43
Finch J D 1984 Aspects of law affecting the paramedical professions. Faber & Faber, London
Fletcher W 1983 Meetings, meetings. Hodder & Stoughton, London
Howard K, Sharp J A 1983 The management of a student research project. Gower, Aldershot, Hants

Katz D 1964 The motivation basis of organisational behaviour. Behavioural Science 9: 131–136
Kingston W, Rowbottom R 1989 Making general management work in the NHS: a guide to general management for NHS managers. Brunel University, Uxbridge
Maddux R B 1988 Successful negotiation. Kogan Page, London
Maxwell A E 1970 Basic statistics in behavioural research. Penguin, London
Murphy C 1987 Clinical audit: measuring the quality of individual clinical performance 50(3): 83–85
Ouvreteit 1986 Organisation of multidisciplinary teams. Brunel University, Uxbridge
Partridge C, Barnitt R 1986 Research guidelines: a handbook for therapists. Heinemann, London
Scott J, Rochester A 1984 Effective management skills: what's a manager? Sphere, London

6

Activity analysis

Sybil E. Johnson

The unique characteristic of occupational therapy is the use of carefully planned activity as a treatment medium.

(Willson 1984)

Man is an active being whose development is influenced by the use of purposeful activity. Using their capacity for intrinsic motivation, human beings are able to influence their physical and mental health and their social and physical environment through purposeful activity . . . . occupational therapy is based on the belief that purposeful activity, including its interpersonal and environmental components, may be used to prevent and mediate dysfunction and to elicit maximum adaptation.

(Representative Assembly of the American Occupational Therapy Association 1979)

INTRODUCTION

A glance at the history of the use of activity and occupation in fostering health and alleviating ill-health and dysfunction (Ch. 2) will show that while occupational therapy is a relatively young profession its underlying concepts had their origin in antiquity. However, in recent times, particularly in the late 1960s and the 1970s the profession lost sight of those roots. It was only as occupational therapists began to challenge their affiliation to the medical model of care and to question the application of much assessment which, for a period, was not followed by therapeutic intervention to alleviate or solve individuals' problems, that therapists again turned to the true philosophy and raison d'être of occupational therapy.

That the profession deals with the activities of everyday living is not questioned, but it still needs to be stressed that the *study* of activity is essential. One of the key skills of the occupational therapist is 'the ability to analyse the component parts of an activity in order to use it purposefully and specifically thereby enhancing individual function' (Finlay 1987).

The use of activity is the basis, or core, of the profession. Activity encourages adaptive behaviour, meets specific objectives and fosters active involvement by the individual in addressing his specific problems and needs. In this context activity is taken to mean all the tasks which form the pattern of a person's life, and which are taken for granted until that individual suffers illness or trauma.

Activity used therapeutically may be drawn from the wide sphere of everyday life, including the arts, leisure pursuits, household and personal care tasks, work, education, sport, hobbies, family and social relationships. If an occupational therapist is to use some or all of these activities in her interventions she must do so in a manner which has meaning and purpose for the individual. Moreover, she must be able to analyse the components of such activities.

Activity analysis is the process of separating any task into its constituent parts. In analysing an activity in detail the therapist must physically participate in it in order to understand its components and complexities. The therapist should, first, learn the 'how' of the activity and then concentrate on the 'why', 'what', 'where' and so on. These latter elements will lead to analysis of physical, cognitive, social, interpersonal, sensory, emotional and behavioural components. Once an analysis is complete the therapist must relate her findings to the individual's identified abilities and needs. Utilising the Occupational Therapy Process (Ch. 4) she will reach the stage in an individual's programme where she has to select activities relevant to that person. Her skills of analysis and her knowledge of activities will enable her to discriminate between appropriate and inappropriate activities and to modify them according to individual needs.

Such analysis is used in conjunction with the assessment and treatment of function and dysfunction whereby the therapist determines the extent to which physical, behavioural and other abilities and skills affect an individual's ability to perform 'normally' and then plans, implements and evaluates appropriate intervention.

This chapter begins by reviewing the importance of activity to everyday life, including its contribution to the individual's roles, cultural and social status, life-style and so on. The distinction between purposeful and non-purposeful activity is explained, with particular reference to the application of both kinds of activity to occupational therapy. In subsequent sections the definition and importance of activity analysis is considered, along with the main features the therapist should look for when selecting activities to use in a rehabilitative programme.

The 'why' of activity analysis, that is, the kinds of information that analysis will yield, is then described, and types of models used in activity analysis are briefly outlined. The chapter then provides a detailed framework by which activities might be analysed and assessed. This includes general factors such as environment, safety, appropriateness and adaptability, and, more specifically, the potential physical, sensory, cognitive, perceptual, emotional and social demands that an activity will place upon the individual.

The next section of the chapter outlines methods by which activities can be graded, that is, how they can be adapted to the changing abilities of the individual during the course of his treatment programme. The final sections take three very different activities — making a cup of coffee; setting a line of type; and participating in a discussion group — and demonstrate in more concrete terms how the preceding frameworks for activity analysis and grading might be applied to each. Finally, the application of activity analysis to the therapist's overall therapeutic procedure is summarised.

THE RELATIONSHIP OF ACTIVITY TO EVERYDAY LIFE

Willard and Spackman (1988) describe activity as necessary to man's survival. In addition to meeting his basic needs, activity may also give him pleasure (Fig. 6.1), ensure he is comfortable, solve his problems, enable him to express himself and to relate to others and allow him to earn a living in order to support himself and his family (Fig. 6.2). Activity is characteristic of and essential to human existence (Cynkin 1979, Cynkin & Robinson 1990). It offers rewards and achievements as well as constraints and frustrations. Through activity a person not only develops skills, but also learns about his strengths and weaknesses.

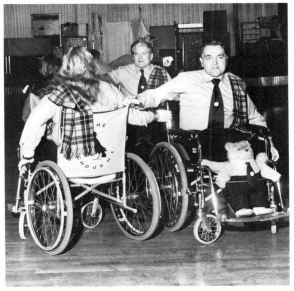

Fig. 6.1 Activity should offer pleasure, as well as physical, psychological and social well-being.

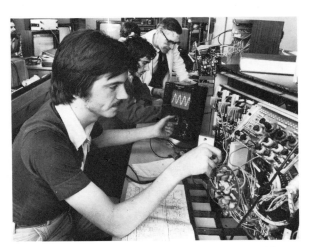

Fig. 6.2 The ability to earn one's living through paid employment is still accepted as a cultural norm in our society.

Activity and routine

Most of the activities an individual performs daily are so routine that he carries them out automatically. For example, a person's set pattern of rising from bed, going to the bathroom, washing, dressing, preparing and eating breakfast and leaving the house to catch a bus or start the car is part of an established routine involving a series of activities. If, however, that routine is disrupted for some reason it will disturb other routines and activities during the day; for example, over-sleeping or tending a sick child may make the person late for work and a vital meeting and result in ill-humour, adversely affecting his usual objectivity and efficiency at work.

Activity and roles

Activity is very closely related to the roles an individual adopts each day. The role of parent, breadwinner, teacher or therapist, for instance, is supported and defined by particular skills, functions and behaviours. Each role requires some activity on the individual's part. The parent role, for instance, involves effective communication, caring for the family home, earning a living, looking after and disciplining the children and setting an example. The individual may pursue some of these activities, such as playing with his children, with enthusiasm and anticipation whilst he finds others, such as spring cleaning, dissatisfying or boring, to be undertaken only as a matter of duty and social norm.

Activity, culture and social status

As well as relating to the roles a person assumes, activities will be significant in terms of culture and social status. They will form patterns which are quite important within the values and norms of the individual's social and cultural group. Hence, if his culture dictates that certain foods should be avoided altogether or at certain times of the year, his activities in relation to food preparation and meals will be adapted accordingly. Each person strives to lead as satisfying a life as possible; therefore, he will endeavour to perform activities which are approved of by his social and/or cultural group, providing those activities also satisfy his personal needs and wants. There are, of course, exceptions and each individual will modify, to a greater or lesser extent, his activity within the parameters of his environment and what he believes is acceptable behaviourally. Envisage the person who enjoys work and leisure to a greater extent than caring for his home. He will work diligently and participate in his leisure interests and hobbies enthusiastically, excluding all but the most basic elements of self-catering and home care. However, if he were expecting relatives for the weekend his behaviours would change, influenced by social and cultural values and norms (which, for himself, he may have discarded). He would tidy, clean, shop and cook to meet the expected needs of his visitors. Therefore, his activity relates to the perceived expectations of his social/cultural group even if *personally* he has modified his own standards and activity levels.

Activity and time

The performance of activities also relates to time. The minutes or hours allocated to a particular activity on a specific day reflects the relative value attached to that task at that time. The value, or importance, of an activity may vary — the family breakfast will be a far more rushed affair on weekdays than at weekends, because family members are routinely preparing for school or work during the week. However, the time allotted to breakfast at weekends enters another time dimension altogether; even with events to attend, shopping to complete or visits to friends to make, the pressure to meet deadlines is relaxed.

Integration of activities

The integration of activities with roles, routines, time, social/cultural groups and the individual's environment will form quite distinctive activity groups relating to work, leisure, recreation, self-care and social interaction. They will also integrate each person's physical, psychological, cognitive and social functions; i.e., the performance of activity will unite the mind, body and will in the actual 'doing' of that task.

All activities which form the daily life pattern of a particular person are taken for granted until illness or accident and subsequent dysfunction intervene. Kielhofner (1985) (Fig. 6.3) describes man's daily functions in terms of a 'function/dysfunction' continuum. That is, whilst man is well he performs at the functional level of exploration, competence and achievement, but when he is handicapped in some way he lapses to the dysfunction level in which he may display helplessness, incompetence or inefficiency in daily activities. Thus, moving from helplessness to achievement, the individual may, in succession, exhibit a complete deficit of skills, an inability to perform a particular skill routinely, a dissatisfac-

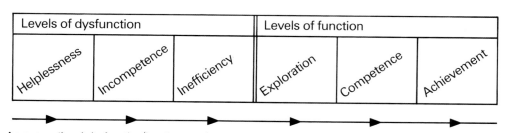

Fig. 6.3 An occupational dysfunction/function continuum. (Adapted from Keilhofner 1985.)

tion with reduced ability, an investigation of skills in a secure environment, a striving to meet the demands of a skill, the development of new skills and, finally, a striving to maintain and enhance his performance.

Cynkin & Robinson (1990) summarise the importance and relevance of activity in daily life thus (Fig. 6.4):

- activity is concerned with the procedures of day-to-day living
- it involves the process of doing
- it is necessary to and characteristic of man's existence and survival
- it is socioculturally and environmentally controlled and/or orientated
- it can be learned.

In the course of her intervention, utilising a very wide range of self-care, work, leisure and social activities, the occupational therapist must fully appreciate man's dependence upon activity if he is to function effectively and to maintain his general mental and physical health while meeting his sometimes complex needs and wants in a manner which suits his life-style and environment.

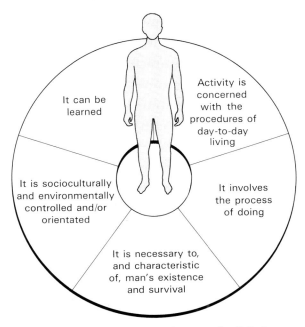

Fig. 6.4 The importance and relevance of activity in daily life.

PURPOSEFUL AND NON-PURPOSFUL ACTIVITY

Thus far, we have considered man's normal daily activities which have directed purpose. However, prior to discussion of activity and its analysis it is important to reflect as well upon non-purposeful activity. In relation to occupational therapy and daily life one could argue that this category includes activity undertaken for its own sake rather than as a means to an end. An example of this might be for an individual to play solitaire for the sake of his normal enjoyment of the game, rather than as a means of improving the range of movement in his upper limb.

Non-purposeful activity might also be understood as that which forms part of a recipe — that is, as activity undertaken because it is standard practice in the circumstances. An example of this would be for a person with a fractured radius and ulna to use a prescribed range of activities in a certain manner at specific stages in his programme. Thus in the early stages he might participate in large remedial games and pottery; in the middle stage he might be offered stool-seating or printing; and in the final stages he might be upgraded to heavy woodwork and wrought iron work. It may be argued that there is nothing adverse in this approach — nor, indeed, is there, *provided that* the activities used mean something to the individual, i.e. that he understands their purpose at that specific stage of his programme.

None the less, the occupational therapist should ensure that she does use specific activities, avoiding those which may be construed as merely exercise-orientated, especially if their purpose is unclear and unexplainable to both the individual and herself.

We might now ask, 'What is *purposeful* activity?' The therapist may argue that activity with some purpose relates as closely as possible to the recipient's work or home life. However, she may also argue that at selected stages in an intervention programme she has to utilise activities that may not relate very closely to general daily life but do encourage, for instance, early reduction of oedema and the return of mid-range movement. The individual himself might also feel that any activity is 'purposeful' for him as long as it improves his function, whether or not it relates to his usual life roles and tasks. Simultaneously, however, there may be occasions when he asks why he is partaking of similar or identical activities in two different therapies, such as transfers or remedial activity to improve his hand–eye coordination.

The debate concerning purposeful versus non-purposeful activity is, perhaps, of little concern to those receiving treatment. It should, however, encourage the therapist to give serious thought to the matter in order that she may clearly define and differentiate her functions as an occupational therapist from those of other team colleagues.

ACTIVITY ANALYSIS

DEFINITION

The study and analysis of any activity is a vital element in the practice of occupational therapy. Analysis provides the therapist with knowledge of how an activity can contribute to the balance be-tween daily living skills, work and leisure and motivate the individual to organise routines and skills into behavioural patterns and roles. Analysis reveals the complexities of an individual's function; it examines his mastery of or ability to learn skills; his possession of integrated concepts (such as size and weight); his neuromuscular control and coordination, sensation and joint stability; his problem-solving abilities and creativity; and his skill in making informed choices.

An activity is a step-by-step process involving a potentially large number of operations in which sequencing is vital. Analysis allows the activity to be broken down into its simplest components, using the actual order or sequence of a task. For example, in relearning to dress after a stroke the individual learns to undress first as this is simpler, and then relearns the skills of dressing his upper half, then his lower half, then of managing fastenings and, finally, his footwear.

Features of activity

All activities utilised by occupational therapists are chosen for specific reasons, as summarised in Fig-

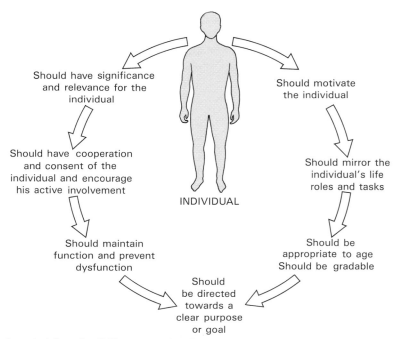

Fig. 6.5 Specific characteristics of activities appropriate for use in occupational therapy.

ure 6.5. In selecting activities, the therapist should bear the following points in mind:

• Each activity must have a purpose. It must be directed at a specific goal, such as enabling the individual to regain confidence and ensure safety when handling kitchen utensils whilst preparing a hot drink (Fig. 6.6).

• The task must be significant/relevant to the individual. Its level of significance may vary with his stage of treatment, but it must be seen, by

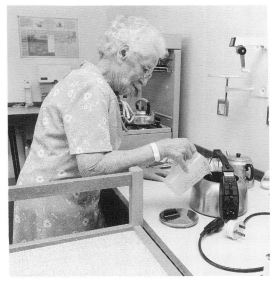

Fig. 6.6 Each activity must have a purpose and be directed at a specific goal.

him, to be of value and use even if its merits may only be fully realised at a later date. Hence, early workshop activity may make it possible for him to aim for a future goal, i.e. the motivation, co-ordination and neuromuscular control which will facilitate his readoption of one of his leisure roles.

• Any activity requires the individual's cooperation and consent to some degree. He must be involved in the actual performance of the activity, but he must also assist in the process of determining which activities are relevant. In this way he receives feedback not only about his physical and mental involvement with the activity but can redevelop and reaffirm his ability to plan, make decisions, initiate action, solve problems, transfer learning and to take increasing responsibility as his programme progresses.

• In addition to maintaining and/or improving levels of function, activity should also aim to prevent any further dysfunction or disability (Fig. 6.7) and to improve a person's quality of life. The specific choice and type of activity used depends initially upon the individual's current functional level, including his ability to participate, but it must also facilitate his progress towards future goals.

• Most, if not all, activities in a programme should mirror an individual's life-roles and tasks, enabling him to achieve or redevelop skills which are vital to him and which assist him to develop the required competence level.

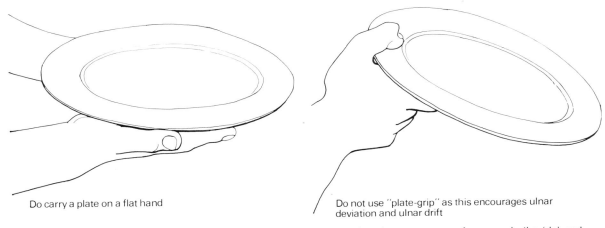

Do carry a plate on a flat hand

Do not use "plate-grip" as this encourages ulnar deviation and ulnar drift

Fig. 6.7 Preventing further dysfunction or disability may require a re-education programme, for example the 'do' and 'do not' of carrying a plate for the person with rheumatoid arthritis.

• If the individual is to demonstrate and fulfil his commitment to his intervention he must be sufficiently motivated. Relating activity to his interests and involving him in the selection of tasks will help both him and the therapist to attain their objectives.

• In addition to the interest element, an activity must be age appropriate. It must also be gradable, i.e. adaptable, in complexity and time in terms of the minutes or hours he performs an activity which aims to increase his range of movement and improve his muscle strength or coordination.

• Activities are selected as potentially appropriate by the therapist based on her professional knowledge and judgement, thereby ensuring that the activity meets the needs of the individual in a meaningful way.

WHY IS ACTIVITY ANALYSIS NECESSARY?

The therapist's skill in activity analysis is essential if she is to utilise any activity with purpose and precision. The step-by-step analysis can be a lengthy and complex process but it can be vital in identifying and meeting treatment aims and objectives. The specific reasons for analysis are summarised in a 'Why?' checklist in Table 6.1 and can be described as follows:

• To observe and understand the numerous elements of an activity, i.e. the individual parts which, when performed in the correct sequence, form the complete task.

• To determine each activity's potential use as a treatment medium in relation to the people receiving occupational therapy, their perceived needs and their life-styles.

• To determine whether an activity is viable in terms of:
— cost
— the space it requires
— whether it needs a particular environment because, for example, it is noisy and dirty
— the availability of materials, tools or equipment
— staff expertise and availability.

• To establish whether or not individuals can perform it. In order for an activity to meet a par-

Table 6.1 The necessity for activity analysis: a 'Why?' checklist

Why?	In relation to . . .
To observe and understand	the numerous elements and sequences which form a complete task
To determine an activity's potential use	treatment, individual's perceived needs and life-style
To establish viability	cost, space, particular environment, materials, tools, equipment, staff expertise/ availability
To establish performance levels required	basic and essential skills required, e.g. coordination, standing tolerance
To identify potential for modification	adaptability and scope for grading
To break down into sub-tasks	learning and teaching purposes, e.g. logical progression, sub-tasks needing simplification
To identify more demanding components	facilitating change in behaviour

ticular person's needs he must possess certain basic skills. If, for example, hand-press printing is used within his programme the skills he requires will include: sufficient coordination to handle the paper, adequate standing or sitting balance and tolerance to maintain his position, an adequate range of movement in his upper limbs to depress and raise the press handle and motivation in order to complete the task set. However, if the intention is to increase his skill level then elements of the activity should be slightly beyond his current ability, thereby offering a further goal. In addition, the elements within the activity which are planned to be of specific use to the individual should form the greater proportion of the whole task in order to make it worthwhile.

• To identify an activity's potential for modification, i.e. for grading and adaptation, thus ensuring that a selected task is a valued experience and applicable to the individual's ability and needs.

• To break down the activity into sub-tasks for learning and teaching purposes. As the therapist undertakes this element of her analysis she can identify the sub-tasks and consider whether they present a logical progression or stages which may need to be simplified or which can be eliminated, or whether the sub-tasks themselves need further sub-division due to their complexity and subsequent required skill levels.

• In order to grade an activity appropriately. To facilitate change in an individual's behaviour the therapist must identify which components are more demanding and why. This will enable her to prepare the individual adequately for the activity and the challenges and problems it may present.

APPROACHES

There are many approaches in the analysis of activity, some quite straightforward, others more complex and lengthy. The form of analysis used by a therapist will usually be influenced by her treatment frame of reference. Models of analysis are described below, but initially the therapist must ask herself certain questions prior to the selection of an activity for therapeutic use:

• How is the activity performed? The therapist must know the basic components and processes involved in the activity and understand its potential. She must undertake the activity herself, under the same or similar circumstances expected or anticipated of the individual. She must be sufficiently competent to teach the person successfully, having considered the media to be used, positioning, movements, reactions, cognitive function required and so on.

• What activity is most appropriate to meet this individual's needs? With him she must select an activity which meets his needs, solves particular problems and relates to his interests and preferences.

• Why is a specific activity selected? The therapist must be able to establish a reason for the choice, which must be consistent with programme aims and objectives. It must be appropriate as well as meeting physical, psychological, cognitive and social demands.

• Where will the activity take place? Whatever the constraints concerning location, the therapist should endeavour to provide appropriate activity in its relevant environment, for example, personal care in the bedroom and bathroom, domestic skills in a kitchen, workshop activity in the therapy department, in the assigned area at home, or in the local community, utilising public services.

• When will the activity take place? Time, in this instance, may relate to time of day or week, season, or stage of a treatment programme. Timing may influence the activity chosen to meet a need, but whatever the task it must take place at its appropriate time or hour, thus confirming its credibility. Therefore, morning self-care will precede and/or succeed breakfast, depending on the individual's normal routine; a seasonal activity such as making a Christmas cake will take place in the autumn.

• Who is involved in the activity? As well as the individual and his therapist, this may include other occupational therapy staff contributing to the programme and to whom the therapist has deployed particular elements. In this latter instance the therapist requires the ability and skill to involve support staff whose expertise in certain creative and practical tasks may far outweigh her own.

Within the question 'Who?', specific factors relating to the individual must be borne in mind. These include age, sex, past or present occupation, social and cultural background, his presenting problems, diagnosis and prognosis, his interests, approximate intellectual level and any disabilities other than the present one(s).

Assembling a 'pen-picture' of the person referred for intervention should precede analysis of potentially suitable activities and the planning of a programme appropriate to his functional and personal needs. Table 6.2 illustrates how the therapist may create such a picture for two individuals.

ACTIVITY ANALYSIS MODELS

An occupational therapist's skill in analysing activity is vital in order to establish valid use of the chosen tasks. She will select a method of analysis which is applicable to the models,

Table 6.2 Assembling a pen-picture prior to activity analysis and programme planning

Factor	Adult	Older person
Age	30	65
Sex	Female	Male
Past/present occupation	Teacher/mother with small child	Miner/retired
Social/cultural background	Settled in UK 20 years ago from Scandinavia. Lives with husband, no other family in area	From mining family, spent whole life in the town. Widower of 3 years, 2 children and grandchildren in same town
Diagnosis/ presenting problems	Depression following birth of child, early signs of rheumatoid arthritis?	Pneumoconiosis, CVA
Prognosis	Uncertain, due to non-confirmation of rheumatoid arthritis	Mediocre due to long-standing pneumoconiosis
Interests	Scandinavian folklore and crafts, wine making, travel abroad	Grandchildren, the local miners' club, gardening (allotment)
Intellectual level	University graduate	Left school at 14, well read
Other disabilities	None	Amputation distal phalanges little and ring fingers dominant hand

Table 6.3 A simple activity analysis method

Question	'Answer(s)'
How is the activity performed?	Potential, basic components and processes involved; use of treatment media, positioning, movements, reactions, cognitive functions
What activity?	Appropriateness related to individual needs, problems, interests, preferences
Why is the activity selected?	Choice must be consistent with programme aims and objectives; must meet physical, psychological, cognitive and social demands
Where will it take place?	Whatever the constraints, choice of environment must be as relevant as possible
When will it take place?	At the appropriate time of day, week, season, year, in order to lend credibility
Who is involved?	Individual, therapist, other staff, carers

approaches and techniques she uses in treatment and one with which she feels most comfortable, i.e. which meets her needs and those of her clientele.

The following section describes two activity analysis models, of which one is quite simple, the other more detailed.

SIMPLE ANALYSIS METHOD

This entails answering the questions How? What? Why? Where? When? and Who? in the manner described above and summarised in Table 6.3. This technique has been used successfully by generations of therapists, often with additional questions

in order to specify more accurately the potential benefits of an activity. For example:

- Does it provide a basic sensory skill?
- Does it need repeated use of the same skill?
- Can it be graded?
- Does it assist tolerance to noise?
- Does it appeal to the individual?
- Does it have any vocational or educational value?

DETAILED ANALYSIS MODELS

These are described in many texts and vary only according to the preferences of the authors. These more complex frameworks itemise analyses in terms of the demands of a particular activity, that is, according to the physical, emotional, social, sensory, cognitive, perceptual and cultural demands of any task.

Common factors

Factors common to all activities and their analysis include:

- The environment in which the activity takes place, including space and equipment, or the environment the activity creates, i.e. the relevance, value, emphasis, priority created by or given to the activity by an individual and his sociocultural group.

- The motivation an activity can evoke. How does it facilitate personal effectiveness and how does it relate to interests, roles, individual values?
- The appropriateness of any activity utilised in a therapy programme to the chronological age of the individual, regardless of his problems, to enable him to learn or relearn age- and role-appropriate skills and behaviours.
- The appropriateness of the activity to the sex of the individual. This will depend, of course, upon the sociocultural background of the person; for example, does his culture accept role-swapping or has it very stringent laws about the roles and behaviour of men and women?
- The adaptability of the activity. This is exceedingly important if optimum use is to be made of it. (This is discussed in detail beginning on p. 169.)
- The degree of vocational application of the activity. The vocational element relates to the potential application of the skills within the activity to work (paid or unpaid), home care, leisure and social relationships.
- The cost implications of the activity. Intervention must be cost-effective and efficient in relation to staff time and departmental/service resources. Factors to consider include whether suitable equipment and materials are available, whether a completed article is to be produced, the time the individual has available and whether there are cost implications for the individual pursuing the activity elsewhere, for example at a sports club.
- The safety of the activity. Whilst everyone lives with an element of risk, the person receiving occupational therapy has to be treated 'safely', i.e. the environment must be as hazard-free as possible, and intervention techniques must be safe for the individual and the therapist. However, the situation will vary according to the treatment venue. Compare, for instance, the individual's home environment with that of a local authority day centre, a sports club or a hospital department. Legislation and regulations will affect the safety precautions taken in specific environments.

- The time required to complete the whole activity. This may or may not have relevance, but the therapist must analyse the time factor, i.e. total time for the activity, time for particular elements or sub-tasks.
- The potential of the activity for individual and/group work. This knowledge is vital when planning individual programmes.

Specific factors

These factors should be applied to analysis as required, i.e. in respect of the individual and his discrete needs. Table 6.4 summarises them.

Prior to initiating her analysis the therapist must establish which treatment approach she will be using, for example, neurodevelopmental, rehabilitative, biomechanical, behavioural, psychotherapeutic. Thus she can facilitate positive change related to a person's presenting functional abilities and clinical and functional deficits. One activity, such as dressing, will be used in different ways and for different reasons with the person with an upper limb fracture than with the individual who has had a head injury (Table 6.5).

Motor/physical demands

These would be selected from the following aspects:

- position — of the activity and the individual. Does positioning remain unchanged throughout (Fig. 6.8) or are changes required at certain sub-stages?
- movement — which large and/or small joints are involved; degrees of range of movement required; specific movements entailed, for example flexion (Fig. 6.9) and extension; grips/grasps needed; muscle groups in action; type of muscle work necessary. What is the unilateral or bilateral involvement and is left and right comparison facilitated if appropriate? What fine or gross movement and coordination, rhythm and speed of movement are required?
- grading/adaptability — may include range of movement, strength and/or precision

Table 6.4 A summary of a detailed activity analysis model

Analysis area	Summary of demands	Analysis area	Summary of demands
Motor/physical			
Position	• of individual and/or activity • does position of both/either change during the activity or not?	Problem-solving	• reasoning • abstract thinking and imagery • decision-making • planning
Movement	• joints involved • range of movement required • specific movements and ranges required • bilateral/unilateral • speed/rhythm	Logical thinking	• concrete/abstract thought • initiating action from thought processes
		Communication	• verbal • non-verbal • relevance of senses
Grading	• range of movement • strength and/or precision required • resistance • endurance • discomfort levels	Organisational ability	• in relation to cognition above
		Perceptual	
Sensory		Agnosia	• non-recognition of familiar objects
Visual	• figure/ground discrimination • spatial awareness • appreciation of form, colour, tone	Apraxia	• loss of ability to perform previously learned task
		Spatial relationship disorders	• relating to figure/ground, form constancy, depth/distance perception
Auditory	• language • cues • selective attention	Self-awareness disorders	• relating to body scheme, unilateral neglect
Olfactory	• relevance in certain activities and environments • compensation for absence of other senses	*Emotional* Activity demands/ offers	• e.g. inventiveness, gratification, expression of mood, exploration of feelings, impulse control, coping with feelings/emotion
Gustatory	• relevance in certain activities • stimulus/pleasure/interest		
Tactile/kinaesthetic	• temperature • texture discrimination • sensations of movement • body awareness	*Social* Activity demands/ offers	• e.g. interaction, communication, cooperation/sharing, competition, role-play
Cognitive		*Independence*	
Motivation	• interest/fun • achievement potential • individual-directed activity	Activity demands/ offers	• opportunity to examine ability to plan, organise, use initiative, make decisions
Learning	• memory • information retention • transfer of learning • attention/concentration span • numeracy/literacy	*Cultural* Activity demands/ offers	• cultural appropriateness in terms of values, roles, life-style

required, resistance offered, coordination necessary, endurance (for example, standing for extended periods of activity) and discomfort level.

Sensory demands

These relate to the sensory and perceptual qualities of an activity and should be considered in terms of sensorimotor integration and proprioception as well as the function of individual senses. All five senses should be considered:

• visual, for example appreciation of form, colour, tone.
• auditory, including comprehension of language, use of auditory cues, use of selective attention.

Table 6.5 Motor and sensory activity demands for a biomechanical and neurodevelopmental approach to intervention

Biomechanical	Neurodevelopmental
Deals with joint range, muscle strength and endurance. Full voluntary control of movement is usually present.	Used in relation to developmental and upper motor neurone disorders and other conditions with neurological deficit, e.g. CVA. Individual may no longer have full control of voluntary movement. Loss of voluntary movement may result from changed muscle tone and/or re-emergence of primitive reflexes. Equilibrium reactions and sensation may be impaired.
Prerequisite of activities used in this approach: movement needed must occur often enough to be therapeutic, and must facilitate grading to maintain pace with person's progress.	The nature of activity and the responses it elicits must be analysed in conjuction with the development sequence of learned movement at the appropriate level for the individual; for example, head control is necessary prior to undertaking activity in a sitting position.
Consider: Position of individual in relation to activity — position must be maintained to effect required treatment outcome Which joints are used? Range of movement through which joints move Which muscle groups are involved? Type of muscle work — eccentric, concentric, static? Degree of muscle strength involved/required Resistance offered Repetition and frequency of movement(s) Degree of coordination required Endurance/stamina required	*Consider:* Does activity encourage control of righting and equilibrium responses? Does it encourage normal/abnormal movement patterns? Does it provide stability/mobility at specified joints depending on the developmental sequence required? What sensory feedback does the activity provide (for example: proprioception, touch sensation), facilitating the learning/relearning of functional movement through sensory feedback?

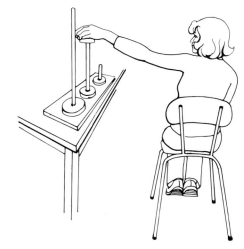

Fig. 6.8 Positioning should facilitate specific movements required, for example shoulder abduction.

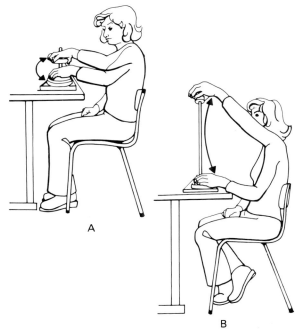

Fig. 6.9 Shoulder flexion. (A) Using a standard span game. (B) Increasing flexion with lengthened dowel rods.

- olfactory — often overlooked but appropriate in home care, workshop and community activities and skills. In addition to offering pleasure, for example in cooking spicy foods, it may alert an individual to potential danger

and it may become a well-developed sense in those with impaired vision.

- gustatory/taste — also frequently overlooked but particularly important for people with severe disability and for whom mealtimes can

be a source of pleasure as well as nourishment. As mentioned above, food can provide a much-needed stimulus and in this case the tasting of food in preparation as well as eating the completed dish can offer interest and pleasure to the cook and to others invited to participate.
- tactile/kinaesthetic — includes temperature and texture differentiation, degrees of touch (light, firm), body awareness and sensations of movement.

Cognitive demands

These concern the level of function the activity requires in relation to:

- motivation — whether the activity promotes interest, fun, potential achievement (see Fig. 3.9); whether the individual perceives it as relevant; whether he is self-directed in performing the activity
- learning-level(s) required — use of memory (short-term, long-term or both); retention of information regarding procedures, stages and changes; transfer of learning; concentration and attention span; numeracy and literacy
- problem-solving — use of reasoning, abstract thought and imagery; judgement and/or decision-making; planning versus trial and error
- logical thinking — concrete and abstract thought; use of imagery; initiation of action from thought processes
- communication — verbal (including written); non-verbal (simple and complex); relevance of hearing and vision
- perception — may be included in cognitive demands or dealt with separately. See Perceptual demands, below.
- organisational ability in relation to all the elements enumerated above.

Perceptual demands

Difficulties with sensory integration can be grouped as follows (see also Chs 16, 17):

- agnosia — inability to recognise familiar objects; can be visual, auditory or tactile
- apraxia — the loss of ability to perform a previously learned task although the motor power, sensation, coordination and comprehension required are retained
- spatial relationship disorders — relating to perception of figure/ground, position in space, form constancy, depth/distance
- self-awareness disorders — leading to uni-lateral neglect, distorted perception of body scheme.

Proprioceptive and stereognostic functions may be included within perception, but some practitioners consider this incorrect. However, it could be argued that as poor proprioception involves a loss of postural or position sense it ought to be considered alongside other general sensory and specific perceptual deficits. Stereognosis describes a person's ability to recognise items by touch; this too is a sensory input, the perceptual element being described by subsequent sensory integration (followed in normal function by motor output).

Emotional demands

Does the activity demand or offer opportunities for: inventiveness and originality; destructiveness/aggression; gratification; expression of a present mood, attitude, perception; exploration of feelings; structured or unstructured time; impulse control; independence or dependence; testing of reality; coping with feelings/emotions?

Social demands

What interaction is required? Is the activity undertaken alone, in a group, or both? What interaction with others is needed vis-à-vis: verbal communication, cooperation, dependence; sharing ideas, equipment, tools, materials; responsibility for others; consideration for needs and safety of co-workers; competition; testing reality; role-playing, e.g. leading, cooperating?

Independence

Does the activity offer the individual an opportunity to examine his ability to plan and organise, to use his initiative, to make decisions and to gradually relinquish dependence on others?

Cultural demands

The activity must be culturally appropriate in terms of values, roles and life circumstances. Some activities, for instance domestic tasks, may have underlying cultural assumptions rendering that activity unsuitable or inappropriate for some people.

Having analysed an activity in order to use it therapeutically the therapist must be an able teacher of the processes and procedures involved. If the individual is to benefit from the activity he must understand what he has to do, with minimum correction, and how and why he is doing it, particularly if he does not see its immediate relevance.

GRADING ACTIVITY

To what degree do the innate properties of any activity permit realistic adaptation relative to an individual's needs and personal style and to activity in the 'real world'?

Whilst it is recognised that activity needs a sequence or routine for successful achievement, it must also possess a structure which facilitates the learning of skills beyond those currently possessed by the individual. An activity must stimulate and sustain eagerness and the will to learn. As well as being relevant and practical it must also be versatile, i.e. lend itself to a variety of processes, end products and environments, and be adaptable to individuals, their needs and environments.

Some activities have more potential for modification than others. The therapist must use her own judgement and ingenuity in deciding when and how it is necessary to change from one activity to another or when to grade or adapt an activity to meet individual needs. She must remember that all activities utilised need to be adjustable so that, with the individual's improvement or deterioration, they can be adapted to suit his maximum capability.

Grading methods

Whatever grading methods she uses, the therapist must adhere to the following rules:

- The activity must foster and maintain a good working posture and position
- The individual should know and understand why he is required to perform an activity in a way which may differ from the norm
- The therapist must ensure that adaptations secure a positive rather than a negative effect on the individual
- The therapist must consider the time required for modification and maintenance of adapted activities.

Additionally, the therapist should decide whether any grading method is activity-centred, in which case the task itself is graded to meet a particular need, or person-centred, in which case the individual's position, cognitive process and so on are 'graded'.

Adaptation

Trends or fashions come and go with respect to activity adaptation (Fig. 6.10) and depend upon a number of factors, such as the personal preference of the therapist, priorities in treatment, the types of problems an individual is experiencing, the therapy service itself and where it is based. Whether the adaptation of an activity relates to a specific skill or to the modification of the environment in which the task takes place, it must meet the specific needs of the individual. It must be simple, both for the individual to manage and for the therapist to implement (Fig. 6.11). It must maintain the value of the activity for the person, i.e. focus on the activity rather than on the movements or processes involved.

Grading

Activities are paced and modified to meet immediate needs — the individual's maximum current capacity. A variety of grading methods are used if the required movements, resistance, creativity and so on are not obtained when an activity

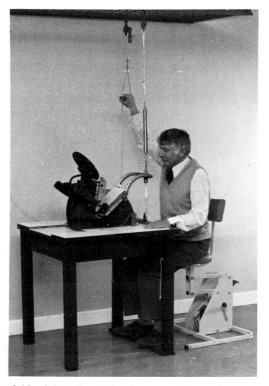

Fig. 6.10 Adaptation to hand-press printing using a rope and pulley circuit to increase the range of movement at the shoulder joint.

is performed in its usual manner. For example, if injury to an individual's hand prevents him from gripping a saw, the saw handle may be enlarged so that he can grasp it sufficiently to perform the correct actions in safety. This enlargement will be decreased as his grip improves.

The following elements may be of importance in the grading of activity:

● *Resistance.* In order to strengthen affected muscles or muscle groups, assisted gravity may be decreased gradually; thus weights and spring resistance may be added to selected tasks so that the individual has to overcome the resistance in order to complete the activity — adapted circuits for hand-press printing illustrate this well. The person may use heavier equipment or tools, e.g. moving from a light plane to a surform. Textures of materials may be modified to offer greater resistance; for example, the person may be given harder wood to work with, cutting with the grain initially and then against the grain.

● *Endurance/tolerance to activity.* This requires careful gradation. The therapist may use light work initially, grading the individual's programme until he can manage heavy work appropriate to his needs. The length of time spent on a particular activity can be increased, as can the number of

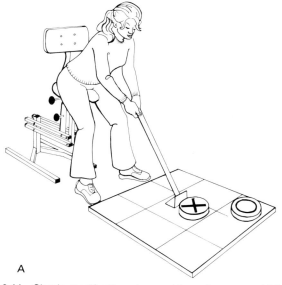

A

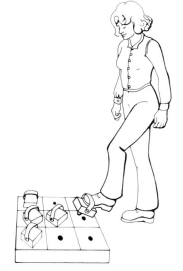

B

Fig. 6.11 Simple modifications to noughts and crosses which, in this example, enhance balance (A) in the early stages and (B) in the later stages.

sessions per week. These latter elements are of particular relevance for individuals whose work tolerance needs to be enhanced.

● *Organisation and integration of activities.* In terms of modifying and grading activity this includes:
— selection of appropriate activity based on needs, age, culture, environment and the individual's own goals
— structuring of activity in such a way as to render that activity therapeutic; the activity should include systematic learning stages, involve sequencing, and allow for modification, the monitoring of progress and the prioritising of goals
— timing of activities so that they are integrated into the individual's daily routine as soon as possible
— interaction between the therapist and individual, the therapist acting as a model of competence.

● *Techniques and tools.* The grading of these also relates to other elements. The 'how', or technique, of an activity must be integrated with the individual's physical and psychological needs; it must 'make sense' to him and interrelate with activities and situations in his environment. Tools encompass: equipment such as daily living aids, adjustable furniture, special crockery or orthoses; the environment, i.e. physical settings, people and objects of relevance to the individual. Tools and equipment, to a greater or lesser degree, will be important in the effective grading of activity for achievement and may be utilised temporarily, for example in the early stages of a programme, and then discarded as function improves.

● *Developmental grading.* This is relatively straightforward in that it adheres to the sequences of normal development; for example, the individual must be able to sit before he can stand, and stand before he can walk. This is of vital importance for people with neurological deficit who may have to relearn normal movement patterns.

● *Positioning.* This is of great importance throughout therapy but can also be utilised to a large extent in grading. The relative positions of the individual, the activity and its accessories can be modified to meet specific requirements, for ex-

ample by positioning paper for printing in such a way as to facilitate spinal rotation or extended reach. Positions will change as ranges of movement increase and joint function improves. Utilising vertical planes and horizontal positions for selected activity can add variety to a task; for example, placing a board game in the vertical plane may facilitate spinal side flexion, shoulder abduction and flexion and coordination.

● *Standing and walking tolerance.* These are vital elements of many individual programmes. The performance of many activities can offer: increases in the time spent standing; practice in transferring weight and balance; progression from static to mobile activity. The degree of physical support required can be decreased, e.g. by a gradual removal of trunk/pelvic supports and seats to facilitate a planned return to independent standing. The amount of walking in an activity can be increased, for example by encouraging free movement about the workshop to select tools and materials, or movement about the garden to select an activity.

● *Coordination and muscle control.* These are achieved primarily through increasing fine movements and decreasing gross ones. As a programme progresses the individual should undertake a large proportion of tasks requiring fine movement, control and coordination whilst gross movement decreases — even though it may not be eliminated from his schedule completely. If in his daily life the individual requires particular skills or unusual movement patterns, such as particular grasps used in handling large or awkward items, these should be introduced as soon as he can attempt them.

● *Dexterity.* Accompanied by *speed* when relevant, dexterity can also be upgraded. Timed activity related to particular objectives as well as tasks requiring greater manipulative skills will be utilised. Composing in printing, computer keyboard work and small table games provide the opportunity to practise fine movements, and speed and accuracy can be added dimensions which enhance potential to return to work. Where appropriate, skills can be transferred to other, more important tasks.

● *Complexity.* The very great variety of activities used in occupational therapy enables the individual and his therapist to select tasks requiring greater skill as his abilities increase. Activities with a large number of stages can be utilised. Printing, for example, involves a progression from a preliminary design to a finished article, thereby fulfilling not only physical needs, but providing opportunities for creativity, originality, achievement and feedback. If the individual has particular cognitive needs the complexity of activity must be developed to increase the demands on the individual. More demands can be made in a particular area of skill by adding more information to be remembered. Also, additional areas of cognitive function can be introduced, such as problem-solving and decision-making.

- *Social interaction.* The individual may begin by working alone, later sitting with one other person, and then with a small group. He might then begin to *work* with another person and, later, to participate in a small and then a larger group. To this type of grading can be added a number of additional functions, for example degrees of responsibility; expected interaction with one or more people; or initiation of a particular stage of the activity for the group.

Passive v. active participation

Passive involvement in activity requires no special effort by the individual, as in watching television or accepting a drink made by another person. Active participation, on the other hand, demands that he contribute. The individual's progress from passive to active involvement can be graded to meet developing needs, moving from straightforward and non-threatening activity which the individual wants to undertake to complex, challenging activity which he needs to be able to carry out in order to fulfil his chosen life-style and particular roles.

Creativity and spontaneity

Creativity and spontaneity are vital elements of the grading process and can be integrated with any of the other elements. The therapist should avoid stereotyped and structured activity when and where appropriate, stimulating the individual's creativity, self-expression, and originality and offering him the opportunity to plan, implement and review his selected actions.

Meaning and relevance

Finally, the meaning and relevance of activity and its grading or modification warrants particular attention. Any activity used in an individual's programme must be meaningful to him. It must relate to time and place and to his life-style. Activities must be acceptable to the individual and enable him to transfer his learning from one skill and environment to another. If activities have meaning then successful completion is more likely; in turn, success promotes the development of competence. The person's interest and involvement will be enhanced by feedback and once he is motivated by this process the therapist can facilitate further development and achievement. Additionally, the individual must be able to understand and interpret his improved function — for example, his greater range of movement or increased coordination; this is essential, as it leads him to perceive the psychological value of success and achievement.

Although the necessity for activity to be relevant or appropriate has been reiterated throughout this chapter, this requirement is so important that it warrants even further attention. Activity needs to be relevant for two key reasons:

1. In relation to personally determined attributes:
   - historical: past experience of activities and the attitudes, feelings and associations these offer
   - symbolic: the meaning of certain activities to the individual, including the process of completion and/or the end product
   - motivation and the variety of unconscious needs, drives and feelings the activity may satisfy
   - the new learning required and/or achieved
   - the retention of former skills or parts of those skills and their relevance now; for example, is it relevant that former skills be sequenced differently in order to achieve the required results?
   - the individual style of each person, his behaviour, his preferred ways, how he

may have modified these in the past to suit his environment

2. In relation to the socioculturally determined attributes of people, relationships, actions and objects which may be based on a person's age, sex, status (e.g. occupational, educational, socioeconomic), past roles, values and beliefs

— cultural background, including religious or ethnic elements and certain activities within this framework

— the history of social trends and attitudes with regard to certain activities in the person's sociocultural environment

— the relationship of activity or parts of activities to the person's current concepts of work, recreation and self-care

— the relationship of the above to other daily living activity and its potential for integration in terms of learning achievement.

The application of all or part of these grading methods may seem potentially complex. However, with practice the therapist masters the elements which are most applicable to her work ethic, environment and speciality and refers to the less frequently used elements when necessary.

ANALYSIS OF THREE ACTIVITIES

The analyses below aim to clarify the essential elements of three areas of activity, i.e. a daily living skill, a creative or work activity and an interpersonal skill.

Daily living skill

Making a hot drink: the purposes of using this activity therapeutically may include assessment of previously learned skills and behaviours; safety in the kitchen; specific cognitive function; specific sensorimotor skills; ability to meet a particular need. Table 6.6 is intended to assist the reader in understanding and applying an analysis of this activity.

Table 6.6 Analysis: making a hot drink. *Task*: To make a mug of coffee, with milk, in the kitchen. The individual is ambulant, upper limb function and senses are intact and all equipment and materials are available (cont'd overleaf)

Component	Demands		Component	Demands	
General factors	Motivation —	thirst, wish for coffee rather than alternative beverage			and maintenance of upright posture
	Relevance —	age appropriate, drinks coffee regularly, acceptable socioculturally, sex inapplicable in this instance, role as provider to self acceptable		Sensory —	proprioceptive awareness; coordination; visual sense to aid mobility
				Cognitive —	motivation (thirst); social; knowledge of activity and where it occurs; decision-making
	Time —	routine, habit	2. Assemble equipment and materials, i.e. kettle, mug, spoon, coffee, milk from cupboard(s), fridge, drawer, shelf	Motor —	walking, standing, balance, weight transfer, bending, reaching/stretching; lower and upper limbs involved in gross movements; upper limbs required to produce finer, skilled movements and grips, for example, lateral, spherical, cylindrical, hook, prehensile
	Risk —	aware of potential risk factors			
	Emotional —	gratification			
	Social —	coffee for two			
	Cultural —	coffee for visitor			
Stages 1. Enter kitchen	Motor —	walk independently; coordination; balance; weight transference; lower limb, pelvic and trunk joints and muscles to enable mobility, balance			

Table 6.6 Cont'd

Component	Demands		Component	Demands	
	Sensory —	coordination and proprioception, visual/tactile senses used in unison and independently		Cognitive —	appreciation of safety, sequencing, memory, concentration, organisation
	Cognitive —	memory and knowledge, logical and sequential thought, organisational skills		Perceptual —	spatial awareness, figure/ground form constancy; visual sense: praxis and gnosis, figure/ground discrimination, spatial awareness, appreciation of form, colour
	Perceptual —	spatial awareness, visual/tactile senses, figure/ground discrimination, praxis, gnosis	4. Putting coffee and milk into mug	As above plus:	
3. Filling the kettle, i.e. unplugging kettle, removing lid, moving kettle to sink, placing under tap, turning on tap, filling kettle, turning off tap, returning kettle to work-top, replacing lid, plugging in, switching on	Motor —	as above and moving in small area; upper limb movements: flexion and extension of joints, shoulder ab/adduction and rotation, forearm pronation/supination, various grips		Motor —	grips: prehensile, spherical, tripod
				Cognitive —	judgement/decision re quantities
				Perceptual —	stereognosis
			5. Making drink once kettle has boiled	As above plus:	
				Sensory —	olfactory
				Perceptual —	tactile/temperature
	Sensory —	coordination, particularly hand/eye; proprioception; tactile sense: degrees of touch, temperature and pressure, body awareness, sensation of movement; auditory sense	6. Drinking coffee	Motor —	mobility, coordination, sip and swallow
				Sensory —	thirst satisfied; olfactory, gustatory and tactile senses
				Emotional —	gratification
				Social —	communication, interaction and social skills

Creative or work activity

Composing type in printing: the therapist may use this particular element of the printing process to assess, enhance and reinforce cognitive function; specific sensorimotor function; use of tools/equipment; organisation; tolerance. Table 6.7 offers an analysis of this activity.

Interpersonal skill

Maintaining a relationship with a co-member of an educational group. Analysis of relationships and allied interpersonal skills may be deemed the province of therapists working with people whose primary problems relate to mental health dysfunc-

tion. This *is not* and *should not* be the case. Physical dysfunction of all degrees of severity may have some effect on an individual's motivation, interests, roles, values, routines and practical skills. Therefore, the therapist should master analysis of these potentially more nebulous areas of human behaviour and function. The analysis in Table 6.8 demonstrates the value such specific activity may offer.

Activity and treatment planning

The analysis of any activity is a prerequisite to the therapist's plan to assist an individual to overcome or manage his dysfunction. The analyses illus-

Table 6.7 General analysis of the demands of composing type. *Task*: To compose a line of type for printing. The individual is seated at a table which supports the type case and is holding the composing stick in his left hand

Component	Demands
General	Good eyesight Sitting balance and tolerance dependent on type of seat used and posture High degree of hand/eye coordination Concentration Literacy and numeracy Ability to follow written, verbal, diagrammatic instructions Memory Clarity of thought Ability to observe and correct errors Accuracy/responsibility Speed, if required Confidence in ability to accomplish task Patience/tolerance to frustration/perseverance Initiative
Holding the composing stick in left hand	Static muscle work: thumb opposition, IP and MCP joints, wrist, elbow, shoulder Ability to maintain static muscle work for required period of concentration/task completion
Selecting and picking up type with right hand	Pincer grip/release thumb and index finger tips in order to select type from case Sensation: degree required dependent on type size High degree of muscle control and coordination to transfer type from case to stick Range of movement required in other right upper limb joints dependent on position of type case, e.g. close, distant, to one side High degree of dexterity

trated above may be required before treating some people, but not all. For instance, the more complex a person's needs the more likely the requirement for attention to detail in activities in order to enhance abilities and to begin to address difficulties. If the therapist is working with an individual who has motor, cognitive, social and sensory deficits as the result of a head injury she may need to sub-divide tasks into component parts, whereas an individual recovering from repair to a severed tendon in his index finger will

usually participate in activity which is sub-divided into motor/physical components only.

The therapist's skills of analysis and her comprehension of activity in its broadest context enable her to define applicable and inapplicable activities and to modify them according to a person's needs. If, for example, a person needs to be able to make himself a hot drink during the course of the day and his dysfunction renders this difficult or impossible at the commencement of intervention, the therapist may initially use the activity as an assessment tool by which she can identify specific problem areas such as cognitive or hand-eye coordination deficits. Having established abilities and problems, the therapist can plan a programme of activity which offers means of overcoming the latter. She may, for example, change the method of performing an activity, use a different technique, reorganise the work area, modify the person's work position, introduce adapted equipment (e.g. tools that are lighter in weight or that have modified handles), suggest an aid to daily living or inject specific treatment to improve particular functions such as memory, coordination, sitting balance, or elbow flexion and extension (see p. 59).

Analyses such as those described will enable the therapist to select activities relevant to a particular individual. In summary, she will carry out the following procedure:

1. Assessment of the person, acknowledging his abilities and identifying his needs
2. Selection of a treatment approach
3. Selection of specific activities matching the individual's abilities, needs, interests, roles and values to activities which have been analysed and evaluated as offering or demanding certain skills such as perseverance, social interaction, hand/eye coordination and problem-solving.

CONCLUSION

The opening paragraphs of this chapter summarise the philosophy of occupational therapy as being founded on the therapeutic use of activity and

Table 6.8 Analysis of a relationship with a co-member of an educational group. *Task*: Identify the relationship and allied interpersonal skills required in an educational group, i.e. living with disability (carers and individuals)

Component	Demands	Component	Demands
General factors		*Specific factors*	
Environment	Suitability for specific needs and purposes of group, including its relevance for programme elements, proximity to other essential facilities, accessibility, comfort, conduciveness to positive group dynamics, value given to it by members, appropriateness of space/equipment, social and cultural acceptability	Motor	What are the specific motor demands? Programme elements may include: safe mobility, handling and moving skills, seating, positioning for particular activities, accessing venue/facilities
Motivation	Facilitation of personal effectiveness including ability (potential/actual) to manage physical, psychological, social and emotional stresses. Programme elements related to interests, values, quality of life, needs, roles (changes, reversal, routines, caring)	Sensory	What are the specific sensory demands? The senses: — visual, eye contact within group, spatial awareness/personal space, need to see for programme elements — auditory, comprehension of language, use of auditory clues, selective attention
Relevance	Programme composition meets age, sex, perceived/identified needs of group members. Orientated to men and women in content and presentation, taking account of sociocultural backgrounds of members		— tactile, spatial awareness, physical touch — olfactory and gustatory, depends on activities but includes refreshments
Vocational applicability	Identified needs include work as a carer, paid employment, leisure interests and skills, home care routines, work-related relationships including communication, roles	Cognitive	Motivation — induces group interest; potential achievement and management of dysfunction and associated problems; group directs programme content Learning — new skills: methods, techniques, activities; transfer of and retention of learning; requires concentration
Cost	Financial implications for group members and facilitators: venue, equipment, materials, speakers Time commitment required by group members and facilitators Future cost implications for individuals to be considered		Problem-solving — logical thinking, reasoning, planning; making choices and decisions actively encouraged Communication — all members encouraged to contribute verbally and non-verbally; specific help available for those with communication handicaps Organisational skills — members control and run group with committee who plan programme
Risks	Programme includes 'living with risk'. Also implications of risks of working with (initially) a group of strangers — trust, honesty, objectivity; physical elements of risk and safety		
Time	Efficient and effective use of time allocated and/or available Group meetings timed to suit members (rather than facilitators) Sufficient time to meet needs and complete programme/series of group meetings	Perceptual	What specific perceptual demands are made? Spatial awareness, appropriate utilisation of senses, perceptions of group dynamics and group objectives
Effectiveness in imparting information	Media used appropriate to group members: language, pace, assumed knowledge level, concentration/attention span. Do the media used facilitate the individual's active participation?	Emotional	Group offers and demands: inventiveness, honesty, gratification, communication, trust, objectivity, display of positive attitudes to fellow members and group purpose, choice. Enables exploration of feelings regarding disability, society, group

Table 6.8 Cont'd

Component	Demands	Component	Demands
Social	Interaction level decided by group with expectation that level will increase within group setting and programme Communication essential in self-help environment and includes cooperation, sharing, taking responsibility		organise with carer; to take decisions on own initiative
		Cultural	Programme flexibility planned by group members taking account of each member's cultural needs as well as individual beliefs, values, roles and circumstances in a mixed socio-economic group membership
Independence	Offers opportunities to analyse own abilities and needs in relation to independent living; to plan and		

on the belief that the performance of activity promotes and enhances physical and mental health. Occupational therapists believe that dysfunction can be modified, changed and reversed through activity. Such activity enables an individual to direct his time, energy, attention and interest productively and in such a way as to offer him opportunities for learning, development and satisfaction.

The analysis of activity which contributes to the productivity and satisfaction of any individual offers the therapist scope to identify how activity may motivate the individual, assist him in organising skills, behaviours and routines and make a contribution to role and task balance.

Analysis also indicates the flexibility, simplicity/complexity and relevance of a task, and enables the therapist to design an effective treatment programme which, building on a person's existing abilities, helps him to achieve the desired results.

The occupational therapist's knowledge and application of the therapeutic use of activity is enhanced through activity analysis. Any activity used in an individual's programme must have certain qualities to enable him to learn, explore, experiment and achieve. These qualities are discovered through thorough analysis of activities which have a wide range of potential as therapeutic media.

REFERENCES

Cynkin S 1979 Occupational therapy: toward health through activities. Little, Brown, Boston
Cynkin S, Robinson A M 1990 Occupational therapy and activities health: toward health through activities. Little, Brown, Boston
Finlay L 1987 Occupational therapy practice in psychiatry. Croom Helm, London

Hopkins H L, Smith H D 1988 Willard and Spackman's occupational therapy, 7th edn. J B Lippincott, Philadelphia
Kielhofner G (ed) 1985 A model of human occupation: theory and application. Williams and Wilkins, Baltimore

FURTHER READING

Allen C K 1987 Activity: Occupational therapy's treatment method. American Journal of Occupational Therapy 41(9): 563–575
Hume C, Pullen I 1986 Rehabilitation in psychiatry. Churchill Livingstone, Edinburgh
Pedretti L W 1990 Occupational therapy: practice skills for physical dysfunction. C V Mosby, St Louis, MO

Willson M 1983 Occupational therapy in long-term psychiatry. Churchill Livingstone, Edinburgh
Willson M 1984 Occupational therapy in short-term psychiatry. Churchill Livingstone, Edinburgh

7

Assessment

Margaret Foster

INTRODUCTION

Definition

Assessment can be thought of as occurring whenever one person, in some kind of interaction, direct or indirect, with another, is conscious of obtaining and interpreting information about the knowledge and understanding, or abilities and attitudes of that other person.

(Derek Rowntree 1987)

Assessment is a conscious task. This means that the assessor must be aware of the process during the performance of the assessment. If this is not so, it is merely a casual observation and will be dependent on the memory of the assessor, who may overlook vital information surrounding the item observed.

The process of assessment is not confined to the gathering of the data, but is dependent upon its interpretation and evaluation. The therapist when performing an assessment must therefore:

- be aware of the task of the assessment
- have the ability and tools to elicit the relevant data
- have the skill to analyse and interpret the findings correctly.

This final stage is vitally important if the assessment is to be purposeful and meaningful and not just a collection of information. The interpretation and analysis will be dependent on:

- the therapist's own knowledge base
- her understanding of the assessment procedures and their correct performance
- her ability to objectively analyse the information gathered, without bias or prejudice
- her ability to apply the findings to the particular needs or circumstances of the individual.

Rowntree's definition states that assessment may be a direct or indirect action. In occupational therapy the majority of information is usually gained through a direct interview or a specific performance measurement. However, some assessment data may be gained as a result of other sources of information which may not involve direct contact with the individual, for example, through the case notes or an interview with another member of the care team. Whilst valuing such additional sources of information, care should be taken to ensure others' opinions do not bias or prejudice the occupational therapist in her attitudes to, or assessment of the individual.

The definition also outlines the nature of the areas of assessment. Knowledge and understanding are familiar areas of assessment. We have all experienced these in the educational field in school examinations. In occupational therapy these areas also commonly need to be assessed to determine an individual's knowledge and understanding of his disability, his understanding of needs, or his knowledge and understanding of the occupational therapist's role and the purpose of the activity chosen. This area may be assessed through interview and questioning. Some information concerning knowledge and understanding may also be gained through observation of the person's non-verbal cues.

Abilities are more commonly assessed through practical or functional task performance tests. This may involve the person's physical capabilities, perceptual abilities or cognitive skills. It is important for the therapist to have a range of practical tests in order to identify the particular abilities or deficits accurately for each individual, as many tasks require a combination of motor, perceptual and cognitive skills in their successful completion.

Attitudinal assessments are most commonly carried out through verbal interchange or observation. This may be in direct interchange between the therapist and the interviewee or it may be through observation of the interchange between the interviewee and others, for example in a discussion group or activity group. Attitudes may also be assessed in individual task performance through identifying how the individual applies himself to the task, whether conscientious or slapdash practices are used, and how the individual perceives the outcome of the task.

This chapter aims to identify the reasons for assessment and the different types, to alert the reader to the stages of the assessment process, and to identify some of the areas and practices of assessment in occupational therapy.

TYPES OF ASSESSMENT

Baseline assessment

This assessment aims to determine a baseline of information regarding the present skills of the person, the difficulties and limitations he encounters and the aspirations and needs of him and his carers, from which realistic aims, objectives and goals can be determined.

It may be carried out at an early stage of contact to gain an overall picture, or it may be necessary to undertake a baseline assessment for a specific reason within a programme if a particular skill or group of skills is being investigated. For example, a person may have had contact with the occupational therapist for some time, practising daily living skills or organising home modifications, but a baseline work assessment may still need to be carried out when the person wishes to consider returning to or taking up employment.

Progress assessment

Progress assessment should be ongoing throughout a programme to determine the degree of change. From this may be gauged the effectiveness of the activity to meet the aims, objectives and goals set. The findings may ascertain the realism of the decisions made from the baseline assessment and the need for adjustment of the programme or plans. This may result in a minor change of activity to reflect the lack of success or a quicker recovery than expected, or there may be a major change in emphasis to meet an unplanned or unanticipated demand from the person or his carer.

Specific assessment

Occupational therapists are sometimes asked to complete specific assessments when they may not in fact be involved with the individual in further therapeutic contact. There are a number of instances where this may occur, for example assessment of a handicapped child for the purposes of reporting for a 'Statement of Education'. Similarly, an occupational therapist may be asked to assess a person to determine whether proposed surgery may benefit the individual's functional capabilities, as in the case of rheumatoid or osteoarthritis. The therapist may also be required to give evidence of the level of a person's functional ability where compensation for disability is being claimed, for example following an injury at work, a road traffic accident or for a brain damaged child.

Final assessment

A final assessment is usually carried out at the end of a period of contact between the individual and the therapist with a view to discharge. This assessment aims to determine how far the aims and objectives have been achieved, and any residual problems or needs which should be noted for future reference or referral to other personnel or agencies. The final assessment is a particularly valuable record if a person is re-referred to occupational therapy at a later date.

Follow-up assessment

Occasionally the occupational therapist may be required to carry out a follow-up assessment, which aims to establish that progress has been maintained and that there is no immediate need for further therapy intervention. It is particularly appropriate where a person is expected to continue to make a slow improvement which does not necessitate regular therapy contact, for example in the later stages following a stroke or head injury. Such follow-up assessments may be monthly, 3 monthly, biannually or annually to monitor progress or possible deterioration. They may be necessary because of a change in circumstances for an individual with whom the therapist has had prior contact, for example a handicapped child moving to a new school, or a person with a progressive condition who has been using a major item of equipment for some time, or whose carer has changed.

In all forms of assessment it is vital that the assessment methods are appropriate, thorough and accurate and that clear, concise records and reports are made and maintained.

THE ASSESSMENT PROCESS

PRELIMINARIES

The referral source

Whether employed in the community, in social services, voluntary organisations, in the private sector, or within the hospital, the therapist may obtain the referral in a number of ways from a number of sources.

From other medical personnel

In the community the therapist frequently receives referrals from other members of the team. They may be from the person's general practitioner, the health visitor, community nurse, home help or social worker to name but a few, and the level of information received will therefore vary considerably according to that person's knowledge of and involvement with the individual and occupational therapist.

In hospital the therapist may similarly receive referrals from a variety of personnel. Other members of the paramedical team, i.e. the physiotherapist, speech therapist or social worker, may identify a need for occupational therapy. In some instances, especially in wards where the majority of residents would benefit from occupational therapy, a 'blanket referral' system may operate. In this instance the occupational therapist has permission to commence treatment with any of the residents when she feels it necessary without having to notify the doctor and gain his permission in each individual case.

It is important for the occupational therapist in all areas of practice to have access to the medical practitioner with overall responsibility for the individual.

The British Association of Occupational Therapists (1990) Code of Ethics and Professional Conduct states that 'Occupational therapists shall undertake treatment either when the consumer has been referred by a medical practitioner or where occupational therapists have access to the consumer's doctor. Blanket referral systems are appropriate, provided medical clinicians are fully aware that this system exists'.

From the general public

In the community the occupational therapist may receive the referral from a member of the public. Requests may be made by the individual himself, or by the family, carers, neighbours or friends. In most instances the referral is with the approval and knowledge of the person concerned but this is not always the case.

From clinics

In hospital it is common for referrals to be received from outpatient clinics, particularly those concerned with rheumatology, neurology, physical medicine or orthopaedic disorders. These referrals may not necessarily be from the directions of the doctor or consultant. In some instances the occupational therapist may attend the clinic to receive direct information on the person referred. If this is not possible it is important to ensure that those in charge in the clinic have a clear understanding of the role of the therapist and the facilities available. Although proportionately fewer referrals in the community are received from clinics, some may be initiated from chiropody, speech therapy or possibly such sources as 'Age Well' clinics.

From case conferences

In many places case conferences have replaced the rigid formal ward rounds because they give the opportunity for fuller discussion in a less threatening environment for the person concerned. Medical and paramedical staff may attend the conference and it is not uncommon for the person concerned and his relatives or carers to be present and contribute equally. These conferences may take place in the hospital setting or in the community and are a common aspect of the social services procedure in many areas. For those with special needs, educational or employment case conferences form part of the programme planning process and the occupational therapist may contribute to such conferences or receive referrals from them.

From ward rounds

Ward rounds are most frequently conducted by the consultant, the team of doctors and the ward sister/charge nurse responsible for the ward. Other paramedical personnel involved with the ward residents may attend. During attendance at such rounds it is possible to gain information about people to be referred and to report on those whom the therapist has already seen. If the therapist is not present at the ward round, she may still receive referrals from this source, if those conducting the round are familiar with the occupational therapist's role.

The method of referral

Occupational therapists may receive either written or verbal referrals, but when there is no formal written referral it is important that formal documentation is completed for the records. This may not necessarily be completed by the person making the referral.

In many departments there are specifically designed occupational therapy referral forms. These vary considerably in design and the amount of information requested. Such forms may be available in the wards, clinics or departments in the hospital, or in the health clinics or general practice centres in the community.

When a written referral is received by other means, for example a letter from a doctor, or a relative, or an entry in a person's case notes, the occupational therapist will usually complete the referral form herself, attaching a letter of referral to it.

If a verbal referral is received, it is also usual to complete a written form, either at the time of the verbal referral, which may be by telephone, or at the initial interview. In some instances, particularly in social services, the referral may not initially be received by the occupational therapist, but may be passed to the intake/duty officer for the day, who may be a therapist or a social worker, for later re-direction.

However, by whatever means the referral is received, certain information is essential. This information will include:

- The person's full name, both surname and forenames
- The full address *where the person may be seen*. Confusion may arise if the home address is given and the person is staying with relatives. If he is resident in hospital, the ward and the hospital record number would be given. The latter will enable the therapist to accurately locate the case notes
- The date of birth
- The consultant/doctor responsible for the person referred
- The date of the referral
- The diagnosis and/or presenting problems and any secondary complications or diagnoses. This is the ideal. However, particularly in a lay person's referral in the community, the diagnosis may not be known and the therapist has then to ascertain this information from any other persons involved, for example the general practitioner, and the initial visit
- The name of the person initiating the referral.

Other useful information will include:

- The persons' religion

- The person's marital status
- The person's next of kin
- A specific reason for referral. This may give some indication of the specific expectations of the therapist but may not in itself be definitive; for example a request may be received for a person who is having difficulty standing up from his easy chair. While this may be so, there may also be many other related mobility problems concerning stepping in and out of the bed or the bath, or going up and downstairs or getting in and out of a car
- The person's occupation. This may be appropriate if the person is of employable age and wishes to return to work. It will also give the therapist an indication of previous functional levels
- School age/pre-school age . . . school attended.

Making contact

It is essential that a good working relationship is established between the person and the therapist if the contact is to be successful. This does not always occur immediately but the first meeting is vitally important as initial impressions tend to colour opinions, and too formal or too casual an approach can hinder the development of a therapeutic relationship. A good relationship will lead to mutual trust so that all parties can feel at ease in future contacts. In some cases it may be advisable to see the person only briefly prior to the first full assessment because:

- the person's situation is not appropriate to carry out the initial assessment. He may be awaiting a meal, a visitor, transport or another treatment — or he may be too unwell — or the venue of the initial contact may not be appropriate, for example a busy clinic or day room.
- the therapist may not be prepared — she may not have the relevant information or be in the middle of a treatment session when she first meets the person. However, in this instance the therapist should introduce

herself clearly and explain the purpose of the proposed interview and how she hopes to help, especially as occupational therapy is a frequently misunderstood label. The therapist should explain the format of the interview and a further appointment should be made. A written explanation of the interview and the date, together with a contact point for the therapist, should be given to the person as a reminder, or to assist him to explain to others. He may also use this to contact the therapist in the event of illness, transport problems or unanticipated inconvenience of the date/time proposed.

The initial interview preparation

The purpose of this interview is threefold. To be successful both the therapist and the interviewee will be required to:

● give information
● receive information
● establish a rapport.

In order to facilitate this, various factors need to be considered.

The venue of the interview

The therapist should remember that most people feel more relaxed and secure if approached on their 'own ground'. If this is not possible, the familiar surroundings of the bedside or a quiet corner of the day centre and day room will usually be better than a strange department or office. The venue should be as quiet and private as possible so that both parties feel free to ask and answer questions.

Positioning

The therapist should ensure that the person is secure and comfortable and does not feel hemmed in, by respecting 'personal space' and not sitting so close that the interviewee feels threatened. The interviewee should be at the same level as the therapist so either person can take the initiative to make or break eye contact. The therapist should

not dominate the interview by standing over him, neither should she lurk behind a large untidy desk with books and telephones creating a barrier to free exchange of information (Fig. 7.1).

Understanding the purpose of the interview

It is vital that both parties clearly understand the reason for the interview. The therapist must know what information she aims to gain from the interview to help her plan further action, and she should ask the appropriate questions to gain this knowledge. The interviewee should understand the reason for referral and the role of the therapist. This may need frequent reiteration by the therapist as interviewees are often confused about the many and varied roles of the host of members of the multidisciplinary team involved with one person. Equally, opportunity should be given for the interviewee to express anticipations or anxieties regarding the outcome of the interview to ensure that they are realistic and not threatening; for example he may envisage complete recovery from a deteriorating condition, or fear admission to a home or the provision of an unwanted wheelchair or home care aid. Such hidden agendas can inhibit free exchange of information and lead to future misinterpretation or mistrust.

The therapist's presentation

The therapist should be neat, tidy, well prepared and unhurried. She should have read any relevant notes and organised the interview at an appropriate time in the person's daily routine. The therapist should be aware of any communication problems such as deafness or language barriers, and take the necessary steps to overcome them. She should also be familiar with the clinical features of the diagnosis and any other routine treatments. She should be able to address the person by name, have any information about the referral to hand, have any assessment equipment prepared and be prompt. The therapist should show empathy, i.e. understanding without over-involvement. This may be shown through:

● her listening and observation skills

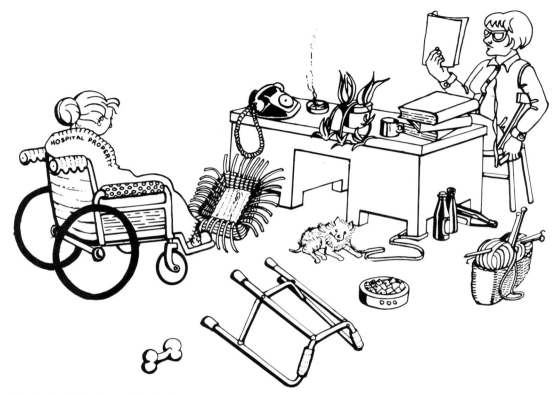

Fig. 7.1 Lurks behind an untidy desk . . . .

- her questioning skills
- her recording method
- her social skills.

Listening and observation skills consist of allowing the interviewee time to express himself and maintaining a positive regard for him. Observation of non-verbal communication is especially important as this may more accurately reflect true responses than the spoken reply. When relatives or carers are present the therapist may have to maintain a balance diplomatically, between respecting their responses and ensuring the interviewee's true wishes or views are noted. She should observe the interviewee's non-verbal cues to the carers' responses. If there is a conflict, she should clarify this by asking the interviewee if there is agreement with the carer and listening carefully to his verbal response while observing the non-verbal cues.

Questioning skills. Using language and ter-

minology which the interviewee understands and asking pertinent questions relevant to the situation are an indication of the therapist's awareness of potential problems and her sound professional knowledge base. Care should be taken to ascertain the interviewee's understanding of his condition and his attitude to it. The therapist should never assume the interviewee is aware of his diagnosis; so such shocked responses as 'Well, the doctor didn't tell me I had multiple sclerosis' or 'Do you mean Billy is a spastic?' are avoided. The therapist should offer the interviewee (and the carer if appropriate) the opportunity to reveal his knowledge of and attitude to his condition by asking, for example, 'How long have you had difficulty walking?' This may disclose an open 'Well the doctor told me last month I have multiple sclerosis but I'd had my suspicions for a year or so' or 'It's been awkward for a month or two, but it's getting better and I'll soon be fully recovered.'

Questions should be clear and concise and free

of ambiguity. They should be delivered in a natural tone which is neither demanding nor patronising. Where possible, open questions should be used which encourage the interviewee to explain or elaborate, as these will yield more information than those requiring a 'yes' or 'no' answer.

Recording method. Most therapists prefer to make notes during the interview, but there should be a balance between writing and paying visual attention to the interviewee. A clear explanation of the need for notes to ensure that the record is accurate should be given to the interviewee. The opportunity for him to either read the notes or agree them verbally with the therapist allays any anxiety concerning their content. Accurate notes and records will enable the interviewee and therapist to plan the outcome of the interview, and will provide a sound baseline from which to measure progress.

Social skills. In most situations the therapist is the interviewee's 'guest'. Whether she is interrupting the interviewee's conversation with a person in the next chair or bed when visiting him on the ward or making a home visit as a guest, she should observe the normal social graces of introducing herself, asking permission to handle an injured limb or measure a toilet height, and thanking the interviewee at the end of the contact.

METHODS OF ASSESSMENT

The following methods of assessment are described in detail:

- interview
- observation
- specific tests
- physical measurement
- self-evaluation.

The interview

Much has already been said regarding the venue of the interview, the understanding of its purpose by both parties and the presentation skills of the therapist. This method of assessment has the advantage of sufficient possible flexibility of content to be appropriate in the majority of situations and enables the therapist to give information, receive information and begin to establish a rapport. In order for the interview to be successful the therapist should respect normal interview progression — the opening of the interview, its development and the method of closing or terminating the interview.

In the opening, following introductions, the therapist should define the reason for the interview, the type of information to be discussed, the time it is likely to take and the use to which the information will be put.

As the interview develops, the nature of the content will depend on the initial purpose. This may be a need to investigate a particular area of difficulty which will be explored in detail, or the interview may aim to cover a range of topics to compile a total picture of the individual's circumstances. The therapist should be aware that the first interview may be an emotional experience for the interviewee as this may be the first occasion he has been asked to face the facts of his situation, let alone share them with the therapist. She must be prepared for emotional outbursts such as crying or aggression which may result from the frustration of adjustment to a residual disability or limitation, or anger at himself or towards the professionals with whose help he expected to achieve a complete recovery. Interviewees may respond unrealistically to some questions, either because they are too embarrassed to acknowledge the problem which they consider to be of a particularly private nature, or because they overrate their skills and are genuinely unwilling to accept the situation. The therapist should endeavour to use her knowledge, her awareness of non-verbal communication and her observation skills to identify such discrepancies, and either raise the topic again at a later time when the interviewee appears more relaxed or check the verbal assurance of ability with an appropriate functional assessment.

The therapist should recognise signs of distress and respect these by (a) allowing the interviewee to share concerns, or, if he does not wish to do so at this time, by (b) giving him the opportunity to continue the interview and discussing another topic, or by (c) terminating the interview. It may be necessary to terminate an interview early if the interviewee is showing signs of fatigue. Over-running the pre-arranged time should be avoided, especially in the initial interview.

The therapist or interviewee may bring the interview to a close. Summarising the topics which have been covered is an accepted way of concluding it. This acts as a check on the information shared during the interview and indicates that both parties have understood the points made. Unless there is a particularly urgent item which has not been addressed, new information should not be introduced at this stage, but a further interview date should be arranged. The interview should be concluded by the participants making shared decisions regarding priorities from the topics already discussed, and identifying the date and format of a further appointment. Occasionally it may be possible to make firm decisions and recommendations from the initial interview, but it is more usual for a number of options to be considered by both parties; or a further form of assessment may be necessary to ensure that the aims and goals are accurate, appropriate and achievable.

Observation

Observation in the formal interview has already been considered. The skills of successful observation are based on the therapist's ability to listen well and to identify relevant observations from the surrounding information. Observation may be an appropriate part of assessment in structured situations, such as the performance of a particular functional task, or in less formal situations, such as having a meal on the ward or talking with a member of the family in the home.

Verbal responses

People communicate in different ways in different situations. Short, terse comments or over-wordy responses may both be signs of anxiety. Only through observation of other non-verbal cues can these verbal responses be categorised as normal for the individual, or indicative of the tension of the situation. The tone of the response may also indicate the emotions or attitudes of the speaker. Similarly, the choice of words may be an indi-cation of the level of cognitive ability, emotion or culture.

Non-verbal cues

Observation of body language and non-verbal responses is equally important. Frequently these embellish the verbal or written responses, but when they contradict each other it is frequently the non-verbal cues which give a more reliable picture of the true response. Non-verbal cues may also indicate mood, cognition or behavioural patterns which may influence the subsequent success of the therapeutic relationship and activity programme.

When observing performance the therapist should consider both the process and the product. In addition to noting the person's physical capabilities in terms of function, the therapist may observe the attitudinal and behavioural factors through the way the task is approached. Facial expression and posture may indicate pain or discomfort, whilst attention to detail and the standard of performance may demonstrate the individual's values. The willingness or hesitancy to participate may be a measure of interest in the activity, personal volition or level of confidence in performance.

Interpretation of observations

Objectivity in observation is based on the therapist's knowledge of the biological and clinical features of the impairment. A child with cerebral palsy may knock over a cup, which could be misinterpreted as naughtiness rather than lack of muscle control by the uninformed observer. An understanding of the behavioural sciences will help a therapist interpret her observations, not only when analysing non-verbal responses, but also in acknowledging the influence of personality, culture and life roles on performance. Recognition by the therapist of her own interpersonal skills and ways of communicating will enable her to more fully understand her observations of others.

It is vital to consider the observations in the context of the situation and the environment. These external circumstances may alter the person's usual behaviour, both in practical performance and in the tone of the responses. Past experiences in similar environments may also influence responses. This frequently occurs in formal clinical situations where the normally relaxed outgoing person may become anxious and hesitant. Environmental influences may also affect the therapist. Her familiarity with the situation and the routine of the assessment may lead her to anticipate the response in the light of previous assessment experience. She may be at risk of overlooking minor details of the person's performance in favour of the more obvious anticipated information. Assessment interpretation is rarely truly objective, but the therapist should endeavour to minimise her own perspectives by checking her observations through other assessments, specific tests or measurements. In this way risk of personal bias in observation can be minimised.

Specific tests

A large number of specific tests are used by occupational therapists to assess function. Some tests have been devised by therapists but many have been designed by others and are used by the occupational therapist to measure a specific function. Many visual perception tests were originally created by psychologists or neurologists, but may now be used by occupational therapists to assess visual perceptual skills following stroke or head injury, or with children affected by cerebral palsy.

Occupational therapists may test motor, sensory, cognitive and perceptual skills and their use in areas of self-maintenance, role duties and leisure activities. Assessment of the environment, the cultural and social situation, and the carers' needs and quality of care may also be part of the occupational therapist's role. In addition, attitudes, volition and motivation, and behavioural and social skills may be assessed. With such a breadth and diversity of areas of assessment it is inevitable that a wide variety of specific tests may be used. Vital factors in determining the value and success of any test are the therapist's skills in:

- identifying the need for the test
- identifying the most appropriate test for the situation

- administering the test accurately and sensitively
- interpreting the results correctly.

Specific tests may be considered in three main groups — standardised tests, non-standardised tests and checklists.

Standardised tests

Some tests used by occupational therapists have been standardised, but unfortunately many have not. Standardisation provides two main advantages to the measurement:

1. It provides a valid and reliable standard or 'norm' against which to measure individual performance
2. It sets out the content of the test and explains how it is to be carried out to achieve maximum validity and reliability.

In order to appreciate the value of standardisation it is important to understand its process and the ways in which validity and reliability may be achieved.

Standardisation involves the establishment of a 'norm' or standard, both for carrying out the test and as a basis against which to measure individual results. This is achieved by using the test with a large sample group which reflects the group for which the test is intended. A standard set of assessment tools and instructions is formulated to ensure the same procedure is carried out under similar conditions each time. Analysis of the results of the sample group will determine the range of variation. The 'norm' or standard will be the result or small band of results which contains the majority of the group. The extent of this may vary according to the sensitivity of the test, the accuracy of control and the nature of the skill being measured. Acceptable variations to each side of the 'norm' are usually referred to as standard deviations.

Validity is the extent to which the test *truly* measures what it is intended to measure. Consideration should have been given to the face validity, construct, content and criterion-related validity of the test.

Face validity is how far the test appears to do what it is supposed to do. This is a lower form of validity as it cannot easily be tested. It is, however, important for the individual participating in the test as he may be less motivated to perform to his optimum if the test procedures do not clearly reflect the skills to be tested. The therapist's own perceptions of face validity may influence her opinion of the test.

The circumstances of the disability and their effect on the test procedure may affect face validity. An example may be seen when testing perceptual function with a person with receptive dysphasia. It may be difficult to determine how far the results truly reflect perceptual performance or how far they have been influenced by the person's difficulty in understanding the instructions. Similarly, the distraction of pain may influence performance; so while the test appears to be measuring a specific function, the results may be biased by other unseen impinging factors.

Interpreting results of tests which have only face validity may involve considerable personal opinion on the part of the therapist. She should confirm them, wherever possible, by carrying out other tests which have greater validity before making clinical judgements.

Construct validity considers the components which act together in the construction of the activity. These may be defined through task analysis to ensure all contributory skills are identified. This may seem a relatively simple logical process for occupational therapists who are skilled in such analysis. However, the true complexity of this task may be realised when they attempt to define the constructs of visual perception, memory, intellect or self-maintenance — all areas familiar to many occupational therapists and included in many therapy tests.

Content validity considers whether the contents of the test adequately measure the areas of the construct and are sufficiently exact to identify variables in performance. Content validity cannot exist without the construct.

Criterion-related validity is how far the findings from one test can be used to make particular inferences. It is derived from the belief that comparison of the results against some other measurements or criteria can be used to interpret particular test findings.

Criterion-related validity has two subdivisions:

1. *Concurrent validity* says something about what *is* at the time of the test. We can say that something is now because this criterion exists now.
2. *Predictive validity*. Because some criteria exist now, predictions can be made about the future.

Rothstein (1985) states that 'criterion-related validity is lacking in many physical tests and measurements'. This may be because of the difficulty in obtaining accurate initial criteria against which to make comparisons. Measurement of a specific factor, for example sensation, may be more easily criterion-related than performance in a functional task such as feeding. Human task performance is frequently difficult to define accurately in criterion-related terms, as successful performance will involve a combination of physical, cognitive and psychological factors as well as social, cultural and environmental influences. Criteria for concurrent or predictive validity would need to accommodate these factors and would therefore result in a vast range of criteria interpretation data against which to make comparisons.

However, attention to the development of criterion-related validity would add to the accuracy of the interpretation of the person's test results, both in the recognition of the present levels of function and in identifying possible future outcomes.

Reliability is the consistency of the measurement when all conditions are thought to be held constant. The same results should therefore be obtained when the test is repeated under the same conditions.

Kerlinger (1973) stated that 'high reliability is not a guarantee of good scientific results, but there can be no good scientific results without reliability.'

Various forms of reliability have been tested in the process of standardisation.

1. Intratester reliability is the consistency of the test over time when the same person measures the same thing on different occasions.

2. *Intertester reliability* is the consistency of the test between testers when different testers measure the same thing.

To ensure that both the above forms of reliability are achieved the actual procedure for performing the test must be *constant*. The test tools and materials must be the same on each occasion, and the test instructions must be described in detail and adhered to. This attention to detail is sometimes viewed as being unnecessarily complex, but is essential to ensure reliability.

Specific tests are frequently used to measure progress, so it is vitally important that the procedure is intratester reliable if the results are to be accurate. Intertester reliability will enable different therapists, or other personnel, to use the same test with an individual to obtain accurate results. This is a useful asset when the person may be seen in different environments during the rehabilitation process.

Intertester and intratester reliability are also necessary when making comparisons between individuals, either for the purpose of a more objective measure of the standard of each person's results, or for comparative research.

3. *Parallel reliability and internal consistency.* In some situations it may not be possible for exactly the same assessment tools and materials to be used with an individual. Where this is so, and more than one assessment tool is used, it will be necessary to consider parallel forms of reliability. These determine how far one method is consistent with the other. An example of this is measurement of grip strength which may be carried out using a vigorimeter, dynamometer or sphygmomanometer (see Physical measurement). Parallel reliability is the level to which all these tools yield the same measurement.

In some tests involving a number of procedures, different parts of the test may be designed to assess the same skill. Internal consistency is the level to which each of these different parts yields the same result. Significant variations in internal consistency may bring into question the sensitivity or validity of the procedure. Consistency within the test will confirm or consolidate a skill measurement about which the therapist may be unsure if it is only measured on one occasion.

4. *Population-specific reliability.* This is the degree of reliability the test has for the specific person being measured. Many tests have been standardised with particular age, sex and disability groups, and nationality and cultural factors may have been considered.

When using and interpreting tests, occupational therapists wish to consider individual performance as accurately as possible. Standardised tests describe the population group or groups with which they were standardised. Obviously not all factors related to the particular person will have been represented in these groups.

The therapist should therefore consider the clinical relevance of the test, i.e. how far the particular person equates to the group or groups for which the test has been standardised. Using her theoretical and clinical knowledge she should consider the reliability of particular findings in light of the person's individual differences from the standardisation groups.

Objectivity and accuracy. It is virtually impossible to achieve total objectivity and accuracy in any assessment involving human performance.

There is usually some subjectivity by the assessor and the person completing the test. The assessor has usually chosen the particular test and will often be responsible for interpreting the results, which may be affected by her relationship with the individual and her view of the actual test.

The individual's volition and motivation when participating in the test will affect the outcome. Intratester reliability is rarely 100%, as most people will experience some change over time. Merely having completed the test on a previous occasion may alter anxiety levels which in turn will affect performance.

Accuracy in intertester and intratester reliability is difficult to achieve in tests involving significant levels of visual observation, or complex test procedures. However, if the need for making some allowance for human subjectivity and individual differences is recognised, validity and reliability are valuable components for achieving optimum accuracy and objectivity when obtaining and interpreting the results of a test performance.

Interpretation of results. Comparison of results against a predetermined 'norm' to enable the individual and the therapist to make a judgement and identify an outcome or need, should not contradict the therapist's basic philosophy of valuing individuality. Deciding actions from the outcomes of tests should be a shared activity, and the person should have the right to accept or reject any suggestions made by the therapist. The person may be content to recognise his lack of ability to perform the task in the normal way and he should not be expected to adjust accordingly (provided the outcome is satisfactory to him). However, by alerting him to his performance he may be able to make an informed, as opposed to an uninformed, choice. The test may have provided an accurate measure against which to evaluate individual performance, but the 'norm' should not be used too rigidly to dictate aims or objectives.

Non-standardised tests

These have been devised to test skills and measure performance but have not been standardised to determine the 'norm'. They may or may not have valid or reliable procedures.

Many occupational therapists devise tests to meet the needs of particular groups or situations. Whilst these may have been developed and refined to improve reliability within a given environment, many lack the detailed preparatory analysis to determine the validity of the construct. Similarly, the precise description of the use of the assessment tools and materials frequently lacks definition, which risks producing discrepancies in both intertester and intratester reliability.

Therapists should not be dissuaded from developing such tests as they may form pilot studies for further developments which may later be standardised. However, the therapist should not 'reinvent the wheel' by duplicating standardised assessments which are already available, but may require more experience in analysing the results to reflect her client group. This adjustment should not take place in the actual test procedure as this will render the results invalid.

A non-standardised test may be an indicator of functional level at a specific time in a particular setting if it is valid and reliable. However, it cannot be used to measure this performance against the population 'norm'. Non-standardised tests may therefore have very restricted use because they are limited to a particular environmental or client situation. Similarly they have limited use in comparative research. Keith (1984) reflects this concern in his article 'Functional assessment in medical rehabilitation' which states: 'Many organisations still prefer to construct measures to fit their particular situations. Since these *ad hoc* methods have not been well developed, many assessment instruments have uncertain validity for clinical, research or programme evaluation.'

Scoring. This is an important aspect of any form of assessment and many different methods are used. Most tests involve the completion of some form of record sheet. This may include a grading structure which indicates outcomes simply in terms of able/not able, or has interim categories. Some record sheets may show times taken to complete the action and have a grading of time acceptability.

Grading scales also have different ranges. Some have 3-, 4- or 5-point scale; others are more dependent on the variations available, for example they grade ability with the variables, not able, able with manual assistance, able with support equipment, able with verbal prompts, able with extra time, fully able. Many such gradings are based on observations which risk the bias of subjectivity on the part of the assessor unless strict scoring criteria are defined.

Weighting. Some test scores are allotted weighting. This is often in number form. When all tasks are given the same numerical range they are all measured as equally important, and any differences between the value of the tasks or their complexity are lost. Equal weighting of activities therefore indicates equal 'disability value'. Therapists recognise that identification of the perceived disability level for particular tasks is very individual and varies considerably from person to person and such variations are lost in equal weighting.

Where unequal weighting or categorisation of tasks does occur, it is not always clear how such differences have been devised. Some tests seem to group the essential or most important tasks in one section, and organise subsequent sections in order of perceived importance, with greater numerical scores allotted to those in the first section, or at the top of each subgroup. Other tests accord different weightings to particular tasks, and it is not always clear whether these reflect the complexity of the demands of the task or its perceived importance in the activity as a whole. Frequently this does not relate to the individual's perceptions of the task's importance for himself.

Dangers may occur when such scores are totalled to identify levels of function or predict outcomes. Individual strengths and needs will inevitably be masked in the total score. A person may score highly in many aspects of the test, but may be totally unable to perform in one crucial area. Unless this area is very heavily weighted the final score is likely to be high, despite the person's inability in a vital area of personal need.

Score totalling may be a useful part of analysis of data in quantitative research. However it has limited application in enhancing the occupational therapist's information for individual problem analysis, or for measuring progress in particular performance skills. Score totals are equally unreliable in predicting outcomes, as much progress is dependent on individual volition and the levels of support provided.

Checklists

These are frequently used by occupational therapists and are sometimes referred to as 'performance checks'. A checklist aims to ensure all areas are addressed and particular aspects are not overlooked.

Most checklists are comprehensive lists of activities or factors to be noted in a particular area. Checklists may be general, i.e. covering a variety of areas or skills, or they may be specific to one particular aspect, for example a home visit or communication checklist.

Whilst it is useful to ensure all areas are addressed, a checklist cannot be considered as an assessment because it does not include tools or procedures for measurement, and it is not tested for validity or reliability. However, it may be used to identify a particular area of concern which requires a more detailed assessment.

Conclusions

When analysing specific tests, consideration should be given to variations in 'normal' human performance. When making clinical judgements there are a number of advantages of tests which have been standardised over those which have not and over checklists. Standardised tests are likely to be more reliable and valid and have a broader application. They may be used by a number of professionals in different situations and the results can be compared against a standard or 'norm'. However, interpretation of results of some standardised tests may require a particular skill level which is confined to one group of professionals or those who have had specific education and training in this area.

Physical measurement

Specific physical measurement may be the most appropriate method of ascertaining the level of function in particular areas. In order to ensure any measurement process is efficient, and as comfortable as possible for the individual, the therapist should make certain preparations:

- All necessary equipment should be to hand and in working order. The therapist should be familiar with the equipment and able to use it accurately and confidently. Accessories such as record cards, or a comfortable stool or chair on which the person can sit while measurements are taken, should also be available.
- Measurement should be carried out in a well-lit warm environment where there is adequate space for both the therapist and the individual to move freely. Privacy is important to avoid embarrassment, particularly in the first measurement session when the required actions are being explained and the individual may be particularly apprehensive.
- The therapist should explain the procedure and the reason for measurement. A simple short explanation of the method and importance of the measurements will put the person at ease and make the procedure quicker and easier.
- The therapist should know the particular measurements required and the methods of

achieving them. She should handle and move the person's limbs with care and confidence, thus causing minimal discomfort. If she wishes the person to perform an action independently, a simple demonstration may clarify the task.

- Any support or tight clothing which may restrict the movements to be measured should be loosened or removed unless contraindicated.
- Whenever possible, measurement of one person should be carried out by the same therapist, as familiarity will increase confidence and minimise the possibility of any minor discrepancy in measurement technique.
- Where possible, measurements should be taken at the same time of day and at the same time relative to any treatment. The importance of this may be illustrated by differences in the levels of hand function in individuals with rheumatoid arthritis between early morning, when stiffness may limit function, and later in the day. Similarly, the movement of a joint is likely to change from the beginning to the end of a treatment session, so measurements should be taken consistently either before or after treatment, but not at random.
- Measurements should be taken regularly and recorded clearly and accurately for further reference.

Areas of measurement

- Muscle power
- Range of movement
- Swelling
- Muscle bulk.

Measuring muscle power. Reduction in power may result from muscle wasting following a period of inactivity, reduced or absent nerve innervation, or a mechanical disturbance such as damage to the tendon or muscle body. In such circumstances it may not be possible to measure muscle power against gravity, but some measurement is necessary to determine the existing level of strength and chart recovery of power. Ultimately, as improvement occurs the therapist may assess power through comparison with the unaffected limb.

A method of manually estimating muscle power around a particular joint, known as the Oxford Rating Scale, has been developed for this purpose.

The person is asked to move the particular joint as far as possible in a given plane, so muscle power around the joint can be noted. The power is graded on a scale from 0 to 5 in the following way (an example is given for the elbow joint in brackets).

O. Zero. No muscular contraction or joint movement is evident. (With the arm supported to compensate the effects of gravity, no muscle contraction or elbow movement is felt or seen.)

1. Flicker. A flicker of muscle contraction is seen or felt, but no joint movement is evident. (With the arm supported as above, a muscle flicker or twitch can be seen or felt, but no elbow movement occurs.)

2. Poor. Movement is only possible with compensation for gravity and no other resistance. (The elbow joint is only able to move in a horizontal plane when both the upper arm and forearm are supported.)

3. Fair. Movement is possible against gravity but no other resistance. (The elbow can be flexed in a vertical plane without support.)

4. Good. A full range of joint movement is possible with some resistance. (The elbow can be flexed in the vertical plane with an object held in the hand, or against the counterforce of pressure on the volar aspect of the forearm.)

5. Normal. A full range of movement is possible against gravity and resistance in comparison with the unaffected limb. If both limbs have been affected, measurements should be compared to that person's previous level of performance. (The elbow can be fully flexed when holding a weight in the hand or against volar counter pressure, consistent with the unaffected limb.)

Grip strength. Occupational therapists are frequently required to assess specific aspects of muscle power, especially grip strength in the hand. A number of pieces of equipment are specifically designed for this purpose.

1. *The vigorimeter or dynamometer.* The bulb-type vigorimeter (Fig. 7.2A) consists of a pressure

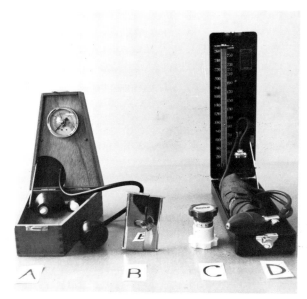

Fig. 7.2 Equipment for assessing grip strength
(A) Bulb-type vigorometer (B) Spring-type vigorometer
(C) Torquometer for measuring twist grip
(D) Sphygmomanometer adapted to assess grip.

gauge to which one of three bulbs of different sizes may be attached. When assessing cylinder or whole hand grip it is usual to choose the bulb which the person can hold comfortably in the palm of the hand. The smallest bulb is usually used to measure pincer or tripod grip. Both needles on the gauge are set to zero and the person is asked to squeeze the bulb securely and then relax. The coloured needle will remain static on the dial at the maximum point reached, from which the reading may be taken. The dial is then reset to zero. Usually the measurement is performed three times and the average of the three attempts is recorded. Vigorimeters produced by different manufacturers have variations in gauge scoring so there is no uniform system of recording. It is therefore important to accurately record the gauge readings in case of equipment changes between assessments.

2. *A spring vigorimeter or sphygmomanometer* (Fig. 7.2B and D) may also be used to measure grip strength. The spring vigorimeter consists of a metal rectangle, or two metal bars, which are spring loaded together and attached to a gauge or dial. By squeezing the bars together the dial or

gauge records the pressure applied to the springs. This equipment offers more resistance than the bulb vigorimeter and is therefore more commonly used to measure stronger grip strength. However, the thumb is involved less in the grip action.

The sphygmomanometer records small pressure changes on a column of mercury and is therefore more suitable for detecting minor changes in the hand which is particularly weak. The equipment consists of a small hand-held bag which is attached to a column of mercury. The bag is inflated to a basic pressure (for example 20 mm mercury) and the column of mercury will rise to detect any pressure change when the bag is squeezed. Pressure should be released on the mercury column when the equipment is not in use.

It is usual to take the average of three readings with both these pieces of equipment in the same way as with the bulb vigorimeter.

Measuring range of movement. Joint range of movement may be measured in a variety of ways. The therapist should check both active and passive range within the joint for each action. When moving a joint through a passive range the therapist should always support the limb above and below the joint. Passive joint movement enables the therapist to demonstrate the movement she wishes the person to perform actively, and she may be able to identify some possible causes for limitation of active joint range of movement. For example, a joint which moves freely through a passive range of movement, but is limited when moved actively, will indicate that muscle weakness is inhibiting the range despite freedom to move in the joint articulation. A joint which is limited in both active and passive range may indicate other limiting factors, such as contractures, oedema, soft tissue or bone damage.

However, the therapist must also be aware that a discrepancy between expected active joint movement, based on its passive range and muscle strength, and actual active movement, may have other causes. These may include a misunderstanding by the person regarding the movement required, pain, or fear of pain on active movement. It may also be due to conscious or unconscious inhibition of joint movement by the individual for further gain — often referred to as 'compensationitis'. This may occur when a person is involved in a formal claim for compensation following trauma when the level of impairment may be a basis for insurance payment. It may be a less obvious desire for attention by the family or carer, or be a means of avoiding a particular situation or responsibility.

When measuring joint range of movement the therapist should never force the joint to move beyond the range which can be easily achieved passively. Apart from causing considerable pain to and loss of trust by the individual, by forcing a joint to move beyond this range the therapist may cause myositis ossificans which will further delay or inhibit joint movement.

Principles of measuring joint range of movement.
- Starting position. The most widely used method of recording joint movement is one in which all joints are measured from a specifically defined starting position which is taken as zero (0°). In the majority of joints this zero starting position is the anatomical position of the joint. For example, at the elbow the starting position is extension (Fig. 7.3(i)).
- Measuring joint movement. The joint movement is measured in degrees from the starting position (0°) to the furthest point of travel. For example, for the elbow joint the measurement is taken from 0 to the point of greatest flexion (Fig. 7.3(ii)).
- Measuring limited range of movement. If the joint cannot be placed in the anatomical starting position (0°), measurement should be taken from the angle nearest to this which the person can achieve. For example, in Figure 7.3(iii) the measurement of movement at the elbow joint would be taken from (a) to (b).

- Measuring a joint which hyperextends. Should the joint fall into hyperextension then this extra movement can be recorded as a 'minus' reading. In Figure 7.3(iv), for example, the measurement at the elbow joint would be taken from the furthest point of hyperextension(a) through to the furthest point of flexion(b).

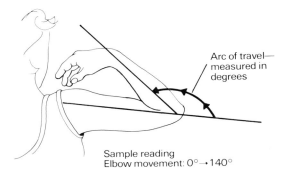

Sample reading
Elbow movement: 0°→140°

Fig. 7.3(ii)   Measuring joint movement at the elbow.

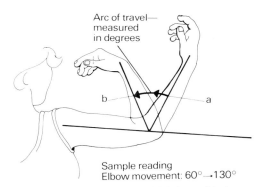

Sample reading
Elbow movement: 60°→130°

Fig. 7.3(iii)   Measuring a joint which is unable to reach the normal starting position.

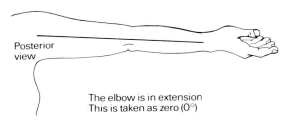

Posterior view

The elbow is in extension
This is taken as zero (0°)

Fig. 7.3(i)   Starting position for elbow measurement.

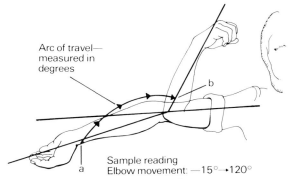

Sample reading
Elbow movement: —15°→120°

Fig. 7.3(iv)   Measuring hyperextension.

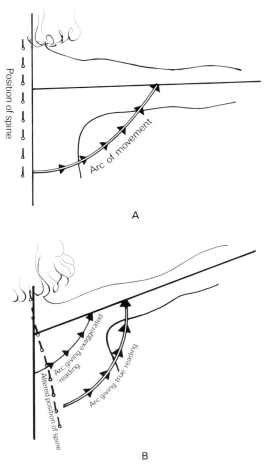

Fig. 7.3(v) Allowing for compensatory movement around a joint (A) Correct movement (B) Compensatory movement of the spine exaggerating shoulder movement. (*Note.* The fixed arm of the goniometer must remain parallel to the spine to give a true reading)

● Measuring a unilateral disorder. When measuring someone with a unilateral disorder, measurements of the unaffected side should always be taken as a guide to the expected level of recovery. Where both sides are affected the average range of movement of the joint should be used as a guide (see Table 7.1.) The therapist should remember, however, that this can only give a rough guide to the expected level of recovery, as this will depend on the age, physical build, race and occupation of the individual.

● Handling the person. Moving an affected joint is often painful and, therefore, all measurements should be made as quickly as possible.

● Compensatory movements. It is important to identify whether a person is making compensatory movements when asked to perform a certain joint motion. This may be conscious or unconscious and usually takes the form of an apparent exaggeration in the movement performed which is the result of a sympathetic movement of a joint close to the one being examined. For example, when the person is asked to abduct the arm he does so in conjunction with side flexion of the spine, thus exaggerating the shoulder movement (Fig. 7.3(v)).

This compensatory movement can be overcome by:

— telling the person he is doing it (frequently he will be quite unaware of this) and correcting the movements he is making
— asking him to perform shoulder movements bilaterally, so that the spine remains static
— supporting the part which is not required to move, either manually or by resting it on a firm surface so that it remains still
— asking him to perform the action in front of a mirror so that he can check his own compensatory movements.

If these methods are not successful the therapist should make allowances for the additional movement when she is measuring the joint.

Joint measurement using the goniometer. The goniometer is the most commonly used instrument for measuring the exact range of joint movement. Several different designs are available but the standard goniometer consists of:

● the central protractor marked in degrees
● a fixed arm
● a mobile arm.

Figure 7.4 shows a standard large goniometer for general use (B), a standard smaller instrument specifically designed for measuring the joints of the hand (C) and a more modern model capable of measuring most joint movement (A). To use the standard goniometer the therapist must first find three points related to the joint to be measured:

1. The axis (or fulcrum). This is the point on the body surface which most closely responds to that around which the joint movement occurs.

Table 7.1 Points of reference for joint measurement

Joint	Starting position	Fixed line	Axis	Mobile line	Average range of movement
Shoulder	Anatomical position	Line parallel to the spine	Acromion process	Shaft of the humerus	Elevation through flexion 0°–158°. Elevation through abduction 0°–170°. Extension 0°–53°
Elbow	Anatomical position (with the shoulder flexed for ease of measurement)	Shaft of the humerus	Lateral (or medial) epicondyle of humerus	Shaft of radius (or ulna)	0°–146°
Wrist	Anatomical position (with elbow flexed) for flexion. Forearm in pronation (and elbow flexed) for extension	Shaft of ulna	Ulnar styloid	Shaft of fifth metacarpal	Extension 0°–71° Flexion 0°–73°
Metacarpal phalangeal joints of fingers	Anatomical position	Shaft of metacarpal	Over dorsum of MCP joint	Shaft of proximal phalanx	0°–90°
Proximal inter-phalangeal joints of fingers	Anatomical position	Shaft of proximal phalanx	Over dorsum of PIP joint	Shaft of middle phalanx	0°–100°
Distal inter-phalangeal joints of fingers	Anatomical position	Shaft of middle phalanx	Over dorsum of DIP joint	Shaft of distal phalanx	0°–80°
Carpo-metacarpal joint of thumb	Anatomical position	Parallel to metacarpal of middle (3rd) phalanx	Base of 'Anatomical snuffbox', that is over base of 1st MCP	Shaft of 1st metacarpal	Extension 15°–45° Abduction 0°–58°
Metacarpal phalangeal joint of thumb	CMC joint of thumb in abduction	Shaft of 1st metacarpal	Over dorsum of joint	Shaft of 1st proximal phalanx	0°–53°
Inter-phalangeal joint of thumb	CMC and MCP joints of thumb in extension	Shaft of 1st proximal phalanx	Over dorsum of joint	Shaft of 1st distal phalanx	0°–81°
Knee	Anatomical position, that is extension (patient seated on plinth with knee at the edge of the plinth)	Shaft of femur (or in line with the greater trochanter)	Lateral condyle of femur	Shaft of fibula (or in line with the lateral malleolus)	0°–134°
Ankle	Anatomical position (patient seated on table with knee bent over edge)	Shaft of fibula (or in line with head of fibula)	Lateral malleolus (or the indentation just below it)	Shaft of the fifth metacarpal	Dorsiflexion 0°–18° Plantarflexion 0°–48°

Note. The reader will notice that several joints/movements are not mentioned in the above table. This is because, in the experience of the author, they are not usually measured with a goniometer by the occupational therapist. The measurement of these joints/movements is discussed later. Those which do not appear at all, for example the movement of the toes, are rarely measured by the occupational therapist.

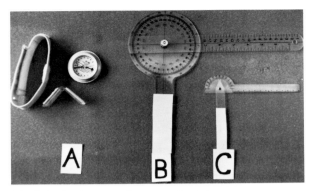

Fig. 7.4 Goniometers for measuring joint movement (A) Swedish OB goniometer 'Myrin' (B) Standard-size goniometer for measuring large joints (C) Small goniometer for measuring joints in the hand.

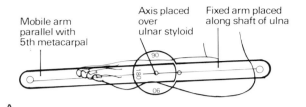

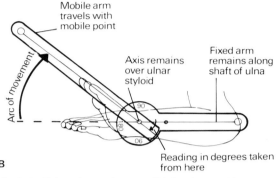

Fig. 7.5 Using the goniometer (A) Starting position (B) Position to read movement.

2. A fixed line. This is the line close to the joint which acts as a reference point from which movement occurs.
3. A mobile line. This is the line close to the joint which acts as a reference point to show the arc of movement of the joint.

For example, at the wrist joint the axis can be the ulnar styloid, the fixed line can be the shaft of the ulna and the mobile line can be the fifth metacarpal. With the joint held in the starting position (see Table 7.1) the goniometer is lined up with the relevant reference points (Fig. 7.5A).

The person is then asked to perform the required movement while the therapist, ensuring the fixed arm of the goniometer remains parallel to the fixed line on the body surface, moves the mobile arm to lie along (or level with) the mobile line when the movement is completed (Fig. 7.5B). The central screw (if there is one) on the protractor is tightened to secure the reading and the person is allowed to relax while the therapist reads and records the movement obtained. Table 7.1 shows the starting position, fixed line, axis, mobile line and average range of movement of those joints most commonly measured with the goniometer by the occupational therapist.

Joint measurement using a tape measure or ruler. In some cases it is difficult or inappropriate to measure the range of movement of a joint or series of joints in degrees, so a tape measure or ruler may be used. An example is the span of the hand which

is a combination of abduction of the fingers and extension of the thumb. This is frequently measured as the maximum distance between the tips of the little finger and the thumb (Fig. 7.6).

Other joints which can be measured in this way include:

- Joints in the hand. Composite movement of finger flexion can be measured as the distance between the palm and the finger tip (Fig. 7.7).
- Joints of the spine. Composite movement of joints involved in forward flexion can be measured by recording the distance between the spinous processes of C7 and S1, first with the person standing erect and then when he is bending forward in flexion.

Visual assessment of joint movement. The person is asked to perform a specific movement whilst the therapist makes a visual assessment of the range of movement at the joint. Under these circumstances, the movement cannot be recorded in specific units of measurement such as degrees or centimetres; it is therefore often expressed as a percentage or fraction of the person's normal range of movement (in comparison with that of the unaffected side). The recording may, for instance, show that a joint can move through 50% (or one half) of the expected range.

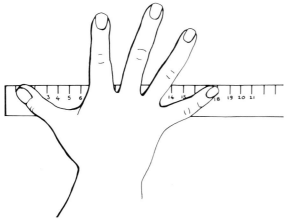

Fig. 7.6 Measuring span of the hand with a ruler.

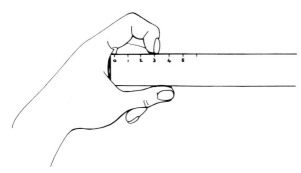

Fig. 7.7 Measuring composite movements of the finger with a ruler.

Visual assessment is often used to estimate movements which are particularly difficult to measure using the goniometer. These movements include medial and lateral deviation and internal and external rotation at a joint. The joints where visual assessments are used most frequently are the spine, the shoulders and hips, the forearm and thumb, and occasionally radial and ulnar deviation at the wrist (Figs. 7.8(i)–(iv)). Whilst visual assessment is a recognised form of measurement, it is very subjective and the results are prone to variable accuracy.

Joint measurement using a joint outline. The range of movement at a joint may be measured either by drawing around the outline of the joint or by tracing the joint outline with a soft thin wire (this latter method is used less frequently).

For the former method the therapist must locate the fixed point, axis and the mobile point near the joint which is to be measured. The fixed point and axis are then placed over the area marked on a prepared piece of card, and the person is asked to move the joint through its maximum range while the therapist marks the furthest point reached (Fig. 7.9).

This method is usually used for measuring the finger joints where a composite reading is required. The visual record enables the person to see changes in range of movement over a series of measurements.

Measuring swelling. It is often necessary to measure swelling around a joint. The therapist should note whether any reduction is occurring

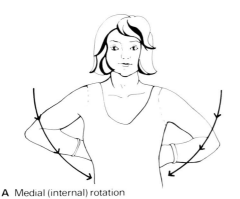

A Medial (internal) rotation

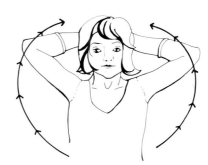

B Lateral (external) rotation

Fig. 7.8(i) Estimating movement at the shoulder. Method 1.

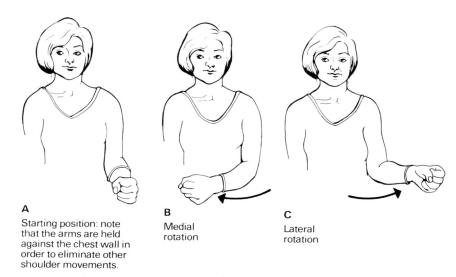

A

Starting position: note
that the arms are held
against the chest wall in
order to eliminate other
shoulder movements.

B

Medial
rotation

C

Lateral
rotation

Fig. 7.8(ii) Estimating movement at the shoulder. Method 2.

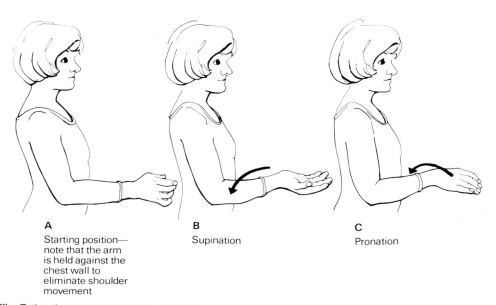

A

Starting position—
note that the arm
is held against the
chest wall to
eliminate shoulder
movement

B

Supination

C

Pronation

Fig. 7.8(iii) Estimating movement in the forearm.

during treatment and the healing process, as persistent swelling is likely to inhibit joint mobility.

Measuring swelling with a tape measure. The simplest method of assessing swelling is by measuring the circumference of the swollen area with a tape measure. The tape must always be placed around the same point of the limb for accuracy. If swelling is present in the hand, this may be measured by placing the tape around the palm, just proximal to the metacarpophalangeal joints.

Measuring swelling by immersion in water. It is possible, though less common, to estimate the amount of swelling in the whole hand (rather than around the level of the palm) by measuring the amount of water displaced when the hand is immersed up to the wrist crease (Fig. 7.10).

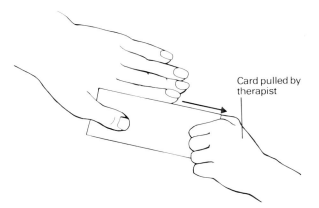

Fig. 7.8(iv) Estimating adduction of the thumb.

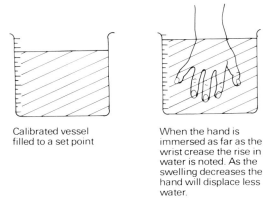

Calibrated vessel
filled to a set point

When the hand is
immersed as far as the
wrist crease the rise in
water is noted. As the
swelling decreases the
hand will displace less
water.

Fig. 7.10 Measuring swelling in the hand by immersion in water.

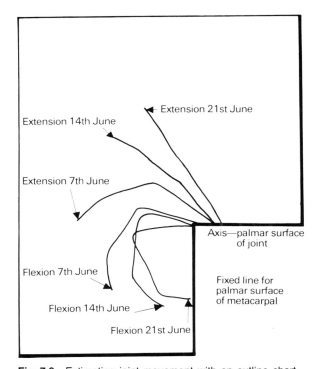

Extension 21st June

Extension 14th June

Extension 7th June

Axis—palmar surface
of joint

Flexion 7th June

Fixed line for
palmar surface
of metacarpal

Flexion 14th June

Flexion 21st June

Fig. 7.9 Estimating joint movement with an outline chart.

Measuring muscle bulk. The muscles most commonly measured in this way are the quadriceps group. These muscles waste very quickly during a period of inactivity and their rate of recovery can be checked by measuring the muscle bulk. The measurement is usually made with a tape measure and the circumference around the thigh is taken at a set point each time (for example 150 cm (6 in) above the proximal border of the patella). Other muscle groups may be measured in this way.

Self-rating

This is sometimes referred to as self-evaluation and usually takes the form of a written questionnaire or a rating scale which requires the respondent to answer statements or prioritise them. The individual completes the questionnaire independently of the therapist who then uses the response to identify the individual's personal perceptions of his achievements and his levels of expectation, or his rating of priority skills or needs. In so doing the individual is actively involved in the identification of his own level of function, which may improve his motivation to prioritise needs. Such an assessment may also indicate an over-optimistic or a pessimistic attitude.

Self-evaluation or self-rating tests are difficult to design to ensure the questions or statements elicit the information accurately and are free from bias. Many such tests lack clarity in the questions and are ambiguous, thereby producing confused responses. Familiarity with the assessment may affect subsequent responses, particularly in the assessment of cognitive or perceptual performance.

Hidden agendas about the purpose of self-evaluation tests may skew the responses. The individual may complete the form in a way which he believes will please the therapist. For example he may indicate an improvement in ability following treatment when this is not so. Alternatively the respondent may deny a problem area if this is likely to necessitate further treatment or delay return home.

However, despite these difficulties this form of assessment does have considerable merit. When used in conjunction with other assessments the therapist is able to identify the individual's personal perspectives in relation to observed or measured performance in more formal assessments. This insight adds to the total picture and will increase the extent of information on which to plan and prioritise intervention. The opportunity for the individual to be actively involved as the assessor as well as the recipient may raise his view of the value of assessment and improve his volition on the possible outcomes.

CONCLUSION

'Assessment is a process in which the occupational therapist identifies in her terms the individual's requirements for restoration and enables him to make an audit of his own needs. Once agreement has been reached, they can move together towards their goal'.

(see p. 769)

A wide variety of methods of assessment are available to the occupational therapist. No one measure will provide all the necessary information. Care should be taken to ensure the most appropriate types and methods of assessment are used to yield the most useful information, and the individual is not subjected to unnecessary, inappropriate tests or measurements.

No assessment involving human performance can be totally objective, and the very nature of the tests, where results are judged against a defined standard or 'norm', frequently conflicts with the occupational therapist's philosophy of valuing individuality. However, without some form of reliable comparative measurement it may not be possible to ascertain individual needs or to identify progress. The therapist should involve the individual with the findings to facilitate a shared understanding of the data so that it can form a basis on which to plan priority needs and therapy intervention. Having acquired such information it should be accurately and concisely recorded for further reference and interpretation.

As the therapist becomes proficient with different facets of assessment she will be able to identify particular strengths and limitations of individual methods. It is important for such expertise to be developed in order to more fully evaluate the use of particular methods in specialist situations, and to improve the quality of assessment and measurement in all areas of practice. Campbell's (1981) comment on research education in measurement and technical skills outlines this well in the statement: 'If therapists want to claim efficacy for their practice they are totally dependent on the quality of the measurement used to show change in patients. As more and more therapists have adopted the role of assessors and treatment planners, as well as that of treatment givers, it is ironic that they have not been more concerned with the measurements that justify this role.' The importance of the quality of assessment cannot be underestimated in the total therapy process.

Successful completion of an assessment should not be an end in itself. It is merely a part of the occupational therapy process and should be used to plan, implement, evaluate and change intervention as necessary.

Whilst respecting confidentiality, the findings may be used as a basis for liaison within the multidisciplinary team. They should therefore be clear, concise and accurate, and expressed in communicable terms without risk of ambiguity.

REFERENCES

British Association of Occupational Therapists 1990 Code of Ethics and Professional Conduct
Campbell S K 1981 Measurement and technical skills — neglected aspects of research education. Physical Therapy 61: 523
Keith R A 1984 Functional assessment measures in medical rehabilitation: current status. Archives of Physical Medicine and Rehabilitation 65(2): 74–78
Kerlinger F N 1973 Foundations of behavioural research, 2nd edn. Holt, Rinehart and Winston, New York
Rothstein J M 1985 Measurement in physical rehabilitation. Churchill Livingstone, New York, pp 23–4
Rowntree D 1987 Assessing students. How shall we know them? 2nd edn. Harper & Row, London

FURTHER READING

Eakin P 1989 Assessment of activities of daily living: a critical review. British Journal of Occupational Therapy 52: 11–15, 50–54
Granger C V, Gresham G E 1984 Functional assessment in rehabilitation medicine. Williams and Wilkins, Baltimore
Hopkins H L, Smith H D 1988 Willard and Spackman's occupational therapy, 7th edn. Lippincott, Philadelphia
Kane R A, Kane R L 1984 Assessing the elderly: a practical guide to measurement, 4th edn. Lexington Books, Massachusetts
Kanfert J M 1983 Functional ability indices: measurement problems in assessing validity. Archives of Physical Medicine and Rehabilitation 64(6): 260–267
Maczka K 1990 Assessing physically disabled people at home. Chapman Hall, London
Open University 1981 Research methods in education and social sciences. Open University, Milton Keynes
Pedretti L W 1985 Occupational therapy: practice skills for physical dysfunction, 2nd edn. Mosby, St Louis
Trombly C A 1989 Occupational therapy for physical dysfunction, 3rd edn. Williams & Wilkins, Baltimore
Wade D T, Langton Hewer R et al 1985 Stroke: a critical approach to diagnosis, treatment and management. Chapman & Hall, London

8

Life skills

Margaret Foster

INTRODUCTION

Life skills constitute a vast subject for study which has implications for all areas of occupational therapy practice. It is impossible in one chapter to provide detailed information on the entire range of life skills and on all the possible rehabilitative options for dysfunction. Whole books have been written on particular areas of living and there is a wealth of reference texts on the assessment and management of particular disabilities related to life skills.

This chapter, therefore, aims to present an overview of life skills. It identifies requirements for success in individual areas of function and illustrates ways in which the occupational therapist may be involved in assisting individuals to address problem areas. Specific techniques and items of equipment are offered only as illustrative examples; the references given at the end of the chapter will provide the reader with more detailed information in specific areas.

The present chapter begins by defining what is meant by 'life skills' and describes their classification into three overlapping categories: self-maintenance, role duties and leisure. The general development of life skills is described, together with the implications for the individual of any disruption in his ability to perform everyday tasks.

Next, the role of the occupational therapist in helping the individual to recover his competence in life skills is outlined.

The chapter then discusses each of the three categories of life skills in turn, describing what types of functional ability each entails, the kinds of assessment appropriate to each area, and ways in which the therapist can help the individual to optimise performance and meet his own priorities for activity. The discussion of self-maintenance activities includes sections on mobility, processing skills, feeding, toileting, dressing, personal cleansing and grooming, communication, and manipulative hand skills.

The discussion of role duties first examines the responsibilities and skills associated with the homemaking role. Next, the role of carer is discussed, with particular attention to the needs of those who provide support to disabled people and to the statutory and other assistance available to them. The special needs of disabled carers are described, as well as the needs of parents of disabled children. Following this, the worker role is considered. This discussion looks at the value of work in maintaining the individual's self-esteem and at the occupational therapist's role in assessing the disabled individual for resettlement in his former job or in alternative employment. In addition, the various kinds of support available to disabled workers and trainees are outlined. Finally, two roles related to the worker role — that of student and of volunteer — are briefly considered.

The final section of the chapter examines the importance of leisure pursuits in helping the disabled individual to achieve a healthy balance of interests and activities, especially where the worker role can no longer be fulfilled. Leisure activities provide an avenue for socialisation, relaxation and mental stimulation and can form a vital component of the rehabilitative programme. Options for leisure activities are described, along with ways in which the therapist can help the individual regain the confidence necessary to take up new interests and make social contacts beyond his family circle.

Throughout the chapter, a problem-solving, rehabilitative approach, by which the individual can finds ways of compensating for loss of function, predominates. It must be stressed, however, that the therapist's approach must be determined by the particular needs of the individual and his carers, and that her treatment plan must, above all, reflect the aspirations and priorities of her client. Other therapeutic approaches may be used to improve performance and overcome rather than compensate for impairment.

WHAT ARE LIFE SKILLS?

Life skills are the abilities individuals acquire and develop in order to perform everyday tasks successfully. As well as varying from person to person, these may change throughout the life span. Evolving roles and responsibilities will influence the individual's balance of activity, his perception of the relative importance of various activities, and the very nature of the activities in which he is engaged (Fig. 8.1). The emphasis given to particular skills in an occupational therapy intervention should reflect the individual's own priorities, taking into account his desires and aspirations and the demands placed upon him by his various roles.

The acquisition or recovery of a life skill depends not only upon the level of its complexity in relation to the individual's dysfunction, but also upon the person's motivation and accustomed lifestyle. The therapist's awareness of the individual's priorities is vital to the success of treatment. For some individuals, independence in self-maintenance activities will be the prime concern. Others may prefer to accept ongoing assistance with self-care tasks in order to conserve energy for other pursuits. For others, the acquisition of skills that will allow them to return to paid employment will be the prime objective.

The occupational therapist must also consider the nature of the skills which she proposes to address in her treatment programme. She will need to analyse each in terms of its sensory, cognitive, perceptual and social components, and consider to what degree these components may be transferable from one area of living to another. Her primary concern will be with how the individual's skills *interrelate* in the performance of activity. Therefore, while she may make frequent use of the

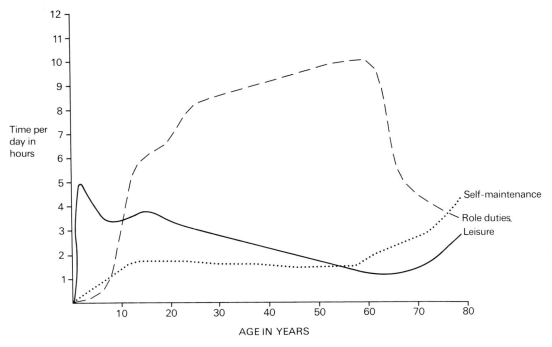

Fig. 8.1 Life skills map for a 77-year-old widow living alone who maintained the roles of housewife, parent and part-time employee until 60 years and nursed her disabled husband until his death when she was 63 years old.

specialised measurements taken by other professionals in order to locate specific areas of functional weakness, her particular contribution will lie in her ability to take a holistic view of the performance of functional tasks and perceive their relative importance in the wider context of the individual's life pattern.

Categorisation of activities

Life skills may be grouped into various categories, such as 'domestic activities', 'work activities' and 'activities of daily living' (ADL). Such categories, although useful, often overlap; money-handling skills, for example, may be related to work or to domestic activity. While bearing this fluidity of categories in mind, this chapter considers activities under three main headings: personal self-maintenance, role duties, and leisure (Fig. 8.2).

● *Self-maintenance.* Skills related to self-maintenance include personal care activities

such as feeding, toileting, dressing, personal hygiene and grooming, mobility skills, communicative skills, fine manual skills and processing skills.

● *Role duties.* Duties which are demanded by the individual's roles and which are not (primarily) related to self-maintenance or leisure may be termed role duties. These may include the domestic duties of the homemaker, the academic duties of the student, the work duties of the employee.

● *Leisure activities* are, of course, those in which the individual participates in order to socialise, relax, or pursue interests and hobbies.

Again, the activities included in each of the above categories will vary from one context to another. A lucrative hobby, for instance, may be classified as work or as a leisure pursuit. Eating a meal may be a matter of self-maintenance, but a business lunch may be seen as a role duty and dinner with friends as a leisure activity. Moreover,

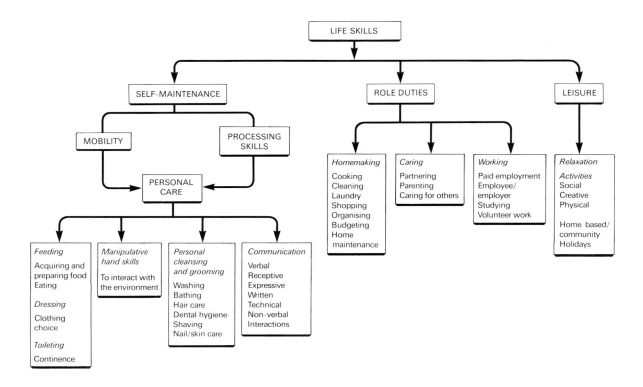

Fig. 8.2 Categorisation of activities.

role duties may be perceived differently from one culture to another. A more extensive exploration of such difficulties of classification may be found in Cynkin and Robinson (1990).

However problematic, the categorisation of activities can provide the therapist with a starting-point for assessment, and help to ensure that the full range of an individual's activities is given consideration. It is instructive to ascertain not only the individual's level of performance of a given activity, but how he perceives and categorises that activity, as this will provide some insight into his attitudes and priorities. In a study of time-use by adults with spinal cord injuries, Yerxa and Locker (1990) identify differences in the perception and classification of activities between the study group, a parallel non-disabled group, and occupational therapists. Their study suggests that the increased

value accorded to some activities by the disabled group may be linked to the loss of the work role and reflect a desire to find alternative occupational competency.

To sum up, although the therapist will need some kind of structure through which she can isolate and assess the various activities which constitute life skills, she should not apply any categorisation rigidly, but should take time to identify the significance that each activity has for the individual concerned.

THE DEVELOPMENT OF LIFE SKILLS

Skills in self-maintenance are acquired gradually throughout childhood. They improve with practice and are finally taken for granted. Consider the process of getting up each morning and preparing to go to work or school. On waking one automatically stretches, gets out of bed and walks to the bathroom and toilet. One washes, dresses and prepares breakfast, all without much thought. But imagine the thinking and preparation required for those who rely on a wheelchair or prosthesis for mobility, or are only able to use one hand, or have difficulty with balance and reach. These simple tasks which are taken for granted by the able-bodied person take on vastly different proportions for the person with a disability.

For some people, the impairment may be short term and advice regarding ways of overcoming temporary disabilities in certain aspects of living may be all that is required. For the person with long-term problems the learning, relearning or modification of techniques may be necessary, and entail considerable practice. The therapist who guides such learning must be able to analyse tasks and adapt their performance to individual needs and capabilities.

When assessing each individual's condition, abilities and limitations, the therapist should consider that the ultimate success of intervention lies in the person's willingness to maintain a programme of strenuous practice and exercise to strengthen weakened muscles, improve coordination and agility, and consolidate skills. Periods of frustration, anxiety and depression may affect motivation and drive. Much will depend upon the encouragement and support that the individual receives. It is also important that *realistic* goals be set. The number and nature of the activities which a person can manage independently will depend on his level of ability, his own standards and those of his family, and the resources available to him.

Consideration should be given to the priorities determined by the individual. If work is a high priority it is pointless to strive for complete independence in a morning self-maintenance routine if this leaves the individual too fatigued to meet the demands of his job. In such a case it might be preferable for the person to accept help. Similarly, for the person living alone, eating breakfast in night clothes may be more acceptable than getting dressed in day clothes only to become too fatigued to make breakfast. The person who is independent only in the self-maintenance activities which are

important to him may be better able to fulfil his role duties and to enjoy leisure pursuits than the person who is totally independent in self-care. The desire for independence should be weighed against the benefits of a good balance between the physical, psychological and social aspects of life.

Skills in role duties develop through education and practice. The schoolchild learns about role expectations in the classroom and playground environment, but he can be prepared for some of these demands before entering school. Similarly, skills learned in the school environment relating to socialisation, adherence to rules, structure and organisation, as well as many of the performance skills related to mobility, communication, reasoning and creative activities prepare the child for adult role duties. Provided that adequate resources are available to enable a disabled child to integrate practically and socially, experience of the normal education system will give him the opportunity to prepare for the rigorous demands of adult living. Additional post-school training schemes may continue this preparation after formal schooling is completed.

Those whose activities as employee or homemaker have been interrupted by illness or disability may need support in regaining the skills and confidence to resume their former role. Similarly, those whose disability has had a significant impact upon performance in their usual role may need help to make the necessary readjustments. Practice in domestic skills in the therapy department, in a training flat or (with support) at home may prepare the disabled person for a return to homemaking. Activities which simulate the working situation may be used to assess or build levels of competence for return to employment. Further training schemes or additional education may also be necessary.

A child learns leisure activities naturally through play. As he develops, his interests expand, in accordance with the opportunities available. Such developments often form the basis of life-long leisure interests. For example, the person who enjoys music at school is likely to pursue it in later life, either actively or as a listener, and the child who is keen on active games or sports may have similar interests in adulthood. Those who enjoy precise or individual activities such as model-building, reading or sewing are more likely to pursue individual rather than team leisure pursuits. For this reason, introduction to play experiences and activities is vital for the disabled child if he is to mature in leisure skills. Frequently, such opportunities are denied because of the limitations imposed by the impairment or because the demands of daily care leave little time or support for play. Family support and introduction to community resources for leisure activities are of great importance for the disabled child's future development.

Disability in adult life may lead the person to devise new ways of pursuing favourite activities or to take up new interests altogether. The therapist should encourage the person's involvement in leisure activities by providing information about the resources available in the local community for both disabled and able-bodied participants.

THE ROLE OF THE OCCUPATIONAL THERAPIST

Habilitation or rehabilitation in life skills involves the individual and his family or carers as well as medical, paramedical, employment and community services personnel. Success will depend upon the ability of team members to work together, understanding and supporting one another's roles, on the drive of the individual, and on the resources available.

The role of the occupational therapist will vary in accordance with her clients' circumstances and needs. As well as providing direct treatment, she may act as facilitator, planner, educator, resource person, advisor and liaison officer. She should know and understand the roles of her colleagues in the medical, educational and employment fields, be familiar with community provision for support in self-maintenance and domestic tasks, and be aware of local facilities and support for leisure pursuits. She should be familiar with legislative provision for disabled people and with the financial support available to them and their carers. She should appreciate the importance for each individual of independence in specific skills

and should also be sensitive to the demands of caring that have been placed upon those close to the disabled person.

The therapist's intervention must begin with a thorough assessment of the person's weaknesses, strengths, wishes and needs. In identifying areas of difficulty and selecting goals for treatment, she must also be able to analyse daily tasks and recognise the specific skills or attributes necessary for their successful performance. In almost all cases, her intervention will be based in a problem-solving approach. However, she will need to be conversant with specific treatments to overcome particular difficulties and improve bodily function. Biomechanical, neurodevelopmental, cognitive and behavioural techniques might all be used to overcome impairment and promote independence in life skills. However, for many people with permanent disability, a compensatory rehabilitative approach may be the most appropriate. This will involve the modification of techniques and the development of strategies to compensate for functional limitation.

SELF-MAINTENANCE

Self-maintenance activities are usually the primary focus of the occupational therapist's intervention, since for most people these are the basic essentials for independence and dignity. Assessment in self-maintenance activities aims to identify which activities the person wishes to perform, those he can and cannot do, how far activities can be improved and the most appropriate methods by which problems can be overcome. 'Baseline', 'progress' and 'final' assessments will be necessary to identify needs and monitor progress.

Assessments may take place in a number of different places, some of which are more appropriate than others. The hospital ward may provide a setting with which the person is familiar and the opportunity to evaluate such activities as dressing at a realistic time of day. However, ward assessments are often unrealistic in the style of furniture they provide and in their lack of privacy for intimate personal activities.

The occupational therapy department or assessment flat may afford a more realistic environment along with many special facilities for testing, but will be unfamiliar to the person being assessed and may therefore raise levels of anxiety or embarrassment.

The home environment is the most familiar setting; here, the assessment can take place using personal equipment and facilities in the presence of relatives and carers. However, for hospitalised clients this may only be possible through a short home visit after considerable practice in basic self-care skills has taken place in the ward.

MOBILITY

Some form of mobility is essential for independence in almost all areas of self-maintenance and for many role duties and leisure activities. The ability to control specific limb movements, to transfer from place to place and to interface with equipment and the environment are vital to success in the wide range of tasks necessary for independence.

The occupational therapist should assess the person's mobility skills in relation to his environment and consider whether he will be able to improve his physical abilities in order to overcome problems or whether it will be necessary to use a compensatory rehabilitative approach to facilitate independent function. The ability to negotiate stairs, for example, may be gained through specific treatment to improve balance and lower limb strength and range of movement. This will usually have greater urgency for the person who is living in a two-storey house than for someone who is living in a bungalow. Where disability is likely to cause long-term difficulties in negotiating steps and stairs, consideration should be given to choosing a more suitable residence or adapting the existing home, either by the addition of downstairs facilities or by the provision of a stair raise or lift.

Additionally, the occupational therapist should consider outdoor mobility — in the garden, in the neighbourhood, at the shops, on the way to work or school — in accordance with the individual's life-style. Chapter 9 describes mobility needs, techniques, equipment and facilities in detail and

should be considered in conjunction with the present discussion.

PROCESSING SKILLS

The ability to be independent extends beyond physical capabilities for performing tasks to the cognitive and intellectual skills necessary for problem-solving and decision-making.

It is impossible to predict and rehearse all of the situations which a person might have to cope with in the community, at home, at work or in a recreational setting. A wheelchair or other piece of essential equipment may break down; a helper may fail to arrive; an unexpected social, educational or business opportunity may arise. It is therefore important to facilitate the development of the independent processing skills that will enable each individual to deal with situations as objectively, positively and autonomously as possible.

For the disabled person who has had previous life experience, the development of processing skills may involve re-education and/or an adjustment of attitudes to take account of the changed situation. Where disability has occurred early in life, opportunity to practice processing skills may have been limited; such skills may have to be learned and developed from a theoretical base rather than from previous experience.

Processing skills enable the person to interpret information and make the most appropriate response in a given situation. They involve the receptive abilities to take in and absorb information; knowledge; understanding; analytical and discriminatory skills to interpret the facts; imaginative, judgemental and evaluative skills to consider possible implications and outcomes; expressive skills to deliver a response; and practical skills to pursue a solution. Processing skills may be developed gradually; the person may progress from simple choices, such as which items of clothing to wear, to more complex decisions in such areas as budgeting or home modification. In each situation, the basic facts should be identified and the pros and cons of the available options explored. The individual should then decide upon and pursue the option he prefers, provided that all the possibilities have been addressed and that there are no major negative factors or health and safety hazards. In some instances, the individual's choice may not be in line with the judgement of the therapist or others, but provided it does not entail unacceptable risk, unnecessary expenditure or an unreasonable burden upon others, the decision should be respected. Where the outcome turns out not to be as the person had anticipated, the therapist can help him to analyse the possible reasons why.

The therapist's objective is to enable the individual to perform such actions practically and independently in his own environment. However, where there are major difficulties with thought processes, such as those which may occur following a stroke or head injury, or where experience is limited and important decisions are involved, it may be best for learning to occur through theoretical exercises before practical action is attempted. Games, problem-solving exercises using case situations or audio-visual materials, individual counselling, and group discussions may be used to promote learning. The therapist may take a guiding or facilitating role in such activities, depending on the needs and skills of the individual or the group.

SPECIFIC SELF-MAINTENANCE ACTIVITIES

Feeding

The consumption of nourishment is the most basic voluntary activity for sustaining life. While those who are unconscious or severely ill may be fed by the artificial means of tubes or drips, the usual way of gaining nourishment is through taking meals. This involves acquiring and preparing food as well as eating and drinking. The hierarchical scale of independent function defined by Katz et al (1963) recognises feeding as the first activity to be regained (and probably the last to be lost) following impairment. Difficulties in eating and drinking involve the acquisition and preparation of food, the structure of the environment in conjunction with the mechanics of feeding, and problems with mouth control, chewing and swallowing.

Acquiring and preparing food

The general level of a person's mobility, the accessibility of shops, and the availability of transport need to be considered here. Large supermarkets with wide aisles and parking space close to the entrance enable the wheelchair user to take an active part in shopping, although the height of shelves and freezer cabinets may make total independence difficult. Some ambulant disabled people cope well in this environment, using the shopping trolley as a substitute walking aid, but many find the hustle and bustle of the busy supermarket frightening and prefer to use a small local shop where personal service compensates for difficulties in reaching and handling foods.

For those who are unable to use supermarkets or small shops themselves, home delivery may be arranged; alternatively, a member of the family, neighbour, friend or home help may be able to shop from a prepared list. It is important for the individual to retain some control over the shopping, even if only by deciding which items should be bought.

Food preparation may involve a wide range of skills, depending on the type of meal to be made, the ingredients necessary and the equipment available in the home. Successful practice in the preparation of simple meals will help to build the confidence to tackle more ambitious menus. Frozen or partly pre-prepared meals will reduce the task demands, as will the use of a microwave. In all situations safety is of paramount importance.

A large variety of small domestic equipment is available for the disabled cook. Many everyday labour-saving items designed for the general user will also be of assistance. Kitchen layout and equipment design should be assessed; modifications may be required to improve manoeuvrability for the wheelchair user or to increase accessibility for the person with limited reach or poor manipulative skills. Impairments of vision, motor control or bilaterality may also restrict the use of some kitchen equipment, but with ingenuity and minor modifications many problems can be safely overcome.

The environment and mechanics of feeding

When assessing feeding difficulties the therapist must consider the accessibility of the family dining area, the choice of tableware and furniture, the positioning of the person's head, arm and hand in relation to the food and the need for any protective clothing.

When considering the dining area and furniture the therapist needs to ascertain whether the disabled person will sit at the table on a dining chair (or in his wheelchair or other chair) or whether he will use a tray attached to his wheelchair. Any of these situations may enable the disabled person to dine in the same room with the family, but for some people this may not be possible and meals will be taken in bed with a stable over-bed table of a suitable height.

When considering whether existing tables and chairs are suitable for the disabled person, the therapist needs to consider balance and stability. A chair with arms will provide more support than one without. A slightly higher table and chair may be required for the person with stiff lower limbs. The wheelchair user requires clearance under the table apron and the table must be stable enough to withstand any inadvertent knocks from the wheelchair. Domestic armrests on the wheelchair will facilitate closer positioning at the table. If the person cannot use the dining table he may be able to use a cantilever table or detachable tray.

A winged headrest on the wheelchair may assist the person with limited control of head and neck movements whilst eating, but if tremors or spasms are severe independent feeding may be unfeasible. Where weakness of the upper arm and forearm are the primary cause of difficulty, stabilising the wrist with a lightweight orthosis and using ultra-light cutlery may help. The technique of pivoting the forearm of the feeding hand on the clenched fist of the other hand, resting on the table, will facilitate greater hand mobility without upper arm movement.

Finger feeding is much easier than using cutlery but is contrary to etiquette in many Western cultures. However, in many Eastern cultures finger feeding is the norm and should be respected. Equipment for feeding should be as similar as possible to that used by a non-disabled person; special equipment which draws attention to the individual's problem should be avoided as far as possible.

Western cutlery is held like a small tool, with the handle pressed into the palm and stabilised by thumb pressure against the middle finger. It is stabilised and guided from above by the index finger and additional downward pressure for picking up or cutting food is exerted by flexion of the wrist joint. If any of these abilities is limited or absent, as in median nerve lesion, rheumatoid arthritis or tetraplegia, efficiency is considerably reduced. The therapist must identify the deficit and either suggest alternative methods of holding cutlery or recommend substitutes or aids, such as clip-on cutlery, cutlery with padded handles, or small orthoses to hold the fingers in the normal grip position.

If cutlery handles are thin and slippery and the person has poor grip, is in pain, or has generalised muscle weakness, one of the many types of lightweight cutlery with or without enlarged or modified handgrips may be used. People who can use only one hand may become very dextrous when using an upturned fork or a spoon, but may need assistance when cutting food. Independence in cutting can be achieved by using a Nelson knife, Dynafork, 'Spork' or 'Splayd', or a sharp, curved cheese knife. Cutlery such as this has a sharp cutting edge incorporated with a fork and the therapist must ensure that the individual and his family are aware of the potential danger of cutting the side of the lips if it is used for taking food to the mouth. Many people with strong Islamic beliefs may prefer to be fed rather than use the 'unclean' hand for one-handed feeding.

For people with limited range of movement and restricted reach in the upper limbs, angled and lengthened cutlery may prove to be a suitable solution. This must be adjusted to meet individual needs. Swivel cutlery is also available for people with limited wrist and elbow movement or slight loss of motor control.

Suitable crockery may enable the person to become independent and retain dignity when eating. Deep, rimmed plates are available to match some ranges of crockery but these are often expensive and quite heavy. Their weight may make them unsuitable for those living alone who have to do their own washing-up. Some specifically designed tableware, such as the Manoy range, includes dishes which incorporate a shaped rim to assist in pushing the food onto the spoon or fork. Plate guards fitted to a dinner or breakfast plate may be used in the same way but these are more obtrusive.

The type of food may affect the success of independent feeding. Such foods as tough meat, spaghetti, peas or meringues cause difficulties for everyone and the disabled person is no exception. Foods which require slicing and cutting may pose problems. Whilst the person should not be restricted to a diet of minced meat, mashed potatoes and yoghurt, particularly difficult foods which draw attention to his disabilities, especially when eating out, are best avoided.

Drinking difficulties may be overcome by only partly filling a cup, mug or glass and by using a lightweight beaker, flexistraws or a small piece of narrow plastic tubing clipped to the side of the cup or glass. Bottle carriers of the type used by cyclists can be adapted for the severely disabled wheelchair user. (The carrier and bottle are attached to the side of the chair and fitted with a longer piece of plastic tubing.) For people who have severe problems with motor control, non-spill beakers may be used. Insulated beakers help prevent cooling of hot drinks for those who are slow to drink and afford protection to the hands for those with sensitivity problems. Modern thermal containers with dispensers may be used make hot drinks available throughout the day for those who are unable to manage a conventional kettle or pan safely.

Crockery can be stabilised with a varnished cork table mat or PVC-coated cloth or mat. These are easy to clean, pleasant to look at and do not draw attention to the person's problem. Other forms of stabilising material include Dycem sheeting or mats and pimple rubber. Even a damp cloth will serve to steady a plate. For people with severe co-ordination problems a rimmed tray with a non-slip surface may be necessary.

Difficulties with mouth control, chewing and swallowing

Children may readily accept bright towelling or plastic bibs to protect clothes during meals. However, these are very demeaning for most adults. A fabric napkin tucked into the neck of a shirt or, in the case of ladies, a large, detachable floppy bow clipped to the front of the garment will absorb drips in a less obvious manner. A plastic-backed fabric bib that matches the person's clothing is less obvious than one made from white towelling.

Choice and presentation of food may obviate some of the difficulties with eating. Severe temporomandibular joint involvement in rheumatoid arthritis may cause pain and difficulty in opening the mouth. Similarly, the person with facial burns may have limited mouth opening, and foods cut into small pieces and which require little chewing will be easier to manage.

For people with a spastic condition, eating can be very difficult. Spasms may occur when anything touches the teeth or gums, so food should be sucked from a fork or spoon with the lips. Others may have tongue-thrust problems. Placing food to the side or back of the tongue will reduce food loss. People who have difficulty controlling head movements should eat from a central forward position. Under no circumstances should the head be tipped back to retain food in the mouth, as this adds to difficulties with swallowing and may cause choking.

Problems with the fitting of dentures should also be addressed, particularly following a cerebrovascular accident (CVA) which has affected the facial muscles.

Obviously, the choice of food consistency and texture will be important. Foods may be minced, shredded or liquidised, but where a number of different foods are treated in this way they should be prepared individually to retain their separate flavours and colours. Small, regular snacks may be easier and quicker to prepare and eat. The diet should be nutritious and appealing and include adequate fibre and vitamins, protein and carbo-hydrates. Difficulties with mouth control and diet may be discussed with the speech therapist and dietician to find the most appropriate solution for all concerned.

In conclusion, feeding is a complex task vital to human survival. Emphasis has been placed on the essential tasks necessary to obtain adequate nourishment. These should be given priority, but it should also be remembered that eating is frequently a social activity with accepted norms of behaviour. Inability to perform such behaviours may cause embarrassment and anxiety for the disabled person, his relatives and carers. The individual may become reluctant to join others at mealtimes or to eat away from home. The therapist has an important contribution to make in identifying the precise nature of the individual's problems, which may be as diverse as an inability to respond to a waiter's questions or a loss of inhibitions in drinking and chewing food, and devising ways in which they can be alleviated or overcome.

Toileting

Toileting is the area where most disabled people first wish to regain or maintain independence. For those with severe impairment it is one of the most difficult areas of self-maintenance and one which is crucial to retaining dignity and remaining independent in one's own home. Difficulties in toileting may be divided into those which are caused by difficulties in coping with the environment and manipulating clothing, and those which are due to medical conditions causing continence problems. Frequently the two aspects are interlinked — the person with problems resulting in urgency may be incontinent because of additional difficulties with mobility which prevent him from reaching the toilet in time.

Environmental problems

The toilet is usually the smallest and most inaccessible room in the home. Generally, the more disabled the person is the more space he will require for manoeuvring. Even when the toilet is combined with the bathroom there is not always adequate or suitable space. Access to the toilet is often hindered by steps and stairs, narrow doorways, corridors and awkward corners. These will often necessitate major structural alterations, particularly for the wheelchair user. Where the toilet and bathroom are separate, the removal of the dividing wall to integrate the two rooms may provide more space for manoeuvring. Access may be improved in some cases by widening the doorway and providing good lighting, a gentle ramp or shallow step, and handrails. Installing a sliding door or rehanging a door to open the opposite way may add space and facilitate mobility.

The positioning of equipment in the room is also important. Wheelchair users often find that sideways transfer is easier if the toilet pedestal is set further forward from the wall than is usual. The majority of less able people prefer a pedestal seat which is higher than usual. A variety of raised toilet seats are available, some of which clip to the toilet bowl and others which incorporate handrails in their design. The type of seat may make a difference to comfort and ability; for example, the horseshoe shape (Fig. 8.3.) makes perineal cleansing easier, but may be less stable for some people. Ideally, there should be a wash-basin close enough to the toilet to save additional movement and exertion.

The size and positioning of handrails is a matter of individual need and preference. Horizontal and

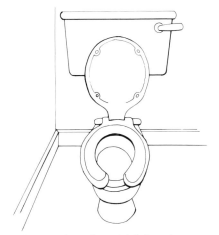

Fig. 8.3 A horseshoe-shaped toilet seat.

vertical rails usually offer more assistance and stability than those which are inclined, although some people find inclined rails of great assistance when rising from the toilet because they support the forearm as well as providing a firm hand grip. A matt finish, either ridged or rubberised, is safer than a chrome finish and a rail 3.75–5.00 cm in diameter is more serviceable than a slimmer one. Texts such as *Designing for the Disabled* (Goldsmith 1984), *Coping with Disability* (Jay 1984) and *Designing Bathrooms for Disabled People* (Kings Fund 1985) are useful sources of reference.

Transfers

Transfer techniques to and from the toilet should be considered, particularly for people who are wheelchair users.

Some people may be able to stand up, take one or two steps, turn around and sit down. The continued use of such abilities should be encouraged, as this will enable the person to be more independent in toileting both at home and elsewhere.

For permanent wheelchair users the most suitable technique will, ideally, be one that requires the minimum of environmental adaptation. Consideration of transfers should be included in the choice of a wheelchair. If the individual is unable to manage a direct sideways transfer, a portable sliding board may enable him to transfer independently by using the mobility and strength of his upper limbs, shoulder girdle and trunk. Detachable wheelchair armrests, chassis design which permits close approach and, occasionally, folding or removable backrests may all facilitate independent transfer. Some people, most commonly those who have double above-knee amputations, will transfer forwards onto the toilet and function sitting back to front (see p. 251).

Sanichairs are available for people who cannot transfer from the wheelchair to the toilet. These can either be propelled by the occupant or wheeled by a helper and positioned over the toilet pedestal.

Management of clothing

Undressing, cleansing, washing and dressing must all be assessed in conjunction with actual use of the toilet. These activities are usually undertaken in a confined space, thereby adding to some people's difficulties. Alteration to clothing, especially underwear, and instruction in alternative methods can enable some people to become independent.

If the person is no longer able to stand and balance, he may be taught to slide forward on the toilet seat and wipe himself from the back, or to slide back on the seat and clean himself with his legs apart. Simple cleansing aids such as paper tongs, Maddak toilet aid tongs or the Sunflower bottom wiper may assist people with limited reach or poor manual dexterity. For the severely disabled person the use of a bidet or electrically operated toilet such as the Clos-o-mat or Medic loo, which dispense warm water followed by warm air, may solve cleansing difficulties.

Menstruation can cause discomfort, embarrassment and sometimes depression. Periods are often painful, with a heavy loss of blood, and the person may seek medical advice to suppress or regulate menstruation. Therapists should assist women to manage as easily as possible and may be able to offer advice, particularly to younger women, about the most suitable and easily managed forms of protection, such as self-adhesive pads which adhere to the inside of the pants. The need for perineal hygiene to prevent odour and secondary skin problems should be emphasised.

Assessment in toileting skills should consider the person's need to use a conventional toilet. Some people may find that using a bottle or commode or chemical toilet is preferable to making major alterations to the home or expending the energy necessary for them to use an ordinary toilet.

Assessment should include both day-and night-time needs. For night-time it may be necessary to make arrangements different from those used during the day, taking account of relatives' and helpers' needs. Carers who are heavily committed to supporting the person during the day will need an uninterrupted night's sleep if they are to continue in this role. Urinals, commodes and chemical toilets may provide safe and convenient alternatives for night-time toileting. Whatever method is suggested and followed, safety is of paramount importance.

Continence problems

Incontinence is symptomatic of various conditions and may be a major contributory cause for admission to care. Elderly people, those with neurological disorders such as multiple sclerosis, CVA, peripheral neuropathy or paraplegia, and some people with cognitive and emotional disorders may require help with the management of continence problems. An understanding approach is necessary for all involved, for incontinence of urine and/or faeces causes the individual acute embarrassment, misery and discomfort. A number of ways of overcoming difficulties can be devised by the occupational therapist, nurse, continence advisor and carers. If a regime has already been formulated, all members of the treatment team should be aware of it and adhere to it.

Training in a particular regime is important, whether the person is wearing an appliance which needs emptying at regular intervals or whether urgency or frequency of micturition is the problem. Worrying only makes the situation worse, and so people need help and reassurance in timing visits to the toilet. This is a very individual matter. Some people may need to empty the bladder every hour by manual expression, while others may have to go to the toilet following meals, and during the mid-morning and mid-afternoon. Curtailing fluid intake throughout the day is not usually advised because of secondary risks to the urinary tract, but some people may be advised to restrict intake in the latter part of the day to avoid nocturnal incontinence. Medical advice must be sought in this regard.

A variety of appliances are available for coping with urinary incontinence. Men are often able to manage problems more readily because their anatomy makes the wearing of condom-style appliances easier. Most women prefer to wear some form of absorbent one-way pad inside protective pants. Several types of pad are available, together with a range of pants which may be pulled up in the usual way, or which have drop front panels or side openings.

Clothing for the lower half of the body should be kept to a comfortable minimum, and made from easy-care fabrics which are not likely to cause secondary friction or sweating problems. Wide openings and concealed zips in trousers will facilitate undressing. Separate upper and lower garments are usually easier to manage and a short upper garment is less likely to be soiled than a longer one. Skin care and odour control are also important for comfort and self-respect. Regular hygiene and skin care, together with the use of products to disguise odour, promotes confidence and reduces the risk of skin breakdown.

It is common for psychological stress to affect urinary habits and control. Discussion, counselling and reassurance regarding any emotional difficulties and anxieties can help to relieve stress. Continence problems may also be associated with confusion, disorientation or loss of memory following neurological damage, with ageing, or with chemotherapy. Identification of the cause of the individual's incontinence, together with the introduction of a regular regime, will help to alleviate his difficulties.

When using a rehabilitative approach to overcome toileting problems, modifications to the home environment or the provision of major items of equipment should be considered only if they are absolutely essential, since their value will be limited to facilitating ability within the home. Modification of techniques or clothing, introduction of a timing regime, and the provision of advice or small transportable items of equipment may be more helpful overall.

It should be remembered that there are many different habits concerning toileting in various cultures and religions, particularly Islam; these should be identified and respected.

The therapist should be able to advise the individual and his carers about the range of help available locally and the advantages and disadvantages of particular equipment and techniques. Detailed information can be gained from the Disabled Living Foundation information service, Equipment for the Disabled booklet

Incontinence and Stoma Care, and texts such as *Coping with Disability* (Jay 1984) and *Incontinence and its management* (Mandelstam 1986). (The reader is referred to Useful Addresses, p. 240 and References, p. 241.) In addition, information on local services may be obtained through the social services community nursing service.

Dressing and undressing

Both able-bodied and disabled people express their personality and sexuality in their choice of clothing. Anyone may draw attention to himself by virtue of his dress and appearance and the disabled person is no exception. Clothing may exaggerate deformity or may disguise it, depending upon the wishes of the individual. Careful selection or adaptation of clothing may help to conceal deformities and to compensate for difficulties with dressing activities.

The ability to undress, dress and make our appearance presentable and pleasing to ourselves and others requires balance and coordination, joint mobility to facilitate reach, dexterity and muscle strength, insight into the task to be undertaken, sensation, and a degree of spatial awareness.

General principles

Everyone should be encouraged to change into day clothes rather than spend every day in night clothes and slippers. This is a primary move to boost morale and initiate the psychological move back to 'normal' living away from the 'sick role'. Full independence in dressing should not be rigidly pursued if such activity is likely to fatigue the person unduly. Assessment of undressing and dressing abilities should be undertaken as soon as possible. Expectations for rehabilitation should be realistic. Assessment will identify those areas in which the individual is independent and those which require teaching or practice.

Undressing is easier than dressing. It is less tiring and should be tackled before dressing in the treatment programme. It is usually carried out at a time of day which is comparatively relaxed, i.e. in the evening. This may contribute to success, but cumulative fatigue from the activities of the day may counteract this.

Garments on the upper half of the body should be removed first, followed by those on the lower half and, finally, the shoes. Footwear is usually left until last in case the person has to stand, when he will be much safer in shoes than in socks or stockings, but with tight trousers footwear may need to be removed before taking the trousers off.

When undressing the individual should be encouraged to think ahead in preparation for dressing. Clothes to be worn again should be left with the right side out, and in the order in which they will be put on.

In most cases, dressing will occur in the bedroom. Clothing should be stored to hand and both the bed and a bedside chair may be used for dressing practice. The chair should be firm and stable, with arms if the person's balance is affected. The seat should be of a suitable height to enable the individual to place his feet flat on the floor. A good level of balance is required to reach up to pull clothes over the head, to lean forward and twist the trunk when managing the lower half of the body, and to reach back fastenings. For some people, sitting or lying on the bed may be easier for dressing the lower half of the body.

The room should be warm, comfortable, and as private as possible, remembering that some degree of privacy may have to be given up in the interest of safety. When planning techniques for dressing and undressing, consideration should be given to the person's level of ability, his choice and style of dress and any habitual techniques which he has retained. It is useful to respect the differences between men's and women's habits in removing jumpers, sweaters or other upper-half garments. Men tend to grasp the upper back of the garment to pull it over the head, while women will more frequently pull it up over the arms and head from the waistband. Such strongly automatic techniques may be retained despite perceptual problems or confusion. Special garments, adaptations or equipment to assist dressing should be used only as a last resort, when alternative manual techniques have been fully explored and found to be inadequate.

The dressing sequence should be considered carefully. Pants and trousers should be put on before transferring to a wheelchair. Prostheses and shoes must be put on before the person stands.

Timing is also important. As far as possible, the person's dressing schedule should fit into the family routine, particularly if he requires help. The therapist should try to fit into the person's normal routine when conducting dressing practice, as this will give her a realistic picture of his level of capabilities at the relevant time of day, and will facilitate normalisation for those who are confused or disorientated. Ample time should be allowed for dressing practice, but the person should not be permitted to become cold or too fatigued. The therapist should decide at what stage help should be suggested, considering the person's pain, stiffness, slowness and weakness. This help may only be required temporarily, as specific difficulties may be overcome with practice.

The person should practise dressing first his upper half and then his lower half, with the therapist observing, advising and assisting when necessary. He should be encouraged to persevere in trying to attain standards which are personally acceptable. Particular methods of dressing or undressing must be suited to the individual's needs; those which have been worked out by the person himself are usually best for him and most likely to be continued without supervision.

Clothing

Where possible, it is best to select clothing which is currently available in high-street shops. It is almost always possible to find ready-made garments which meet the person's taste, are suitable for his age and capabilities, and conceal deformities, appliances and wasted muscles. Each person's needs, circumstances and disability must be considered in the choice of garments. Particular attention should be paid to comfort, as some disabled people have to spend many hours in the same position. Any specially made clothing should be skilfully designed to disguise the problem and should be produced in contemporary materials, styles and colours.

Shopping for clothes is often difficult and frustrating. Many people find that the larger stores are more accessible, have larger fitting rooms and offer a wider choice. If shopping locally is not possible, reputable mail-order firms may provide a solution, as clothes can be tried on at home and returned if unsuitable.

Ideally, garments should be simple and loose fitting, with a minimum of fastenings and with ample openings and gussets. Elasticated waists, cuffs and shoulder straps are easy to manage if they are not too tight. Because of limitations on their physical activity, many people with disabilities need warmer clothing than others do. They should be advised to choose warm fabrics rather than to wear many layers of clothing which will require considerable effort in dressing and undressing.

Personal cleansing and grooming

Personal cleansing comprises the generalised activities involved in washing all or part of the body. Grooming includes such activities as hair care, dental hygiene, shaving, nail care and make-up. Some of these activities are essential to the maintenance of good hygiene and the prevention of infection, but personal cleansing and grooming also affect general well-being, morale, and confidence in social settings.

Habits vary considerably from person to person. Some people wash the whole body daily while others wash only certain parts daily and bathe the whole body weekly. Hair care and methods of washing may be determined by religious practices and cultural norms, or by familial habits.

Washing and bathing are areas of self-care where most people have a desire to be independent for reasons of privacy and dignity, whereas grooming activities are generally less private in nature.

Washing

Most people are able to wash the hands and face, provided they have access to hot water, soap, a flannel and a towel. If the bathroom wash-basin is inaccessible it may be possible to use a bowl of water on a stable over-bed table. Tap turners, flannel mittens or soap holders may make manipulative tasks easier.

The whole body may be washed in a bath,

under a shower, by means of a 'strip' wash or, for those who are unable to attend the bathroom, in bed.

Bathing is a difficult task for many people with a disability. Considerable strength, agility and balance (including the ability to stand on one leg) are required to step in and out of the bath safely in the conventional manner. The provision of suitably placed fixtures and equipment, such as rails, boards, seats, non-slip mats, stools and hoists, may make the task easier and safer. The use of these aids is described in Chapter 9.

Taps and other fittings should be of a design and in a position that facilitates their use. People should be discouraged from using taps, inset soap dishes and the wash-basin as additional grab rails, for the stability of these fittings may not be adequate to take extra weight. For those who are unable to operate conventional taps, lever taps or a tap turner may be of assistance. Soap, flannels, sponges, nail brushes and other accoutrements should be within easy reach; suitably positioned bath bars, trays and shelves will assist.

It may not be possible for the person with upper limb dysfunction to reach all parts of the body without assistance. Long-handled sponges, brushes or loofahs may facilitate greater reach. Trick methods are often helpful — for example, using one foot to put soap onto the other. It should be remembered that sitting on a board or seat over the water can be cold if the room is not adequately heated. Deeper water which enables the person to be immersed will be soothing and relaxing for those with painful muscles or joints.

For many people, a well designed and positioned shower provides a more suitable and safer method of washing than a bath. Showering may be easier to manage, more hygienic and more economical, but it can be an uncomfortable task if the room is cold. The person's capabilities should be carefully considered before a shower installation is recommended. Shower sprays attached to taps may be easy to manage but thermostatically controlled showers are generally safer for elderly and disabled people.

The position of the shower rose is important; those fixed overhead are generally unsuitable for the disabled person, who is likely to have difficulty balancing in either a standing or a sitting position when bombarded with water over the face and head. The rose should be at chest height, and it should be moveable to allow all-over washing from a seated position.

In the case of an independent shower unit, the choice of tray is important. Those who are ambulant may be able to use a lipped shower tray, but a fixed handrail may assist when stepping over the rim into and out of the shower. A shower tray flush with the floor and with sloping drainage will facilitate the use of a wheeled shower chair, on which the individual can move into the cubicle.

Shower stools or chairs should have rubber ferrules, similar to those attached to walking aids, to prevent the seat slipping or damaging the shower tray. Some cubicles have built-in seats and others may have seats attached to the wall. These should be positioned at a height and depth to suit the person's needs for transferring and sitting comfortably. Some seats may be hinged so that they can be hooked back against the wall when other members of the family are using the shower.

If it is not possible to install a separate shower cubicle, a shower spray attached to the bath taps may suffice. Care must be taken to control the temperature of the water. Sitting on a bath board or seat, the individual may be able to use the shower to wash himself, with or without the bath filled with water.

Drying the body requires grip and coordination to control the towel, to reach the extremities and to apply sufficient pressure to dry the skin. A warm room and facilities on which to warm a towel or bathrobe are most useful. The person who is wrapped or wraps himself in a warm robe or bath towel will dry with a minimum of effort. A length of towel with handles or tape loops at each end facilitates drying of the back or legs (Fig. 8.4), and thick, soft, towelling mittens may be used by people with severely impaired grip.

In all instances safety is of paramount importance. Heat, condensation and steam may make surfaces slippery and may cause light-headedness and fatigue. Floors should have a non-slip surface and any mats or unneccesary clutter should be removed. Care should be taken when making transfers, and where appropriate the individual

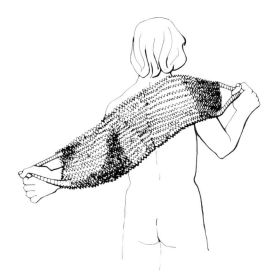

Fig. 8.4 A towel with tape loops.

should be advised not to lock the door, and to bathe only when someone else is in the house, in case he should need assistance. The community nursing service may provide assistance for people who live alone or whose relatives are unable to help.

Some people may prefer to have a strip wash seated or standing at the washbasin for reasons of safety or because of difficulties with transfers to the bath or shower. Problems in reaching the lower parts of the body or the back may be overcome with a long-handled sponge or brush. The room should be warm, as this method of washing can be very cold.

Washing the body is a very important ritualised activity in some religions. Every effort should be made to ensure that cultural norms are understood and that the wishes of the person and his family, particularly regarding privacy and techniques, are respected.

Hair care

If it is not possible to wash the hair independently at the handbasin, it may be possible to wash it when bathing by using a shower attachment. For people who are unable to attend a local hairdresser, a mobile service can usually be engaged to attend the person at home. If the disabled person is confined to bed, a hair-rinsing tray may be used.

Hair washing, setting and drying is often difficult. Short, simple, minimum-care styles which do not require regular pinning, setting or plaiting are easiest for the disabled person to manage independently. A more complicated style may be managed with the cooperation of a willing carer if the person is not able to cope alone.

Dental hygiene

This is important for everyone but is particularly vital for those who take regular medicines which may affect the tooth enamel. Tooth-brush handles can be enlarged to assist people with weak grip. Handles may be lengthened and/or angled to assist people with impaired upper limb mobility in reaching the mouth. An electrically operated tooth-brush may be essential for the person who wishes to maintain independence in oral hygiene despite serious impairment in hand function.

Shaving

While women may be able to use a depilatory to remove underarm or leg hair, this method is not acceptable for removing men's facial hair. Wet shaving with a hand razor is a hazardous business which can only be performed satisfactorily with a steady hand. A battery-operated or electric razor is safer. If the disabled person is unable to hold the razor it may be fitted into a holding bracket angled at the required height or may be attached to the hand with an elastic or leather strap.

Shaving may be particularly problematical for the person who has suffered facial burns. The skin may be sensitive and uneven; great care should be taken when shaving. Growing a beard might not be a suitable solution as many hair follicles may have been destroyed, resulting in uneven growth.

Nail care

Proper care of finger- and toe-nails is essential for reasons of hygiene and appearance, and the care of toe-nails is closely linked with mobility. Nail-files and clippers may be attached to small boards to assist stability and grip when cutting finger-nails. Toe-nails often present insurmountable problems and it is advisable to obtain help from the family, the community nursing service or a chiropodist, particularly if the feet and toe-nails need professional attention, for example for the person with diabetes.

When cleaning the finger-nails the person with weak grip may find a curve-handled nail-brush which clips around the fingers easier to manage. Suction pads which attach the nail-brush to the side of the basin may be helpful for those who are only able to use one hand.

Make-up and skin care

A person may have had previous experience of skin care and the use of cosmetics, but due to the present disability the former regime may be difficult or impossible. Alternatively, changes in the condition of the skin may necessitate a change in skin care.

Provision of adequate lighting and easily managed containers for beauty preparations may ease the problem for people with limited hand function. A suitably placed mirror (which may have a magnifying facility for the person with poor vision) may be of assistance. Extended handles for powder pads, make-up brushes or lipsticks will enable the person with limited reach to apply make-up.

People who have suffered skin damage may benefit from the advice of a trained beauty therapist on types of cosmetic preparations and their application. Some baby products or non-allergenic skin preparations can be recommended. Camouflage make-up may be used to boost the confidence of those who are particularly conscious of facial or hand disfigurement. Those who have had skin damage should be particularly careful in bright sunlight, as their skin may be more sensitive than prior to the injury.

Personal cleansing and grooming are essential parts of everyone's daily routine. It is important to encourage the person to take a pride in his appearance, for the sake of morale and hygiene

and in order to be acceptable to carers, friends and workmates.

COMMUNICATION

Communication may be defined simply as the 'passing of information, ideas and attitudes from person to person' (Williams 1968). Communication is an extremely important life skill. We may need to move, to eat and to toilet in order to survive, but we also need to communicate from birth to death in order to gain assistance with any of these activities, and to become accepted members of society. The baby or young child laughs or cries to express feelings, the adult modifies and refines communication skills according to his environment and personal wishes, and the elderly rely on communication to maintain contact with others in the face of many losses. Whatever our age, our success in communicating with others determines a large measure of our quality of life.

What is communication?

The spectrum of communication methods is vast. Communication may be direct or indirect: it may take place face to face or via an intermediary, in verbal, written or expressive form, or through the use of technical appliances. Messages may be conveyed by a smile or frown across a room, or by a fax transmission across thousands of miles. Whatever its form, communication consists of the same creative and receptive processes: a message or idea is initiated, formulated and presented, to be received, decoded and understood. This process becomes circular as messages are transmitted and responses given (Fig. 8.5). Problems may occur at any of these stages; some difficulties will be directly attributable to impairment, others to factors related to learning, culture or social context. The interpretation of messages is not always straightforward. A smile, for example, may be a sign of friendship or welcome or a signal of ridicule or disrespect. The receiver's interpretation may depend on his previous contact with the sender, on the formality of the situation, or on his self-image and self-esteem.

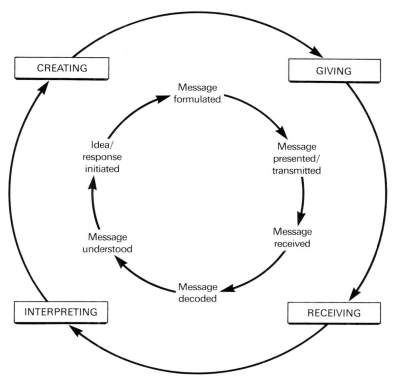

Fig. 8.5   The communication circuit.

Communication problems related to impairment may occur in both the receptive and expressive domains; these are discussed below.

Receptive problems

These are usually caused by sensory or perceptual impairments, but may also reflect a limitation of intellectual capability resulting from, for example, head injury or some types of cerebral palsy. Receptive problems may also be the result of lack of experience, orientation or cultural understanding.

Sensory impairments affecting communication are predominantly those associated with limited hearing or vision. Visuo-perceptual problems and receptive dysphasia also affect communication. Limited cognition may impede learning and understanding of the verbal and written language, as well as the interpretation of non-verbal communications.

Hearing difficulties may be overcome in a number of ways. A hearing aid or voice amplifier, for example, can improve reception of sounds and various forms of apparatus can be used to compensate for a lack of hearing. The latter may include flashing lights on door bells or alarms, and such equipment as a vibrator pad placed under the pillow to act as an alarm clock. In all cases, instruction in the maintenance and use of such equipment must be given. Alternative communication techniques such as sign languages and lip-reading require considerable education and practice and are frequently acquired more successfully by those who developed their hearing impairment early in life. The Royal National Institute for the Deaf, speech therapists, audiologists, social workers for the hearing impaired and equipment suppliers such as British Telecom may provide assessment of needs and specialist support.

Some visual impairments may be overcome

through the use of optical aids such as magnifiers or large-print books. Where these are not adequate, more specialist means of communication such as braille texts, sensory maps and taped books or scripts may be of assistance. The Royal National Institute for the Blind and social workers for the visually impaired are the experts in this field.

Perceptual deficits should be identified by the occupational therapist through specific assessments. Once the problems have been identified, her role is to inform the person and his carers of the deficit, to help the person practice techniques to overcome particular difficulties, and to find alternative ways through which he can communicate.

Problems with reception or understanding may be due to purely linguistic barriers, that is, difficulties in translation, differences in dialect, or even a lack of familiarity with technical jargon. The therapist should be aware of language or dialect difficulties and every effort should be made to facilitate interpretation by spoken or written means. Professionals tend to use jargon; this should be avoided when discussing issues with the disabled person or his carers because it further accentuates any perceived disadvantaged role.

Expressive problems

A number of expressive communication problems occur as the direct result of impairment. These problems may be with verbal or non-verbal expression or with the practical management of communication equipment.

Verbal problems may be the result of damage to the speech centres of the brain resulting in difficulties with remembering and formulating speech. Problems may be due to damage to the mechanisms for articulating speech, e.g. the muscles of the mouth, the tongue, the larynx or the trachea. This can occur with neurological disorders such as multiple sclerosis, cerebral palsy or motor neurone disease, or may be the result of surgery (for example, laryngectomy). The occupational therapist should liaise with the speech therapist to identify the specific problem and the most appropriate ways of overcoming it. Rehabilitation may include practice in speech sounds or words in conjunction with visual stimuli, the introduction of aids such as letter or word boards through which the individual can indicate a request or response, or instruction in the use of more sophisticated means of communication such as voice synthesisers or electronic communicators.

Non-verbal expression may be limited by impairments which affect the control of the muscles of the face or upper limbs. Limited mobility of the facial muscles, such as that which occurs with Parkinson's disease, affects the ability to show emotions or responses facially. Where hypermobility of the facial muscles occurs, as in some people with athetoid cerebral palsy, the control of a facial response may be difficult. Speech may also be impaired in both situations, further adding to communication difficulties. The listener or 'receiver' should be attentive to any response and check its validity. (In this the 'sender' should, where possible, employ an alternative method of communication, for example head-nodding, pointing or a written response.)

Uncontrolled movements of the upper limbs also hinder non-verbal communication. A hand or arm may be used to point, gesticulate, initiate contact by beckoning or emphasise a point. A sudden spasm of an upper limb may be misinterpreted as an invitation or a rejection. It is important for the therapist to explain such problems to the relatives and carers and to encourage them to verify the meaning of the person's non-verbal cues with him, thus ensuring understanding.

Written communication may be affected by limitations in hand function or by visual impairment. Various modifications may be made to pens to assist with grip and control. For those who are not able to write, alternative means of communication by word such as an electric typewriter with modified keyboard, a word processor or the possum system (Patient-Operated Selector Mechanism) may be considered. The use of a tape recorder to transmit the spoken rather than written word may be more appropriate for people with visual impairments who are unable to use a keyboard. Impairments of hand function may also affect the use of other pieces of communication equipment such as the telephone. A number of modifications are available from British Telecom.

Communication problems may also occur because of difficulties with language, or as the result of limited mobility or social experience. These difficulties may affect anyone, but often are an additional handicap for the disabled person.

People with mobility problems have difficulty keeping in touch, even with other members of the family in different rooms in the house. A simple intercom system may facilitate room-to-room communication. Where there is a need to make contact outside the home, either for pleasure or in the case of an emergency, a portable telephone or alarm system may be used to alert neighbours, family or friends. A large number of systems are available and careful choice should be made, bearing in mind the needs of all parties involved.

Limited social experience can impede the development of communication skills. This may lead to anxiety in social situations because of uncertainty regarding the most appropriate type of behaviour. In some instances inappropriate behaviour may lead to embarrassment and further handicap the individual. Every opportunity should be made for the disabled person to gradually integrate in a number of social settings; appropriate instruction and support should be provided so that he can build confidence in social communication skills.

MANIPULATIVE HAND SKILLS

In order to regain or maintain independence in self-maintenance and other life skills, it is necessary to be able to perform a number of manipulative hand functions. These manipulative skills may be used in verbal or written communication to handle papers, books or writing implements; in mobility to manage keys, locks and door handles; or in maintaining a comfortable environment through the use of heating, lighting or window controls. Dexterity skills are required to operate a telephone, to wind an alarm clock, to turn taps and to flush a toilet. All or any of these tasks may be crucial to safety, comfort and independence in self-maintenance activities.

Detailed assessment of manipulative skills, dexterity, grip strength, sensation and coordination, together with analysis of needs and of existing equipment and environmental controls, may be necessary to determine levels of function and dysfunction. Some problems may be overcome by adopting alternative methods when performing activities, for example using the elbow to depress the toilet flush. Modifications to tools or controls may be necessary to overcome some difficulties. An immense number of variations are available, ranging from simple alterations to knobs, switches or handles to facilitate grip to sophisticated electronic devices to operate such items as door locks or heating controls. Careful assessment and practice with a number of different options will enable the individual to make the most appropriate choice for short- or long-term needs.

ROLE DUTIES

Throughout life we all adopt a number of different roles, for example, as child, friend, employee, partner, carer. Each role imposes a range of duties and tasks in order to be fulfilled successfully, either by our own standards or in line with the expectations of others. Most people have a number of different roles at one time and may need to consider the demands of each and to prioritise activities in order to retain a healthy balance in life. While the skills and attributes necessary to each role often overlap, some roles demand very specific skills (Fig. 8.6).

Individual role demands vary considerably, depending on the person and his relationships with others in the fulfillment of the role. In some situations, duties may be carried out entirely by one person, who may adopt an almost servile compliance to the demands and wishes of others. In other relationships the same roles may be perceived as shared partnerships, each person contributing equally to the completion of tasks.

Individual perceptions of roles influence priorities. Some people value the role of the homemaker above that of the worker and gain satisfaction and pleasure from the achievements and freedom it holds, while others regret the restrictions on career opportunities imposed by the

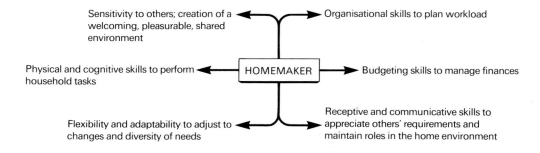

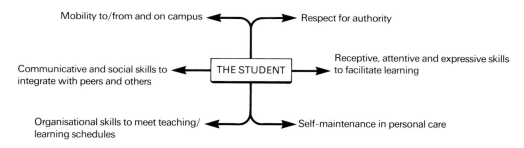

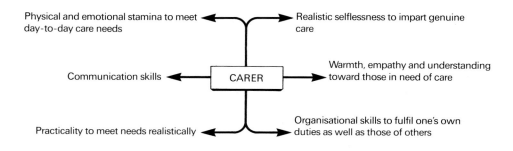

Fig. 8.6 Some aspects of role duties.

homemaking role. Severe disability frequently restricts the range of roles which may be pursued; in such cases considerable effort, ingenuity and support are required to maintain old roles and build new ones.

The following discussion considers the roles of homemaking, caring and working in their broadest sense. Caring includes the parenting role; the role of the worker includes that of the student, employer and volunteer.

HOMEMAKING

Skills for homemaking include planning, organising and budgeting; shopping; preparing, cooking and serving meals; laundry, sewing and mending; and basic home maintenance. Obviously there will be considerable differences in the demands of this role depending on the occupants of the home. A person living alone may need to be independent in all activities because of the lack of help available, but will only have himself to look after. The homemaker who is responsible for a number of people will require many additional organisational and negotiation skills to maintain a home environment physically and emotionally suited to the needs and wishes of all the occupants. This will vary, depending on the other occupants and their roles in the homemaking process. Sharing responsibilities for the planning and execution of activities may ease the burden of homemaking for each individual, whereas responsibility for young children, disabled or elderly relatives or members of the family who take no part in domestic tasks will add to the demands placed on the homemaker. Many homemakers also have a worker role and must manage the essential demands of employment alongside their domestic tasks.

Assessment and training or retraining of the disabled homemaker is an area in which the occupational therapist can make an important contribution. Assessment should include details on the type, design and organisation of the person's home, on how many there are in the family, on what help is available from the family and/or other agencies and on whether the appropriate reorganisation of any of these will make the person more independent or the homemaking role less demanding. When selecting specific areas for intervention the therapist should take account of the person's level of disability, his personal wishes and priorities and other roles he is pursuing.

Intervention must be realistic and practical. The therapist can assist the person who has been in hospital for some time to regain confidence and reestablish a routine. She may help in organising tasks so that each family member has his own duties, for example bed-making, cleaning his own bedroom, shopping, or preparing vegetables for a meal. For the disabled person, training in specific areas may be necessary, such as balancing on a kitchen stool, safe mobility in the home, optimum working positions or lifting techniques. The therapist can help the person to build up physical stamina and to improve physical and organisational skills, and can recommend appropriate and safe labour-saving techniques.

If the disabled person is not able to perform homemaking tasks other avenues should be explored. Trombley (1984) states that the 'severely disabled homemaker may be an effective home manager, directing the efforts of other family members or paid household help. She can manage the finances and oversee the shopping.' Trombley states that the experienced householder may manage this with little training but the 'inexperienced homemaker may need practice in hypothetical financial management and in directing others effectively by words alone'. Others may prefer to retain a more active role in home management through modification of methods or techniques or changes to equipment or the domestic environment, only accepting manual assistance in a small number of activities. Whichever role is pursued, careful planning is important to ensure that the work-load is evenly distributed and needs are met appropriately. Forward planning of the week's activities and organisation of tasks, labour and equipment are essential prerequisites to successful completion of activities. Where the person is an active participant, it is important to plan the day so that necessary tasks can be completed comfortably, allowing for rest periods and leisure time with family members or friends.

A compensatory approach may be used where previous methods are no longer possible. New techniques may be tried and the most appropriate ones adopted. Practice in these new techniques will, of course, be necessary. Reorganisation of the home layout to minimise difficulties and facilitate mobility, modification to storage, selection of major items of equipment such as cookers, cleaners and washing machines, and the provision of suitably sited power sources and small items of specialist domestic equipment may all assist the disabled person in many household tasks.

When tasks cannot be completed independently or with the assistance of family members, other sources of help may be sought. Local authority home-help provision varies from area to area in the duties the helpers are permitted to carry out. Some may only provide assistance with shopping, food preparation, cooking and serving meals, while others will do laundry and cleaning. The local Meals on Wheels service can meet the needs of the disabled person who has difficulty shopping and preparing food, but this is usually not available every day of the week. Various voluntary organisations in many localities also provide assistance with domestic tasks in the person's home. Specific individual requirements for the disabled person and his family may be financed in some instances by the Social Fund or the Family Fund. In many areas, local privately organised services exist to help with domestic care. These may be engaged through the use of benefits such as attendance allowance, income support or severe disablement allowance. The therapist should be aware of local facilities and services and should advise the disabled person and his family on how to make applications and gain the most benefit from such services.

CARING

In many instances the occupational therapist is involved in assessing the disabled person for community living. This may be with a view to an individual's return to the community following hospitalisation. It may also be undertaken to find the most appropriate environment in which the home-based disabled person can continue in community living. It is therefore vitally important that the therapist be conversant with the needs, demands and resources for successful community care for both the disabled person and his carers.

Emphasis is often placed on the needs of the disabled person in the assumption that a partner or member of the family will take an active part in his care. Such assumptions infringe upon the rights as individuals of those concerned. Open, informed discussions should take place to identify the resources and options available; each person's wishes should be considered before decisions are made regarding future care. In many situations the outcome may have to be a compromise by both parties in light of the limitations of available resources. However, where compromise decisions

are made they should be considered as sensitively and positively as possible to limit any feelings of anger and bitterness which may mar personal relationships between the carer and the disabled person. Information should be provided on services and personnel available to cope with unexpected pressures or crises in caring and, where possible, regular appraisal or reviews to monitor the situation and any changes in needs should be carried out.

The carer

Care may include help with any aspect of life skills. It may be given in the form of advice, guidance and stimulation to support the disabled person in learning how to safely perform a given activity himself, or it may extend to practical assistance to compensate for the person's inability to do the task independently. Each of these forms of care has its own particular strains. The former requires genuine respect and unflagging patience in promoting the person's achievement according to his own wishes and without the imposition of the carer's own standards. The latter type of care may be physically demanding, for example in terms of lifting and moving the disabled person, and may impose impossible or unrealistic physical strain on the carer. In either case, care is time consuming, either in terms of the total number of hours devoted to the care of an individual or by virtue of an ongoing commitment to a daily or weekly schedule.

The Disabled Persons Services, Consultation and Representation Act 1986 extended the provision of the Chronically Sick and Disabled Persons Act 1970. Section 8 of the 1986 act recognised the rights of carers to request an assessment of needs for the disabled person for whom they are caring which takes account of their ability to continue to provide care. For the purposes of the act, carers are those who provide a substantial amount of care without remuneration on a regular basis for a disabled person who is living at home.

Many carers are themselves elderly or disabled and the burden of caring for a loved one who is also disabled, over and above managing their own problems, can cause considerable physical, mental, social and financial strain. Successful caring requires a partnership in which each party recognises and respects the wishes and needs of the other. This should be viewed not just in terms of the demands each places on the other when they are together, but should also be considered in terms of the need for personal space, privacy and periods of freedom from the patient or carer role. Much will depend, therefore, on provision of and access to resources for support to permit respite periods to occur on a regular basis, without feelings of guilt or bitterness and without any sacrifice of safety.

Where the carer has a close relationship with the disabled person, changes in this relationship precipitated by disability may place heavy demands on both partners in their emotional and/or sexual interactions. Sensitive discussion of each other's feelings and needs may enable each partner to come to terms with his own and the other person's wishes and roles, and to find ways of modifying and continuing the close relationship.

Caring also includes child care and parenting. The stresses of looking after a disabled child may affect the entire family physically, emotionally, financially and socially. In addition to the pressures on parents, those imposed upon siblings must be considered. Siblings may feel jealous of the attention given to their disabled brother or sister, angry at the limitations imposed on the family or burdened by their extra duties toward the disabled child. These feelings should be shared and discussed and the family should be encouraged and supported in finding ways to achieve an acceptable balance of attention and activity for all its members.

Where a parent, particularly the mother, is disabled, practical difficulties may arise in caring for the children, especially when they are very young. Specialist equipment and practical assistance with caring duties may enable the disabled person to fulfil the parenting role safely. Where possible, such assistance should be home based; this will enable the children to develop in their own environment and permit the parent to retain maximum contact with them. Day nurseries should be considered only when home care is not possible, or where it seems to be necessary for the social development of the older child, as early separation of the child from the parent may affect emotional bonding. As children grow older they should be encouraged to take responsibility for their own personal care but should not be overburdened with unrealistic domestic duties over and above those normally expected of children their age.

On a more positive note, it should be emphasised that caring can be a pleasure. It can provide friendship and companionship for both parties. Maintenance of abilities and small achievements can be a source of pleasure and pride to the disabled person and to the carer, adding to a fuller appreciation of life and living.

Needs for caring

The support required by carers in order to successfully fulfil their role includes:

- Information about the services available, how to make an application, how decisions are made and how to make an appeal against unfavourable or unsuitable decisions. This information should be given in easily understood terms in the languages of the local community.
- Separate assessment of needs for the disabled person and the carer. Both parties are entitled to this service and the legitimate interests of both parties should be considered equally.
- Consultation: this should occur at all levels *before* care plans are formulated. This should extend beyond the disabled person and the carer to include appropriate external agencies, for example voluntary organisations, social services or housing agencies, before decisions are made for future care.
- Practical help, which may include assistance with self-maintenance or domestic activities, mobility, employment or home adaptations. Practical help may also include financial provision in the form of benefits, or emotional support through counselling, befriending or self-help groups.
- Relief from care for both parties. Both short and long spells of relief should be

considered, ranging from the occasional social or shopping trip to holiday periods. The type of relief should be compatible with each person's needs. However short the relief may be, a regular, predictable service is usually valued most.

Sources of information

These include the National Council for Voluntary Organisations, which provides a directory of voluntary agencies and their roles; DIAL UK, Disability Alliance and the Citizens' Advice Bureau, all of which provide information on rights and services; the Equal Opportunities Commission; the Department of Social Security and the appropriate acts of Parliament, which provide information on statutory provision; the Association of Carers and the Association of Crossroads Care Attendant Schemes, which consider specific care provision; and many other agencies which provide information and assistance for specific groups of disabled people and their carers.

WORKING

Work may be defined as the purposeful application of effort. Over the century work and work patterns have changed considerably. Whereas in previous decades many people spent long hours in heavy manual labour, employment in less physically demanding tasks and more flexible, shorter working periods are now becoming the norm. Advances in technology have enabled tasks to be completed by push-button control, which in some instances has led to a need for fewer employees to meet production demands and higher levels of unemployment. Despite this relatively high unemployment amongst all sectors of the population, many people with disabilities feel inadequate if they are not able to work. This may be linked to the perceived status of the worker and the gains which employment brings.

Gains from working

Independence

Work may provide the means to be self-sufficient.

Many people work to earn sufficient income to sustain independence in daily living for themselves and their dependents. It is important to consider that those in low-paid employment may not benefit financially from work. Equally, statutory benefits do not usually provide sufficient funding for holidays, outings or other luxuries.

Additionally, many illnesses carry added expense; special dietary requirements, extra heating and transportation costs, and expenses for personal care and home cleaning can add to the strain for those on a low income.

Self-esteem/status

It is interesting to note that social class may be determined by occupation (Box 8.1). Some jobs have a status image attached to them which affects the ways in which the individual is perceived by society. The work people do may determine the type of house in which they live, the area in which they live, the people they meet, the items they can afford to buy and, in some instances, the opinions they hold.

Work carries with it a sense of purpose and worth, a role in life, and a responsibility to or for others. Unemployment, by contrast, is still commonly associated with an image of laziness. Many people who cannot work feel a 'burden on society'. Some lose their self-respect and feel they cannot contribute to the society in which they live. Some still think of themselves as living on charity when receiving benefits or other services to which they are entitled and for this reason (as well as others) they may not apply for the help available to them.

Box 8.1 Work and social class
(Registrar General, Somerset House, National Records Office)

Category	Occupation
Social class I	Professional occupations
Social class II	Intermediate occupations
Social class III (N)	Skilled occupations: non-manual
Social class III (M)	Skilled occupations: manual
Social class IV	Partly skilled occupations
Social class V	Unskilled occupations

Group membership

Man is a naturally gregarious animal and his need to be part of a group and to have a defined role in society is a constant pull. People can gain support and social contact from those with whom they work. For many people, the primary focus of work is not financial gain, but the benefits of meeting others, getting out of the house and being a useful member of society or part of a social and employment circle.

Structure

Everyone enjoys the freedom to do what he wants to do, when he wants to do it, for a limited period, but for many people this freedom may lose its attraction after a time, as they lapse into apathy because of a lack of variety or purpose to the day. Work, on the other hand, can provide structure to the day, week, month and year. It may determine the individual's allocation of time, type of dress and social behaviours. In so doing it may add to his appreciation of non-work time — in the evening, on weekends, or during holidays — because of the change and freedom it brings.

The duties of the worker

In order to sustain employment the worker must be able to meet the demands of the job adequately. These may be many and varied, depending upon the type of employment and the work situation.

Physically, employment demands extra effort and in some cases a sustained level of strenuous physical activity during the working day. Considerable effort may be required by the disabled person in order to travel to and from work, in addition to fulfilling the demands of the actual work tasks. Some work, such as computing or fine assembly tasks, demands a high degree of coordination and dexterity. For some people these demands may prove too great if such skills are unpractised or if illness has resulted in a residual manual disability.

Psychologically, any work demands a degree of concentration and adherence to routine. Certain rules and regulations must be followed; acceptable dress, language, social habits, timekeeping and personal hygiene must be displayed. Skills of communication and organisation are required to perform adequately in many situations.

Work tolerance, which may include the ability to tolerate noise, heat, cold, heights, dust, outdoor work and long hours, may actively need improving in some people whose physical and psychological fitness have been seriously impaired. People who have been unemployed for a substantial period of time may need help in achieving the correct level of skills in budgeting, in adjusting their personal life around a work routine, and in using public transport, work canteens or specialist equipment. Social skills necessary to relate adequately to workmates and employers and independence in all activities of self-maintenance may require attention. The person may need practice to acquire the confidence to work unsupervised or to attain the level of accuracy necessary for the job.

Additionally, awareness of current trends and societal opinions may assist the individual to gain personal acceptance by workmates in both work and social contexts.

The use of technology in the form of computers, programmers and word processors linked directly to the employer enables many people who have difficulty with mobility, self-maintenance activities or verbal communication to work from a home base. In this situation the psychological demands for concentration and adherence to routine are particularly important to maintain the work pattern in the domestic environment. In the past, home employment has frequently been in poorly paid assembly or packing tasks but advances in information technology have raised job status and the level of remuneration for some people who work from a home base.

The role of the occupational therapist

In some cases, work assessment will be a part of the individual's comprehensive programme of treatment; thus, the occupational therapist will already be familiar with the person's skills and limitations. In other instances, the individual will be referred to the therapist specifically for work assessment and thus may have had no previous contact with her. In either case a good rapport is important so that the purpose of the assessment is understood by both parties and the person being assessed feels able to talk through any fears or anxieties with the therapist. Depending on the nature of the individual's impairment, the occupational therapist's role may involve any or all of the following:

• Teaching independence in self-maintenance activities. Where personal independence is limited the therapist must aim to restore this by suitable means before full work resettlement can be attempted. If a person is severely disabled and/or needs to attend an assessment or training centre, it will be necessary for him to become independent in self-maintenance activities before he can be accepted for such a scheme.

• Improving physical ability. The occupational therapist will be concerned with helping the person to regain or optimise function when this has been lost or limited. This may include activities to improve range of movement, strength, dexterity, coordination, balance, etc., to enable the person to function at work.

• Improving psychological skills. If concentration, perception or other mental processes have been affected, the therapist may devise activities to help the individual improve these skills. Similarly, if speech is affected the occupational therapist will support and complement the work of the speech therapist.

• Teaching or improving basic skills. Where confidence or ability in the performance of basic skills is limited the therapist will be concerned with improving the person's level of function in these areas. This may include practice using public transport, handling money or relating to workmates. Driving a car may require specific assessment and practice, which may be available through a disabled driving centre or a driving school such as the British School of Motoring.

• Building or improving work tolerance. Following illness and a long period away from work, many people have difficulty in regaining a work habit or sufficient stamina to cope with a full day's work. In such a situation the occupational therapist can begin to build up the person's work tolerance by gradually increasing the amount of time, effort and concentration required in the activities he is performing. Similarly, it may be necessary to accustom the person to specific working conditions such as noise, dirt, outdoor work or bench work, where this is deemed appropriate. It is often difficult for the therapist to simulate the demands imposed by a full day's work in industry or commerce but, where work tolerance is lacking, improvement in this area can certainly be initiated whilst the person is attending the hospital or centre regularly.

Assessment of the person's potential for return to work

Frequently, the occupational therapist is asked to assess a person specifically to see if he will be able to return to his former occupation or, where this is not considered feasible, to discover his ability to undertake assessment and training for a new job. The activities performed in a work assessment vary. Many self-care skills should be assessed and improved if found lacking, for a person may not be accepted for open employment if he is not personally independent. In addition, certain specific assessments may be necessary, depending on the nature of the job and the area of impairment. For example, it may be necessary to note the ability of a clerk to sit for long periods, use a typewriter or computer, and write legibly. Lifting, climbing and carrying skills may need to be assessed for the bricklayer

When assessing a person's ability to return to work the therapist should ensure that she is well aware of the skills demanded by the job; this will entail making an ergonomic job analysis. This can usually be done by asking the person himself what his job involves, but where this is not possible the therapist should ensure she receives accurate information by contacting the person's employer or another reliable source. In some situations there may be opportunities for the person to practise in simulated work tasks, either in the occupational therapy department or in other areas of the hospital or community, before returning to full-time employment or making application for alternative training.

Many occupational therapy departments devise their own work assessment and report forms for use with people undergoing this type of assessment. Standardised assessments may be used to determine abilities in specific areas of function; these include the Raven's Progressive Matrices, which assess diagrammatic reasoning abilities; the Mill Hill Vocabulary Scale, which assesses linguistic intellectual performance; the Rivermead Perceptual Battery, which determines perceptual function; and particular dexterity, strength, and clerical skills assessments.

The occupational therapist may complete the DPl work assessment report for the Disablement Resettlement Officer (DRO) to assist him in advising the individual on employment opportunities, or she may present the report to the consultant, general practitioner or other personnel concerned with the person's future or with his compensation claims.

Giving information and guidance

Frequently, people whose employment prospects are doubtful have little idea of the type of help available to them either for building up fitness for return to work or for retraining for alternative employment. It is often a source of great concern to the person that his future employment prospects seem poor. The occupational therapist should be able to supply accurate and appropriate information on the sources of help available (Fig. 8.7) and on what benefits the person may receive. The therapist may be a member of the team which assesses the person's capabilities and makes direct referral to the DRO or other appropriate agency.

Ordinary further education courses provide pathways for some disabled people to gain experience and qualifications at an academic and social level which may enhance employment opportunities.

The resettlement clinic

In some hospitals or specialist rehabilitation centres a resettlement clinic may be held regularly to determine the future work prospects of individuals undergoing treatment. Such clinics are usually run by the doctor in charge of the unit or the consultant responsible for rehabilitation services. They are usually attended by the occupational therapist, physiotherapist, social worker, a senior nurse attached to the unit (where appropriate) and the DRO. Occasionally, the psychologist or the person's relatives may also attend. The person's case is presented, his progress charted and his future prospects and options discussed. Where further intensive medical treatment is considered advisable, he may be referred to a medical rehabilitation centre. Alternatively, it may be considered that he has reached his maximum potential and that referral to employment training or support services would be more suitable.

Medical rehabilitation centres

These provide an intensive programme of rehabilitation following serious illness or injury. Individuals may be referred to such centres following initial assessment and treatment in hospital. Such centres have the facilities to build up a higher degree of physical fitness and work tolerance than is possible in most hospital departments. Treatment is provided under medical supervision by a team comprising physiotherapists (who may conduct hydrotherapy and gymnasium work), occupational therapists, speech therapists and social workers. The centres offer a non-hospital atmosphere. Some centres are residential on a weekday basis; residents are encouraged to be personally independent and make their own arrangements for transportation and entertainment during their stay.

Sources of assistance for the disabled worker

The Disablement Advisory Service (DAS)

This is part of the Employment Service Agency and is usually based at the Employment Service area office or Job Centre. The DAS exists to assist both employers and people who are already in employment or are seeking work. It can provide advice on developing and implementing a sound

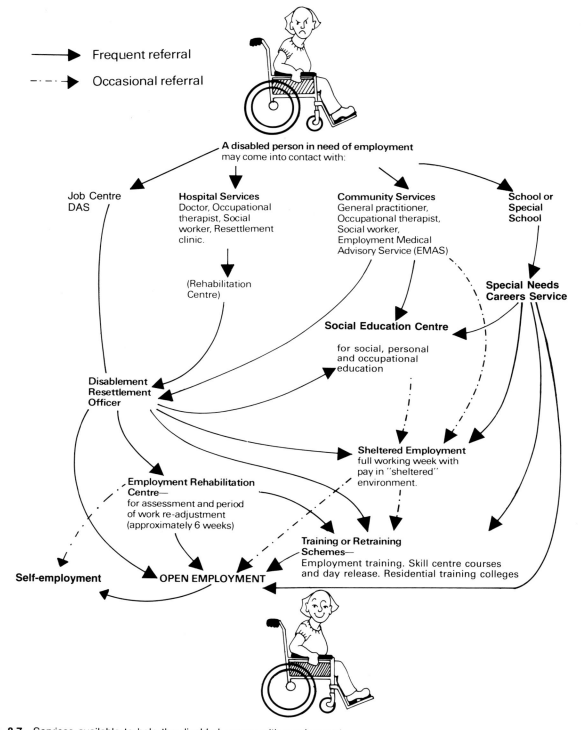

Fig. 8.7 Services available to help the disabled person with employment.

company policy on the employment of people with disabilities, as outlined in their *Code of Good Practice on the Employment of Disabled People*. Specific advice may be given regarding the recruitment, career development and retention of workers with disabilities. A number of special schemes exist to overcome particular difficulties. These include the Job Introduction Scheme, the Special Aids to Employment Scheme, the Adaptations to Premises and Equipment Scheme, the Personal Reader Service for the visually impaired and the Working at Home with Technology Scheme.

The Disablement Resettlement Officer

The DRO deals specifically with individual problems regarding employment and is a vital member of the DAS. His role, for which he has undergone specific training, involves advising the disabled person about and introducing him to open employment, vocational or professional training schemes, assessment centres and sheltered or alternative work. The DRO will keep the person informed of any suitable jobs available for him in the area and will contact local employers on his behalf.

Where it is felt appropriate the DRO may help the person to enlist on the Disabled Persons' Register, which is held by the Department of Employment. This is a voluntary register for people over 18 years of age and is designed to help disabled people obtain and keep a suitable job as determined by the Disabled Persons (Employment) Act of 1944. The DRO is conversant with job training opportunities in the locality and the types of employment available. He may meet clients through the local hospital by referral from the doctor or therapist or through the Job Centre where they have gone to find work.

Employment Rehabilitation Centres (ERCs)

These centres provide opportunities for people who have not been employed for some time following illness or injury and who need a chance to adapt themselves gradually to normal working conditions. The ERCs also assess people's employ-

ment capabilities. Courses vary according to individual needs and the facilities offered aim to simulate working conditions and a realistic work atmosphere.

During the stay at the centre individuals are paid a tax-free maintenance allowance which is at a higher rate than basic unemployment and sickness benefit. Each person's programme is regularly discussed and reviewed at a case conference.

Employment training

A number of employment training schemes are available for the disabled person on a residential or daily basis. Residential colleges provide training courses for disabled people in a range of commercial and vocational skills. Trainees receive an allowance whilst on the course. Applications should be made through the local DRO. Local employment training initiatives vary from area to area and information is available through the DRO at local employment training or skill centres. Some further education establishments provide day release courses and other employment training courses suitable for disabled people.

Sheltered work

Where the disabled person is unable to work in open employment sheltered work provides an opportunity for him to offer a productive day's work under realistic conditions. Sheltered employment, established under the Disabled Persons (Employment) Act 1944, can be provided through Remploy Ltd, local authority workshops or schemes organised by voluntary organisations. Remploy provides jobs for severely disabled people under sheltered yet realistic commercial conditions. Products include furniture, leather goods, textiles and equipment for disabled people. Employees are paid a wage for their work. Local authority workshops and those run by voluntary organisations such as the Royal British Legion and the Spastics Society also provide work, usually under contract with local firms. In most workshops people must be capable of putting in a standard working week even though their output is low.

Social education centre

For those who are unable to cope with either open or sheltered employment, social education centres run by the local authority offer social and occupational education. As well as simple work tasks performed in a realistic work atmosphere (again, usually under contract with local firms), these centres provide education in life skills such as self-maintenance, homemaking and social interaction. Trainees receive standard state benefits while attending the centre and a small remuneration for the work they produce. Some people may progress to further courses after a period at the centre.

Other initiatives

A variety of local community programmes are available to help the less disabled person who has not worked for some time to regain confidence. These differ from region to region and rely largely on local initiatives.

Some specialist training courses are offered for people with particular impairments; for example, training schemes for visually impaired people are offered by the Royal National Institute for the Blind.

The Rehabilitation Engineering Movement Advisory Panels (REMAP) will also design and provide special items of equipment to assist the disabled person to overcome a particular problem at work.

The Job Introduction Scheme from the Employment Service Agency gives both the employer and employee an assessment period during which a grant may be paid to the employer to fund the trial introduction period for both parties to assess suitability for the job.

In addition to specific equipment for employment and training courses, assistance may be provided by the Employment Service Agency for travel to and from work and for adaptations and modifications to the workplace.

Self-employment

Able-bodied and disabled people alike may wish to become self-employed, using their skills in a creative or consultative capacity. Starting one's own business can seem very attractive but there are many factors to consider before embarking on such a venture. Realistic, reliable advice regarding available resources and potential pitfalls is of vital importance. Consideration should be given to the viability of the skill or product in question, and to financing the venture in terms of materials, premises, marketing and production costs. The physical, psychological and social demands of such a project should be assessed realistically in light of the person's impairment and the stress that self-employment is likely to cause to the individual and his carers should be considered. The DRO may be able to advise the disabled person regarding the opportunities and schemes available to him, and advice from banking and business agencies will be invaluable.

The disabled employer

Many people are able to maintain their role as employers despite substantial levels of physical disability. Much will depend on the type of work involved. Cognitive and communication skills are usually the disabled employer's most important personal assets. Modern technology and good support staff have enabled people with limited mobility and very restricted physical skills to continue in the managerial role, using their knowledge and experience to organise and negotiate effectively, and retaining their pride, dignity and the respect of employees and customers.

The Employment Service Agency may provide advice concerning specialist equipment or other resources available to the disabled employer.

THE STUDENT

Studying is included here under the work role because many of the skills necessary for successful schooling are similar to those needed in employment. Both roles require adherence to the rules or regime of the establishment, social skills to communicate with those in authority and with one's peers, practical skills to meet the demands of set tasks, and mobility skills to travel to, from and within the school or campus.

The occupational therapist's role is also similar in both situations. She may be involved in assessing and developing skills in relation to the demands of the role, reporting to others about individual needs, and providing advice, guidance and liaison between the individual and the establishment to facilitate successful integration.

The 1981 Education Act encouraged increased placement of disabled children in mainstream schools. The occupational therapist may be involved in detailed assessment of the child's abilities for the Statement of Special Needs (form F.A.2). Areas evaluated may include independence in personal care tasks, fine and gross motor skills, and perceptual, cognitive and social skills. The Statement aims to ensure that the necessary provision is available for the child at school. The therapist may be involved in the development of these skills in readiness for school and she may also be required to provide advice to parents and teachers. This may include recommendations on site modifications, handling techniques, and special equipment to promote mobility or facilitate teaching and learning.

For the older student, the therapist may assist with the assessment and development of skills for future study, employment and community living.

Many adult and elderly disabled people who are unemployed or retired may consider study as a means of purposefully filling the day without the direct objective of attaining gainful employment.

THE VOLUNTEER

Some disabled people who are not in paid employment use their knowledge and skills in a voluntary capacity to assist others. The range of voluntary activities is extensive and provides assistance to all age groups. People who have skilled knowledge and experience in managerial activities may be valued members of voluntary groups, while others who have particular physical skills or communicative abilities may be able to use these in teaching or assisting others. Personal experience of problems often promotes greater understanding of the difficulties others may be facing. Some people with disabilities become active members of disability organisations or pressure groups which aim to improve recognition and facilities for disabled people in general.

Many people who do not wish to join the paid work-force find that their volunteer 'work' provides structure, satisfaction, pride in their abilities and recognition. In some instances, volunteer work has led to paid work in open employment or to educational or managerial roles in charitable organisations.

In conclusion, purposeful occupation — whether as homemaker, carer, worker, employer, student or volunteer — is a vital component of the disabled person's quality of life. Many disabled people are able to fulfil some if not all of the duties associated with their roles, and the occupational therapist may assist them in recognising, maximising, and utilising their skills and in identifying techniques, equipment and resources that will help them to overcome particular areas of difficulty.

LEISURE

Leisure-time pursuits are an important part of any person's daily life. These may include hobbies, sports, exercise, entertainment, holidays, relaxation, and play. For the disabled or elderly person who is not able to work, leisure plays an even more important part in living. Leisure activities and involvement in local organisations are a substitute for work and provide opportunities for participation in creative activities and for maintaining or increasing social contacts. They may introduce the person to broader areas of interest and compensate him for the lack of status associated with unemployment.

Initially, leisure activities may help the more severely disabled or elderly person to adjust to a new life-style, but later these activities may become more than a time-filler. They may encourage the individual to strive for more knowledge and skills than he had time for previously.

Individual needs differ considerably, depending on the temperament, personality, interests and level of intelligence of the person, as well as on the impairments and disabilities he may have. The therapist must be aware of such factors before she can guide the person towards fulfilling his needs. She needs to take into account previous interests, for these may still be pursued to advantage by some people; however, for others who have a significant level of disability, returning to previous activities may cause frustration and accentuate functional losses. Much will depend on the person's desires and the facilities and resources available locally to meet his requirements.

EXPLORING LEISURE OPTIONS

The most important task is to identify what the disabled person would like to gain from leisure pursuits. For some people socialisation may be the prime objective, while others may see creativity as the most important aspect. Socialisation may involve active participation with others in a social setting or group; alternatively, the individual may be a passive receiver in a social environment such as the cinema, theatre or at a football match. The range of possible creative activities is immense. Some people may wish to join others in classes or groups, while others may prefer to be creative in their home environment if the facilities and materials are available. Others may wish to expand their education and knowledge through adult classes or independent learning methods.

Leisure pursuits may be explored individually, giving an opportunity for the development of relationships away from the carer or family. Such wishes should be clearly identified and discussed to avoid any feelings of rejection on the part of the family or carers. Alternatively, the disabled person and the family may wish to identify activities that all members can participate in together. This may be particularly important for holidays.

Issues such as travel, transport, cost of materials or activities and any special equipment should be explored. Some financial assistance may be available either through reduced attendance fees or through grants or loans from charitable organisations such as the British Sports Association for the Disabled or the Royal National Institute for the Blind. Jay (1984) suggests that many disabled people do not participate in the wide range of leisure opportunities available to them because of:

- lack of confidence in their ability to participate, which reduces motivation to explore options
- lack of knowledge of how or where to find information about leisure activities.

Confidence

Some people do not wish to join activities specifically for disabled people. They would prefer to participate in activities with people who are not disabled, but are concerned about others' attitudes to them and whether they will be able to participate equally. Unfortunately, many may have suffered rejection or over-protection by their non-disabled peers because of their disability.

The therapist can help such individuals to discuss their anxieties and societal attitudes and can provide opportunities for assertiveness training and confidence building. Where he lacks confidence in his practical abilities to pursue the activity, the disabled person may be able to explore the activity in a day centre before joining a local group or club. Many centres provide a wide range of social and leisure activities with help and guidance from centre staff or peers. Books and reference texts may be obtained from the local library to assist learning.

If communication skills are impaired they may be improved through regular practice in communication techniques in a safe environment in one-to-one and group activities. Social skills training may be based in discussion groups, role play, video exercises and organised excursions. Cognitive skills may be developed through reality orientation, problem-solving games and simple quizzes or through activities or exercises that involve following verbal or written instructions.

A one-to-one introduction may assist both the organisers and the disabled person to share concerns and discuss any special arrangements which may ease anxieties about participation in a club, class or group. In some instances a relative or carer may be able to a accompany the disabled person; this may reassure him, particularly on the first visit. However, if he is happy with his choice of activity he may not wish the relative or carer to continue attending, as this may impede his social integration. It is possible in some instances for the occupational therapist to fulfil this introductory role.

Sources of information and range of options

Nationally, information may be obtained from a number of sources. Many charities provide information on the range of activities available to their members. Additionally, the Disabled Living Foundation information leaflets, the Equipment for the Disabled booklet *Leisure and Gardening* and the *Directory of Sports and Leisure for the Disabled*, as well as many other leaflets and books, provide a wide range of information on organisations and equipment specifically for disabled people (see Further Reading, p. 241). On a local basis, information can usually be obtained from the Citizens' Advice Bureau, leisure or education services departments of the local council and from the social services department. Access information and details of facilities available in particular areas can be obtained from city information and access guides, and organisations such as the National Trust provide their own information booklets.

Information about travel can be obtained from the Department of Transport *Door to Door* booklet, RADAR publications on holidays and travel, and from RAC and AA publications. A number of holiday organisations have details of access and mobility facilities in holiday accommodation in resorts in Britain and abroad. Some organisations provide holidays specifically for disabled people and their families.

The range of leisure options available to a disabled individual may include:

- practical pastimes such as model-making, gardening, photography, cookery and needlework
- intellectual pursuits, including further or higher education, adult education classes, study and appreciation of music, art, literature, computing and many other areas of interest which may be used for intellectual stimulation or pleasurable appreciation
- active participation in sports or games, ranging from card or board games to more active pursuits such as archery, swimming, riding or skiing
- specific interest collections such as stamps, coins, books, records and many other collectable items
- interests requiring little or no active participation, such as theatre, cinema, television and radio, music or spectator sports
- social clubs which organise particular social activities or outings, either specifically for disabled people or as a broader facility for all.

In conclusion, a wide range of opportunities are available for the disabled person to pursue leisure activities at home or in the community. The occupational therapist may introduce leisure interests through therapeutic social activities or may provide information on where to obtain details of services or equipment. She may stimulate the disabled person to explore old skills or interests or encourage him to consider new leisure pursuits. For those who are not able to obtain paid employment, leisure activities provide structure to the day and enhance self-esteem.

Satisfaction, pleasure or achievement in recreational activities can add quality to the day or week and promote a sense of purpose and well-being for the disabled person, and may ease some of the emotional burden on relatives and carers.

CONCLUSION

This chapter has attempted to outline the life skills necessary for successful community living. Of necessity, the coverage of each particular area has been superficial. The chapter has addressed the main aspects of self-maintenance, role duties and leisure, but the reader will need to explore particular areas in more detail to meet the specific needs for a given individual. The practice chapters in this volume will identify some of the problems resulting from specific diagnoses, but other texts which provide detailed information on equipment, techniques or particular life skills should be explored.

Many of the techniques used by the occupational therapist in helping the disabled individual to develop life skills are based on the rehabilitative approach, and thus explore ways of compensating for loss of function. However, these techniques should not be used in isolation as many problems may be minimised or overcome by the use of other therapeutic approaches to enhance physical, intellectual or social performance, and thereby improve function.

Realistic consideration of the individual's personal wishes in the context of his present physical, social, psychological and environmental situation is the crucial factor in devising a strategy which will meet his needs and those of his relatives and carers in developing life-skills.

USEFUL ADDRESSES

Association of Carers
29 Chilworth Mews
London W2 3RG

Association of Crossroads Care
Attendant Schemes Ltd
10 Regent Place
Rugby, Warwickshire
CV21 2PN

Banstead Place Mobility Centre
Park Road, Banstead
Surrey SM7 3EE

British Sports Association for the Disabled
34 Osmaburgh Street
London NW1 3ND

Centre on Environment for the Handicapped
35 Great Smith Street
London SW1P 3BJ

DIAL UK
Dial House
117 High Street, Clay Cross
Chesterfield, Derbyshire

Disabled Living Centres Council
c/o Disabled Living Foundation
380–384 Harrow road
London W9 2HU

Disabled Living Foundation
380–384 Harrow Road
London W9 2HU

Disability Alliance
25 Denmark Street
London WC2 8NJ

Equal Opportunities Commission
Overseas House
Quay Street
Manchester
M3 3HN

Equipment for the Disabled
Mary Marlborough Lodge
Nuffield Orthopaedic Centre
Headington
Oxford OX3 7LD

Kings Fund Centre
126 Albert Street
London NW1 7NF

Mobility Advice and Vehicle Information Service
Department of Transport TRRL
Crowthorne
Berks. RG11 6AU

National Council for Voluntary Organisations
26 Bedford Square
London WC1B 3HU

Rehabilitation Engineering Movement
Advisory Panel (REMAP)
25 Mortimer Street
London W1N 8AB

Royal Association for Disability
and Rehabilitation (RADAR)
25 Mortimer Street
London WIN 8AB

Royal National Institute for the Blind
224 Great Portland Street
London W1N 6AA

Royal National Institute for the Deaf
105 Gower Street
London WC1E 6AH

REFERENCES

British Telecom 1989 Action for disabled customers. British Telecommunications, London

Chronically Sick and Disabled Persons Act 1970. HMSO, London

Cynkin S, Robinson A M 1990 Occupational therapy and activities health: toward health through activities. Little, Brown, Boston

Department of Transport 1989 Door to door. A guide to transport for disabled people. Department of Transport, London

Disabled Persons (Employment) Act 1944. HMSO, London

Disabled Persons Services, Consultation and Representation Act 1986. HMSO, London

Education Act 1981. HMSO, London

Goldsmith S 1984 Designing for the disabled, 4th edn. Royal Institute of British Architects, London

Jay P 1984 Coping with disability. Disabled Living Foundation, London

Katz S, Ford A B, Moskowitz R W, Jackson B, Jaffe M W 1963 Studies of illness in the aged. The index of ADL: a standardised measure of biological and psychosocial function. Journal of the American Medical Association 185(12): 914–919

Kings Fund 1985 Designing bathrooms for disabled people. Kings Fund, London

Mandelstam D 1986 Incontinence and its management. Croom Helm, London

Trombly C A 1987 Occupational therapy for physical dysfunction. Williams & Wilkins, Baltimore

Williams R 1968 Communications. Penguin, London

Yerxa E J, Locker S B 1990 Quality of time use by adults with spinal cord injuries. American Journal of Occupational Therapy 44(4): 318–326

FURTHER READING

British Association of Occupational Therapists. Occupational therapists reference book. Parke Sutton, Norwich in association with the BAOT, London (Published annually)

Charities Aid Foundation. Directory of grant making trusts. Charities Aid Foundation, London (Published annually)

Countrywide Publications 1989 Sports and leisure for the disabled. Countrywide Publications, Peterborough

Darnborough A, Kinrade D 1988 Directory for disabled people: a handbook of information and opportunities for disabled and handicapped people, 5th edn. Woodhead Faulkner, Cambridge

Hale G 1983 The new source book for the disabled. Heinemann, London

Maczka K 1990 Assessing physically disabled people at home. Chapman Hall, London

Mandelstam M 1990 How to get equipment for disability. Disabled Living Foundation, London

Roper N, Logan W W, Tierney A J 1990 The elements of nursing: a model of nursing based on a model of living. Churchill Livingstone, Edinburgh

9

Mobility skills

Ann Turner

INTRODUCTION

Independent mobility is a skill which develops throughout normal infancy and childhood into adult life. From the baby's first attempts at lifting, moving and controlling his head to the adult's proficiency at dancing, cycling, running and climbing, many forms of independent mobility are practised, improved upon, and mastered.

Alongside this increasing ability to move and control our bodies we develop our cognitive and social abilities. Together, all these abilities allow us to explore and control our environment and to create and maintain our personal, social and working lives. Our ability to move, therefore, becomes an integral part of our lives, and something we take for granted. Not until it becomes affected in some way do we realise the wide-reaching consequences that the loss of independent mobility may have on all aspects of our lives. Stepping on a nail, for instance, may cause a relatively minor injury, but can temporarily render someone unable to walk without the assistance of sticks or crutches, climb up stairs, get into a bath with ease, drive to or at work, dig the garden or play with the children. Not only may the person's activities be limited, but any activity he does perform may take twice the time and energy that it did before. In the short term this interruption to daily activity may be viewed as an enforced 'holiday', an opportunity to rest, sit back and let others take on the work and responsibility for a while. However, should such a state of restricted mobility continue for whatever reason, the person will view his loss of independence, role, income and leisure pursuits in quite a different light. When a person loses spontaneous independent mobility even the most basic tasks need more planning and time and, possibly, assistance from equipment or a helper.

It can be seen, therefore, that interruption to, or loss of, independent mobility can have a wide-ranging effect on all aspects of a person's life. For the occupational therapist a knowledge of the methods, equipment and help available to maintain and/or increase a person's level of mobility is an essential part of being able to help restore him to as high a functional level as is practicable. Where independent mobility is considered to be an inappropriate goal, the therapist needs to impart her knowledge to both the disabled person and his carer(s) so that they can work together and make the carer(s)' help as effective as possible.

This chapter, therefore, will present the methods, equipment and other help available to increase a person's level of mobility devoting a section to each of the following areas: (1) transfer techniques; (2) hoists; (3) walking aids; (4) wheelchair mobility; (5) outdoor mobility; (6) mobility within the home.

PART 1: TRANSFER TECHNIQUES

In order to reach even the most basic level of independence a person needs to be able to transfer himself to and from bed and chair/wheelchair and on and off the toilet/commode. The therapist's role, therefore, is to enable the person to achieve independence in transfer techniques where at all possible. Where this is not possible an assisted transfer, which should be taught to both the person and his assistants, may be the most satisfactory alternative. Where neither of these is possible, or where they prove inappropriate, methods of lifting

the person, either manually or by means of a hoist, should be explored.

In the following pages various techniques by which a person can move, with or without assistance, from one place to another are described. There is no 'correct' way for any particular person or circumstance, nor are all methods suitable for any one person and/or his helper, so the choices should be considered by the disabled person and his helper with the therapist, whose detailed knowledge of the person's abilities and of the methods available should enable the most appropriate choice to be made.

During the teaching of transfers, methods should be selected with an eye to progression from assisted to independent manoeuvres, where this is considered feasible. It is also worth considering that, as ours is an ageing population, many people may have a short memory and poor retention of new knowledge. It follows, therefore, that once a suitable method has been found, it should be used consistently, and its teaching accompanied by simple commands given one at a time. Similarly, where assisted or lifting techniques are necessary, it is important to explain to the person how best he may help (by positioning his body or maintaining his posture, for example) and also what is unhelpful. Where more than one assistant is necessary, one of them should be 'in charge' in order to give the instruction of when to lift, where to turn and so on.

Three types of transfer will be described in turn:

- Independent transfers
- Assisted transfers
- Lifting techniques.

INDEPENDENT TRANSFERS

PRINCIPLES

- The surfaces for transfer should be stable and as equal in height as possible. Where a wheelchair is used the brakes must be applied before the transfer is attempted. It may also be necessary to remove one or both arms from the chair and to lift, retract or remove the foot-rests.

• The surfaces should be as close together as possible. Where a gap exists it may be bridged with a transfer board.

• Although there is no 'correct' method of transfer for any one person, that which is easiest and safest for the individual should be employed.

• When teaching transfers, the therapist must be sure that her instructions are clear and she should satisfy herself that she has been understood.

• Balance must be maintained throughout the transfer.

• Independence in transfer must be taught at the most appropriate stage of rehabilitation. It is important not to attempt it too soon, lest the person feel he may fall or fail. Nor should help be continued for so long that he loses the desire to move independently.

• It is important to show the person how to use his body weight to advantage by, for example, leaning in the direction of travel or 'rocking' in order to increase momentum before pushing off.

METHODS

Chair transfers

Sitting to standing (Fig. 9.1)

For those with difficulty rising from or sitting down on a chair the following points may help:

• A high-seated chair is easier to transfer to and from than a low-seated one. A chair that is too low can be raised either by a chair raise or, if this is more appropriate, by lengthening its legs.

• The chair seat needs to be firm. Chairs that are too soft can be improved by placing a wooden board under the cushion.

• Any loose or additional cushions should be removed from the chair.

• A chair with arms is easier to push out of when rising. Arms also provide a support to hold on to when sitting.

• An 'ejector' seat or chair can give the extra impetus needed to help the person rise independently, but, for safety's sake, should be used with caution. The weight of the user

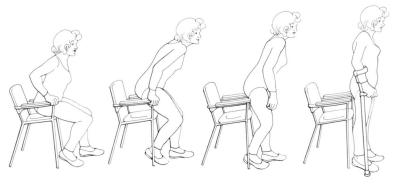

Sit well forward on the chair with both feet on the floor and the weight taken through the stronger (rear) foot—if this is applicable. Hold the arms of the chair firmly. Keep the head up.

Push up with the hands and feet, with the head well forward.

Transfer weight evenly onto both feet, and adjust balance.

Collect aids

Fig. 9.1   Transfer from sitting to standing.

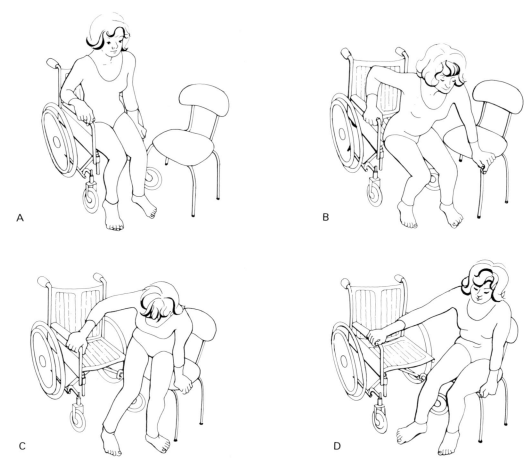

Fig. 9.2 Corner transfer.

determines the amount of spring assistance built into the chair. Different types of controls are also available to suit individual needs.

Chair to chair

Types of independent transfers from one chair to another are:

- Corner transfer (Fig. 9.2)
- Side transfer (Fig. 9.3)
- Transfer using a sliding board (Fig. 9.4)
- Front transfer (Fig. 9.5).

Bed transfers

Transfers onto or off a bed can be made easier if the following points are borne in mind.

- *The bed frame.* For many disabled people a standard divan bed is too low to allow easy transfer. Where possible the height of the bed, i.e. the distance from the floor to the top of the mattress *when compressed*, should be as near as possible to the height of the seat of the chair onto which the person will transfer. For a standing transfer onto or up from a bed the compressed mattress should be at the optimum

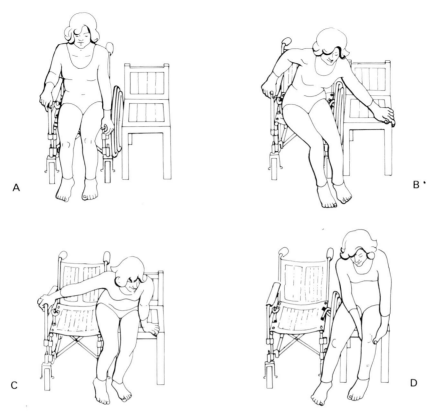

Fig. 9.3 Side transfer.

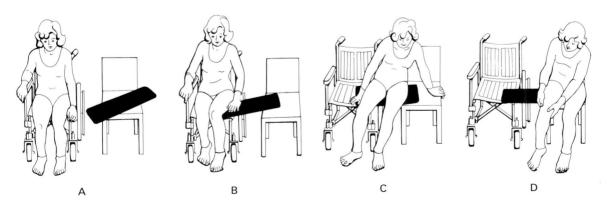

Fig. 9.4 Transfer using a sliding board.

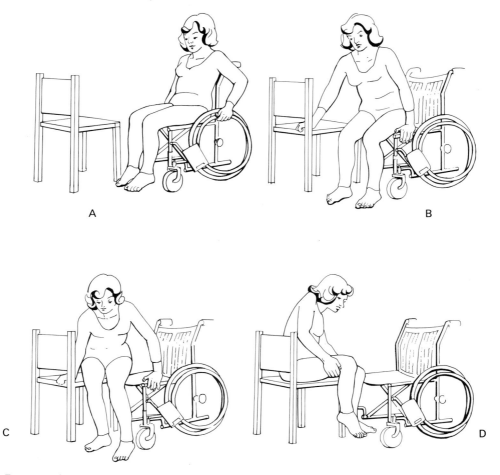

Fig. 9.5 Front transfer.

height to allow easy transfer. The height of the bed can be altered by lengthening or shortening the bed legs or by the use of *secure* bed blocks. In some cases it may be advantageous to remove the castors from the bed legs, as these may cause the bed to move during transfer.

- *The mattress.* This should be the same width as the bed frame. A firm-edged mattress is easier to rise from. If the mattress edge is soft, boards can be placed between the mattress and the bed frame to provide a firm base for transfers. Ideally, the boards should cover the whole width of a single bed and at least half the width of a double bed so that the individual does not have the additional problem of negotiating a ridge in the mattress.

- *Positioning.* When the person needs to transfer to a chair or walking aid there must be sufficient space at the side of the bed for these manoeuvres.

Sitting up in bed

See Figure 9.6.

Sitting over the edge of the bed

See Figure 9.7.

Getting up from the bed

The same principles apply here as for getting up

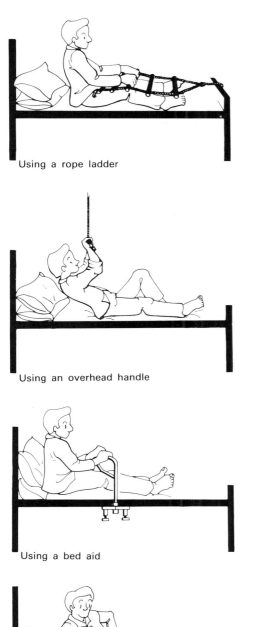

Using a rope ladder

Using an overhead handle

Using a bed aid

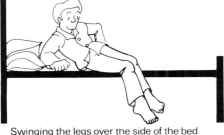

Swinging the legs over the side of the bed
and pushing up with the arms

Fig. 9.6 Sitting up in bed.

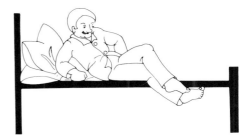

Hooking the weak leg over the strong leg

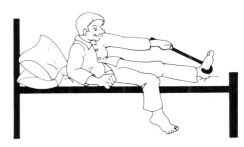

Lifting the weak leg with the aid of a stick handle

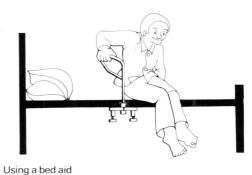

Using a bed aid

Fig. 9.7 Sitting over the edge of the bed.

from a chair. If additional support is needed
a bed aid, head or foot board, or *stable* piece
of furniture, such as a chest of drawers placed permanently by the bed, can be used for the person
to push up on.

Sitting down on a bed

The same principles apply here as for sitting down
on a chair.

Lifting legs onto the bed

This can often cause a problem if legs are weak and/or oedematous. It may be possible to hook one leg over the other or to use a walking stick handle (see Fig. 9.7). Alternatively, a stool or a low chair may be used as a 'half-way house'. Leg ladders and other commercial equipment are also available and may be tried to see if they help an individual where the above methods do not.

Bed to chair, chair to bed

The transfer used depends on the person's ability and the space available around the bed. Consequently, a standing, corner, side, or sliding board transfer, as already described, may be used. If none of these is appropriate one of the following may be tried:

- Forward transfer (Fig. 9.8)
- Backwards transfer (Fig. 9.9).

Toilet transfers

When transferring to and from a toilet several points should be borne in mind:

- Many toilets, especially modern ones, are quite low and the seat may, therefore, need raising to allow easy transfers. Various designs of seat raise are available and the therapist must ensure that a raise fits *securely* before issuing it. Ejector and sloping seats are also available.

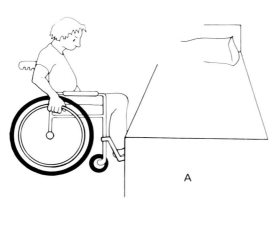

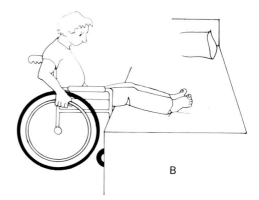

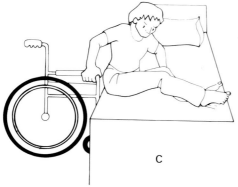

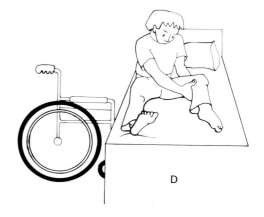

Fig. 9.8 Forward transfer onto a bed.

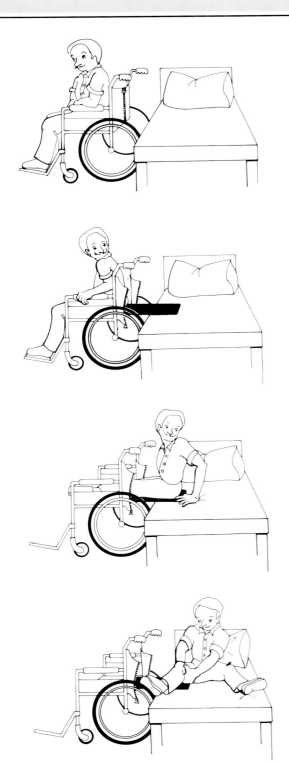

Fig. 9.9 Backward transfer onto a bed.

• Grab rails fixed to the wall near the toilet, or frames fixed around the toilet will provide a firm grip for transfer. Again, many designs are available, including some which combine a toilet frame and raised seat.

• An individual must be able to cope with clothing, toilet paper and flushing the toilet as well as with transferring on and off the toilet.

• Where transfer onto the toilet presents great difficulty because of the person's disability, lack of space, distance to the toilet or other barriers, alternatives such as commodes, urinals, sanichairs, or sanitary facilities combined with wheelchairs or hoists must be considered.

• If a wheelchair is used the type selected should allow easy and close access to the toilet.

Standing up from and sitting down onto the toilet

The same principles are applied as for 'standing from sitting' and 'sitting from standing'.

Chair to toilet

The following methods may be employed:

• Corner transfer (see Fig. 9.2).
• Side transfer (see Fig. 9.3).
• Front transfer (see Fig. 9.5).
• Forward transfer (see Fig. 9.8). Note that for this transfer (for example, for a double lower limb amputee) the person uses the toilet facing the cistern with his legs on either side of the seat. Toilet rails are essential to assist transfer.
• Backwards transfer (see Fig. 9.9). Note that for this transfer the sliding board is not used. A chair with the large wheels at the front is best as it can be wheeled right up to the toilet. For both forward and backward transfers, chairs with a single cross-brace frame can be pushed nearer to the toilet.

Bath transfers

Independent transfers into and out of the bath will require much practice and, frequently, considerable upper limb strength. Whenever bath transfers are being attempted it is advisable that the person be supervised until he is quite certain of his ability, so that assistance may be given if necessary. Where the bather, understandably, wishes to maintain his privacy it is advisable that someone remain within earshot in case the bather needs to shout for assistance. Alternatively a pull-cord alarm may be installed.

Where bath transfers create major problems that cannot be overcome by bath aids, an alternative method such as a shower, all-over wash or bed bath may be preferable for the sake of ease and safety. Where major expenditure is feasible, a specially designed bath such as one with opening sides may be considered as an alternative for, or in addition to, the existing bath. It may be necessary to consider whether the person would prefer to expend the considerable time and energy required by bathing on activities which he sees as having greater priority.

Where aids such as bath boards, bath seats or grab rails are needed these should always be checked for security and safety and should, if at all possible, have a non-slip surface. It is also advisable that either a non-slip bath mat or some non-slip patches be placed in the bottom of the bath. Other bath transfer aids, such as those that work on an electrically operated bellows system, or a hoist, can also be considered. The therapist must also ensure that any aids selected will not cause damage to the bath/shower tray — especially if these are made of fibreglass.

Getting into and out of the bath from standing

Many types of grab rails and poles are available for those who need a little help getting into and out of the bath. Three types are illustrated in Figure 9.10. Additionally, grab rails may be attached to the wall by the side of the bath. Some baths are designed with integral grab rails.

Getting into and out of the bath from a sitting position

Transfers from a chair, stool, wheelchair, extended

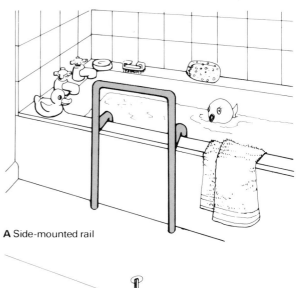

A Side-mounted rail

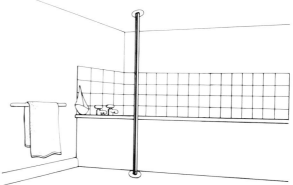

B Safety pole

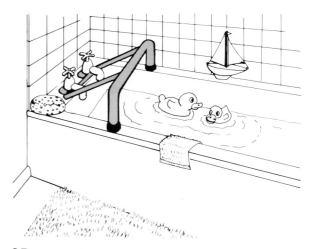

C Tap-mounted rail

Fig. 9.10 Grab rails for the bath.

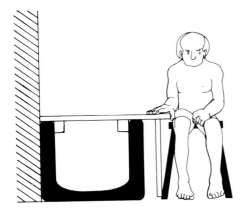

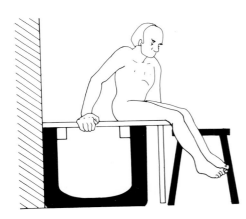

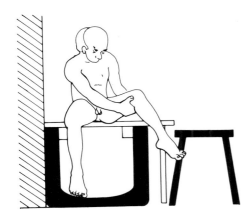

Fig. 9.11 Side transfer using a board.

bath board, bath side or other seated position will now be described. For side transfer techniques with and without bath aids, see Figures 9.11–9.13. The following points should be noted:

- For those with a unilateral weakness it is advisable to have the stronger side nearest to the bath when getting in.
- The person may take an over-all wash or shower while sitting over the bath on the bath board.
- For many, the provision of a seat by the side of the bath, plus an inside bath seat, will suffice.

ASSISTED TRANSFERS

PRINCIPLES

For those whose disability does not allow them to move independently, assistance with transfers may be necessary. The therapist must be aware that, under these circumstances, both the disabled person and his assistant must have confidence in one another. Such confidence will come from the knowledge that each is sure of the moves the other will carry out and that each person is sure of his own role in the procedure. The principles listed below apply to any type of assistance with transfers which may be given by the helper or therapist.

- Before giving assistance the helper must be aware of the amount of help the disabled person is able to give and the type of help that is required.
- In some cases the disabled person will be able to tell the helper how he is usually moved.
- The disabled person should assist the helper as much as possible, when and where he is able.
- Giving assistance during transfer often demands considerable physical effort and the helper, therefore, should learn, practise and cultivate skill and technique rather than rely on strength.
- The 'force' for assistance comes from the leg muscles. The helper should ensure that

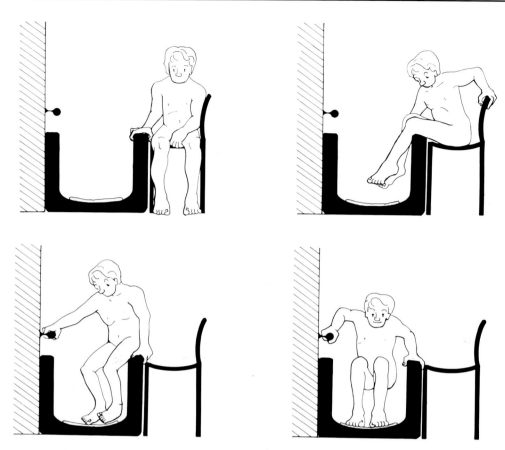

Fig. 9.12 Side transfer without aids.

before and during the manoeuvre her hips and knees are flexed, her spine straight, her head erect, her feet well spaced to give a firm base, and that balance is maintained throughout.

● The helper should prepare the way, ensuring that any aids necessary are to hand and that the place the person is transferring to is prepared. There should be an obstacle-free passage through which both people can move.

● The helper should prepare herself, know exactly what help she is going to give and stand in the appropriate place to give it. She should ensure that she is suitably dressed — that shoes give firm support, that clothing allows adequate movement and that hair or jewellery do not dangle across the disabled person. The helper/therapist should also ensure that personal hygiene does not give offence!

● The helper should prepare the person, telling him what she is going to do and how he can help. She should ask him to move into the position required to start the transfer or move him into that position if he cannot manage alone. She should ensure that he understands where he is transferring to and what method will be used to get him there.

● To initiate movement the helper may rock the person backwards and forwards in the chair to help him gain enough impetus to stand.

As with independent transfers, there is no 'correct' way of giving assistance. When deciding which transfer to use the therapist should consider:

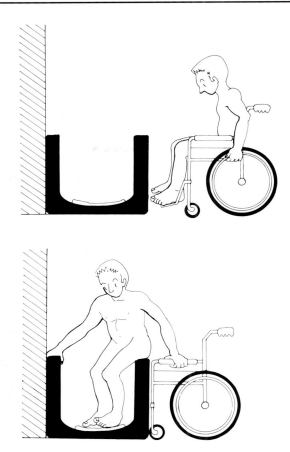
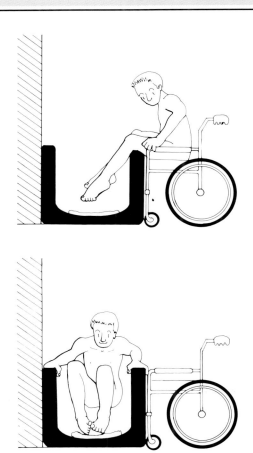

Fig. 9.13 Forward transfer without aids.

- the person's abilities — balance, ability to bear weight, upper limb strength, cognition and whether the situation is static or changing
- the helper's abilities — her strength, fitness and cognitive ability
- the relative builds of the helper and disabled person
- the environment in which the transfer will be executed, including the relative heights and positions of surfaces, the space available and the floor covering.

Some basic holds are illustrated in Figures 9.14–9.17. The pelvic hold is described in some detail to explain some of the principles that apply to all assisted transfers.

METHODS

The pelvic hold (Fig. 9.14)

- The person prepares for transfer by sitting towards the front of the chair, leaning slightly forward and placing one foot (the stronger where this is applicable, or the dominant) slightly behind the other. His feet should be apart.
- The helper faces the person and places one foot and knee against the person's forward leg and knee in order to 'block' the leg and prevent it from slipping. The other foot is placed so that her feet are well apart, giving a firm base. She may block both feet if required.
- With knees bent and back straight the

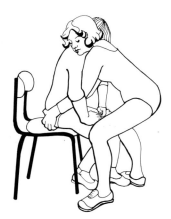
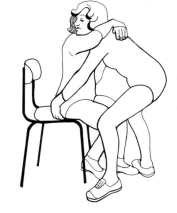

Fig. 9.14 Pelvic hold.

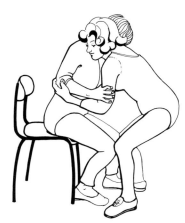
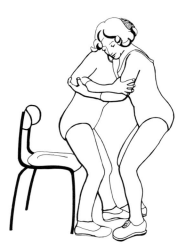

Fig. 9.15 Forearm hold.

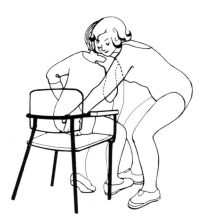
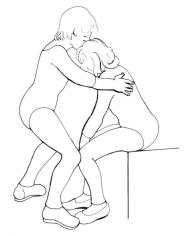

Fig. 9.16 Arm-link hold.

Fig. 9.17 Scapular hold.

helper passes her arms under the person's arms and places her hands under his hips, as shown. If she cannot reach this far she may prefer to place one hand under the hips with the other grasping firmly onto the person's clothing at waist level. For the person's comfort the lift should *never* be attempted by holding clothing only.

• To execute the lift the helper and the disabled person stand together on command from the helper. When transfer to another seat is required the person is helped to swing his hips towards the second seat before he sits down.

There are several variations to the pelvic hold:

• The helper places one hand on the person's hips and another over his scapula.
• The helper places both arms round the person's ribcage and locks them together behind his waist.
• The disabled person holds across the helper's back with both hands during the lift.

Other basic holds include:

• The forearm hold (Fig. 9.15)
• The arm-link (Fig. 9.16)
• The scapular hold (Fig. 9.17).

LIFTING TECHNIQUES

PRINCIPLES

Where the person's disability does not allow him to support his own weight during transfers he may be lifted from one place to another by two helpers. The same principles used when transferring apply to lifting. However, when two or more helpers are involved in lifting, one must take overall charge and give commands to the others. Good timing is essential during lifting so that effort is synchronised.

Before executing the lift the person should be asked to:

• relax, have confidence in the helpers and not 'fight' against them during the lift
• look ahead, not at the floor or the lifters

• endeavour, if at all possible, to maintain his body in the position in which it has been lifted.

In order to prepare for the lift the lifters should:

• decide who is going to give commands in order to synchronise proceedings
• ensure that both the disabled person and the lifters are confident about what is expected of them
• check that there is ample clear space in which the lifters may manoeuvre during the lift.

There are several different ways of lifting a disabled person. The lift chosen should depend upon:

• the number and abilities of the helpers
• the physical condition of the disabled person, including his ability to maintain his posture, whether any particular movement or position will cause him pain, and the state of his muscle tone
• the distance and frequency of lifting required.

Two of the most frequently used methods are the through-arm lift and the shoulder or Australian lift. Both methods can be adapted to move a person up a bed or up from the floor.

METHODS

The through-arm lift (Fig. 9.18)

1. The person prepares himself for lifting by sitting as upright as possible, crossing his arms in front of him and grasping his own forearms if possible.
2. One lifter stands behind the chair (or kneels behind the person on the bed), passes her arms under the person's axillae and then grips his forearms. The second lifter, standing beside the person, places her hands under his legs, one under his thighs and one under his calves, in order to support them during the lift.
3. On command from the lifter in charge (preferably the one holding the person's arms) the person is lifted and moved to the required position.

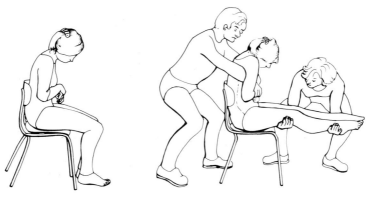

The patient crosses her arms
in preparation for lifting

The helpers lift as shown

Fig. 9.18 The 'through-arm' lift.'

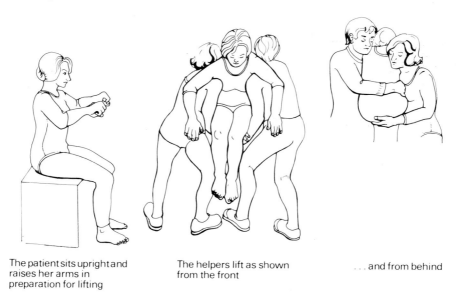

The patient sits upright and
raises her arms in
preparation for lifting

The helpers lift as shown
from the front

...and from behind

Fig. 9.19 The 'Australian' lift.

N.B.: The arm-lift alone is especially useful for lifting a person back into a more upright position if he has slumped down on a bed or in a chair.

The shoulder or Australian lift (Fig. 9.19)

1. The person prepares himself by sitting as upright as possible and holding his arms out to the side, as shown.

2. The lifters stand to either side of the person, facing towards his back, with their knees bent, feet apart, backs straight and heads erect. They each press the shoulder nearer to the person against his chest wall under his axilla, so that his arms rest across their backs. The helpers then reach under the person's thighs (again using the nearer arm) and they grasp each other's wrists.

3. The lifters' free hands can be used to

support the person's back, to push up on the chair/bed during the lifting process or to open doors if the person is being moved over a long distance.

4. Both lifters rise on command from the lifter in charge. Once upright, the helpers can use this lift to transport a person over a considerable distance.

PART 2: HOISTS

A hoist is a mechanical lifting aid designed to lift and/or transport an individual, by means of suitable slings or a static seat, from one place to another. A hoist is usually supplied in a person's home because:

- the person is unable to transfer himself independently. This inability may be total or may apply to just some situations such as transferring into and out of the bath
- assistance with transfers from a carer is not feasible, perhaps because of the carer's limitations of strength and/or stamina
- the carer and the disabled person prefer an alternative method of transfer to be available for all or some occasions.

SUPPLYING A HOIST

It is essential that an accurate assessment is made before a hoist is supplied, and that adequate training is given to all users once it is installed. Hoists and slings that are not suitable for a particular situation can be uncomfortable and, quite possibly, dangerous to use. Equally, if people are uncertain of how to use a hoist this may cause damage to the disabled person, the helper, or the hoist itself. A bad experience when using a hoist can damage the users' confidence and make them apprehensive about, or unwilling to use the hoist again. In order for a hoist to be used competently and regularly it must meet the needs of the disabled person and his helper to the extent that daily life is simpler

with rather than without it. When a hoist is supplied it is essential that a maintenance contract is established so that both hoist and slings are checked regularly and assistance is readily available should the hoist break down. The users must be aware that they must *never* tamper with a hoist or try to adapt its slings.

ASSESSMENT

The therapist needs to consider the following when assessing for a hoist.

The user

- *Need for a hoist.* Is a hoist really necessary? Can the inability to transfer be overcome by other means, such as a new transfer technique, a different wheelchair or an alteration to the environment?
- *Physical abilities and limitations.* These will influence the type of hoist supplied and the type of sling/seat to go with it. The therapist should look specifically at the user's head control, sitting balance, limb control, muscle tone and sensory abilities especially related to visual and tactile appreciation. Do his physical abilities enable him to use a hoist or not?
- *Height and weight.* This must be taken into account in selecting the most suitable size of hoist and sling.
- *Clinical condition and prognosis.* This may indicate the period of time for which the hoist may be required and can be important when considering the feasibility of a permanent or temporary arrangement.
- *Cognitive abilities.* Can the person learn to use the hoist independently if he is physically able to do so? If not, has he the ability to cooperate with the carer by controlling his limbs and posture?
- *Specific needs.* For what purposes will the hoist be used? Do the slings need to be used for transferring on/off the toilet or in/out of the bath? Does the hoist have to transport the person from one place to another or is a static/fixed type more suitable?

The environment

- *Space available for use and storage.* This may dictate the size of the hoist chosen and whether it will be a mobile, floor- or ceiling-fixed or gantry type.
- *Construction of the building.* Certain types of building cannot support a fixed-track hoist. Similarly, if a hoist has to move the person from one room to another at different levels a mobile hoist would be unsuitable.

The carer/helper

- *Physical abilities and limitations.* These may affect decisions about the controls and sling attachments on the hoist, whether a mobile or track hoist should be supplied and how frequently a transfer can be carried out.
- *Cognitive abilities.* Is he able to learn to use the controls and slings safely?
- *Attitude.* Is he prepared to learn to use a hoist? Is he reluctant or over-confident?

Once the most suitable hoist has been chosen the therapist must ensure that the disabled person and his carer are instructed adequately in its use and care. Teaching the use and care of a hoist should convey a sense of confidence and security so that the new users trust both the hoist and the therapist. The therapist must emphasise the importance of not trying to adapt or alter the slings or hoist in any way and to report any faults or problems as soon as possible. Any therapist, user or carer who wishes to try out a range of hoists and/or receive objective help in choosing the most suitable one should contact the nearest Disabled Living Centre (see p. 290).

TYPES OF HOIST

When the assessor has established the needs of the user and his carer and examined the features of the environment a choice of hoist must be made. The therapist needs to decide:

- which *type* of hoist is most appropriate
- which *model* of hoist within that group is most suitable.

The assessor must be aware, however, that a compromise may have to be made. Where necessary, she must decide which of the features and functions required in a hoist take priority. She may also, of course, be limited by factors such as existing contracts, cost and local policies.

Mobile hoists (Fig. 9.20)

These are the most commonly supplied type of hoist for home use and a wide variety is available. They are generally supplied where it is necessary to move a person over a distance, i.e. across a room or from one room to another, or where, for whatever reason, an overhead hoist is not appropriate. Whilst a range of features is offered within the different models, all have certain features that need to be considered.

- *Castors.* These enable the hoist to be manoeuvred from place to place and vary in size on different models. Large castors will be easier to move over carpets or small thresholds but will require more clearance under a bed or car with which the hoist will be used.
- *They are helper operated.* The helper needs

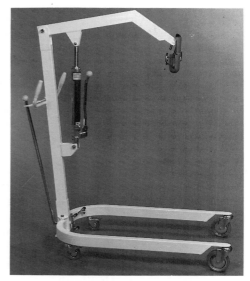

Fig. 9.20 The New Oxford Hoist — an example of a mobile hoist (by kind permission of F. J. Payne (Manufacturing) Ltd.)

to be reasonably fit if he is to manoeuvre the hoist over carpets or around furniture.

• *Hoisting mechanism.* The boom may be raised or lowered by means of a hydraulic system, a pump handle, or a hand screw mechanism. A few mobile hoists are operated by means of an electric motor. These add weight to the hoist but may make possible the use of a hoist by a frail carer who could not manage a hydraulic or pump control.

• *Safe working load.* All mobile hoists will safely lift people up to 127 kg (20 stone) in weight. Some models will guarantee to lift heavier weights.

• *Storage and/or transportation.* All mobile hoists can be dismantled for storage or transportation; however, some models are lighter and smaller than others.

Hoists fixed to the floor (Fig. 9.21)

These hoists may be permanently fixed to the floor or may be of a mobile type whose upright can be detached from the chassis and inserted into a floor socket as required. They are invariably used to transfer a person into and out of the bath. They are useful where space is limited or where the bath is unsuitable for use with a mobile hoist. Some models can be operated by the user or helper whereas others can be operated only by the helper.

Fixed overhead hoists (Figs 9.22, 9.23)

These hoists are fixed to an overhead mechanism by means of a retractable strap. Points to take into account when considering an overhead hoist are:

• *Long-term or short-term need?* Most overhead hoists are supplied where a long-term need exists for assistance with transfers. Both practically and aesthetically a hoist fixed to the

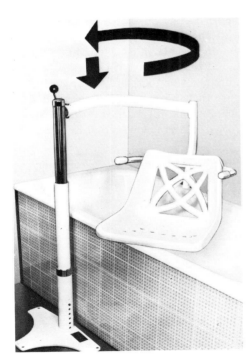

Fig. 9.21 Hoist fixed to the floor: Autolift. (Photograph reproduced by kind permission of Mecanaids Ltd.)

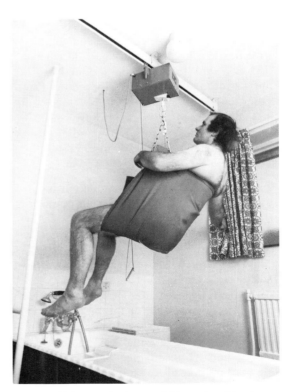

Fig. 9.22 Hoist attached to straight overhead track. (Photograph reproduced by kind permission of Wessex Medical Equipment Co. Ltd.)

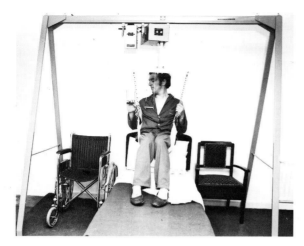

Fig. 9.23 Hoist attached to a free-standing gantry. (Photograph reproduced by kind permission of Wessex Medical Equipment Co. Ltd.)

ceiling, either at a single point or on a track, will usually prove the most desirable means of help in the long term. Overhead hoists fixed to the ceiling occupy no floor space and the control box can be moved to one side when not in use. A ceiling track can be designed to run to one or more points specifically required by the user.

In some instances, however, an overhead hoist may be attached to a free-standing gantry. Such an arrangement may be appropriate in cases where:

— The structure of the accommodation is unsuitable to take a ceiling fixing point or a track.
— The user may shortly be moving house or is being rehoused.
— The user/carer wishes to try out an overhead hoist before committing himself to a permanent arrangement. He may, for example, be uncertain of the best layout of the room and wish to test his options.
— The user may be terminally ill and/or a mobile hoist is unsuitable.
— He may only need to use the hoist in one room, using a wheelchair or shower chair, for example, to transport him to living areas or bathroom.

- *Fixed point or track?* An overhead hoist may be fixed at one single point such that the person can be lifted straight up and down, or onto a track that enables him, additionally, to move sideways. The track may be short, for example to enable a transfer from bed to wheelchair, or it may run from one room to another on a straight or curved track to assist transfer from, say, bed to toilet. This, however, involves considerable alteration to the building, such as leaving gaps above the doors to allow for the passage of the track, and may, for this reason, prove impractical or unacceptable. A fixed-point hoist may be used to lift a person from the ground to the first floor.

- *Operation.* Overhead hoists are usually controlled by means of cords, using one cord for each direction of travel, and these may be colour-coded. These cords may be made easier to operate by attaching parrot perches or knobs (Fig. 9.24). Consideration should be given as to who will operate the hoist. In some circumstances people who are unable to transfer themselves independently by other physical or mechanical means can do so by using an overhead hoist.

- *Installation.* If an overhead hoist is being considered the building will need to be assessed by an architect or the manufacturer of the hoist to ensure that the hoist can be used. A track must be attached to weight-bearing beams or joists or, if this is not possible, to bearers

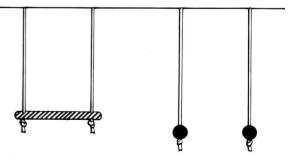

The parrot perch links the two control cords, facilitating hoist operation

Knobs are attached to the end of each control cord

Fig. 9.24 Cord control systems with electrically operated hoists.

inserted between the joists. Electrically operated hoists will need a conveniently situated electricity supply. If such a hoist is to be used in a bathroom or toilet an isolating transformer is necessary so that it can be operated safely in a wet or damp area. The Electricity Board must be consulted in such circumstances.

Car hoists

These are fixed to a car roof by steel clamps and are helper operated. When considering the use of a car hoist the assessor must check that the car door is wide and high enough to allow easy access. Information about the suitability of the design of the car to take the hoist must also be obtained.

SLINGS

It is important that the assessor has a comprehensive knowledge of the slings available so that the most suitable type can be selected, taking into consideration the height, weight and physical and mental capabilities of the user.

Slings are available in a variety of materials, sizes and designs and are all washable. Manufacturers design their own range of slings to fit their particular hoists and it is important not to try to mix and match different manufacturers' slings and hoists. Most manufacturers now supply a range of slings which can be quickly fitted to the hoist without the use of metalware, as well as the more traditional types which use metal hooks and chain fittings. Three basic types of sling are described below. All are available in small, medium and large sizes, or can be made to specific, individual requirements.

All-in-one slings

These are the most popular type of sling as they give overall support to the user. Manufacturers produce a wide variety of all-in-one slings and whilst they all have their own particular features they can be regarded under the following headings:

Universal type (Fig. 9.25)

These slings are usually of the 'quick-fit' type and are used mostly to move a person from one seated position to another. They do not, generally, offer as much support as the hammock type and may not offer head support.

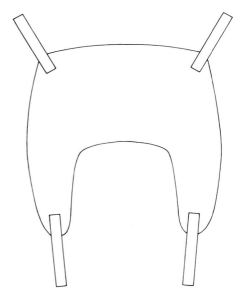

Fig. 9.25 A universal sling. (Reproduced by kind permission of Carters (J. & A. Ltd), Trowbridge.)

Hammock slings (Fig. 9.26)

These slings give maximum support and security to more disabled users. They offer full support to the body and can also be ordered with a head support if required. They can, therefore, be used to lift a person from a lying position. Most manufacturers offer commode aperture and/or divided leg options to assist with toileting.

Two-piece slings (Fig. 9.27)

These slings are occasionally used for less disabled people who have some control over their sitting balance. Two-piece slings comprise a back and seat sling and attach to the hoist with a sling bar and chain mechanism. It is vital to ensure that

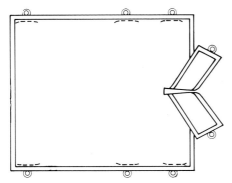

Fig. 9.26 A hammock sling. (Reproduced by kind permission of F. J. Payne Manufacturing Ltd, Oxford.)

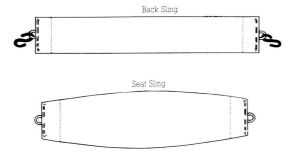

Back Sling

Seat Sling

Fig. 9.27 Two-piece slings. (Reproduced by kind permission of F. J. Payne Manufacturing Ltd, Oxford.)

they are correctly positioned, with the person seated properly on the seat sling and his arms out over the top of the back sling, and that he has sufficient physical capability to reduce the risk of 'jack knifing' or sliding off the seat sling.

PART 3: WALKING AIDS

Where the mechanism of walking is impaired due to disease or injury a variety of mechanical aids is available, ranging from large, stable aids such as gutter frames, to less stable ones such as walking sticks.

This section aims to describe the walking aids in common use, how to measure and check them, and the walking patterns which can be used with

them. In Great Britain most people who need walking aids obtain them either through the National Health Service or their local Social Services department. Aids may, of course, be bought privately.

The occupational therapist will notice that in most hospitals walking aids are supplied by the physiotherapy or outpatient department. However, it is essential that she knows how each aid should be used, in order that good walking patterns can be encouraged, as well as how to check the suitability of an aid for use in the person's home. Occupational therapists working in the community are frequently required to assess for and issue walking aids, and to teach their correct use.

THE ISSUE AND CARE OF AIDS

The main parts of a walking aid are illustrated in Figure 9.28. All aids should be checked before issue, and at regular intervals thereafter. The therapist should take particular notice of the following points:

- Is the ferrule complete? If the tread is badly worn or the ferrule perished or split it should be replaced immediately, as the aid is unsafe to use in this state.
- Does the ferrule fit properly? Many different sizes of ferrule are available to fit the wide variety of aids available and it is important that the ferrule is the correct size for the aid. A ferrule that is too large and has been padded with sticky tape wound round the stick, or one that is too small and has been split to fit the stick, is not safe for permanent use.
- Does the adjusting mechanism work easily? With the spring-knob type of mechanism it is important that both knobs should spring out easily and that the outer shaft move freely over the inner one.
- Is the padding complete? Padding which is split, perished or missing should be replaced in order to avoid discomfort or injury to the user.
- Does the aid stand square and upright if free-standing?

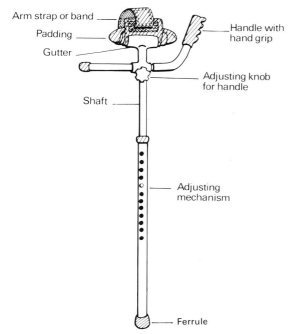

Arm strap or band

Padding

Gutter

Handle with
hand grip

Adjusting knob
for handle

Shaft

Adjusting
mechanism

Ferrule

Fig. 9.28 The main parts of a walking aid.

- Are the wooden parts of the aid free from splinters?
- Are all the joints secure?
- Where there are handgrips are they complete and not too loose? Handgrips which swivel round the handle can be difficult to hold securely.
- Does the user understand how to check the aid for safety, or does he have a relative or friend who can?

HOW TO CHOOSE THE CORRECT WALKING AID

As with many mobility aids there is neither a 'correct' aid to issue for a particular situation, nor a 'correct' time to issue an aid. Some people whose mobility is restricted or unstable prefer to walk unaided for as long as possible whilst others prefer to have an aid for what may seem a relatively minor difficulty.

Walking aids can be used for a variety of reasons. When deciding which aid is most suitable,

therefore, the therapist must bear the following points in mind.

1. The user's physical needs

- *Balance*. Does the aid need to be free-standing, offering a high degree of stability, or is the user's balance sufficient to be able to use a 'stick-based' aid?
- *Weight-bearing capacity*. Is the user non, partial or full weight bearing? Is the aid needed to relieve pain?
- *Gait*. Has the user the capacity to use a normal heel/toe gait with an aid or do his physical limitations demand another style?
- *Strength*. How much support must the aid give him?

2. The user himself

- *Grip*. The strength and type of grip he can achieve will dictate the style of aid he is able to use. Related to this is the strength in his upper limbs and shoulders.
- *Height, weight and age*. These will dictate the size of aid required.
- *Diagnosis*. Is his condition static, progressive or improving? i.e., over what period of time will the aid be used before it needs reviewing?
- *Environment*. Where is the aid to be used and how frequently? Does it have to fit any restricted areas such as between furniture or through gateways? Does it have to be stored or transported? Does it have to be available up and down stairs?
- *Lifestyle*. How active is the user? Does he use the aid in combination with any other mode of mobility such as a wheelchair or a car?
- *Cognitive ability*. Has he the ability to learn to use the aid correctly? Is he aware of any dangers inherent in its use, e.g using a wheeled aid on a slope or using crutches on stony ground, and can he adjust accordingly? Will he notice if the aid is faulty?
- *Reason for using the aid*. Is he using the aid to overcome a specific physical problem or is he

using it more as a 'prop' or a warning to others that he is unsteady on his feet?

THE MEASUREMENT AND USE OF WALKING AIDS

Walking aids can be divided into two main groups:

1. Aids based on a stick. Most of these aids are not free-standing. They include walking sticks, quadrupeds/tripods, forearm (gutter) and axilla crutches.

2. Aids based on a frame. All these aids are free-standing. They include wheeled and non-wheeled frames based on a 3- or 4-legged frame.

WALKING STICKS (Fig. 9.29)

There are several types of walking stick available; these include:

- a crook handle wooden walking stick
- an adjustable metal walking stick
- a 'Bennett' type walking stick

- a 'Fischer' type walking stick
- those of individual design.

To measure the aid

Walking sticks can be measured:

1. By asking the user to stand erect with his weight evenly distributed on both feet, looking forward and with shoulders and arms relaxed. The therapist should ensure that he is not leaning forward or to one side and that he is wearing shoes of similar height to those he normally wears. If he requires support to stand the therapist must check that he is standing symmetrically. With the wooden or Fischer type walking stick the ferrule is removed, the stick turned upside down and the handle placed on the floor. Holding the stick vertically the shaft is marked at the point level with the ulnar styloid (Fig. 9.30). The shaft is then sawn off at this point and the ferrule replaced. For the adjustable walking stick the measurement is taken as above, but there is no need to turn the

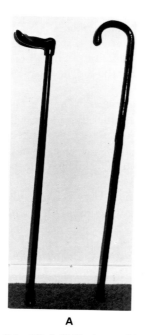

A

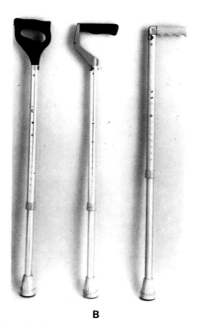

B

Fig. 9.29 Walking sticks (A) (left) Fischer walking stick (right) Standard wooden stick. (B) Adjustable metal sticks (left) Bennett (centre) Swan neck (right) Standard.

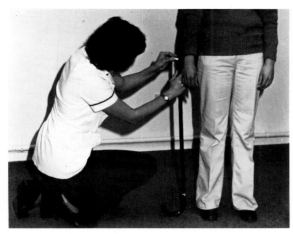

Fig. 9.30 Measuring a walking stick. The stick is held vertically and a mark is made on the shaft at the level of the ulnar styloid.

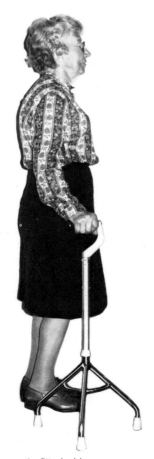

Fig. 9.31 A correctly fitted aid.

stick upside down as the adjustable shaft allows alterations to be carried out in situ.

2. By asking the user to lie straight with his hands at his side and measuring the distance between the ulnar styloid and the bottom of the heel. An inch is then added to this measurement in order to allow for the height of the shoe. The measurement obtained will give the overall height of the stick.

With the stick measured correctly the user should be able to maintain an upright posture with the elbow slightly flexed. In this way he is able to lift his weight when walking by fully extending his elbow as he pushes down on the stick (Fig. 9.31).

Points of use

The user's wrist and grip must be strong enough to allow him to bear weight through this area when using the stick. If this is not possible an alternative aid, such as gutter crutches, should be chosen. When using the stick the person should be taught to look where he is going rather than at the ground and an even heel-toe gait should be encouraged.

Occasions when walking sticks may be used

Walking sticks are used for a variety of reasons and may be required:

- to supplement power where there is muscular weakness, for example in cases of poliomyelitis or nerve injury to the lower limb
- to relieve pain, as in osteoarthrosis or following a fracture within the lower limb
- to widen the walking base in conditions of impaired balance, for example following a head injury or for those with multiple sclerosis
- to protect weak bones or damaged joints, for example in cases of osteoporosis or following a meniscectomy
- to compensate for deformity, for example where there is scoliosis or limb shortening
- as a feeler, for example for blind people or some with hemianopia
- for social reasons, for example to warn others of the user's slowness or lack of confidence

in walking or — occasionally — as a 'fashion aid'.

THE QUADRUPED (Fig. 9.32)

This is a more stable version of the walking stick, having a four-footed base. Tripods with a three-footed base are also available but are considered by some to be rather unstable.

To measure the aid

These aids are measured in the same way as an adjustable walking stick. The therapist should ensure that, when the aid is in use, the open end of the handle is facing backwards and the flat side of the rectangle made by the feet is nearest the user; see Figure 9.31 for a similar example.

Points of use

These are as for the walking stick, but it is particularly important to ensure that the aid is neither so close to the user that he leans over it to balance when taking weight, nor so far away that the aid will tip inwards when weight is taken on it.

Occasions when quadrupeds may be used

These are usually issued singly for a weakness of one lower limb or a unilateral weakness of the whole body where more support is needed than can be obtained from the use of a walking stick, for example in some cases of hemiplegia.

N.B. The therapist may note that, where the 'bilateral' approach to treatment is followed the use of such aids is discouraged by some practitioners, who feel that they raise muscle tone in the hemiplegic side by virtue of the effort involved in using them. Others, however, feel that where the rise in tone is slight, or if the provision of an aid offers independent mobility where this would not otherwise be possible, its value outweighs any disadvantages. The therapist, therefore, must weigh each situation individually and use her professional judgement as to whether to issue an aid or not. Quadrupeds may also be issued in pairs following bilateral amputation of the lower limbs or to young sufferers of cerebral palsy or spina bifida.

CRUTCHES

Elbow crutches (Fig. 9.33)

These aids, which are usually issued in pairs, provide an armband support which fits round the forearm thus bracing the wrist when the aid is in use.

To measure the aid

The height of the aid from the floor to the handle is measured as for the adjustable walking stick. The forearm band should be neither so tight that the aid is difficult to remove, nor so loose that it does not give enough support. The band should hold the forearm at a point slightly above midway between the wrist and elbow, for if it is too low it will not give sufficient support and if too high it may block the action of the elbow and/or rub on

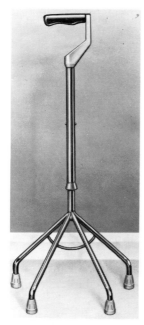

Fig. 9.32 A quadruped.

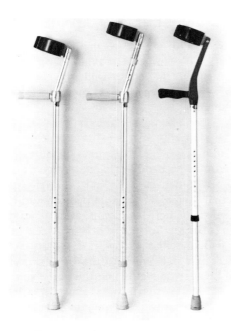

Fig. 9.33 Elbow crutches.

the ulnar nerve, causing bruising and subsequent tingling or loss of sensation in the fourth and fifth digits.

Points of use

The points of use of these aids are as for those of the walking stick. However, as elbow crutches can be awkward to handle, the user may need some practice in putting on and taking off the aids as well as in walking with them. It is essential that the user has good strength throughout his upper limbs as they support much of the body weight when walking on these aids.

Occasions when elbow crutches may be used

As elbow crutches offer a great deal of support to the lower limbs they can be used when the user's strength or balance has been severely affected. Elbow crutches may be issued in cases of:

- bilateral weakness and/or incoordination of

the lower limbs, for example following spinal injury or in some cases of spina bifida
- unilateral weakness of a lower limb when the user is not permitted to bear his full weight through the injured limb, for example in the early stages following an ankle fracture or meniscectomy
- bilateral severe weakness and/or incoordination affecting the whole body and/or where the upper limbs are unable to provide sufficient support using walking sticks. This may occur in some cases of a progressive paralysis such as muscular dystrophy, or following brain damage.

Forearm or gutter crutches
(Fig. 9.34)

This is another variety of a single stick aid, but one in which the weight is borne along the length of the forearm rather than through the wrist and hand.

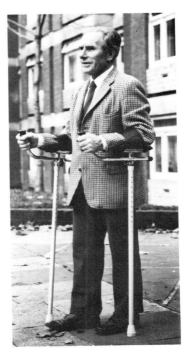

Fig. 9.34 Forearm or 'gutter' crutches.

To measure the aid

The user should stand as upright as possible with his arms and shoulders relaxed, looking forward and with his weight evenly distributed on both feet. Measurement is taken from the floor to the olecranon process. In some cases the user may have to be measured lying down, as he may have difficulty in standing without the use of an aid. The measurement should then be taken from the olecranon process to the bottom of the heel and an inch added to allow for the height of the shoe. In both cases the measurement obtained will give the distance required from the ferrule to the bottom of the gutter padding.

When adjusting the handle the therapist should check that there is sufficient space between the front of the gutter and the handle to leave the wrist free from pressure, especially over the ulnar styloid. Similarly, she should check that the elbow is free at the back so that the gutter does not press on the ulnar nerve which, at this point, lies just under the skin with little protection from pressure.

Points of use

The crutches should not be placed too far in front of the body as this can unbalance the upright posture. It is important to ensure that the user's balance and coordination are adequate before he attempts to walk unsupervised, because the aids are strapped over the forearms and so cannot be discarded quickly in a crisis.

Occasions when forearm crutches may be used

These are usually issued in pairs and can be used for unilateral or bilateral weakness in the lower limbs in cases where the upper limbs are unable to bear weight through the wrists and hands. The most common example is the person with rheumatoid arthritis. Other examples include persons who, because of injury to both the lower and the upper limbs, find weight-bearing through the wrists and hands impossible.

Axilla crutches (Fig. 9.35)

These are aids in which weight is borne through the wrist and hand. The axilla pad, which is pressed against the chest wall, is not an area through which weight is taken but helps to stabilise the shoulder.

To measure the aid

The height of the hand grip is measured as for the walking stick, that is, it should be level with the user's ulnar styloid. The axilla pads should be adjusted so that there is a gap of approximately 2 inches (or three fingers' width) between the top of the pad and the axilla. If the aids are too long there is a danger of putting pressure on the brachial plexus, thus affecting the nerve supply to the upper limb. If they are too short, posture will be affected during walking and the user will have difficulty in keeping the pads pressed against the chest wall, for they will tend to slip out.

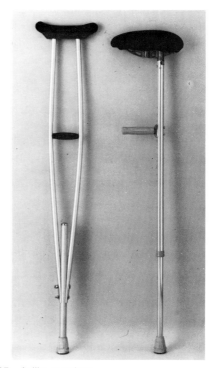

Fig. 9.35 Axilla crutches.

Points of use

It is essential that the user appreciates the importance of bearing weight through the handles of the aids and of not leaning on the axilla pads because of the danger of putting pressure on the brachial plexus. The axilla pads should be pressed against the chest wall in order to give support by bracing the shoulder and upper limb. The crutches should be used at an angle of approximately 15° to the side of the body.

Occasions when axilla crutches may be used

These aids are issued in pairs and may be used where there is unilateral weakness of the lower limb through which only partial or no weight may be taken, for example following a fracture of the tibia and fibula or after a bone graft to a previously un-united fracture. The aids may also be used where there is bilateral dysfunction of the lower limbs for which a reciprocal gait is inappropriate, for example if the hips or spine are fixed in a hip spica plaster or if other supports fixing the hip are worn.

WALKING FRAMES

The lightweight walking frame (Fig. 9.36)

This is the simplest style of walking frame and may be referred to as a 'pulpit' or 'Zimmer' frame. A hinged version, known as a reciprocal walking frame, is also available.

To measure the frame

The height is measured as for the walking stick.

Points of use

It is important to ensure that the user does not step too closely into the frame as there is a danger that he may tip backwards. Where this is a persistent problem it may be practical to tie a piece of coloured tape or elastic across the back legs of the frame at knee level (not below, as this may trip

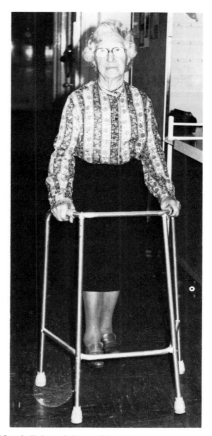

Fig. 9.36 A lightweight walking frame.

those with poor sight or a high stepping gait) to prevent the user stepping in too closely to the frame. Similarly, the frame should not be placed too far in front of the user when walking, for this may not only upset his balance but can also cause the frame to tip if all four legs are not placed firmly on the floor when weight is taken onto it.

Occasions when a lightweight walking frame may be used

This is a very popular aid and can be used for:

- unilateral weakness or amputation of the lower limb where general weakness or infirmity makes the greater support offered by the frame necessary, such as in osteoarthritis or a fractured femur in an elderly person

- bilateral weakness and/or incoordination of the lower limbs or whole body, whenever a firm, free-standing aid is appropriate, as for example for those suffering from multiple sclerosis or Parkinsonism.
- general support to aid mobility and confidence, for example following prolonged bed-rest or sickness in elderly people.

Although not as commonly used as the standard walking frame, the reciprocal frame is useful for those who require a firm, free-standing aid for use with a reciprocal gait. Where there is additional weakness in the upper limbs the use of this hinged frame frees the user from having to lift the whole weight of the frame at once.

Folding frames such as the three-point walking frame (Fig. 9.37)

This is a compact, folding variety of the light-weight walking frame and may be referred to as an 'Alpha' frame.

To measure the frame

The height is measured as for the walking stick.

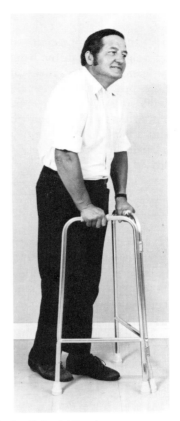

Fig. 9.37 An Alpha folding frame.

Points of use

See lightweight walking frame.

Occasions when the three-point frame may be used

This aid is issued for the same reasons as the light-weight walking frame, but in cases where space is restricted. For example, it may be more appropriate in a small house or flat; if the standard frame will not fit into the user's car; or for especially small users who find the standard frame too cumbersome. Owing to its design this aid requires a little more balance by the user.

Wheeled frames (Fig. 9.38)

This section includes aids such as the Rollator, which is a frame-type aid with two wheels at the

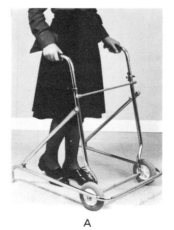 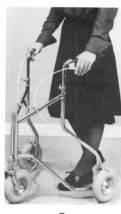

A   B

Fig. 9.38 Wheeled frames (A) Rollator (B) Delta aid with brakes.

front and two ferrules at the back which act as brakes. Several versions are available, including those with seat or carrying baskets attached. A similar aid is the three-wheeled or 'Delta' version of the Rollator which, on some models, has a brake-system attached to the handgrips.

To measure the frame

The height is measured as for the walking stick.

Points of use

Although simple to use, most wheeled frames can be awkward to manoeuvre in confined spaces as they require a fairly large area in which to turn. This is especially true of the rollator. When issuing such an aid the therapist should ensure that the user is able to control the braking system so that the aid presents no hazard when used on a slope or camber. Because of its design and mode of use, the rollator is not easy to use out of doors.

Occasions when the wheeled frames may be used

• *The rollator.* Because this aid does not require the user to remember any particular walking pattern or to have sufficient strength and/or balance to lift it off the floor during use, it can be issued to those who cannot use a lightweight frame. Although useful, therefore, for the elderly infirm or for those with spina bifida, it needs a large turning area and the therapist must make sure that enough space is available for this.

• *The three-wheeled aid.* This aid, like the rollator, is used where a 'pick-up' aid is unsuitable and also where space is restricted.

Frames with forearm rests (Fig. 9.39)

Of this group, the forearm walker and the standing aid are the most widely used. The forearm walker is a chest-high version of the walking frame which has gutter attachments fixed to the upper bars of the frame. The frame is usually moved on castors. The standing aid is another chest-high walking

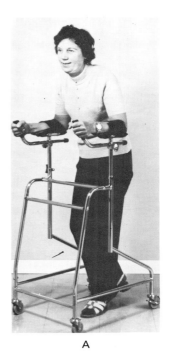

A

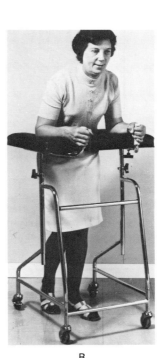

B

Fig. 9.39 Forearm resting frames (A) Forearm walker (b) Standing aid.

frame which has a padded resting platform on which the forearms are placed when walking.

To measure the aids

Both aids are initially measured as for the forearm crutches. However, depending upon the severity of disability of the user, some adjustment may have to be made in order to allow the most appropriate and comfortable posture.

Points of use

As both aids are rather cumbersome they can be difficult to manoeuvre in confined spaces or out of doors. However, many users are restricted to them as their only means of mobility and, therefore, will be obliged to adapt their activity to the limited manoeuvrability of the aid.

Occasions when forearm rest frames may be used

The forearm walker can be used in cases where a lightweight frame or gutter crutches are appropriate, but where weakness of the lower limbs, combined with weakness and/or incoordination of the upper limbs, make them impractical. The aid is suitable, therefore, for some people with advanced rheumatoid arthritis or where injuries to both upper and lower limbs have been sustained, making weight-bearing through the wrist or hand impossible.

The standing aid may be used instead of the forearm walker when gutter attachments are inappropriate, for example in cases of upper limb deformity.

The therapist will notice, when looking through manufacturers' catalogues, that many variations and combinations of these aids are produced.

WALKING PATTERNS

All walking aids must be used correctly in order to provide adequate support and allow the user to maintain good posture, balance and gait. Walking aids, like all other aids, should never be issued unless full instruction for their use is provided. The walking patterns illustrated below cover the use of aids already discussed. The therapist may find that the names given to the gaits vary from place to place. The types of aid with which each gait can be used are given in brackets.

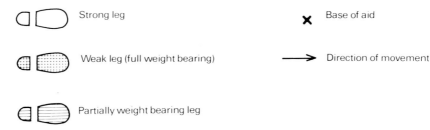

Fig. 9.40 Key to diagrams of walking patterns.

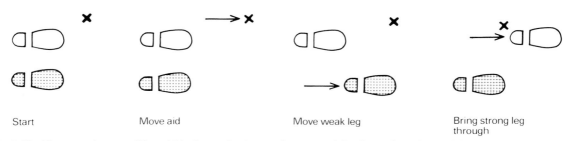

Fig. 9.41 The use of one walking aid in the early stages of recovery (tripod, quadruped or walking stick).

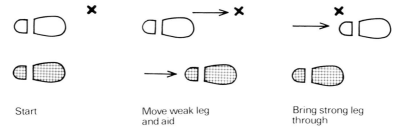

Start

Move weak leg
and aid

Bring strong leg
through

Fig. 9.42 The use of one walking aid in the later stages of recovery (tripod, quadruped or walking stick).

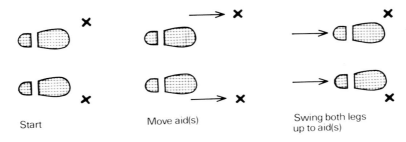

Start

Move aid(s)

Swing both legs
up to aid(s)

Fig. 9.43 The swing-to gait (axilla crutches or pick-up frame).

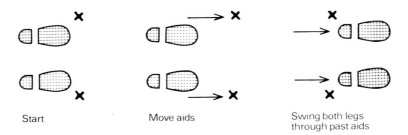

Start

Move aids

Swing both legs
through past aids

Fig. 9.44 The swing-through gait (axilla crutches).

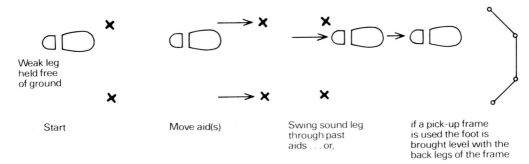

Weak leg
held free
of ground

Start

Move aid(s)

Swing sound leg
through past
aids . . . or,

if a pick-up frame
is used the foot is
brought level with the
back legs of the frame

Fig. 9.45 The non-weight-bearing gait (axilla crutches or pick-up frame).

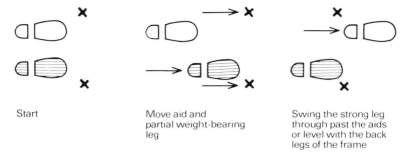

Start

Move aid and partial weight-bearing leg

Swing the strong leg through past the aids or level with the back legs of the frame

Fig. 9.46 The partial weight-bearing gait (axilla crutches, pick-up frame or elbow crutches).

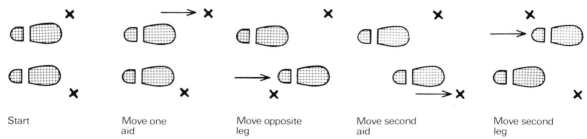

Start

Move one aid

Move opposite leg

Move second aid

Move second leg

Fig. 9.47 The four-point gait used in the early stages of recovery (gutter crutches, axilla crutches, elbow crutches, walking sticks or reciprocal frame).

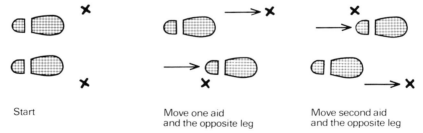

Start

Move one aid and the opposite leg

Move second aid and the opposite leg

Fig. 9.48 The four-point gait used in the later stages of recovery (gutter crutches, axilla crutches, elbow crutches, walking sticks or reciprocal frame).

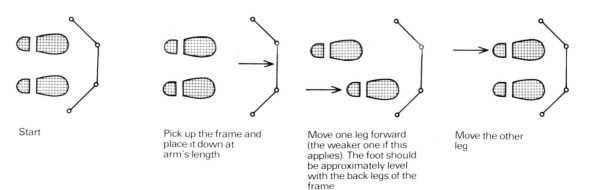

Start

Pick up the frame and place it down at arm's length

Move one leg forward (the weaker one if this applies). The foot should be approximately level with the back legs of the frame

Move the other leg

Fig. 9.49 Using the pick-up aids.

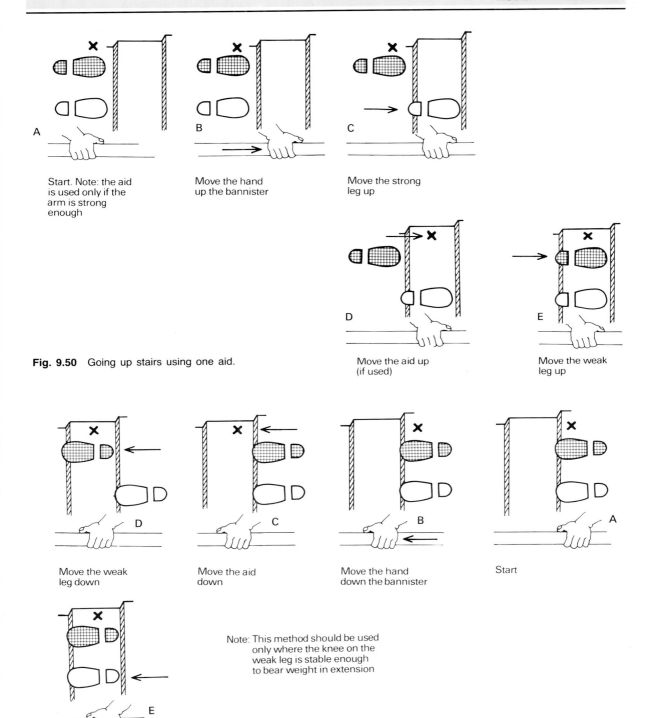

Fig. 9.50 Going up stairs using one aid.

A. Start. Note: the aid is used only if the arm is strong enough

B. Move the hand up the bannister

C. Move the strong leg up

D. Move the aid up (if used)

E. Move the weak leg up

Fig. 9.51 Going down stairs using one aid.

A. Start

B. Move the hand down the bannister

C. Move the aid down

D. Move the weak leg down

E. Move the strong leg down

Note: This method should be used only where the knee on the weak leg is stable enough to bear weight in extension

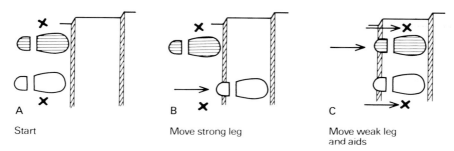

Fig. 9.52 Going up stairs using two aids (partial weight-bearing).

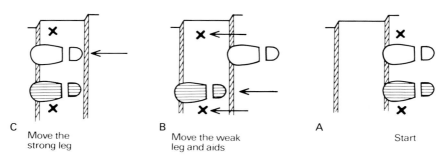

Fig. 9.53 Going down stairs using two aids (partial weight-bearing).

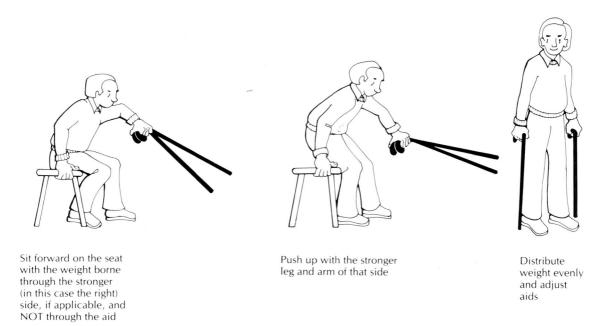

Sit forward on the seat with the weight borne through the stronger (in this case the right) side, if applicable, and NOT through the aid

Push up with the stronger leg and arm of that side

Distribute weight evenly and adjust aids

Fig. 9.54 Standing with a non-free-standing aid.

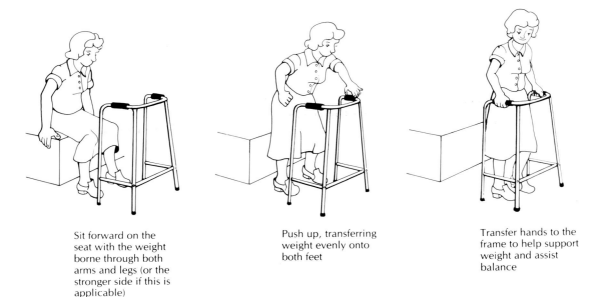

Sit forward on the
seat with the weight
borne through both
arms and legs (or the
stronger side if this is
applicable)

Push up, transferring
weight evenly onto
both feet

Transfer hands to the
frame to help support
weight and assist
balance

Fig. 9.55 Standing with a free-standing aid.

PART 4: WHEELCHAIR MOBILITY

There is more to wheelchairs than meets the eye. When, early in their training, occupational therapy students are asked to spend a day in a wheelchair in order to gain first-hand experience of disability their initial reaction is usually one of eager anticipation. However, the reports of their experiences invariably show that the novelty soon wears off (often around lunchtime when fellow students tend to get fed up with their slowness and incompetence) and they often sheepishly confess that their 'day' finished around 6 p.m. when they could stand the confines of the wheelchair no longer. Some have been ashamed to admit to wanting to throw the chair into the nearest river; others have been asked to leave restaurants, refused entrance to pubs, patted on the head, given sweets by elderly matrons and stared at by children and adults alike. Some have been infuriated to find, upon trying to buy a pair of shoes, that the shop assistant asked their partner what size feet they had!

Despite this love/hate relationship with an object that frequently provides mobility at the cost of anonymity and dignity, the occupational therapist needs to be aware of the wide variety of models that are available, their features and accessories, and how to assess for and obtain the most suitable model for the person in need of a chair.

AVAILABILITY AND SUPPLY

Wheelchairs can be prescribed for people who have limited walking ability and whose ability is likely to be permanently affected. A person does not need to use his wheelchair as his only means of mobility in order to be eligible for one. For the person to obtain a wheelchair from the DoH an application has to be made on his behalf and sent to the local wheelchair supply centre (sometimes called the Disablement Services Centre). This may be made on form AOF 5G, but some centres design and use their own forms. Where the AOF 5G is used, practice regarding signatures varies. Some regions still prefer a medical practitioner to sign, but others prefer the assessing therapist to complete and sign the form. Wheelchair clinics may be held in some areas in order to help streamline the assessment for and supply of wheelchairs within a local area.

The time taken for the chair to be delivered will depend, in part, on the type of chair ordered. A standard, popular model of wheelchair may be held in stock at the Centre and be available for immediate delivery, whereas a less commonly ordered chair, or one that requires additional features or alteration, will not be available straight away.

Wheelchairs may, of course, be bought privately and the disabled person may choose to use his Mobility Allowance to fund such a purchase. Objective assessment, information and guidance can be obtained from the person's nearest Disabled Living Centre (see p. 290).

People who require chairs for a short period, for example following an accident, whilst on holiday, or while awaiting their DoH chair, should be able to borrow one from their local Red Cross Society. In some areas the local hospital or social services department may operate a loan system.

ASSESSMENT

The therapist must be aware that a poorly prescribed wheelchair can cause deformity and discomfort by affecting the user's posture and not offering correct support or distribution of weight. In order to find the most suitable type of wheelchair for an individual, she should take the following factors into consideration.

1. The user

• *Age.* If he is young is he likely to outgrow the chair in the near future? How much wear and tear is he likely to give the chair?

• *Height and width* (Fig. 9.56). When seated, the user should find that his hips are comfortably flexed at 90°; there should be room to place a flat hand vertically between the back of his knees and the front edge of the seat/cushion and also space to place a flat hand between the back of his knees and the top of the seat/cushion at the front. His feet, with

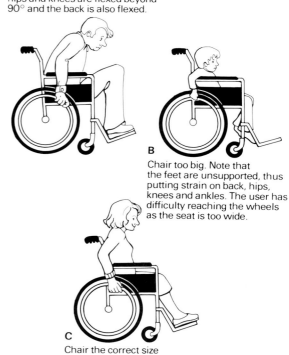

A
Chair too small. Note that the hips and knees are flexed beyond 90° and the back is also flexed.

B
Chair too big. Note that the feet are unsupported, thus putting strain on back, hips, knees and ankles. The user has difficulty reaching the wheels as the seat is too wide.

C
Chair the correct size

Fig. 9.56 Fitting a wheelchair.

ankles at 90°, should rest securely on the footrests. He should be able to reach the wheel-rims with ease whilst maintaining an upright position when seated with his usual cushion in place. The backrest should offer sufficient support for his spine but not hinder his ability to manoeuvre the chair. The 'correct' height of the backrest will vary according to the strength of the person's trunk, i.e. the amount of support his back needs to maintain a good posture, and the use to which he puts the chair, (e.g. if he needs to twist his trunk to reach behind him in the office or kitchen, or if he is an active sportsman).

The seat should be wide enough to allow a flat hand to be placed between either side of the user's thighs/hips at their widest point and the sides of the chair, remembering that if the user is frequently going to wear bulky clothing when using the chair this should be taken into account.

- *Weight*. Different sizes of chair within each range are available to take people only up to a certain weight. If the user is too heavy for the chair it will be under too much strain and will wear out more quickly. However, if the chair is too heavy for the user it will be hard and exhausting for him to push and manoeuvre.

- *Diagnosis*. Whether the condition is static, progressive or likely to improve may determine how long the chair will be in use, and indicate how frequently it will be used. If the condition is progressive is it possible to determine how long the person will be able to control, manoeuvre and use the chair before it will need to be modified or replaced? Does the diagnosis point to the fact that the person is, or may become, incontinent and can the model be fitted with appropriate features to cope with this?

- *Physical abilities*. The user's ability to physically cope with a chair should be carefully considered. Can he propel a chair himself, and if so, can he do so over carpets, paths and rough ground or only some of these? Can he cope with slopes, tight corners and thresholds? Can he balance sufficiently to open and close doors and reach objects from a table or shelf? What type of brakes can he operate? Can he remove armrests, and swing and remove footrests?

If he cannot propel with standard hand-rims can he manage a capstan type, or gain more force if the propelling wheels are larger? If self-propulsion is beyond him, has he the physical and mental ability to cope with an electrically propelled chair and what method of control is most suitable?

How will the user transfer into and out of the chair? Do armrests and footrests need to be removable to allow this? If a hoist is needed to assist transfer are the two compatible in size and lifting height? Are the user's bed/bath/toilet of the appropriate height to facilitate transfer from the wheelchair?

Can any deformity, or any abnormality in posture or balance, be accommodated in the chair? For example, if the person suffers from scoliosis will the chair being considered permit adequate support to be added?

- *Attitude and reason for supply*. Has the person asked for a chair or has one been considered advisable? In the latter case, is the person prepared to accept a wheelchair? If he is reluctant to accept a chair can he explain why?

- *Cognitive ability*. Can the user understand when and how to use and maintain the chair? If not, will the attendant be confident in its use?

2. The place of use

Does the user need more than one chair to suit the different environments in which he will be using it, for example a self-propelled chair indoors and an attendant-propelled one outdoors?

- *In the home*. Consider the widths of the doors and corridors and the space for manoeuvring within them. Are there any steps that need to be negotiated and can they be ramped? If so, can the person manage the gradient of the slope? The angle and space available for transfers onto toilet, bed and easy chair should be noted. Can grab rails be fitted or will a hoist/assistant be needed?

Is there room to store the chair when not in use? Is the store dry and access to it easy?

Is there someone who can carry out routine maintenance to the chair? If an electrically propelled chair is being considered are battery charging facilities easily available and are these in a well-ventilated area? If the chair is to be charged overnight for a person who uses the chair constantly is there someone who can take it from the bedroom to the charging area and back?

Will the users' knees, when seated, fit under the sink, basin, desk or table as required?

- *Outside*. Are paths, steps, gates and doors suitable for the chair or can they be made so? Does the user require a separate chair for outdoor use?

- *At work or school*. Is the chair suitable for use here? Can it be manoeuvred within the environment in which the person works? Is it compatible with any furniture or equipment he may need to use there?

3. Other transport facilities

Is the chair going to be used in conjunction with any other transport such as a car or adapted transporter? If so, can the user transfer in/out of the vehicle and can the chair be folded, lifted and stored in it, either by the user himself, an assistant or a roof-mounted hoist?

Will a hoist or any other equipment be necessary to help with transfer? Can the car be parked in a suitable place at home to allow room for (preferably sheltered) transfers?

4. Carers

Are carers able to accept the chair or will their attitude prevent the individual from using it? If carers do not accept the chair is it possible to ascertain why?

If help is needed for pushing, transfer or maintenance of the chair are carers willing and able to do this?

5. Stability

Several factors can alter a chair's stability and, therefore, make it less safe to use. Contributing factors include:

- excess movement, as when the user suffers from an athetoid or choreic condition or is an active sportsman
- an altered centre of gravity, for example when the user is a double lower limb amputee or has severe postural deformity
- the fitting of an angled backrest and/or cushions
- inappropriate controls on an electrically propelled chair which prevent the user from operating the chair smoothly
- an uneven environment such as an excessive camber on a pavement, drive or road, or a steep slope.

The user should be assessed using the chair in as wide a variety of circumstances as possible in

order that stability can be checked before a final decision is made.

6. Cushions

Both the needs of the user and the chair in which it will be used should be carefully considered when deciding on a suitable cushion. The sitting posture and stability of the user can be helped or hindered by the cushion, and its height and firmness must be taken into account when considering transfers in and out of the chair. The therapist must also be aware that the use of a cushion will alter the internal dimensions of the chair and so it is imperative that the two are chosen together.

Additionally, the appearance, durability, weight, comfort, cost and purpose of the cushion, together with the user's continence and ability to care for the cushion should also be taken into account.

When all those points have been considered the best size and model of chair, together with any additional features and accessories, can be decided upon. It is important to remember that the more standard the chair the more quickly it is likely to be delivered. (For further information on types of cushions available see p. 284.)

TYPES OF WHEELCHAIRS AND FEATURES TO CONSIDER

Whilst it is beyond the brief of this chapter to look at individual models of wheelchair it is essential that the therapist understands the different types of chair that are available and the main features to consider during assessment for the most suitable model.

Types

1. Hand-propelled chairs

These may be either:

- occupant-controlled, generally having two large wheels (usually fitted with hand rims) for pushing and one or two small wheels which swivel to allow the chair to be manoeuvred. Standard, lightweight and

high-performance (sports) chairs are included here; or
- push chairs with four smaller wheels.
  Children's buggies are included in this group.

2. Electrically operated indoor chairs

These chairs can be operated by the user from one of a variety of different controls, such as a chin switch, joystick or suck-blow control, the most suitable of which is attached to the control box and fitted on the chair at the place most convenient for the user.

3. Electrically operated outdoor chairs

These may be either:

- attendant controlled. Only one model (28B) is available through the DoH and is supplied for outdoor use only. Other models may be purchased privately. Or:
- occupant-controlled. Many models are suitable for both indoor and outdoor use and can include special features such as kerb-climbing capability.

Generally, no attempt has been made here to indicate whether chairs are available through the DoH or not. With the devolvement of budgets to local Centres, rigid guidelines as to what may or may not be available would be misleading. The therapist must be aware of the policies that operate in her own local Centre.

Features

Frames

Frames may be folding or rigid. Rigid-framed chairs tend to be sturdier and more comfortable for prolonged periods of use but are, of course, more difficult to store and transport. Several models of sports and children's chairs have rigid frames.

Folding frames may have a single or double cross-brace. A single cross-brace chair can be pushed nearer to a toilet, bed, etc. to facilitate forward transfer, whilst a double cross-brace chair is

slightly sturdier, though heavier. Folding frame chairs may vary greatly in the degree to which the chair will fold.

Stand-up frames are available on a few models. These are generally for private purchase only.

Wheels

Large wheels for self-propelled chairs can vary in size. Whilst bigger ones are easier to reach if the user has limited upper limb mobility, they do make side transfers more difficult as they protrude higher above the seat. They also take up more space when the chair is folded.

Castors are also available in different sizes. Small castors make a chair more manoeuvrable whereas larger ones will enable the chair to cope more easily with uneven surfaces and are less likely to get caught in ruts.

Solid tyres are easier for indoor use and ease of maintenance whilst pneumatic tyres absorb jolts from uneven surfaces more easily if maintained at the correct pressure.

Hand-rims are a standard feature on most, although not all, self-propelled chairs. Variations include capstan rims for those with weak grasp; one-arm drive, where both hand rims are fitted to the wheel of the non-affected side; and those of small diameter, especially on sports chairs to aid speed and manoeuvrability.

The position of the large wheels may be set back 3" for double lower limb amputees to counterbalance the loss of weight at the front, thus preventing the chair from tipping backwards.

Backrests

Backrest angles vary in their degree from the vertical. A greater angle helps the balance of those with weak or fixed hips or spines. Extensions are available for those who require head support. Horizontally folding backrests enable the chair to be stored in a smaller space, such as the boot of a car. Zipped and reclining backrests are also available. Shallow backrests, especially on sports/high-performance chairs, aid trunk mobility and are especially useful for active chair users.

Footrests

Footrests are available in a wide range and should be chosen carefully. They can be of a single, platform type which will accommodate both feet, or divided into individual footrests. They may be fixed or else capable of being swung/retracted or detached to facilitate transfers and storage. Elevating legrests can be ordered, as can heel/toe loops, leg straps and footrest extensions, all of which give extra support. Foot steering mechanisms are also available.

Armrests

These may be fixed or detachable. Different heights are available to suit individual variation in upper limb length and mobility, and to accommodate a deep cushion. Armrests can be cut away at the front to enable the chair to fit up to a table, or at the back to accommodate mobile arm supports. Armrests can also be fitted to take a tray.

Brakes

Brakes are generally fitted to both sides of a chair but a single lever action can be fitted. Brakes may have a push-on or pull-on action or can be foot-operated by the attendant. Lever extensions are also available.

Cushions

These should be chosen with great care as their individual properties can have a wide-ranging effect on the user. The purpose of a cushion is to distribute pressure evenly and thus prevent, or help alleviate pressure sores. It also makes a chair more comfortable to sit in for a prolonged period. They should not be used to compensate for a poorly fitting chair. Cushions may be of the following types:

• Foam. These are readily available both from local centres and private manufacturers. They are lightweight, relatively cheap and available in a wide variety of thicknesses and shapes. They must comply with the Furniture and Furnishings (Fire and Safety) Regulations 1988.

Hardwood bases or foam crescents are available to provide a firmer, more stable base for prolonged sitting and/or transfers and can compensate for seat sag. The hardwood bases make the user sit higher in the chair and this should be taken into consideration when ordering the chair and cushion and when estimating heights for transfers.

• Solid gel. These cushions are relatively heavy and are cool to the touch but have the advantage of distributing weight efficiently and of not leaking if punctured. The Reston Flotation Pad and the Spenco Omega 5000 are included in this group.

• Gel and foam. These are more supportive than all foam cushions and lighter than all gel ones. The SuMed 83 is an example.

• Gel and air, for example the Seabird Medical.

• Water-filled, for example the Jobst Hydrofloat or the Aquaseat.

• Air-filled. The pressure in these lightweight cushions can be adjusted to suit the individual although this must be done with care and altered for each user. The Roho dry flotation cushion (Fig. 9.57) is an example of this type of cushion. It consists of rows of black, air-filled balloons, which can look strange without a cover, but does provide a good distribution of pressure. It can be difficult to transfer to and from if not covered. These

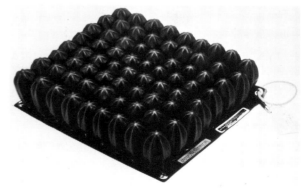

Fig. 9.57 Roho cushion.

cushions are relatively expensive and place the user approximately 12 mm ($\frac{1}{2}''$) above the chair seat, thus effectively altering the seat height. An electric pump is attached to the chair to maintain air pressure within the balloons.

- Silicore, for example the Spenco Silicore cushion.
- Flow form. The Jay cushion has an oil-based fluid 'flow form' sack which provides conformity on top of a moulded foam base.
- Sheepskin. Natural and simulated sheepskins are available in various sizes. They help to prevent pressure sores by distributing weight more evenly and also absorb water vapour, thus preventing accumulation from sweating. Sheepskin is also extremely comfortable to sit on. By trapping air between the user and the seat, sheepskin is also warm to use — an important factor for those with limited mobility.

Other features

Other features may be available on limited models or from particular manufacturers. Whilst these are, individually, inappropriate to mention here it is worth noting that wheelchairs specifically designed for use by people with cerebral palsy are available. Their particular features include a foot-box, ankle straps, a pommel to help reduce adductor spasm, side wings to the back-rest and a restraining harness.

Commode facilities can also be added to certain models as can moulded or matrix seats to improve posture. Lap straps/restraining harnesses should also be considered.

MODIFICATIONS AND ADAPTATIONS

Chairs supplied through the DoH can be modified according to need by the manufacturer. Such arrangements are made through the local Disablement Services Centre. Where such adaptations cannot be carried out locally, or where a specially designed 'one-off' chair needs to be built, specialist centres such as Mary Marlborough Lodge at the Nuffield Orthopaedic Centre, Oxford, can be approached.

USE, CARE AND REPAIR OF WHEELCHAIRS

As with any piece of equipment, the user must learn how to use and maintain his wheelchair. Not only should he and his carers be shown what and what not to do, they should also be given written instructions. The DoH publishes a small booklet on how to use and maintain chairs, 'Personal handbook for users', which should be ordered at the same time as the wheelchair. The booklet varies for each group of chairs and the occupational therapist should ensure that the user receives his copy when his chair is delivered. Another very readable booklet is published by the British Red Cross Society: *People in Wheelchairs — Hints for Helpers*. The booklet is simply written and amusingly illustrated. Also available is 'How to Push a wheelchair', by Griffiths and Wynne, from the Disabled Motorists' Club.

These booklets give, amongst other information, basic hints on use and these include:

- *Maintenance.* When receiving the chair, and at regular intervals thereafter, the user should check that it is in full working order. Brakes, tyres and footrests are particularly important.

Ensure that pneumatic tyres are kept at the correct pressure (a pump is provided) and that the battery is fully charged.

Once the seat canvas sags or is split it should be replaced immediately.

- *Brakes. Always* put the brakes on fully when the chair is stationary and before transferring. Release them fully before moving.
- *Footrests. Always* swing and/or retract the foot-rests before transfer and *never* attempt to stand up on them.
- *Folding the chair.* Remove any cushion first and fold the chair by pulling up on the centre of the seat canvas.
- *Opening the chair.* Push with the heel of the hands on the bars at the side of the seat, keeping the fingers towards the centre to avoid squashing them (Fig. 9.58).
- *Self-propelled chairs.* The user should sit well up and back in the chair, with his feet squarely on the footrests. He should reach back and push the wheels from 90° behind the

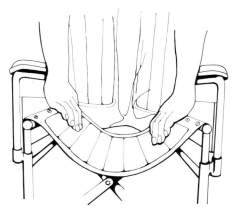

Fig. 9.58 Position of hands when unfolding a wheelchair.

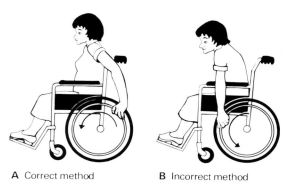

A Correct method   B Incorrect method

Fig. 9.59 Propelling a wheelchair.

vertical to 90° ahead of the vertical, thus keeping a good posture, and not push from the top of the wheel forwards (Fig. 9.59).

● *Repairs.* The DoH issues and maintains its own chairs free of charge to the user. There are lists of approved repairers and when a chair needs repair the user should contact his local centre to have the repair arranged. In an emergency, or in the case of small repairs, the user should have the chair repaired at his own expense and send the bill to his local centre. Owners of chairs purchased privately are responsible for the care and repair of their chairs.

SOME DO'S AND DON'TS FOR ATTENDANTS OF WHEELCHAIRS

A comprehensive list is given in the Red Cross handbook. It includes such common sense hints as:

● *Helping the chair down a kerb/step.* Warn the occupant what you are going to do. Hold the handgrips firmly and tip the chair back onto its rear wheels by pushing a foot on the tipping lever. Lower the chair down gently, ensuring that both rear wheels reach the road together. Lower front wheels.

● *Helping the chair up a kerb/step.* Warn the occupant what is going to happen. Hold the chair firmly and tip it back using the tipping lever. Place the front wheels on to the pavement and push the rear wheels on behind.

● *Helping the chair up and down a flight of steps.* This requires two helpers, one holding the chair by the handles at the back, one holding the front below the armrests (not on the footrests as these are liable to lift off). First warn the occupant what is going to happen and then tip the chair and manoeuvre one step at a time, balancing the chair on its rear wheels. One helper should take command to ensure that the lifting is done simultaneously. *Note.* Whether going up or down stairs the occupant always faces towards the bottom of the stairs.

● *General points.* Make sure that clothes, rugs and so on are tucked out of the way of the wheels. Talk with, not above, the occupant. Always warn the occupant before any move is made. Don't run when pushing the chair. Don't push the chair out into the road without looking. Beware of pushing the footplate into glass doors, walls, kerbs and shins.

THE ROLE OF THE OCCUPATIONAL THERAPIST

The role of the occupational therapist in assessment and advice regarding wheelchairs and outdoor transport will vary from area to area but she should be able to:

- Give concise and accurate reports on the person's physical and mental state with regard to his ability to handle the chair or vehicle.
- Report accurately on the areas in which the chair or vehicle will be used and arrange for any adaptations which may be necessary to aid its use.
- Know which chairs (and other help) are available. From her own knowledge she should be able to suggest the most suitable chair for the individual. This may be done with the full support of an organised wheelchair clinic or with the responsibility resting almost entirely on the occupational therapist, for example when ordering a chair for a person living at home.
- Teach the user (and/or his attendant) as soon as the chair is delivered how to use and maintain it, and how to transfer in and out of it, ensuring that the user is confident about its use and routine maintenance and knows where to get help if necessary.
- Give advice about facilities available, both on prescription and privately and try to find out what help/services the user may qualify for. It is unfair to raise his hopes by letting him feel he may get a Mobility Allowance or electric chair, for example, when this is not so.
- Always be aware of people who may benefit from the facilities or equipment available, especially a person who has:
(a) suddenly become disabled, for example through a stroke or spinal injury, or
(b) deteriorated to a point where help with mobility will save unnecessary struggle or further advance of conditions such as multiple sclerosis, heart or chest diseases or rheumatoid arthritis.

PART 5: OUTDOOR MOBILITY

The various types of assistance available to help a disabled person with outdoor mobility include:

1. THE MOBILITY ALLOWANCE

This allowance is now the major statutory assistance for most people who have mobility difficulties. It is a weekly, tax-free cash benefit intended to help with extra transport costs.

In order to be eligible for the allowance a person must fall under one of the following categories. He must be:

- unable to walk; or,
- virtually unable to walk out of doors; or,
- able to walk but the exertion needed would risk life or lead to a serious deterioration in health; or
- likely to remain in this state for at least a year and must be capable of going outdoors.

To be eligible, individuals must be five or over and under sixty-six years of age at the time of applying. The allowance stops at age seventy-five. A person can apply whether he lives at home or in an institution. Additionally, any car registered to a person in receipt of a Mobility Allowance is exempt from Road Fund Tax.

Applications are made on form MY1, which is attached to the Mobility Allowance leaflet NI211, available at post offices. Further information is provided in the leaflet.

2. DISABLED PERSON'S BADGE (Orange Badge Scheme) (Fig. 9.60)

This national scheme allows local authorities to issue car badges which provide parking concessions to disabled people who are travelling as drivers or as passengers. It aims to assist physically disabled and blind people to park closer to their destinations. This scheme is open to those who meet one of the following criteria, that is, who:

- receive the Mobility Allowance (or War Pensioners' Mobility Supplement); or,
- use a Department of Health motor vehicle; or,
- are registered blind; or,
- have a permanent disability which is so severe as to cause inability to walk or extreme difficulty in walking; or,
- have a very severe upper limb disability and regularly drive a vehicle but cannot turn a

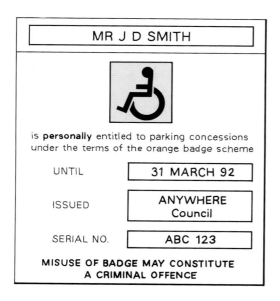

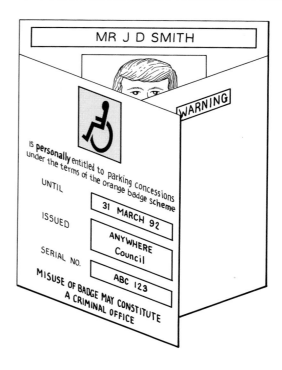

Fig. 9.60 Disabled Persons' Badge (Orange Badge Scheme). (Artist's conception, courtesy of the Department of Transport.)

steering wheel by hand and are unable to put money into parking meters or pay-and-display equipment.

A person must apply to the social services department of his local authority on form DP9. A certificate from his doctor is also necessary (form DP10) and the local authority will then decide whether a person is eligible or not. If eligible the person will be supplied with a front and rear window sticker and a parking disc. The badge is issued to the disabled individual, not to a particular vehicle, and can be displayed in any vehicle (including taxis) in which he is travelling. The concessions should not be exercised when the disabled person is not travelling in a vehicle, even if the badge remains on display. Badges are supplied for three years, after which the holder must re-apply. An institution concerned with the care of disabled people may also apply for a badge.

The badge, when displayed, allows the following on-street parking concessions to the badge holder:

- To park free of charge and without time limit at parking meters, or in designated parking bays (unless local limits are in force)
- To park for as long as he wishes in areas where parking time is restricted
- To park on single or double yellow lines for up to 3 hours within England and Wales, and without time limit in Scotland, except, in each case, where there is a ban on loading or unloading.

However, the badge holder must not park in places where he will cause danger or obstruction to other road users, or in other specified places such as zebra or pelican crossings, bus or cycle lanes or clearways.

Other benefits, such as the exemption of vehicles displaying a badge from being wheel-clamped, and various local concessions and restrictions at the discretion of the local authority, also apply.

3. MOTABILITY

This government scheme aims to help disabled people use their Mobility Allowance to become mobile. It gives people special terms when hiring or purchasing cars, purchasing wheelchairs or obtaining car insurance.

Within this scheme the person may choose to:

- hire a particular model of new car for 3 years, using all or most of his Mobility Allowance. All maintenance and repair costs and an AA membership are included in the scheme. On cheaper car models insurance may also be included. These cars are also exempt from car tax (not to be confused with Road Fund Tax)
- buy a new or used car at a discount price from certain manufacturers on a hire-purchase basis, using all or part of the mobility allowance. Maintenance, repairs, insurance and other extra costs are additional to scheme
- purchase a powered or non-powered wheelchair or an electric vehicle at discount price from certain manufacturers.

The person needs to be aware that:

- cars bought or hired under the scheme can be adapted to suit him but adaptations on hired cars are limited as they have to be returned as 'normal' vehicles at the end of the 3 years
- they do not need to be able to drive to take advantage of the scheme. A car may, indeed, be bought or hired to benefit a child if someone else receives the Mobility Allowance on his behalf
- different arrangements operate for war pensioners or those who possess a government tricycle or DoH vehicle
- as Motability is a registered charity, additional financing may be available from a special fund to help with the expense of putting the car on the road, such as that incurred for adaptations or for driving lessons
- he must have been awarded the Mobility Allowance for a long enough period to cover the period required for the hire or hire-purchase agreement to be completed.

Further details and application forms are available from:

The Information Department
Gate House, West Gate
Harlow, Essex CM20 1HR

4. ADAPTATIONS TO MOTOR VEHICLES

There are many companies that will supply and/or fit adaptations to cars for disabled people, for example hand controls to automatic cars or a hand clutch to a gear lever. A full, though not definitive list of companies offering this service is available, free of charge, from the Motability Information Department (see above).

5. ASSESSMENT CENTRES

There are assessment centres located throughout the country where a disabled person can be assessed for his ability to drive and the adaptations he will need to his vehicle. There are few physical limitations to driving but adapting a car to meet an individual's needs may be expensive. All adaptations for disabled people are exempt from VAT. Some centres may charge a fee for their assessment. A list of centres is available, free of charge, from the Motability Information Centre (see above).

6. LEARNING TO DRIVE

The British School of Motoring offers an assessment and teaching service to disabled people. The company has specially trained instructors, at certain branches throughout the country, who will visit a disabled person, assess his needs and teach him to drive. BSM has several cars that have been adapted to cope with a wide range of disabilities. Where a disabled person's needs are not met by a BSM car he may, of course, be taught to drive in his own adapted car.

7. ELECTRICALLY POWERED OUTDOOR CHAIRS

Only one electrically powered outdoor chair, the model 28B, is made for outdoor use by the DoH (Fig. 9.61). It is attendant propelled and supplied where the user needs to be pushed outdoors but where the usual attendant is unable, because of age, infirmity, the user's weight or local conditions, to push a non-powered chair. A wide variety of outdoor chairs are available for private purchase. For impartial advice the disabled person may visit one of several Disabled Living Centres that stock a wide range of electrically powered chairs/vehicles (for further details see below). The disabled person can also obtain information and advice from exhibitions of equipment for disabled people such as Naidex, where many manufacturers display and demonstrate their chairs/vehicles. Alternatively, of course, he may approach a manufacturer directly for advice and information.

As a result of the recent reorganisation of the supply of wheelchairs through the NHS, Disablement Services Centres are empowered to supply chairs that they feel best meet the needs of the disabled person. It may be possible, therefore, to obtain a non-DoH electrically powered outdoor chair from this source. Where demand outstrips budget such a facility may not always be available, but staff, often occupational therapists, at these centres will be able to offer help and advice about suitable chairs for private purchase and also offer ideas on how funds may be raised.

8. FINANCIAL ASSISTANCE

Where the Mobility Allowance and/or the Motability scheme do not cover the needs of the disabled person it may be possible for him to approach local businesses or local, charities and organisations such as the Lions Club for specific help with fund raising.

9. DISABLED LIVING CENTRES

These centres are located throughout the country. They are open for disabled people, their families, carers and professional workers to inspect and try out a wide range of equipment related to all aspects of independent living. Run by professionals, many of whom are occupational therapists, the centres give disabled people information on all aspects of help available with outdoor transport plus the opportunity to try out outdoor wheelchairs and vehicles.

Further details can be obtained from:

The Disabled Living Centres Council
380/384 Harrow Road
London W9 2HU.

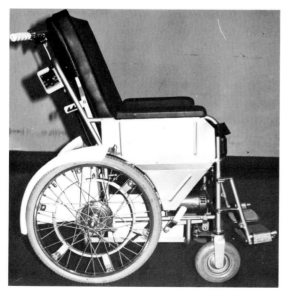

Fig. 9.61 Model 28B: an outdoor electric chair.

PART 6: MOBILITY WITHIN THE HOME

The early sections of this chapter have described permanent limitation of mobility and its far-reaching effect on all areas of life. When focusing on the effects of limited mobility within the home, the therapist needs to assess how the individual is affected in the way he copes directly with his home environment, that is, with the physical structure of the home, the access to and within it and the problems posed by its design, layout, features, fitments, furniture and equipment. In addition she must consider both the overt and covert effects on the person's role within the family, his personal independence, energy level and relationships with other people living in the house.

A temporary period of limited mobility is usually easily absorbed by the individual, his family, friends and workmates. People 'rally round' — they give lifts, do the shopping, mow the lawn and take the children to school. But where this state is permanent both major and subtle changes take place. If the person is no longer able to carry out his functions in the running of the home, be it meal preparation, car maintenance or child-minding, the whole family needs to make major adjustments to ensure that these tasks can continue. More subtle changes, however, may occur over a period of time as people's roles, attitudes, confidence and skills change. Where one partner has to begin to care for another, or where a different family member, through necessity, becomes proficient at a skill that was previously the province of another, the changes in confidence and attitude amongst the family members can radically alter the family's dynamics and bring guilt, frustration and resentment.

Similarly, if a person lives alone, or has been the main carer within the household, major problems can arise and will often reach a crisis point if there are no other immediate household members to absorb the changes taking place.

This chapter, however, whilst written in the knowledge that the reader will bear these psychosocial aspects in mind, focuses on the problems a person with limited mobility may have with the physical structure and features of his home and works on the premise that where these physical barriers can be overcome the disabled person may be able to resume, or continue, at least in part, his role within the home and family.

APPROACHING MOBILITY PROBLEMS WITHIN THE HOME

The principles of approaching a person's mobility problems within the home are the same as those that the occupational therapist adopts when approaching and solving any other problem. These principles are discussed in Chapter 4.

The therapist should be aware of the wealth of literature and information available relating to equipment designs and methods dealing with specific problem areas, but as these are constantly changing and improving it is not within the brief of this chapter to mention any of them in particular. However, she should bear in mind certain principles and guidelines before deciding on her course of action.

Minor alterations or adaptations

These include all non-structural alterations to the building such as putting up handrails or lowering light switches. The cost of these alterations is usually borne by the Local Authority or by the person himself. There is usually a (locally defined) limit per alteration below which the therapist may authorise work herself and above which she is required to refer to a person in higher authority.

Major adaptations

These include structural alterations to a building, such as widening doorways or adding an extension. The occupational therapist will not usually be able to authorise such work herself but will be involved in decision-making and work alongside architects, builders, environmental health officers and other local authority representatives who are also concerned with the work.

Payment for such adaptations may cause difficulties. Under the Chronically Sick and Disabled Persons Act 1970 (and reinforced by the Disabled Persons Act 1986 and Part VIII, Sections 101–138 of the Local Government and Housing Act 1989), Social Services departments are obliged to assess the needs of people with disabilities within their area if asked to do so by the person himself or his representative. They then have to make arrangements for the provision of certain services (included in which are 'aids and adaptations') if they are satisfied that the services are needed by anyone who is permanently or substantially handicapped. However, since budgets are invariably limited it is essential to ensure that sufficient finances are available to cover costs before embarking on any major work. Both discretionary and mandatory grants may be available to help cover the cost of such work, although often the person may be required to contribute at least part of the cost himself. As both Central Government and Local Authority rules related to the availability of these grants is constantly changing, the therapist must ensure that she is aware of the financial 'state of play' in her local area when considering such major work.

Each Local Authority is responsible for adapting its own housing stock as necessary. Such adaptations do not now alter the tenant's 'Right to Buy', unless the property concerned is part of a complex to which special services, such as those given by a warden, are provided.

Supplying equipment

The cost of supplying equipment necessary to help the person become more mobile within his home is, again, usually borne by either the Local Authority, the local health authority, or the person himself. Equipment which is needed to help the person to walk may be issued either by a community occupational therapist or physiotherapist or by the hospital, in which case the cost may be borne by the Health Service.

Within the community, whether employed by their local social services or by the health authority, most therapists have to work within a very limited annual budget allocated to cover the cost of equipment and minor adaptations. Therefore, the therapist must carefully balance the needs of all of her clients together in order to ensure that the budget is spent to its best advantage. The therapist must also be aware of how necessary monies may be acquired. For example, when considering the supply of a stair lift she may find that the cost of the lift itself may come from the 'equipment' budget whereas the money to cover the work involved in fitting it — which may or may not entail structural alteration to the property — may come from another source.

The therapist will need to keep abreast of not only the huge range of equipment available to help the disabled person become more mobile in his

home but also of any local regulations relating to the supply of equipment through special contracts, particular manufacturers or other specific arrangements.

Alternative solutions

Before embarking on major adaptations or expensive alterations it is wise for the disabled person and his family to explore with the therapist the various options that may be available to him. Where extensive work may need to be carried out to create a 'user-friendly' environment various alternatives should be discussed. These can include the possibility of buying or renting a more suitable property; of applying to the local Council for allocation of Wheelchair or Mobility Housing, or of ground-floor accommodation; of considering either private, housing association or Council warden-controlled (sheltered) accommodation; or exploring the feasibility of the individual moving to a Young Disabled Persons' Unit or into residential care.

However, for social, personal and financial reasons the disabled person's preference is often to remain in his present home and it should be the therapist's aim to meet this wish in the most cost-effective way if it is at all practically and/or financially viable.

Creating a 'user-friendly' environment

Where mobility is limited the creation of a 'user-friendly' environment can increase, or even restore, full independent mobility to the disabled person within his home. This in turn can restore or maintain the person's role within the home and family, improve relationships and reduce the stress suffered by both the person himself and his carers.

As she considers adaptations to the environment and the supply of equipment, the therapist must remember that the provision of financial benefits, voluntary and statutory services and appropriate education, information and specific therapeutic intervention are equally important in encouraging and supporting the family's present life-style.

Access

Access to a property requires the ability to move from the public highway, usually a pavement, into the house itself. Difficulties may arise at the following points:

1. The gate

The catch on the gate may need exchanging or repositioning and the spring may need to be replaced with a lighter one. The gate may need to be held open by a catch or magnet to allow a person with a walking aid/wheelchair to pass through more easily. The gate may need to be replaced by a lighter one if it is too heavy to manage, or to be removed altogether.

2. The path

Some surfaces, such as gravel, can cause problems and may need replacing or recoating. Where the gradient of the path is too steep a grab rail at the side can help, as can the provision of shallow steps

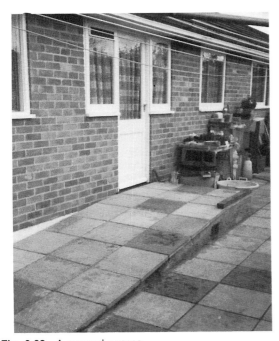

Fig. 9.62 A ramped access.

within the path. If the path has steps that the person is unable to negotiate the provision of small, half-steps may help. Alternatively, a ramp might be installed (Fig. 9.62). Should access via the main pathway still prove impossible then the use of other entrances to the house, for example through a French door or via the back garden, may need to be explored. It may be necessary to consider making a new entrance from the highway, for example through an existing side hedge, in order to obtain access via a suitable gradient.

3. The outside door

Can the individual cope with the locks, handles and any other door furniture? Is there shelter over the door to protect him in bad weather if coping with the door takes a long time? Is the threshold too deep and, if so, can it be made shallower? Is there a flat area immediately outside the door on which a wheelchair or walking aid can rest safely whilst the person opens the door? Would an outside light help? Is the door wide enough to take the wheelchair/walking aid?

GENERAL FEATURES TO AID MOBILITY WITHIN THE HOME

Halls, landings and other rotation areas

1. Easy access

Are there any items in the hall that hinder free mobility? Halls and landings often suffer from a surfeit of coats, telephones, umbrellas, buggies, plant stands and storage chests, all of which can hinder easy mobility. Whilst it is not always easy to relocate such articles it may be worth exploring this option, along with other possibilities such as installing a wall-mounted telephone or hanging coats on wall-mounted hooks rather than on a free-standing rack. Plants may be moved onto a windowsill or, again, onto a hanger fixed to the wall.

2. Circulation

If a hall or landing is narrow there is often little

that can be done to improve the space available. It may be worth considering rehanging doors that open into a hallway so that they open into the room/cupboard instead, or replacing them with a sliding door. Alternatively the therapist may need to consider supplying a narrower mobility aid, for example an Alpha walking frame rather than a standard four-legged type, that will take up less space.

3. Lighting

Halls and landings may be poorly lit and this can hinder the person's mobility considerably, especially when negotiating stairs or steps. A wall-mounted mirror may help to reflect light, as would lighter decorations and/or curtains. Solid doors can be replaced with full or half glass ones and additional lighting can also help. Colour, particularly yellow, can be used to highlight hazards such as a single step.

Doors

1. Width

Where a mobility aid is used the door width needs to accommodate both the aid and the user's arms as he passes through the doorway. Optimum widths for easy access for adults are: 900 mm for an ambulant person to allow for use of walking aids and 775 mm for the passage of a wheelchair.

To ensure that all available space can be used, check that access is not hampered by furniture or other moveable items. It may be possible to rehang the door to help access, or to replace it with a sliding or folding type. Alternatively, if the door is not really needed, e.g. between kitchen and hallway, it may be appropriate to remove it altogether to make the best possible use of available space.

The threshold may also be causing difficulties and may need to be removed, lowered or ramped.

Lastly, of course, the doorway may need to be widened. In some cases this may be a fairly straightforward task but in others it may necessitate structural alteration.

2. Door furniture

Doorknobs may need replacing with lever-type handles if they are difficult to cope with at the same time as a walking aid or wheelchair. Alternatively they may be easier to use if the height is adjusted or if the door is rehung to open from the opposite side. Door handles may be removed and the door fitted with self-closing springs and a kick-plate if necessary; a full width push-bar can also be fitted. Heavy springs can be replaced with ones that offer less resistance, or by 'rising hinges' that lift the door free of the carpet as it opens. Heavy doors may be replaced by lighter ones.

Stairs

Where difficulties are encountered when climbing stairs the therapist needs to consider not only the physical barriers that exist but also how the person's life-style can be adjusted so that the need to use the stairs is reduced or eliminated.

1. Reducing or eliminating the need to use the stairs

The therapist, the disabled person and his family need to look at the reasons why the person needs to use the stairs, how often he needs to do so, and whether these trips can be reduced or eliminated. Most trips upstairs relate to using facilities, such as the bedroom or bathroom/toilet, or to collect items that are required downstairs. In this latter case some forward planning or relocation of items may avoid unnecessary trips. Books, spectacles, tissues or other small items can be taken down in the morning in the pocket of an apron or shoulder bag, or duplicate items can be kept downstairs.

In addition, the cost of assisting the person to get upstairs needs to be weighed carefully against providing the same facilities downstairs, not forgetting that major alterations to arrangements can often affect family dynamics and relationships and may, in the long run, prove detrimental.

● *Temporary solutions.* The therapist must be aware that solutions that prove feasible in the short term may become quite untenable in the long term. However, temporary arrangements that may be considered can include:

— Bath. A strip wash downstairs in a warm room; the use of the facilities within a day hospital or a friend's/relative's house that has an accessible bathroom.
— Toilet. The use of a commode or chemical toilet may suffice if a suitable place can be found for it. The therapist needs to consider the user's privacy as well as the odours caused by such an arrangement. She also needs to consider who will empty the commode.
— Bed. If the disabled person's home has a separate room downstairs that can be used as a bedroom then this arrangement often eases the problem of coping with stairs, and may even prove to be a permanent solution. However, many homes do not have this convenience and whilst it may be possible for the disabled person to sleep on a Put-U-Up or other type of fold-away bed for a short while it is often not only uncomfortable but inconvenient for both the person and other family members. Lack of privacy, disruption of routine and loss of 'living space' can bring additional stresses to a family already coping with extra difficulties.

• *Permanent solutions.* Permanent changes in response to the difficulties encountered in climbing stairs need careful consideration in order that the full impact of such changes on the person and his family is appreciated. Solutions which reduce or eliminate the use of stairs can include the conversion or construction of downstairs areas to provide sleeping and hygiene facilities for the disabled person, the building of an extension to provide similar facilities, or moving to more convenient accommodation.

2. Assistance in climbing the stairs

Permanent solutions can include the installation of additional banisters, a stair lift (that will take the person either in a standing or seated position or in his wheelchair), or a through-floor lift, or obtaining help from another person who may be able to cope if, for example, the disabled person's day is planned so that he only uses the stairs to come down in the morning and go up again at night.

Electricity supply

The positioning of sockets and switches can hinder mobility around the house or the person's ability to use its facilities to the full.

1. Sockets

These should be sited for accessibility and safety

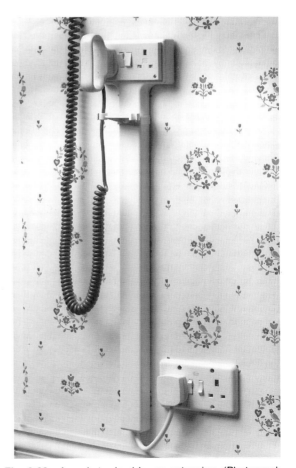

Fig. 9.63 A socket raised by an extension. (Photograph courtesy of Keep Able Ltd, Wellingborough, Northants.)

and should be of the switched variety if possible. It is often a relatively straightforward job to raise a socket from floor to waist level. Alternatively, an extension lead can be plugged into the existing socket and attached to the wall to relocate the socket as required (Fig. 9.63).

2. Switches

A disabled person's passage and safety around the home may be hampered by poor light. Switches should be positioned by the most frequently used entrance to a room and placed at the most convenient height for the disabled user. If several family members are to use the switch then a pull-cord type may be the most convenient for people with different abilities. Several varieties of switches are available for disabled persons whose hand function is poor. Alternatively, the need to operate a switch can be eliminated by the use of an infra-red detector device that will turn on a light when movement is detected in an area after dark.

Storage (Fig. 9.64 A and B)

Various principles applied to the storage of any item can help reduce the person's required level of mobility. These include the following:

• Store items close to the area in which they are required. For example, all items required for making a hot drink, or for having a wash, should be kept close together.

• Items most frequently used should be stored between the person's waist and shoulder height. This may be on a work-top, in a drawer or on a shelf of the most convenient height for the person.

• The use of rotating shelves, storage units fixed to the backs of doors or under shelves,

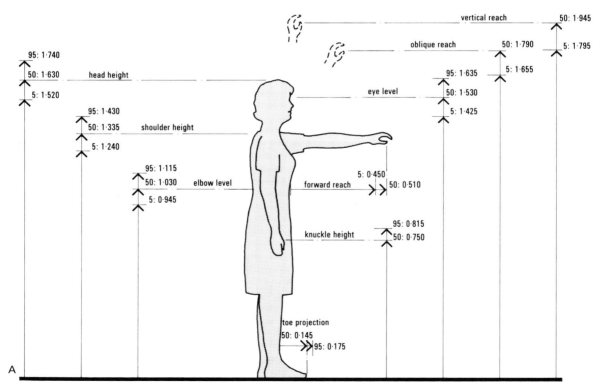

Fig. 9.64 A and B. Contrast of storage and working heights between ambulant and disabled women. (From Goldsmith 1984, Courtesy of RIBA Publications Ltd.)

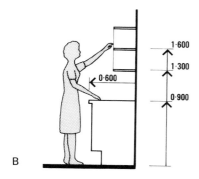

racks inside cupboards and hooks at a convenient height all reduce the need for extra mobility.

Windows

Ventilation controls should be as accessible as possible to avoid having to lean over dressing tables, around television sets, through potted plants, and so on. Being able to open and close windows is a problem that is frequently over-looked, especially if there are other people living in the house and, indeed, the disabled person him-self may rank its priority very low. None the less, if the therapist tackles the problem she needs to find out exactly where the difficulty lies.

The problem may be solved by increasing access, as mentioned, or by seeing whether the type or position of the handle(s), the stiffness of the window (often a problem if the window is rarely opened) or its design (it may be very heavy or require a movement the person cannot ac-complish) are causing the difficulties. Other solutions may involve the use of a fan or louvred ventilation panel within the existing window (con-trolled in such a way that the person can manage), the provision of a handle extension or, possibly, redecoration and lubrication of the window's hinges.

Flooring

Uncluttered access within the house is essential, as is open access to areas and items used by the dis-abled person in order to enable him to move as safely as possible.

1. Surfaces

The surface over which the person moves can, in itself, inhibit mobility. Various points need to be considered:

- Non-slip polish should be used on wooden, vinyl or similarly smooth surfaces.
- Deep pile carpet can cause a problem for those using mobility aids. Carpets are, of course, expensive to replace but it may be possible to lay a strip of a more suitable fabric over the passage most frequently taken by the person, or to exchange one carpet for another from a room the person rarely uses.
- The edges of mats can cause a hazard. The family may consider removing or relocating a mat or fixing the edges so that they do not curl up and so that the mat does not 'creep' across the floor.
- Washable floor coverings are extremely useful if a wheelchair or other indoor/outdoor mobility aid is used.
- Heavy-duty carpeting, woodblock, vinyl, cork or ceramic flooring are useful for heavy-use areas such as kitchens or halls.
- Man-made fibres can cause static on mobility aids and this can be extremely uncomfortable.
- Where mobility aids are used it may be worth protecting the lower part of the wall against knocks and scratches by extending the carpet to cover this area or by using a protective cover or constructing a deep skirting board.

2. Ramps

The provision of a ramp is not the universal answer to the problem of a step. Ramps take up room: a rise of 1 in 20 is preferable (though this can sometimes be reduced, depending on the ability of the person) and sufficient space may therefore not be available, especially inside the person's home. The use of a half step and/or grab handle may suffice for an individual step, but, again, this may not solve the problem. An internal step may often prove an insurmountable problem for a person using a mobility aid and if this blocks off a large part of the house to him major changes may have to be considered.

Where a ramp is being considered the therapist needs to take into account not only the slope of the ramp and the space it takes up but also its surface, width, safety edges and the provision of a flat area at top and bottom to allow for manoeuvring or for opening and closing doors.

SPECIFIC ROOMS

Bathroom

If access to the bathroom is difficult consideration needs to be given as to whether use of the bathroom is essential. Various ways of dealing with difficulties in climbing stairs have been investigated above. Further, more space for access may be made by rectifying the problems posed by doors and by narrow or small entrances.

If getting into the bath is a problem for the disabled person the therapist needs to consider various transfer techniques and aids such as hoists, bath boards and grab rails, which have also been discussed in this chapter. Equally, she may discuss

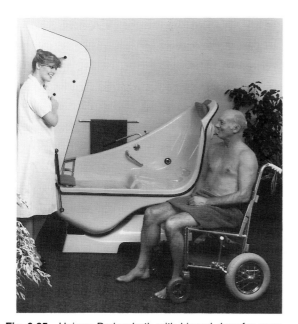

Fig. 9.65 Unique Parker bath with hinged door for easy side entry and exit. (Reproduced by kind permission of Parker Bath Developments.)

alternatives to using the bath (see p. 295) or explore such expedients as the provision of a shower, a specially designed bath (such as the Parker bath, Fig. 9.65) or a bath assistant.

The therapist must also remember that use of a bathroom requires space for dealing with clothing, mobility aids, towels, toiletries, shaving sockets and mirrors. If another person may be assisting with bathing, space can be at a premium, especially if equipment such as a hoist or wheelchair is needed in the room as well. As many bathrooms are small in modern houses this may not prove a feasible alternative.

Specific additional information can be obtained from the Equipment for the Disabled (Bathrooms) publication or the Housing Design Sheet 3 (Bathrooms) published by the Centre on Environment for the Handicapped.

Toilet

Use of the toilet is a basic need. Independence and privacy in using the toilet are top priorities for most people and the therapist should endeavour to facilitate this as far as she is able. She should also bear in mind that in order to ensure privacy the toilet must be insulated against the sounds and smells that the user may create. She must also remember that people with mobility problems often take a long time to use the toilet and that this may have implications for a busy household or carer.

Space and access are often very limited, especially if the toilet is a separate room. When considering making more space available, for example by converting a downstairs storage area or lobby, the therapist needs to be aware that public health regulations stipulate that there must be two doors between a toilet and any room used for habitation. In effect, this means that a toilet must open onto a hall, landing, lobby or other circulation space and must not open directly off a kitchen or living room, for example.

It may be possible to knock down the wall between the toilet and bathroom in some houses in order to create more space. Alternatively, or additionally, doors may be rehung or replaced, as already mentioned above.

The space available within the toilet often dictates the type of transfer used by the disabled person (and his helper), and this in turn may relate to how the disabled person will manage his clothing. For example, if the person is going to use a forward transfer onto the toilet from a wheelchair because of limited space, then the design of his clothing must be appropriate for him to do so. Similarly, if he is going to require the assistance of a helper to make a standing transfer then, when this is being taught, thought must be given as to how and when the person's clothing will be adjusted.

People with limited mobility can often be helped by equipment and/or adaptations to the toilet. By raising the height of the seat (either by use of a raised toilet seat or by raising the toilet pan itself) and providing grab rails, handles or frames, transfers can often be made simpler and safer. Finally, the therapist also needs to address associated problems that may arise, such as cleaning the perineum, flushing the toilet, and dealing with feminine hygiene, stoma care or catheter bags.

Kitchen

When looking at mobility within the kitchen the therapist needs to consider the following:

- What is the 'role' of the kitchen within the household? Is it used solely for meal preparation or also for eating, laundry or other activities? Is it the hub of the house, as it is in many homes, so that the individual without access to it would be isolated from much of the social intercourse that often takes place in a kitchen? Is it a separate room or part of a larger room?
- What is the 'role' of the disabled person within the kitchen? Is he the main or sole user of the kitchen; an occasional user (for example, heating a meal or preparing a sandwich for lunch, other meals being provided for him); or a 'visitor' who uses the kitchen for eating and socialising? The person's role within the kitchen is important to understand as it will relate to the priority given in time, expenditure and effort when dealing with his mobility problems. Additionally, if he is the sole or main user of

the kitchen then it would be more reasonable to adapt the area specifically for his use, whereas if he shares the kitchen with others each user's needs must be considered.

Limited mobility affects:

- The ability to move from one area to another with ease and speed. Consideration, therefore, should be given to:
  — Rearranging items to group facilities where possible, for example keeping together all items needed for washing up close to hand. It is also useful to have storage facilities near the sink and draining board (so that clean items can be put away with ease), and a work surface near the cooker.
  — Adding surfaces to create a primarily enclosed work area in order that items can be reached with the minimum of movement.
- The ability to work at or to reach items stored at different heights. Consideration needs to be given to:
  — Adjusting the height of all, or the main, work surfaces to that most suitable for the individual.
  — Storing the most frequently used items at the optimum height for the individual. The therapist needs to be aware of the ergonomic data related to those with limited mobility.
  — Using narrow shelves for storage rather than deep cupboards.
  — Adding additional storage space of the appropriate height by means of shelves; wire storage units on wheels or on the backs of doors; hooks or magnets.
- The ability to transport items from one place to another. Consideration needs to be given to:
  — Whether the layout of the kitchen or the storage of items within it allows items to be moved whilst the person remains still; for example, can he put crockery and cutlery away in a cupboard within reach of the draining board after washing up?
  — Whether items can be slid along surfaces

or 'rested' on their journey, for example on a chair, shelf or table.
— Whether the item needs to be moved. For example, can washing up be left on the drainer.
— Using a trolley or an apron with large pockets to move some items.
— The fact that 'Small is beautiful'. Small, lightweight items are often easier to move (although they may be more difficult to use). The more compact the working area in the kitchen the less the person has to move within it. Consider, for example, the design of kitchens in spaces which are, by necessity, severely restricted, such as submarines and caravans. Such kitchens make use of all ergonomic and storage principles and are, whilst very small, extremely convenient to use.

• Energy and stamina. Consideration needs to be given to:
— The kitchen layout in order to reduce the need for moving around — see above.
— Prioritising essential activities and looking at how these can be carried out most easily.
— Planning when activities should be carried out to make best use of the person's energy or activity level. For example, people with rheumatoid arthritis take a while to 'get going' in the morning and so their peak activity time would most probably be at midday. Having, or at least preparing, the main meal at this time will make best use of his energy and mobility levels.
— Reducing the need for activity by using labour-saving equipment and prepared or easy-cook foods; by instituting role changes within the family; or by having meals prepared by non-family members, such as Meals on Wheels, day centres, luncheon clubs, neighbours or friends, cafés or restaurants or other voluntary or paid help.
— Whether eating habits can be changed to help save preparation, for example eating pasta occasionally instead of potatoes, or raw vegetables instead of cooked.
— Training other household members (or the person himself) to put things away after use, wash up their own dishes, eat out occasionally, and develop a liking for take-aways and fish and chips (in moderation) without feeling guilty.

Bedroom

Most mobility problems here relate to:

• The ability to transfer into and out of bed. For suggestions on this see pp. 246–251. Consider also the bed's height and its position in the room, especially in relation to any equipment such as mobility aids, commodes or hoists.
• Access to storage areas. Consider changing doors to sliding or folding types or replacing them with curtains; using shelving or pull-out baskets rather than drawers for storage; or using wheeled storage units or those which fit under a shelf or behind a door.

Living area

Most points that need to be considered when helping the individual to move more easily within his living area have already been covered. Principles related to access, flooring, electricity, ventilation, transfers and room usage have been discussed in previous sections.

Within the living room, however, particular attention needs to be paid to the person's ability to reach and use any items and equipment he particularly needs to, especially if his limited mobility means that he spends a great deal of time at home. The possibility of creating storage space next to 'his' chair in order that his books, radio, magazines, telephone and drinks can be readily to hand will save unnecessary moving around. Additionally, his ability to control his environment from his chair by use of remote control switches or an environmental control system will give him more options and control over his activities than he may otherwise enjoy.

CONCLUSION

As can be seen, restricted mobility can severely affect the life of a person and that of his family and friends. Whilst it is not always possible to return the person to full mobility, the teaching of new techniques, the consideration of roles and dynamics within the family, the rearrangement of the environment, the supply of equipment and the alteration or adaptation of the home can go a long way towards reducing the impact such a disability may have. No one solution will be applicable to every circumstance, but careful consideration of priorities, needs, emotions and finances by the therapist, the individual and his family should enable the best solution to be found for a given situation.

ACKNOWLEDGEMENTS

My thanks to Mary Brewin, Occupational Therapist, formerly of the Disabled Living Centre, Medical Aids Department, Leicester; Maryanne Cook, Occupational Therapist, Warwickshire Social Services; Chris Menhinnick, Occupational Therapist, Disablement Services Centre, Wellingborough, Northamptonshire; Sue Morris, Occupational Therapist, Independent Living Centre, St Loyes' School of Occupational Therapy, Exeter; Nancy Wright, Occupational Therapy Tutor, St Andrew's School of Occupational Therapy, Northampton; and Jon Wrightson MD, British School of Motoring, Exeter.

REFERENCES

The Chartered Society of Physiotherapy 1975 Handling the handicapped. Woodhead Faulkner, Cambridge
Griffiths D, Wynne D 1986 How to push a wheelchair, 7th edn. Disabled Motorists Club, London
Goldsmith S 1984 Designing for the disabled, 3rd edn. Royal Institute of British Architects, London
Jay P 1988 Coping with disablement. Consumers' Association, London
Lockhart T 1981 Housing adaptations for disabled people. Architectural Press, London
Maczka K 1990 Assessing physically disabled people at home. Chapman and Hall, London
Tarling C 1980 Hoists and their use. Heinemann and the Disabled Living Foundation, London
Thorpe S 1985 Housing design sheets. Centre on the Environment for the Handicapped, London
Wilshere E R 1985a Hoists and walking aids. In: 'Equipment for the disabled' series. Oxfordshire Health Authority, Oxford
Wilshere E R 1985b Wheelchairs. In: 'Equipment for the disabled' series. Oxfordshire Health Authority, Oxford
Wilshere E R 1986a Hoists. In: 'Equipment for the disabled' series. Oxfordshire Health Authority, Oxford
Wilshere E R 1986b Housing and furniture. In: 'Equipment for the disabled' series. Oxfordshire Health Authority, Oxford

BOOKLETS AND LEAFLETS

Disabled Persons' Act 1986 HMSO, London
The Housing Act 1988 and disabled people — seminar report 1989 Centre on Environment for the Handicapped, London
Housing adaptations and severely disabled people — seminar report 1988 Centre on Environment for the Handicapped, London
Manual wheelchairs — Disabled Living Foundation Information Service handbook 10A 1990 Disabled Living Foundation, London
Mobility Allowance — leaflet NI 211 1988 DSS, London
Motability form CP1B 1989 Motability, London
New cars 1988 Motability, London
The new Disabled Facilities Grant: delivery prospects — seminar report 1989 Centre on Environment for the Handicapped, London
The Orange Badge Scheme leaflet 1989 (plus information handout 1990) Department of Transport, London
Powered wheelchairs, scooters and buggies — Disabled Living Foundation Information Service handbook section 10B 1990 Disabled Living Foundation, London
Used cars 1989 Motability, London

10

Workshop activities

Ann Turner
Charlotte V. MacCaul
(Section on Microcomputers)

INTRODUCTION

Many occupational therapy departments established several years ago were designed around a light workshop, a heavy workshop, and an Activities of Daily Living (ADL) unit. These were the main treatment areas that backed up work done on the wards and provided facilities for outpatient treatment.

In recent years, however, with the increasingly shorter stay of people in hospital, the rising costs of outpatient treatment, the improvement in surgical techniques and the changing demands put upon the occupational therapy service, the use of these areas has undergone quite a radical change. The increased pressure on the therapist's knowledge in self- and home-care techniques, the shift towards greater holistic care and a deeper understanding of neurological dysfunction within general hospital departments, and the many changes in both technology and society have led to changed emphases in the selection of activities for use as treatment media. Additionally, as medical and surgical techniques improve and people are discharged from hospital more rapidly, the opportunity for, and priority of, 'traditional' creative-activity-based treatment programmes have decreased. This apparent shift has implications for the core of our professional practice, i.e. the use of purposeful activity as the basis of therapeutic intervention (see Ch. 1), for whilst the importance of activity has not diminished it is not always easy to see it manifest within a workshop setting.

For various reasons, light and heavy workshops now often can appear under-used, with equipment pushed into corners and cupboards full of neglected materials. 'Traditional' programmes have made way for computer-based activities, an increased use of orthotics, and participation in support groups. These shifts in emphasis are often accompanied by changes in attitude and expertise among therapists. Less time is given in training, now, to the traditional skills and activities around which many departments were established. Many newly qualified therapists have only a hazy idea of how to adapt a printing press, seat a stool or position someone on an electronic cycle. Whilst their training has given them good grounding in areas such as keyboard skills and self-care techniques, they lack confidence in, and therefore rarely use (or perhaps use badly) facilities such as wood- and metalworking equipment that are still available within many departments.

Moreover, long-established activities have risen disproportionately in cost. Wood, which was once a reasonably cost-effective material to use in treatment, is now relatively expensive. As many therapists do not possess the skills to organise and run a woodwork store and workshop they must rely heavily on a technician or helper whose resources of time may already be overtaxed. Similarly, substantial resources in staff knowledge, time and management skills are required in order to run a printing area effectively. From a clinical point of view the number of people who would benefit from these (primarily) biomechanically orientated activities has also dropped and so it has not always been seen as appropriate for therapists or support staff to spend time acquiring the knowledge needed to run such areas efficiently.

On a more positive note, however, workshops can provide an invaluable area in which treatment based around activity (in its widest sense) can take place. With increasing emphasis on, and knowledge of, the role of 'purposeful activity' in healthy living (Ch. 1), and the therapist's skills in analysing activities to meet needs, a workshop,

regardless of the media used for treatment through activity, can remain a lively, supportive and well-used activity area. Similarly, the therapist needs to consider that, if she is abandoning existing equipment on the grounds of her own shortfall in knowledge, or because the activity is considered too time-consuming to be run effectively, or too old-fashioned to appeal to present-day tastes, she must replace it with alternative *purposeful* activities. She should not 'throw out the baby with the bathwater' in favour of squeezing therapeutic putty into ever more inventive shapes or sanding a biro mark off a piece of wood, only to replace the mark with another when the first has been painstakingly removed!

The therapist who, because of the pressures put upon her, sees domestic and self-care functions as the main (if not exclusive) area of concern of the people she is treating, is surely only addressing a somewhat narrow aspect of their lives. People will always require occupational therapy activity programmes following disease or injury. It is true that the group of people we treat, and their needs, are changing, that modern medical technology has eradicated the need for many of the traditional workshop programmes and activities, and that new treatment approaches and techniques compete for the therapist's time and expertise. But it is also true that good management practice requires a staff group to look objectively at what its workshop offers — to evaluate and, where necessary, change its facilities to meet the current requirements of the service. If this does not happen, time-honoured equipment, materials, expertise and ideas will become poorly used as they become more and more inappropriate, and, as they become more difficult to use effectively, will ultimately compromise our basic purpose of providing treatment through the use of meaningful activity.

This chapter, therefore, aims to look at some of the equipment, both 'traditional' and 'modern', available in many departments, with a view to examining its role in the treatment of a person through the means of purposeful activity. The first section of the chapter describes two remedial games, solitaire and noughts and crosses, which can be adapted in various ways for application to a wide range of disabilities. The second section describes the use of the rehabilitation lathe in the treatment of (primarily) lower limb dysfunction. Useful adaptations that can be made to the lathe for special applications are described, and correct safety procedures are set out.

The third section of the chapter describes in detail the OB Self-Help Arm as an example of the application of overhead sling support systems to the treatment of upper limb disabilities, spinal injuries, neurological dysfunction, and so on. The fourth section discusses the importance of adjustable tables as basic equipment for the workshop setting, describing their use in faciliting a range of activities in a standing, sitting and lying position.

The final section of the chapter turns to a newer addition to the occupational therapy workshop: the microcomputer. The rapid growth of electronic technology in recent years poses a stimulating challenge to the occupational therapist, who must now become familiar with the wide array of computer applications now available to her. The chapter describes specialised hardware and software that has been developed for therapeutic use, and offers guidance on evaluating its suitability for particular treatment programmes. Specific applications of the microcomputer to occupational therapy are then described, including its use in treating locomotor, sensory and neurological dysfunction and in helping individuals to improve or regain skills for work and for daily living.

REMEDIAL GAMES

A remedial game is an activity designed to treat a specific disability or problem while, at the same time, being amusing to use. The games described in this section are well known but have been adapted to be played in such a way as to provide very specific treatment for a particular dysfunction.

In addition to using standard commercially produced games many occupational therapy departments make their own adaptations to traditional games or, indeed, invent new games in order to treat a wide variety of disabilities. How-ever, the therapist must remember that any activity presented must be well made, professionally finished and, above all, suited to the purpose for which it is intended. A remedial game which is broken, badly made and finished or clearly designed to be played by an infant is an insult to an adult.

In recent years remedial games have received a 'bad press' because they are easy to misuse. It is important to remember that a remedial game should be used as *part* of a specific treatment programme, not as a mainstay activity. When treating, for example, a person with a hand injury, it is easy to become distracted from the use of *purposeful* activity and establish a programme which consists of a series of repetitive exercises on therapeutic putty; remedial games which are not really *played*, but simply provide an excuse for removing pegs from a board or discs from a pole, and unproductive actions such as turning a handle of a non-productive wire-twisting machine or FEPS (Flexion, Extension, Pronation, Supination) apparatus. Such practices are not only demoralising for the player but do nothing to enhance the interest of either the occupational therapist or other professionals in their work. Correctly used, remedial games can offer an enjoyable challenge both physically and mentally to the player; badly used, they can demonstrate some of the poorest of occupational therapy practice.

Two of the more common remedial games are described in this section. There are very many more in use but the therapist who can understand the basis of analysing and adapting a traditional game to suit a specific remedial purpose can use this knowledge to widen the selection of activities she has available.

SOLITAIRE

Construction

Solitaire is played using a square or round board on which a series of holes is made to conform with the pattern illustrated (Fig. 10.1). A set of 'men' is supplied to fit into the holes. As its name implies, the game is played by one player.

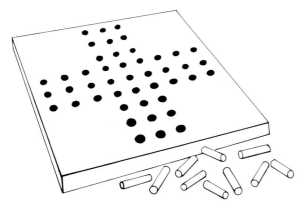

Fig. 10.1 The layout of the solitaire game. (Note: On some boards the outer line of holes is omitted.)

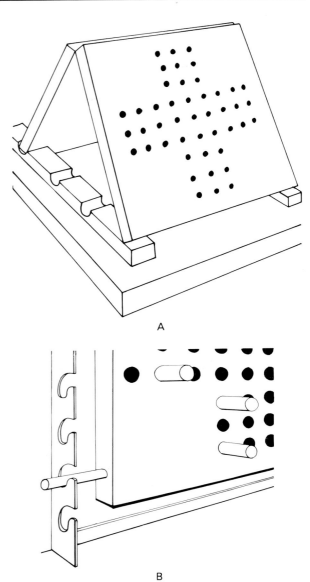

A

B

Fig. 10.2 The board adapted for (A) elevated use on table top (B) wall mounting on a slotted bracket.

Starting position

The game is usually played with the player seated at a table. However, if suitably constructed, it can be elevated either on its own stand (Fig. 10.2A) or on a wall-mounted bracket (Fig. 10.2B). A man is put into each hole except the central one.

To play

The aim of the game is to eliminate all but one of the men from the board and to leave the final man in the central hole. Men are eliminated by being jumped over as shown in Figure 10.3. A man can only jump one piece at a time and moves can be made vertically or horizontally. When a piece has been jumped it is taken off the board.

Source

The game is available commercially through sports shops or department stores. Adapted games are usually made as required in the department.

Therapeutic value

Solitaire can be used therapeutically to improve the following:

Spinal movements

• *Extension.* This is achieved using a large, wall-mounted game placed so that the top line of men is level with the highest point the player can reach. He can stand or sit on a stool or bicycle seat. This latter method also encourages

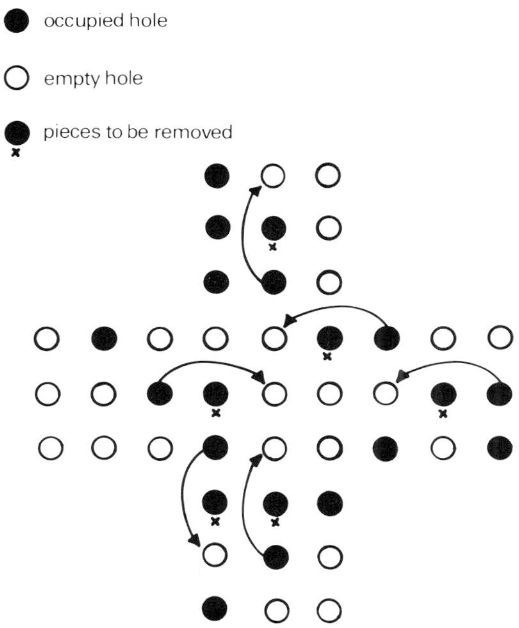

● occupied hole

○ empty hole

● pieces to be removed
x

Fig. 10.3 To play solitaire, moves are made as indicated by the arrows. Diagonal moves are not permitted.

balance and partial weight bearing in the early stages of lower limb treatment.

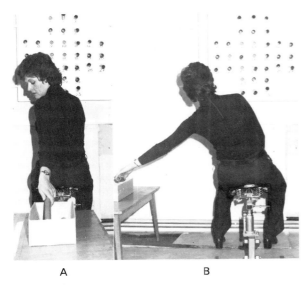

A   B

Fig. 10.4 Wall-mounted solitaire to encourage (A) spinal rotation (B) spinal side flexion.

● *Rotation.* The game is wall mounted at eye level with the player standing or seated on a stool or bicycle seat. When a man has been removed from the board the player twists round and places it in a box behind him. If his hands are used alternately to remove the men he can be encouraged to twist first to one side and then the other (Fig. 10.4A). This can also be done with the game on a table top and the player seated on a stool or bicycle seat.

● *Side flexion.* Again, the game is wall mounted at eye level with the player standing or seated on a stool or bicycle seat. Alternatively it can be placed on a table. When a man has been removed from the board the player leans over to the side to place it in a box beside him. As before, if alternate hands are used then flexion to both sides can be encouraged (Fig. 10.4B).

Shoulder movements

● *Forward flexion.* This is achieved by placing the game on a table so that in order to reach the row of men furthest away from him, the player must use maximal forward flexion.

● *Abduction.* The game is wall mounted or placed on a table and the player is seated sideways to it so that when reaching for the men his greatest range of abduction is used.

● *Extension.* The game is wall mounted or placed on a table and the player faces the game. When a man has been removed from the board the player reaches behind him and — without twisting his spine — places the piece in a box behind him.

● *Medial and lateral rotation.* The game is wall mounted and the player may sit or stand. When a man is removed from the board with one hand the player passes it behind his neck (lateral rotation) or behind his waist (medial rotation) to the other hand. It is then placed in a box.

● *Elevation.* The game is wall mounted and placed so that in order to reach the highest row of men the player is required to use his fullest range of elevation. The player may stand or sit.

● *Elbow movement.* The board is placed flat on the table in such a position that the furthest

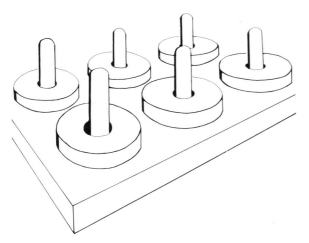

Fig. 10.5 Disc-shaped men and peg design.

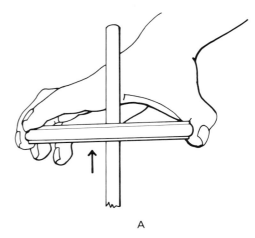

A

row of men requires the player to extend his elbow as far as possible in order to move them.

• *Pronation and supination.* A game in which the men are made of discs which fit over rods is required (Fig. 10.5). The men are picked up with the player's forearm in pronation and replaced with the forearm in supination (Fig. 10.6).

• *Wrist movement.* To treat wrist extension a board in which holes are drilled to take peg-shaped men is required. The holes and pegs should be far enough apart to allow the hand to be placed between them. The game is played with the men held as illustrated (Fig. 10.7A).

Wrist flexion can be treated by using the board with disc-shaped men as shown in Figure 10.5, and placing it at eye level so that the player has to reach up for the discs.

Thumb movement

• *Opposition* is treated using a board with peg-shaped men. These are held as illustrated in Figure 10.7B. *Note.* In the early stages of treating thumb opposition wide pegs are required. The pegs can be held between the thumb and furthest finger tip possible if the grip illustrated cannot yet be achieved.

• *Adduction* is treated using a board with

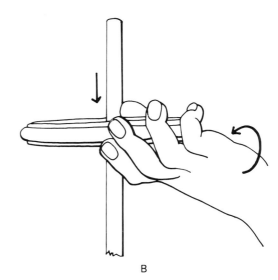

B

Fig. 10.6 To encourage forearm movement the disc is raised with the forearm in pronation (A) and replaced with the forearm in supination (B).

peg-shaped men. The men are held between the straight thumb and second metacarpophalangeal joint.

• *Flexion* is treated using a board with peg-shaped men. The men are held as illustrated in Figure 10.7C. Again, in the early stages of treatment wider pegs can be used, progressing to smaller ones as thumb movement improves. *Note.* Some people, especially those with short or large thumbs, may find this

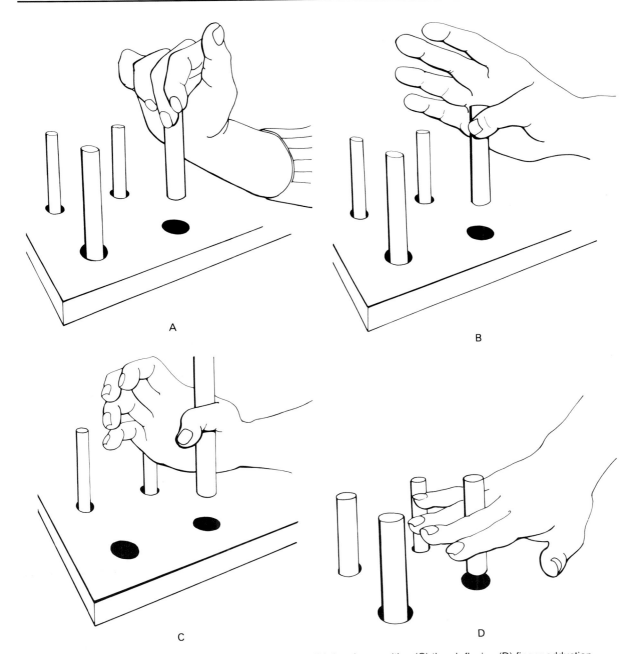

Fig. 10.7 Peg-shaped men held to treat (A) wrist extension (B) thumb opposition (C) thumb flexion (D) finger adduction.

movement difficult to perform normally. Their ability should be checked by asking them to perform the movement with the unaffected thumb where appropriate.

Finger movement

● *Metacarpophalangeal* flexion is treated by asking the player to hold the peg-shaped men as

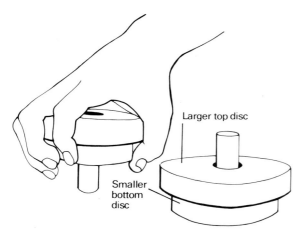

Fig. 10.8 Two disc-shaped men held to treat interphalangeal flexion.

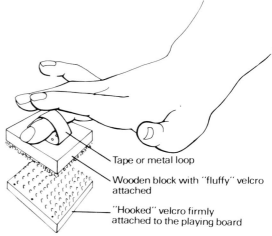

Fig. 10.9 Velcro men held to treat finger extension.

shown in Figure 10.7A. Again, in the early stages of treatment, wide pegs are used, progressing to thinner ones as the range of movement increases.

• *Interphalangeal flexion.* To treat this a board with men shaped as in Figure 10.8 is needed. The men can be made by gluing two discs together. Alternatively, the two discs can be left unjoined so that the size of the top disc can be altered to suit the size of the player's hand and the bottom disc can be changed to suit his level of active flexion. The discs are held as illustrated. *Note.* If only the distal interphalangeal joints are to be treated the disc will need to be enlarged so that these are the joints mainly concerned with grasping. The lower disc would not then be necessary.

Metacarpophalangeal and interphalangeal flexion can be treated together by using tall, peg-shaped men (see Fig. 10.7) which are held in a cylinder grip.

• *Adduction.* This can be treated by asking the player to grasp the peg-shaped men between the two fingers to be treated as shown in Figure 10.7D.

• *Metacarpophalangeal and interphalangeal extension* can be treated by using a board and men constructed as shown in Figure 10.9.

Other conditions which can be treated include:

• *Incoordination.* Upper limb coordination is encouraged by using this activity in most of its forms, as the limb has to be positioned and controlled while grip and release actions are performed. Where coordination is poor a large board with large peg-shaped men which fit securely in position is preferable, as these will not be knocked across the board if touched accidentally. For finer finger coordination a board with small pin-shaped men can be used, or one in which the men are made from dressmakers' pins and the board of a material such as Plastazote.

• *Upper limb weakness.* A large table top board in conjunction with a sling support system can be employed to treat upper limb weakness. Initially, when the limb and grip are weak, the men should be large and lightweight so that they are easy to handle (balsa wood blocks or empty painted containers may be used, for example). They can be lifted bilaterally if required. For those whose strength is improving, resistance can be increased in several ways. The following have been found successful:

— Painted containers filled with sand, lead weights or similar heavy materials.
— Wooden blocks with 'fluffy' velcro attached to the base. The 'hooked' velcro is attached

to the playing positions on the board so that the player must pull against the resistance of the velcro to release the men.
— Magnetic men on a metal board.

- *Pinch grip and opposition.* These can be treated by using a board on which the men are made of clothes pegs and bulldog clips which slip onto pegs on the board secured in the playing pattern. A series of clips of different strengths should be available. The player is asked to grasp the men between the thumb and whichever finger is appropriate for his particular disability. *Note.* In the early stages of treatment standard peg-shaped men, which offer little resistance, can be used.
- *Mental processes.* Concentration, perseverance and patience are encouraged with this game. If the positions are numbered and instructions written down, the therapist can also assess the player's ability to follow instructions. Solitaire can be used for both assessment and treatment in these areas.

NOUGHTS AND CROSSES
(Fig. 10.10)

Construction

Noughts and crosses is traditionally played by two players using paper and pencil. However, many sets are now available commercially or can be constructed for specific treatment.

Starting position

A grid is laid out as illustrated. Each player is given a pen with which to draw his symbol on the paper, or is provided with a set of symbols to place within the grid.

To play

Each player adopts either the noughts or crosses symbol. The aim of the game is for each player to complete a line of three of his symbols vertically, horizontally or diagonally across the grid before being stopped by his opponent placing one of his symbols in the way. Players make alternate moves (Fig. 10.10).

Sources

Noughts and crosses can be played wherever there is a flat surface and a means of making a grid, for example on a blackboard, in a sandpit, using paints on paper or chalk on the floor or drawing on an outdoor surface.

Games of noughts and crosses are available commercially from toy, games and department stores.

Therapeutic value

The various forms of noughts and crosses can be adapted to treat a wide range of disabilities:

Upper limb disabilities

For shoulder, elbow, forearm, wrist, hand, as well as spinal disabilities the noughts and crosses game can be constructed and used in the same way as solitaire.

Lower limb disabilities

With a large grid drawn on the floor, noughts and crosses can be used to treat the lower limb in the following ways:

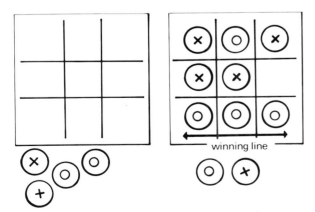

Fig. 10.10 A noughts and crosses grid and counters (left). Each player requires five counters. Game in progress (right).

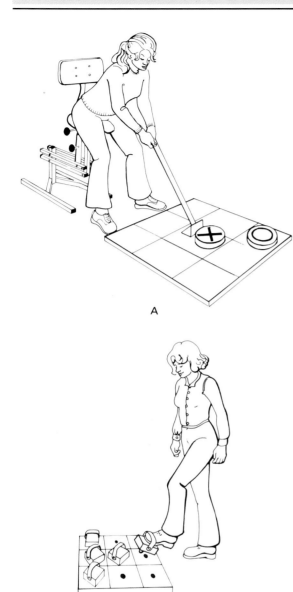

A

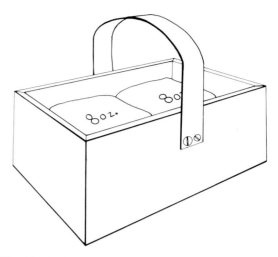

Fig. 10.12 A box-shaped counter with toe loop to take weights.

B

Fig. 10.11 Treating balance in (A) early stages (B) later stages.

● *Balance.* In the early stages the player either stands supported (for example by his walking aids) or sits on a bicycle stool with some weight taken equally through both feet. The game is played using large counters which he pushes into position on the grid using a long-handled pusher (Fig. 10.11A). As balance improves the player stands unsupported. In the final stages of treatment the player stands unsupported and uses counters with toe loops attached which he hooks over his foot and places on the grid while balancing on one foot. (Fig. 10.11B). The game may also be played whilst kneeling or crouching.

● *Ankle and foot movements.* To treat inversion the player sits on a bicycle stool and picks up large, cylindrical counters between the soles of his feet and places them on the floor grid. To treat dorsiflexion the counters with toe loops can be used. As strength in the dorsiflexors improves, resistance can be increased by adding weights to the counters. *Note.* If counters are to be used in this way they should be constructed in a box shape so that the weights can be securely placed inside (Fig. 10.12).

Mental processes

The game aids social contact because it is played by two people. Similarly, concentration can be encouraged, especially if three-dimensional noughts and crosses is played, as this is a longer game and involves more possible moves.

Writing

Noughts and crosses is a useful precursor to writing practice if played with pen and paper or on a blackboard, as the player has to hold the writing implement and draw simple figures with it.

THE REHABILITATION LATHE

The lathe (Fig. 10.13) is based on a treadle action for use with either leg. It has a large footplate which can be easily altered to take an extension plate. The table can be used for wood turning or sanding. The flywheel has three gears, with the resistance wheel attached to the spindle, to allow gradual increase of resistance.

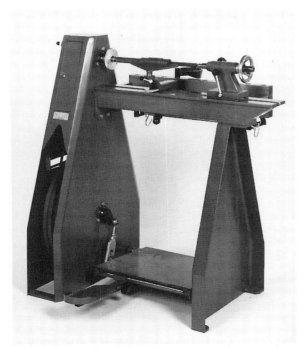

Fig. 10.13 The Larvic rehabilitation lathe. (Photograph reproduced by kind permission of NOMEQ.)

The lathe is primarily used in the treatment of lower limb dysfunction, e.g. following fractures, meniscectomies and soft tissue injuries and in cases of quadriceps lag. It is a useful activity to build up muscle bulk statically, therefore quickly, whilst also improving strength and range of movement. It can be used in the treatment of upper limb injuries to improve joint stability, muscle strength, and grip.

PARTS OF THE LATHE (Fig. 10.14)

The parts of the lathe are indicated in Fig. 10.14. Some parts which are of specific importance to the therapist when adjusting the lathe for use in treatment, are described below.

The pitman

The pitman is attached to the treadle and can be altered to three different heights to give three different ranges of movement. This enables greater or lesser hip and knee flexion to be gained although at each height the range of movement remains the same. The treadle is secured to the pitman by a collar, thus making alterations quick and easy.

Gears

The flywheel is on the side of the lathe and has three gears: low, middle and high. The belt can be adjusted by a handwheel to take up any slack. The low gear is the easiest to use and is the smallest pulley wheel at the base; the largest is at the top and is the hardest to use.

The resistance wheel and weights

The resistance wheel is attached to the flywheel spindle. It is only effective when the wheel revolves anticlockwise and enables the therapist to give a gradual increase in resistance more accurately. Resistance is gained by use of a grades scale from A to F, A being low resistance. A large, weighted metal block is pushed to the appropriate letter on the scale.

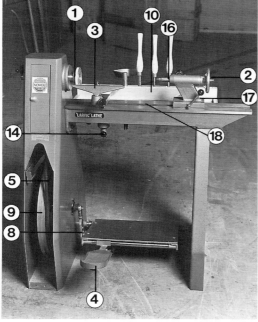

A

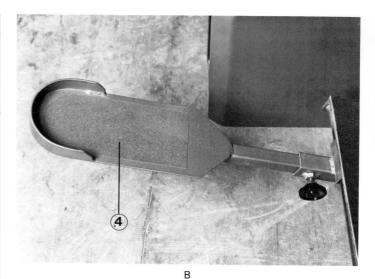

B

C

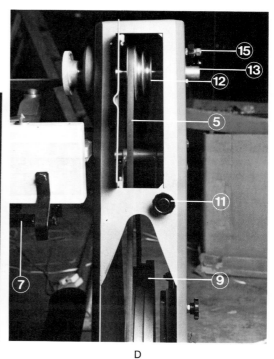

D

Key

1. Faceplate
2. Tailstock
3. Toolrest
4. Footrest extension on treadle
5. Driving belt
6. Resistance weight
7. Leg suspension bar
8. Adjustable pitman
9. 3-speed flywheel
10. Toolrack
11. Belt tension handwheel
12. Driving pulley
13. Hollow headstock spindle
14. Toolrest locking arm
15. Spindle lock
16. Tailstock barrel with central cone fitted
17. Tailstock barrel locking lever
18. Facebed

Fig. 10.14 Parts of the lathe.

The treadle

There are two types of treadle platform: a divided foot board and a single, flat board with footplate extension. The platform is used as a base to increase hip and knee movement.

Footplate extension

This extension is 61 cm long, 11 cm wide and has a safety lip at the heel end. The footpiece has a non-slip surface. The extension is made of box section steel which fits just under the treadle platform and is secured by a knurled, plastic wheel. The extension footpiece can be adjusted in 11 × 2.5 cm gradings. It can be slid along the platform and fixed in a wide variety of positions according to the individual needs of the user.

Leg suspension bar

This runs along the width of the facebed and is sited under the toolshelf. It is used during leg suspension exercise (static quadriceps). The user is seated on a Camden stool and the affected leg is placed in a sling which is attached to the suspension bar. The user then treadles with the other foot. The bar is adjustable to three positions according to the needs and size of the user. The facebed is formed from the steel bars that run the length of the lathe and along which the tailstock runs.

USES OF THE LATHE

As has been stated, the role of the occupational therapy workshop has changed in recent years due to a number of factors. These include shorter hospital stays for many people, the rising cost of outpatient treatment and the changing demands put upon the occupational therapy service. These changing demands are not, however, confined to occupational therapy. Physiotherapy, amongst other professions, is also experiencing these changes. However, as the work of these two departments in the treatment of people with limb injuries and other conditions requiring biomechanical intervention is complementary, prioritising the services available from them makes the most effective use of their facilities to the maximum benefit of those requiring treatment. The lathe, along with other heavy workshop equipment, can be used in the occupational therapy department as a complement and adjunct to the facilities in the remedial gymnasium in the following ways:

- To increase the range of movement (ROM) at the hip, knee and ankle joints
- To increase the strength of:
  - extensors of the hip
  - extensors of the knee
  - plantarflexors
  - extensors of the spine
  - grip and wrist stability
- To increase work tolerance
- To improve hand/eye coordination
- To assess noise tolerance and tolerance to revolving machinery.

When planning treatment on the lathe, the therapist must always examine the person fully *before* starting treatment. This has a two-fold purpose: (a) to assess his primary needs and (b) to make sure that there are no abnormal contraindicatory clinical signs and symptoms.

Before each treatment session, the person should be asked whether there have been any additional problems since the last session.

Hip joint

The main treatment aims are to increase range of flexion and improve the power of the extensors.

- *Flexion.* The user stands on the unaffected leg, the height of the treadle being determined by previously taken measurements. The amount of flexion can be increased in two ways:
  - raising the treadle by moving the notch on the pitman
  - using the foot extension plate. The further the extension plate is pulled out, the easier it is to treadle, so this should be counteracted by increasing the resistance at the same time.
- *Extension.* The user stands on a block on his unaffected leg, with the pitman on the treadle at its lowest point. Care should be taken that the lowest point of the treadle is not below the level of the block. The extension plate can

be either left off altogether or at the 'in' position. To increase resistance, the drive belt should be moved to the large wheel as soon as possible, and the resistance weight moved up the scale.

Knee joint

- *Full extension*. The user stands with his unaffected leg on a block, and works with the affected leg on the treadle to promote full extension. Resistance is not usually required, but fairly long sessions at this activity are indicated.
- *Strengthening quadriceps*. This is the most vital aspect of treatment on the knee.

There are two methods of improving quadriceps strength. The first is used if the person has an extension lag. He sits at the lathe on a Camden stool seat, with the affected leg slung under the facebed (the foot being held in maximum dorsiflexion and eversion), and the unaffected leg treadling. In this way the muscles on the affected leg work statically by reciprocal innervation. Three to four treatment sessions should see a dramatic improvement.

With the second method, the person is positioned as for full extension, with the resistance weight being moved along the calibrated bar as soon as possible, and the drive belt moved to the large flange of the flywheel. He should be encouraged to treadle some of the time with his unaffected leg, bracing his affected leg well back. He will thus build up his quadriceps statically, as well as exercising the glutei on that side.

- *Knee flexion*. At the beginning of treatment of the knee joint, flexion is not the most important aspect. Before treatment commences, it is essential that the knee is examined carefully. Effusion, pain or a hot knee are regarded as contraindications for working towards knee flexion. However, knee flexion can be increased by adding the foot extension plate. The condition of the knee should always be checked after treatment and prior to the next session.
- *Non-weight-bearing treatment*. There are some conditions where weight-bearing is not allowed (i.e. in the early stages of fractured shafts of femur, fractured tibia, or while the leg is still in plaster of Paris or a functional brace) but where treatment is intended to assist the venous return in an oedematous lower limb. It is also important to maintain tone in the quadriceps. In this instance, the static quadriceps exercise is given, by sitting the person on a Camden stool, and placing the affected leg in a long sling. This is suspended from the static quadriceps bar, and the person treadles with the unaffected leg, making sure that he does not hold onto the lathe. Thus the quadriceps and glutei have to work statically to keep balance, and the muscles contract rhythmically as they stabilise the pelvis.

The therapist should always explain to the person why she is giving him this particular type of treatment. It may help to let him feel the contractions of the quadriceps so he will have a better understanding, and therefore cooperate fully.

Ankle joint

- *Plantarflexion*. Powerful and well-controlled plantarflexion is the key to a good walking pattern. It is therefore essential to assess the function of the ankle joint when a person is referred, even though it may not have been the primary reason for referral.

The user should treadle with both affected and unaffected legs. When using the toe block (see Adaptations) and treadling with the unaffected leg, the posterior and anterior tibials work on the ankle joint, while the long flexors exert the downward pressure on the toe block. It is important to keep the knee joint braced in the 'locked' position. This is a very strenuous activity to start with and should therefore be graded carefully.

- *Inversion/eversion*. These movements can be encouraged passively when the person's foot is placed on a triangular wedge fitted to the footplate.

Other possible uses of the lathe

- Head injuries — to assess balance, hand/eye coordination, noise tolerance, and reaction to revolving machinery.

• Back injuries — general strengthening, working in the mid range and building up resistance, provided that the pain level is carefully watched. Equal time should be spent treadling with each leg.

• Hand injuries — later stages of treatment, for general toughening up, to improve grip and increase stability at the wrist. It can also be used to desensitise the stumps of amputated fingers when working with the tools (as they vibrate).

• Lower limb amputees — providing a hollowed out block is used to keep the bottom of the pylon in position. Full extension of the knee should not be attempted as the pylon will lock. This activity will help to keep the other joints mobile.

Conditions treated with the lathe

• Fractures and dislocations of the acetabulum, slipped epiphysis, fractured neck of femur or greater trochanter: to increase stability of the hip joint and improve ROM and strength.

• Fractured shaft of femur, tibia and fibula, patella, condyles and tibial plateau: to reduce oedema, remove extension lag, increase stability of the knee joint and improve ROM and strength.

• Fractured malleoli, calcaneum, talus, ankle (Pott's fracture) and other bones of the foot: to reduce oedema, increase plantar and dorsiflexion and in/eversion. To improve general strength, walking pattern and ROM.

Note. Remember, if the person has been in traction or in plaster, to check the joints above and below the affected joint or the site of fracture.

• Other orthopaedic conditions. Meniscectomy, lateral releases, chondromalacia, osteotomies, arthrotomies, removal of loose bodies, internal derangement of the knee and ruptured tendons (quadriceps and Achilles) — aims as above.

• Arthritic conditions, osteoarthritis, knee replacements: work gently in the mid-range, building up resistance gradually. The aim is to build up muscles as far as possible, reduce pain, maintain adequate function for independence,

prevent joint deformity and stimulate a good reciprocal walking pattern. (In some older people lathe work is contraindicated as the movement can be too jerky.)

• Peripheral nerve lesions, especially of the common peroneal nerve: to help promote regeneration of nerve tissue, prevent muscle wasting/contractures, maintain full ROM and increase returning strength.

• Amputation of the lower limb once pylon or prosthesis is fitted: to maintain and improve balance and coordination of the lower limbs and encourage a good walking pattern. To strengthen muscles of both lower limbs and prevent flexion contractures of the hip joint. To increase ROM and maintain good circulation. For work assessment.

• Head injuries and conditions producing general weakness and incoordination: to increase general strength and ROM in lower limb. To improve balance, hand/eye coordination, concentration and noise tolerance, as well as tolerance to moving machinery. For work assessment.

• Spinal injuries, if there is partial lower limb function and/or weakness in the trunk: to strengthen the muscles of the lower limbs and the back extensors. To increase ROM and improve balance. To stimulate returning movement (sanding or wood turning).

Some people may need to sit at the lathe, especially those with an extension lag, or partial paraplegia; in such cases a Camden bicycle seat can be used. This then becomes a partial weight-bearing activity.

Possible activities

Sanding

Bingo pieces, draughtsmen, solitaire sticks, quoits, rocker bases, bag handles, towel holder ends.

Any sanding activity provided the article is large enough to be held and sanded safely.

Turning

Fruit bowls, table lamp bases, egg cups, salt and

pepper pots, rolling pins, mug trees, candlestick holders, handles, round boxes, skittles.

Points of use

The Health and Safety at Work Act 1974

This Act demands that all moving parts of machinery be guarded. Hence the belt on the lathe has a guard on later models.

Clothing

Suitable clothing must be worn by lathe users — preferably shorts and a T-shirt or a tracksuit. Footwear is also important — gym shoes or training shoes are safest as they usually have a rubber non-slip sole. Long hair should be tied back, ties and jewellery removed or tucked out of the way and cuffs rolled up to prevent flapping.

Positioning

It is important to position the user correctly on the lathe to gain maximum benefit from treatment:

- When treadling, the user should put the ball of the foot on the treadle platform to prevent the knee hitting the base of the facebed on flexion. The push down required in this position is stronger than with the whole foot on the treadle, and also uses the gastrocnemius in addition to the quadriceps.
- When using the foot extension plate, the user should make sure the heel is right back in the guard, to help gain the range of movement required. He should keep the feet as parallel as possible.
- When not using the extension plate, the user should place the standing leg as near the footplate as possible without hitting it on the down movement.
- The user should stand on a block in the early stages of treatment, if knee flexion is poor.

Posture

- The user should be encouraged to stand upright and to keep the standing leg braced back when treadling.
- The user should not hold onto the lathe when treadling; this is to increase his balance, and strengthen the standing leg. It also helps him to avoid touching moving parts.
- The therapist should be alert to compensatory movements.
- When setting up the machine, the therapist must make sure the person is comfortable.

Range of movement

When the person first uses the lathe, the therapist should adjust this to gain the maximum ROM at that time. As the ROM increases, the machine should then be adjusted accordingly, but should never be set beyond the person's range.

Upgrading

The ROM and the resistance can be increased in the following ways:

- increase time
- increase weight load
- alter belt drive to harder pulley
- tighten belt by adjusting hand wheel
- start sanding, then turning
- ROM:
  — use extension plate
  — alter pitman.

Charts

When the person's treatment programme on the machine is altered, adjustments must be recorded. The quickest and most efficient way of doing this is to have charts near the machine, on which are marked the following details:

- name
- time (in mins) — for each leg as appropriate
- (footplate number; in/evertor block (large or small); sling (if used); resistance A–F.

The use of charts is a great help in a very busy department. It helps the therapists and students covering for absences to alter the machine for each person quickly and correctly.

Safety precautions

- When a person is sanding or wood turning, he should be closely supervised. He should also be informed that goggles and aprons are essential.
- The person should be told about moving parts on the lathe before he starts to treadle, each and every time he attends for treatment.
- The person should be told that the injured limb may swell up and ache more than usual after the first few treatment sessions because it is unused to the increased activity. This should be checked prior to the next treatment session.
- The therapist should check that long hair is tied back, ties are removed, and that the person is not wearing unsafe clothing.

Maintenance

Regular maintenance of equipment is essential for good and efficient running, especially when it is in heavy use. Nuts and bolts should be checked, screws tightened, and oiling carried out weekly. Servicing by the manufacturer or on a planned hospital maintenance scheme should be carried out at least once a year, and more often if the equipment is under heavy use.

Adaptations

Several useful adaptations can be made to the lathe to enable quick alterations in the minimum time when the department is busy.

The block

Two blocks, one 7.5 cm and the other 5 cm high can be made. When a person has limited knee flexion, a block is used to stand on. Both blocks can be used together to obtain full knee extension with the pitman in the lowest position, should this be needed.

Numbers on footplate extension

These enable the therapist to put the footplate in position quickly and accurately, providing the information is recorded on the appropriate charts.

Toe block

When standing on this, the user is on tiptoe; this helps to strengthen the gastrocnemius, improve balance, and help to improve the heel-toe gait.

Non-slip surface on treadle

A sheet of rubber is attached to the treadle to prevent the foot slipping.

Availability

Nottingham Medical Equipment Company (NOMEQ).

OVERHEAD SLING SUPPORT SYSTEMS

The OB Self-Help Arm (Fig. 10.15) is described here as an example of an overhead support system. It consists of a mobile stand with a fixed overhead yoke and movable forearms. Each of these forearms holds an adjustable bar and slings which, by a series of counterweights, can be altered to support the weight of weak upper limbs. One limb or both may be treated at a time. The OB Self-Help Arm can be used while standing, sitting or in bed.

PARTS OF THE OB SELF-HELP ARM

The work unit

- *The mobile stand*. This is made of lightweight metal and stands on four castors, the back two of which can be braked. From the fixed overhead yoke two movable forearms protrude which can be adjusted for length, horizontal movement and tilt on the long axis. Each of these adjustments is measurable on the scales provided (Fig. 10.16). The stand contains a clip on which the storage box containing spare slings and cord is stored.

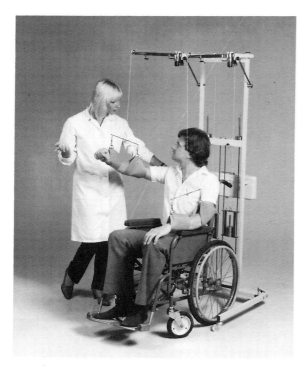

Fig. 10.15 The OB Self-Help Arm. (Photograph reproduced by kind permission of NOMEQ.)

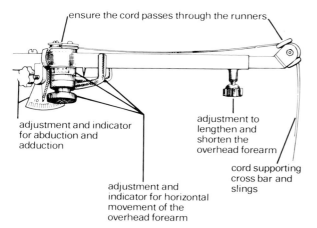

Fig. 10.16 Adjustments on the overhead gantry.

• *The slings*. Each machine is supplied with slings to fit the wrist, elbow and hand. The slings are attached to either end of a crossbar which, by adjusting the weight distributor, can be altered so that the person's forearm can be correctly positioned in the slings. The crossbars are attached to a nylon cord which runs over the forearms and yoke and down to the weight basket.

• *The weights and weight basket*. The weight of the person's upper limbs is supported by the counterbalance of disc-shaped weights which fit inside the weight basket. When the machine is not in use, or while the person is being set up in the machine, the weight box is locked in position on the back of the stand. The weights are stored on a stand fixed to the back of the unit.

The seat

The Help Arm is designed to be used with any static or mobile seat. The machine can also be used for bed-bound people or those standing at a work table.

Transfer to and from the machine

It is most important that the therapist is able to set the person up in the OB Self-Help Arm correctly and easily. The following sequence should be used.

1. The user is seated at a work top. For the bed-bound person a work top is placed over the bed in front of him.
2. The OB Self-Help Arm, with the weight box and forearm bars locked and the cords looped over the forearm bars, is wheeled up behind the user. The brakes are then secured.
3. The user's arm is supported (by the therapist, her helper, on the table top or by the user's other hand if possible) while the slings are put around the elbow, wrist and, where necessary, the hand. They are then clipped to the crossbar.
4. The cords are unlooped and attached to the crossbar.
5. Whilst supporting the user's arm with one hand the therapist unlocks the weight box and lowers it with her other hand. This will take up

the slack on the cord, but will not yet support the user's limbs.

6. Weights are added to the weight basket until the user's limbs are in a good working position.

7. The forearm bars are adjusted for horizontal movement, length and tilt as required.

8. Finally, the crossbar is adjusted by moving the butterfly screw along it until the forearm is correctly positioned for work.

USES

The OB Self-Help Arm is used to support the upper limb or limbs if weakness prevents them from being used for independent actions. Because the weight of the limb is counterbalanced by the machine any power remaining in the limbs can be used to grasp, coordinate and move during work without having to be expended on holding the limb up against gravity. In this way minimum power can be used to maximum advantage.

Additionally, because the user is able to work bilaterally, good upper limb patterns of movement can be retained even if one limb only is affected, such as in a brachial plexus lesion. Sling suspension is *not* helpful where spasticity is present, as the spastic tone may be increased.

Therapeutic value

The following conditions may be treated using the OB Self-Help Arm:

• Fractures or other orthopaedic conditions of the upper limb: to relieve the weight of the plaster of Paris, thus enabling the free joints of the limb to be used while the fracture is immobilised. To support the limb in the early stages of recovery from injuries affecting the shoulder joint, e.g. fractured humerus or dislocation of the shoulder.

• Spinal injuries resulting in upper limb weakness: to support the limb, allowing maximum functional use of weak muscles. To aid coordination.

• Progressive neurological conditions such as

multiple sclerosis or motor neurone disease; the purpose for treatment is the same as above.

• Peripheral nerve injuries affecting the upper limb: to support the upper limb, thus allowing maximum functional use of weak muscles. To prevent joint deformity and muscle shortening by maintaining a full range of movement. To encourage any returning strength.

• Other lower motor neurone conditions such as polyneuritis: the purpose for treatment is the same as above.

Possible activities

Almost any activity can be performed with the OB Self-Help Arm. Those most commonly required include:

• personal care activities: feeding, washing and hair care.
• communication activities: writing and keyboard skills
• activities to increase the functional use of the upper limbs: stoolseating, sanding and remedial games.
• leisure activities: painting, reading and craft work.

Points of use

Because the OB Self-Help Arm is mobile and compact it is suitable for use in the department, on a ward or in home.

The facility to control the horizontal movement of the forearm bar allows the therapist to limit the range of shoulder abduction and adduction within the arc required.

As the strength in the upper limb returns the balancing weights are reduced so that the user begins to support the limb against gravity using his own muscle power.

Availability

The OB Self-Help Arm is available from the Nottingham Medical Equipment Company (NOMEQ).

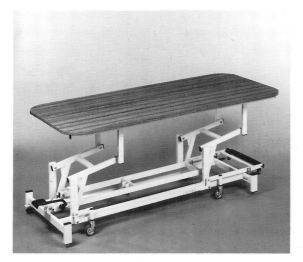

Fig. 10.17 Twin-lift (hydraulic) table. (Photograph reproduced by kind permission of NOMEQ.)

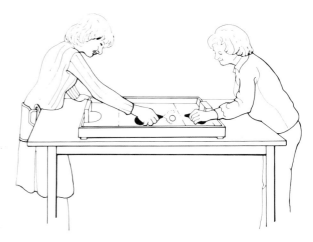

Fig. 10.18 Standing at an adjustable table supported by a hip sling.

ADJUSTABLE TABLES (Fig. 10.17)

A wide variety of tables should always be available within a department to fulfil different treatment needs. Various heights, surfaces, sizes and angles are necessary at different times and such demands cannot be met by a single design. However, a range of adjustable tables has been designed specifically for use by occupational and other therapists. These tables have the advantage of being stable and adjustable in height. Many of them are wheeled, and therefore mobile for easy use within a busy department, and some have additional features such as adjustable tilt. Their potential uses in a workshop are considered below.

STANDING

A person may stand at the table, which has been adjusted to the required height, in order to perform an activity. He may stand unsupported or may be supported by a hip sling, the therapist or a standing frame (Fig. 10.18). Where the person has the ability to stand unaided, but lacks either confidence or stamina, a high stool or chair may be placed immediately behind him.

Positioning

- The person may stand square on to the table to encourage equal weight-bearing through both lower limbs. A widely spaced activity will encourage him to lean from side to side if this is necessary (Fig. 10.19).
- The person can stand at an angle to the table so that activity encourages active weight transfer from one lower limb to the other (Fig. 10.20). Activities such as planing, sanding, collating or pastry/clay rolling can be used from

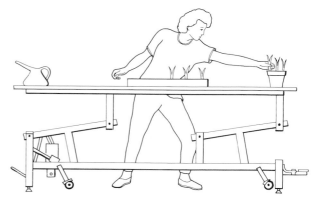

Fig. 10.19 Standing square on to an adjustable table using a wide-based activity to encourage weight transfer.

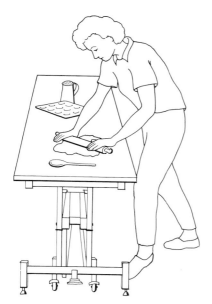

Fig. 10.20 Standing at an angle to an adjustable table, transferring weight rhythmically between the forward and backward leg while rolling pastry.

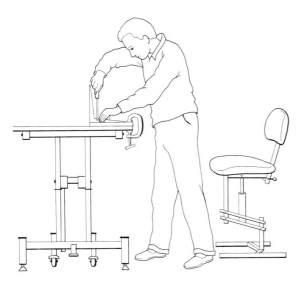

Fig. 10.21 Standing unaided at a table with a stable, high-seated chair (Camden stool) immediately behind for security.

this position to build up a rhythmical motion that will encourage this transference.

● A person can be encouraged to stand from sitting if he is unable to stand continuously. If a stable, high-seated chair with arms (such as a Camden stool) is placed immediately behind him, an activity that requires short periods of work and that can be readily left without causing difficulty can be undertaken. Activities such as composing type, playing a remedial game or working on a computer keyboard may be appropriate (Fig. 10.21)

SITTING

Sitting *at* the table

Heights of both chair/stool and table can be adjusted to give the required working position or range of shoulder/shoulder girdle movement. Spinal position and movement should also be considered when the person is being positioned.

Positioning

● A person may be seated face on to the table and the activity chosen can encourage a static or more mobile posture as required, depending upon the range of movement required to carry it out.
● A person can sit sideways to the table in order to encourage spinal flexion/rotation and wide shoulder/shoulder girdle movement (Fig. 10.22).

Sitting *on* the table

The therapist can use the table in such a way that it gives a wide base for sitting and activity whilst individual height adjustment allows the person's feet to be placed flat on the floor to aid balance and encourage good posture. Whilst sitting on the table the person can be encouraged to:

● Increase sitting balance by using activities that require forward and side flexion and/or rotation of the spine. Lightweight, repetitive movements, such as those required by fabric or potato printing, painting, or some remedial games may be used (Fig. 10.23).
● Where the person needs to weight bear

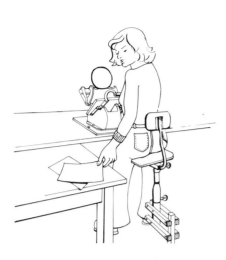

Fig. 10.22 Sitting sideways to a table to encourage spinal rotation and shoulder/shoulder girdle movement.

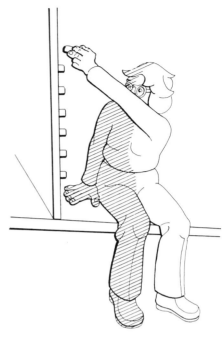

Fig. 10.24 While sitting the person can bear weight through the affected arm, using the non-affected arm for purposeful activity. Leaning to the affected side ensures weight-bearing through the affected hip, knee and foot.

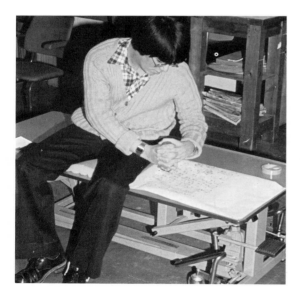

Fig. 10.23 Bilateral stamping to practise trunk rotation. The patient sits on a lowered table with his feet flat on the floor and turns from the ink pad on one side to the paper on the other side.

through the upper limb whilst sitting, i.e. to prop himself up, such a table provides an excellent treatment area. Its adjustability, size and stability enable it to be set up to meet each individual's needs. A non-slip pad may be placed under the palm of the supporting hand to prevent it slipping on a smooth, shiny surface (Fig. 10.24).

LYING

It may be appropriate in the treatment of people with certain conditions in which shoulder movement is limited against gravity, or where the therapist wishes to encourage passive extension of the hip and/or knee, for the person to lie prone on the table. The table is lowered so that the individual can participate in an activity placed on the floor or other low surface (Fig. 10.25).

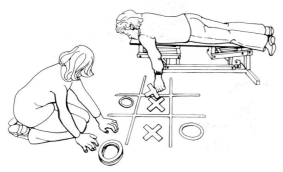

Fig. 10.25 Lying on a table to promote shoulder flexion and abduction and passive extension of hip and/or knee.

USING MICROCOMPUTERS IN THE TREATMENT OF PHYSICAL DYSFUNCTION

Technological advances have gathered momentum over the past decade and the occupational therapist is now familiar with a wide range of electronic aids and equipment. The microcomputer is increasingly part of our everyday experience and the therapist needs to become fully acquainted with it as a therapeutic medium (Clark 1986, Green 1989, Ottenbacher 1986, Roberts 1986a, Rugg 1986). The government provision of microcomputers for evaluation by occupational therapists via the Department of Trade and Industry (DTI) in 1983 gave the necessary impetus to their use by the profession. A national occupational therapy Special Interest Group (SIG) was established in 1984 to continue and expand this initiative.

The computer is a powerful and versatile tool and its applications are limited only by the therapist's knowledge and expertise. The therapist entering this field may at first be overwhelmed by the rapidity and extent of recent technological advances. This discussion, therefore, serves as a guide to the beginning therapist. It assumes a basic knowledge of computer terms.

In using the microcomputer as a professional tool the therapist needs to be able to evaluate its relevance to clinical practice. This discussion will therefore follow Reed's (1986) proposed investigatory model (the who, what, when, where, how and why) as used by Spicer and McMillan (1987) in their American study of computer usage in occupational therapy. Computer applications (why, when) will be discussed in relation to occupational performance dysfunction (West 1984) and the appropriate frames of reference rather than disabilities. This approach emphasises the central role of activity and associated theories in occupational therapy intervention rather than relying on the medical/reductionist model. Other sections will address present clinical usage (who); types of microcomputers, peripheral devices, and software (what); choice of equipment and factors facilitating or hindering the use of the microcomputer (why).

Clinical usage of computers in occupational therapy departments

Computers are now well established as a treatment tool in all areas of occupational therapy practice. However, whilst the assessment and treatment applications are relatively well documented, research comparing computer use to more traditional methods is still lacking (Weiss 1990).

The SIG's membership database, whilst it does not give a complete overview of the profession, identifies usage trends in occupational therapy departments. As of August 1990 the database yielded the following profile of computer usage:

Area	Number of centres
Neurology	57
Elderly	54
General physical	44
Mental handicap	38
Psychiatry	29
Orthopaedics	28
Paediatrics	28
Young chronically sick	14

The following models were identified as being in use in occupational therapy departments as of August 1990:

Model of computer	Number of centres
BBC 'B', B+ and Masters 128	90
PC & PC Compatibles (Amstrad PC, Opus, etc.)	13
Apple Mac & IIe (II comparable with BBC)	11
Amstrad PCW (dedicated word processor)	4
Amiga 500	1

However, it should be borne in mind that the DTI project supplied over 40 computers, all BBC 'B's, to various occupational therapy departments in the United Kingdom. This may have temporarily skewed the numbers of these computers in use in occupational therapy departments but it has also led to the development of hardware and software for use specifically by occupational therapists. A parallel scheme, also using BBC computers, in special needs education enabled the development of many switches (together with software) which occupational therapists have been able to use with disabled people.

HARDWARE

Hardware consists of the physical parts of the computer system: the microcomputer itself, the monitor or visual display unit (VDU), the disc drive and peripheral devices (Figs 10.26, 10.27). Alternative input devices (e.g. switches, concept keyboards) and output devices (e.g. speech syn-

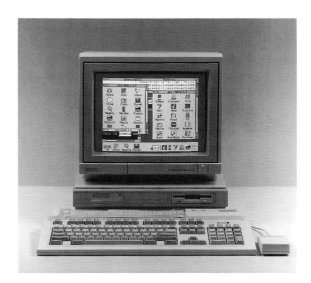

Fig. 10.27 A basic computer package: computer, monitor, disc drive and mouse (Reproduced by kind permission of Acorn Computers Ltd.)

thesisers) are also part of the hardware. Full descriptions of the microcomputer, disc drive and printer can be found elsewhere (MacKenzie 1989, Reid 1990).

Basic package

A basic package for use in an occupational therapy department will need to include the following:

- microcomputer
- colour monitor (VDU)
- disc drive
- printer
- alternative inputs such as joysticks, concept keyboard, touch screen (as necessary, depending on users' needs and treatment objectives)
- slomo (screen speed controller) or equivalent
- accessories (e.g. braked trolley, preferably adjustable)
- suite of programs

In selecting the most appropriate system the therapist should ask the following questions:

- What is the computer required to do?

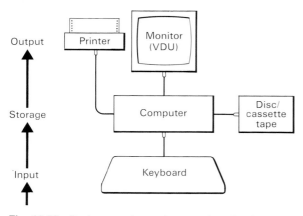

Fig. 10.26 Basic computer package and mode of operation.

- Is there sufficient power and memory in the system?
- How easy is it to connect peripheral devices, etc?

- What suitable software is available? (It must be remembered that the computer is only as useful as the software that runs on it.) (Hope 1987)

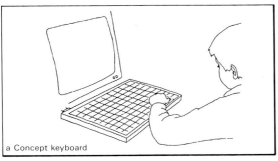

a Concept keyboard

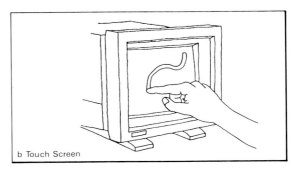

b Touch Screen

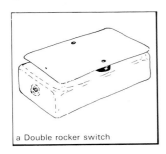

c Joystick

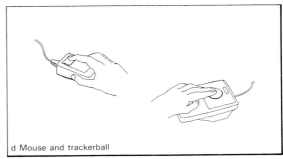

d Mouse and trackerball

Fig. 10.28A

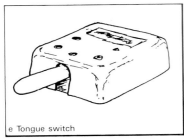

a Double rocker switch

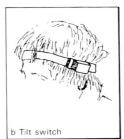

b Tilt switch

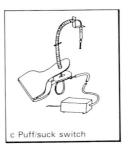

c Puff/suck switch

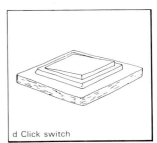

d Click switch

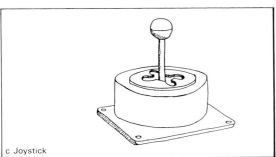

e Tongue switch

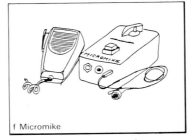

f Micromike

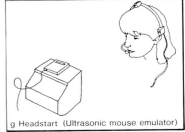

g Headstart (Ultrasonic mouse emulator)

Fig. 10.28B

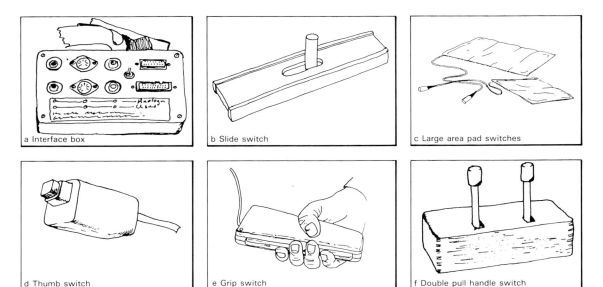

Fig. 10.28C

Fig. 10.28 Input devices. (A) Devices frequently used by occupational therapists. (Examples a, b, d from Colven & Detheridge 1990. Example c from Ace Centre, *Switches and Interfaces*, 2nd edn) (B) Types of switches for accessing the computer. (Examples a–f from Ace Centre, *Switches and Interfaces*, 2nd edn. Example g from Colven & Detheridge 1990.) (C) Interface box and therapeutic switches. (From ACE Centre, *Switches and Interfaces*, 2nd edn.)

Peripheral devices

These include the input and output devices that connect to the computer. Alternative input devices which simplify computer operation are used if the person cannot operate the standard QWERTY keyboard. Those the therapist might commonly meet include switches, joysticks, concept keyboard, light pen, mouse, trackerball and touch screen. All these devices connect to the computer via a cable to a socket. An interface box enables the therapist to connect devices without lifting the computer each time and saves considerable wear and tear on the connections (Fig. 10.28). The output devices most commonly used by the therapist are the screen display (VDU) and the printer.

Input devices and accessories

Information can be entered into the computer by three methods: direct selection, scanning, and encoded selection (Table 10.1). The method chosen

Table 10.1 Methods of putting information into the computer (Colven & Detheridge 1990)

Direct selection	Scanning	Encoded selection
QWERTY keyboard Light pen Touch screen Mouse Trackerball	Switch controlling highlighter moves around the screen from item to item. Two types: • automatic scanning with single switch operation • user controls scanning rate using two switches, one to scan, the other to select	Switch-encoded selection, e.g. Microwriter that uses 5 switches in various combinations (learnt by the user) to select letters of the alphabet Timed, encoded selection e.g. Morse code using one or more switches

will depend on the user's ability and preference.

Simple aids like mouthsticks or head pointers will often allow access via the QWERTY keyboard.

For those with poor coordination, keyguards provide a simple and effective solution as they allow access only to the target keys. Keyguards may have a keylock option. This holds down the control or shift key to enable keys to be pressed by a pointer or one finger. Keylocks can also be obtained without a keyguard. An expanded keyboard with large, well-spaced keys may also be considered for those with poor coordination. These adaptations, together with the incorporation of delay features, will largely eliminate unintended key presses. Another solution for incoordination is to stabilise the forearm and/or wrist and use a miniature keyboard.

The concept keyboard is also a popular input device. With larger key-press areas it has many applications, particularly when coordination or motor control is impaired.

However, for those who cannot use the keyboard, special switches are available for which careful and thorough assessment is required, taking account of the following aspects of the person's level of function:

- Physical: range of movement, coordination consistency and reproducibility of movement, strength (enough force to operate the switch) and tolerance (how quickly the person becomes fatigued)
- Cognitive: attention, concentration, memory, ability to follow instructions
- Sensori-integrative: sitting balance, motor planning
- Psychological: whether the switch and its operation are acceptable to the person.

The final choice of switch can only be made after consideration of all these factors. Switches may be operated by gripping, hitting, tilting, touching, blinking the eyes, sucking, blowing or using tongue pressure (Fig. 10.28). The force needed to operate them is measured in grams. Seating and posture must be correct to avoid undue strain and fatigue and only when seating and posture are correct can the therapist and the person decide where and how the switch should be mounted. Velcro and non-slip mats may be sufficient to mount some switches. Clamps, bendy poles, goose-neck mounting kits and so on may be needed in other situations. The ACE Centre's *Switches and Interfaces* booklet offers further detail (see References).

The voice may also be used to input information through devices such as the Micromike which respond to voice volume — an ideal way to encourage vocalisation. Voice input systems are also available which operate the computer by speech commands alone. However, current systems are still being further refined and developed. Keyboard emulators allow access to standard commercially available software via any one of a variety of switches, as the computer does not then distinguish between the QWERTY keyboard and the alternative input device. Adaptive firmware cards are another means of achieving an emulator for the Apple II computers.

Output devices

The printer is useful for obtaining hard copy of the user's work and records of treatment progress. It can be used not only for ordinary text but, with the relevant programs, can produce large, bold text for the visually handicapped person. Braille input and output devices are also available. Voice output devices (speech synthesisers) for the non-speaking person are well established (about 30 types are presently available in Britain alone).

Other devices

Modems are devices which, when connected to the computer via the telephone network, allow access to remote databases; one example is British Telecom's Prestel (Saul & Saul 1986). The SEND (Special Educational Needs Database) is one of those on Prestel. Such systems greatly increase the amount of information which disabled and non-disabled people can access.

Devices such as Slomo which slow down the speed of program execution are particularly useful in relation to arcade games.

SOFTWARE

Software is the term used for the electronic

Program Name ..... CROOK'S CORNER ....

Source .... LOCHEE PUBLICATIONS LTD. ....

Computer .... BBC MASTER .... Input ..KEYBOARD........

Skill Level: Pre-school .... Primary ..✓...(10-12).....

            Secondary .... Adult ....

Program Categories: (Tick all that apply)

    Cognitive Skills ..✓... Living Skills ..✓.. Utility ....

    Motor Skills ......✓.. Social Skills ..... Education ....✓.....

    Percep/Visual Skills . Work Training ..... Individual ..✓.....

    Balance/Posture ...... Communication ..... Group ....✓.....

Program is intended to assess/improve:

    Monetary skills
    Forward planning
    Decision-making
    Consequences of decisions made

Description:

    Shopping program designed for cognitively impaired adults.
    Person given shopping list plus money to buy desired items.
    Always provided with many prompts if desired.

Documentation (tick all that apply)	Good	Satisfactory	Poor
Written instructions - manual	✓		
screen		✓	
Verbal instructions -			
Recording/scoring in program:		✓	

Ease of Use:

Comes with instruction manual. Disc also carries a tutorial option.
Fairly easy to use. Instructions on screen can be too many for
some people to take in. Good reading ability required to work
independently of therapist. Program uses red function keys.

Comments (including strengths/weaknesses of program; user's reactions;
        ideas for improvement)

STRENGTHS: Stimulation value, graphics good. Sound volume can be
altered. Fairly realistic 'real-life' task.

WEAKNESSES: Often too many graphics on screen at one time; can be
confusing. Only food shops dealt with.

IMPROVEMENTS; More complex shopping lists can be given but it
would be good to have different shops too.

Overall Opinion (including value for money)

Useful program for head-injured adults or those with limited
intellectual skills. However, there is a basic mismatch between
the complexity of the task (fairly simple) and the amount of
cognitive ability required to read and understand all the
instructions and function keys (fairly difficult)

                              Lynne MURRAY 25/9/90
                              Southern General Hospital
                                    Glasgow

Fig. 10.29 A software evaluation.

instructions that make the computer work. They are stored most usually on discs (floppy or hard) but can also be stored on cassette tape. A single item of software is called a program.

Program suites

A suite of programs could address the following:

- *cognition*: programs that build up speed of cognition, concentration, decision-making, memory
- *perception*: right/left discrimination, spatial orientation, figure/ground discrimination, visual scanning, sequencing and matching
- *motor ability*: games or programs of general interest which are at the user's ability level, since the choice and placing of the equipment will lead to the desired movement. Typing programs have also been found useful for improving fine finger control
- *life skills*: ADL: home finance program, money management, shopping
- *work skills*: typing programs, stock control programs, and other work-based programs
- *education*: basic numeracy and literacy programs.

Software evaluation

It is not sufficient to merely locate the software supplier. The therapist also needs to know the skill level of the program and its age-appropriateness; points to look for in design and content; whether documentation is available; and what hardware and peripherals are required to run it. Such evaluative criteria are well-documented elsewhere (Clark 1986, Cromwell 1986, Ross 1987, Okoye 1989). A sample software evaluation is given in Fig. 10.29.

Creating new programs

Whilst it is not necessary for the therapist to learn programming it is very useful to be able to specify program requirements since there is still a need for more specific clinical software for all age groups, and particularly for adults. Programming guide-

lines are available (Smart et al 1985, Aggleton 1987) to help therapists to do this. Authoring systems, such as Microtext, enable the therapist to write her own programs in everyday language without needing to know a programming language (Roberts 1986b). This still, however, requires skill in program planning and design.

Newell (1985) specifies the points to cover in software development as:

- knowing what you want to do
- knowing how to do it efficiently and effectively
- evaluating whether it has been done correctly.

He also points out that in software development there needs to be a threefold assessment covering quality of the program, function of the program and effect of the program in a treatment setting.

Terminology, particulary for switch-controlled software, can be confusing. Colven and Detheridge (1990) propose a common terminology to overcome this problem.

'Content-free' programs allow the therapist to design her own programs within a given framework; for example, VETAS (Versatile Therapeutic Software by Locheesoft) enables the therapist to design a variety of maze-type board games and exercises.

Copyright

It is essential to make back-up copies of the programs used in the department. However, copyright should always be respected and if there is any doubt, the supplier should be contacted.

THERAPEUTIC APPLICATIONS OF THE COMPUTER IN OCCUPATIONAL THERAPY

This section will address evaluation, treatment strategies, frames of reference, and areas of use within occupational therapy intervention. However, it should be clearly stated that the computer should be used in occupational therapy as part of a comprehensive, individualised treatment programme alongside other interventions.

It should also be remembered that while the computer is a useful tool for assessment and measurement any personal details relating to the people seen in the department which are stored on the computer will be subject to the regulations of the Data Protection Act (1984).

EVALUATING A COMPUTER FOR USE IN OCCUPATIONAL THERAPY

As with any treatment medium, a full activity analysis is a prerequisite to discovering its therapeutic potential. In the case of the microcomputer this involves not only the hardware and software but also the physical, cognitive, and sensori-integrative requirements of the system (Okoye 1989).

The various physical parts of the system (monitor, disc drive, inputs and outputs) may require separate evaluation in order to determine their relevance to a particular treatment setting.

In evaluating software the therapist should give particular attention to presentation (screen format, instructions, responses and timing) (Ross 1987), making sure that the presentation is appropriate to the cognitive and perceptual demands of the program. Skill level and gradability should also be noted.

TREATMENT STRATEGIES

The process of formulating a treatment strategy begins with determining the person's level of baseline functioning. In accordance with this assessment, successive challenges are then provided to engage the person in the activity and increase his competence and functional independence (Rogers 1982). The type of challenge offered will influence the character of the therapeutic environment; three types of treatment setting are described in Table 10.2 as they relate to computer applications.

Table 10.2 Occupational therapy settings applied to computer use

Play (safe) environment

Situations will be organised to ensure an experience of success. Sessions will be fairly short. The work area will be quiet, distraction-free, and the equipment set up and 'ready to run'. Wires and equipment will be as neat and unobtrusive as possible. Anxiety will be reduced to a minimum as the therapist will be nearby to give help as soon as it is required. Programs will be menu-driven with as little jargon as possible on the screen. Discs may be coloured for easy recognition. Only simple instructions will be required to be obeyed — maybe only one, or just two, chained commands.

Competency (simulated) environment

The person takes increasing responsibility for his own learning and skill development according to the therapist's breakdown of steps within the task. Simulated and/or job trials are given. The therapist gradually withdraws support and the person is responsible for switching on equipment, putting in discs, using manual to fault-find, etc. There is a limited risk of failure.

Self-achievement (real-life) environment

The therapist is the facilitator only. People demonstrate mastery in computer operation, e.g. writing letters, handling data, writing programs for other people, using the computer in a work or leisure capacity. The situation becomes potentially more stressful, with risk of failure.

FRAMES OF REFERENCE

In using the computer in the treatment of specific dysfunctions, the therapist will need to apply the relevant frames of reference (see Ch. 12). For physical dysfunction these will include the biomechanical, neurodevelopmental, rehabilitative and occupational behaviour approaches. The trait–factor approach used in work assessment may also be appropriate (Creighton 1985). This approach is concerned with identifying an individual's abilities and interests in relation to the requirements of various jobs and thus provides a useful basis for matching abilities with computer skills. Creighton reminds us that work samples or skills checklists (e.g. punctuality, work speed, cooperativeness, attention to task) were used to assess employability. The use of trial jobs (such as a stock control program) or simulated work situations are other methods used in this approach.

AREAS OF USE WITHIN OCCUPATIONAL THERAPY

Physical dysfunction

Whether using the computer to help the individual to maintain or to improve existing function, the therapist must first check: the positioning of the equipment; the positioning and seating of the user; and the cognitive and sensori-integrative demands made on him (Okoye 1989). Separate, lightweight portable units make this task much easier. For those with limited muscle power and range of movement, the therapist will probably find that traditional means such as slings, orthoses and work surfaces or equipment that can be raised, lowered or tilted will enable her to facilitate the movement required. Once the desired positions are obtained the therapist should note them down so that equipment can be easily arranged for the next session.

Tables 10.3, 10.4 and 10.5 give an indication of how occupational therapists are currently using the computer in the treatment of locomotor, sensory and neurological problems and in the enhancement of life skills (Crofts & Crofts 1988, Dickey and Shealey 1987, MacKenzie 1989, Roberts 1986, Stoneman 1985, Wright 1990).

As indicated in Table 10.3, the recently developed MULE Exerciser (Microprocessor Controlled Upper Limb Exerciser) has particular application to the improvement of wrist movement and of extension and flexion in the metacarpophalangeal, proximal interphalangeal and distal interphalangeal joints of the hand. The Exerciser is now commercially available from Nottingham Rehab (Fig. 10.30).

Table 10.3 Computer applications for locomotor and sensory problems

(a) LOCOMOTOR DYSFUNCTION
   Objective: Assess/improve upper and lower limb function

Required function	Equipment/ method	Suggested software
Fine finger control	Keyboard	Typing program
Individual finger function	Keyboard	Multi-key game
Thumb IP flexion/extension	Thumb switch	Games program
MCP/PIP extension and DIP flexion, (also incorporating pronation/ supination)	Span handle of MULE Exerciser*	Games devised for MULE Exerciser
Grip/hand function	Grip switch	Games program
Wrist movements	Roller handle of MULE Exerciser Concept keyboard (angled)	Program for MULE Exerciser Games program
Pronation/ supination	Spade handle of MULE Exerciser (elbow stabilised)	Program for MULE Exerciser
Skill in using upper limb prosthesis	Upper limb Activity Board (collection of everyday handles and controls)	Program for Board — go through rooms of house using relevant items
General mobility	Pressure pad switches	Get fit set program
Dorsi/plantar flexion	Pressure pad switch and fraserbar	As above
Weight-bearing through affected leg or prosthesis	Pressure pad switch or concept keyboard used as pressure pad	Games program As above
Upper and lower limb muscle re-education	Myolink (biofeedback device) and plotter	Modify existing software

(b) SENSORY IMPAIRMENT/DEFICIT
   Objective: To assess/improve hyper- and hyposensitivity

Required objective	Equipment/ method	Suggested software
Desensitise finger/thumb stumps	Concept keyboard or touch screen (Concept keyboard offers more resistance)	Games software Paint program
Resensitise fingers/thumbs	Feely board (textured overlay for concept keyboard)	Program incorporating sounds

*The MULE Exerciser (Microprocessor Controlled Upper Limb Exerciser, Fig. 10.30) is the result of a joint project between the Microcomputer Centre at Dundee University and the Southern General Hospital, Glasgow.

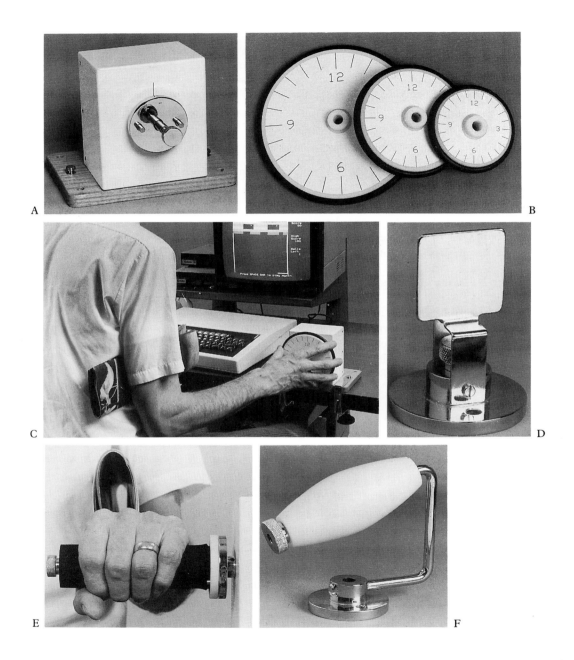

Fig. 10.30 The MULE Exerciser and attachments. (A) Device without handle. (B) 3″, 4″ and 6″ span handles. (C) Mule Exerciser with 5″ span handle. Markings on span handle guide hand positioning. Compensatory movements are avoided by holding magazine close to the ribs. (D) Key handle. (E) Cylinder handle (padded). Unpadded handles can also be used. (F) Spade handle. (Acknowledgements: Southern General Hospital, Glasgow.)

Neurological dysfunction

Neurological dysfunction gives rise to physical, cognitive, perceptual and behavioural problems (Stoneman 1985) and may be of a static or deteriorating nature. However, a deteriorating condition is no bar to using the microcomputer but the therapist will need to take account of the person's prognosis, especially if he is to use the computer on a long-term basis. A decision may be taken, for example, to use a Microwriter with its 5-key ergonomic keyboard from the outset rather than the QWERTY keyboard (Table 10.4).

Table 10.4 Computer applications for neurological problems (cont'd overleaf)

(a) NEUROLOGICAL DYSFUNCTION — physical problems
Objective: Assess/improve postural control incorporating neurodevelopmental techniques

Required function	Equipment/ method	Suggested software
Head and back extension	Raise monitor	Any software of interest to user, e.g. games, numeracy, reasoning, etc.
Sitting/standing balance	Reach forward with hands clasped together to reach touch screen/concept keyboard Position user further away so bottom gradually comes off stool	As above
Weight-bearing	Stand with hands clasped using touch screen Pressure pad switch Weight-bear through affected arm/elbow to operate concept keyboard positioned for maximum reach Position user to one side of midline	As above
Passive movements	Using touch screen with hands clasped	Paint program
Ataxia	Keyguard	Typing program

(b) NEUROLOGICAL DYSFUNCTION — cognitive problems
Objective: Assess/improve cognitive skills

Required skill	Equipment/ method	Software to enable user to learn/play
Short-term memory	Dependent on user's ability Most likely input devices to be used are: • touch screen • concept keyboard • joysticks • expanded keyboard A vertical monitor stand will enable joysticks to be used in the correct orientation (Fig. 10.31)	A new game A cake recipe Puzzle (e.g. find a route through a layout of streets that does not lead down the same road twice)
Long-term memory	As above	Simple to complex quizzes General knowledge quizzes Educational retraining programmes
Concentration	As above	Simple to more complex games
Speed of cognition	Joysticks	Arcade games slowed initially with Slomo
Problem-solving and decision-making	As appropriate	Logical quizzes, questions, problems, jigsaws, maths packages, typing and word-processing (may involve working from manuals), Microtext programming
Forward planning	Keyboard or concept keyboard	Computerised version of Connect 4

(c) NEUROLOGICAL DYSFUNCTION — perceptual problems
Objective: Assess/improve perceptual skills

Required skill	Equipment/ method	Suggested software
Scanning	As appropriate, e.g. spacebar, keyboard, joysticks, simple switches, concept keyboard, touch screen	Programs with moving dots/objects Wordsorting tasks

Table 10.4(c) Cont'd

Required skill	Equipment/ method	Suggested software
Hemi-neglect	Position equipment to encourage head-turning Use only one side of keyboard	Typing program with large print
Colour, shape, size and form differentiation and recognition	As appropriate	Shape matching Colour matching Sorting sizes
Figure/ground discrimination	As appropriate	Word hidden in matrix
Directional and spatial skills	Joystick, simple switches and interface box	Maps mazes for right/left discrimination Jigsaws
Body awareness deficit	As appropriate	Jigsaw of person
Hand/eye coordination	Simple switch	Software requiring user to operate switch at right moment

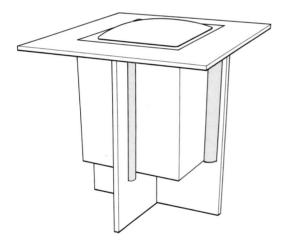

Fig. 10.31 Vertical monitor stand. This can also be used with a touch screen. (Acknowledgement: Brilliant Computing.)

Life skills

With practical activities such as ADL, the com-puter is used to reinforce and recall skills which are being practised either on the ward or in the department (Table 10.5).

Severely handicapped people, such as those with high spinal cord injuries, may wish to learn com-puter skills for application in future work or to

Table 10.5 Computer Applications for life skills

(a) LIFE SKILLS — self-care
    Objective: Improve/reinforce skills in self-care
              Increase independence for the severely handicapped person

Required skill	Equipment/ method	Suggested software
Activities of Daily Living	As appropriate to user's ability and program requirement, e.g. switch, spacebar, keyboard, concept keyboard	Dressing/washing routines Money management, home finance Use of telephone, shopping and budgeting
Health and safety	As above	Games with street signs Quizzes educating on aspects of health and self-help, e.g. joint protection program
Independence in self-care	Computer linked to environmental controls Special switches, e.g. headstart (ultrasonic mouse emulator with puff/suck switch replacing mouse click), useful for those with high spinal cord lesions (Fig. 10.28)	Switch-operated software

(b) LIFE SKILLS — work
    Objective: assess/develop skills in computer use

Required skill	Equipment/ method	Suggested software
Pre-work skills	Keyboard or switch input according to user's ability Assess accuracy as well as speed before progressing to work skills	Typing program

Table 10.5(b) Cont'd

Required skill	Equipment/ method	Suggested software
Work skills	Keyboard or switch input according to user's ability	Word-processing, databases, desktop publishing, programming with and without Microtext

(c) LIFE SKILLS — leisure
  Objective: To provide fun and recreation

Place of use	Equipment/ method	Suggested software
Ward for those on prolonged bed-rest	Equipment placed on over-bed trolley	Games, drawing packages, music, word-processing
Department	As appropriate for user and program used to give reward after rehabilitation session	As above

(d) LIFE SKILLS — social skills
  Objective: Assess/improve skills lost as a result of disability

Size of group	Equipment/ method	Suggested software
One-to-one	Switch or keyboard	Chess and other board games
Larger groups	Consider VDU or touch screen with vertical monitor stands, or large TV screen rather than monitor	Problem-solving and decision-making games, quizzes, topics, e.g. home finance

(e) LIFE SKILLS — communication
  *Objective: Increase interaction skills/reduce isolation of speech-impaired people
  Assess/improve written communication of blind/visually handicapped people*

Problem	Equipment/ method	Suggested software
Speech impairment	Augmentative communication systems of various types are available (ACE Centre 1990)	Word-processing including converting VDU text to speech
Blindness/visual handicap	Screen/printer	Program to enlarge text
	Speech synthesiser	Program to convert VDU text to speech

Table 10.5(e) Cont'd

Problem	Equipment/ method	Suggested software
	Braille keyboard	Program to convert braille to text
	Braille embosser	Program to convert text to braille

(f) LIFE SKILLS — education
  Objective: Continue education whilst in hospital

Problem	Equipment/ method	Suggested software
Cognitive impairment	Switch, touch screen or keyboard according to user's ability	Basic numeracy and literacy
Disability interrupted education	As above	According to subject of interest to user

continue their education. In such cases the therapist will need to liaise with the Disablement Resettlement Officer (DRO) as well as with statutory and possibly voluntary agencies to assist the person in obtaining the necessary training and equipment. Detailed assessment and progress reports enable the therapist to identify precise requirements with the person and to present a well-reasoned argument to support his case.

PSYCHOLOGICAL CONSIDERATIONS

The therapist should introduce the user sensitively to the computer and allay his fears. In switch assessment, for example, the switch in question may initially be connected, rather than to the computer, to a less intimidating piece of equipment such as a tape recorder.

The computer gives strong motivational rewards. Feedback is consistent and non-judgmental. User-friendly software is not only important in this respect, but also in reducing frustration and anxiety. The therapist should look for programs which allow more than one attempt to get the right answer, have different levels of difficulty, give appropriate rewards, and so on.

Computer technology enables disabled people

to achieve tasks for themselves, thus increasing their self-esteem and sense of achievement. Self-expression and creativity are increased with the use of the word-processor, desktop publishing, graphics and music packages.

Table 10.6 Factors that hinder or facilitate the application of computers to occupational therapy

Factors hindering application	Factors facilitating application
Equipment	
Relatively costly in terms of occupational therapy budget	Offers exciting new possibilities and technology is seen to increase the profession's credibility
Requires maintenance, security, space to run it	Maintenance contract Movable trolley and cupboard Negotiated schedule of use in identified areas
Staffing	
Staff not trained in computer use don't know 'how to begin', feel overwhelmed	Computer literacy courses including therapeutic applications available via SIG
Time taken for staff to familiarise, themselves with system, including new staff Staff who received initial computer training have moved on	Appointment of 'specialist' occupational therapist for department or district to develop strategy and schedule of computer use in treatment programme, clarifying aims and objectives related to computer use and being responsible for organising training, carrying out inservice training as necessary and appropriate
Rapid development in the field can make parts and servicing of equipment unobtainable	
Difficulty in keeping up to date	Opportunity to share ideas via magazines, workshops, exhibitions, computer SIG'S, etc.
Lack of acceptance of new role	Liaison with occupational therapy staff and speech therapists, physiotherapists, special needs teachers, etc. Use of 'management of change' skills by District or Head Occupational Therapist
Research	
Lack of research comparing computer use to traditional methods	Beginning to appear but, as Hall (1987) points out, there is a time lag between availability of knowledge and society's ability to understand and use it
Lack of time and money	Research is made part of the job description

FACTORS HINDERING OR FACILITATING COMPUTER USE IN OCCUPATIONAL THERAPY

These factors are summarised in Table 10.6 under the headings of equipment, staffing and research (Green 1989, Spicer & McMillan 1987, MacKenzie 1989). As Weiss (1990) reminds us these are dependent on time, money and attitude, the most important of which is attitude.

Allocation of time and financial resources will only follow if managers are convinced that microcomputers are a useful tool in occupational therapy. In the same article she points out that although research is still in its early stages, there are many advantages which can be put forward in support of their use, which she sees as:

- 'suitability for standardising assessment presentation (Wilson & McMillan 1986)
- increasing availability of high-technology adaptations (Vanderheiden 1987)
- providing self-directed, instruction-based activities
- improving employment potential of disabled people' (Szeto et al 1987).

CONCLUSION

In selecting activities for therapeutic intervention, the occupational therapist now has more options available to her than ever before. Ideally, she will incorporate the best from both traditional and new technologies into her programmes. Both tried-and-true equipment such as the rehabilitation lathe and the latest in computer technology have their place in the occupational therapy workshop.

The therapist must always bear in mind that the specific needs and interests of the individual should guide her selection of one type of activity or equipment over another. As always, careful evaluation of the individual's capabilities and a thorough analysis of any proposed activity provide the vital groundwork for intervention planning. The therapist should also be aware of the limitations of any given activity or piece of equipment; since no single activity or apparatus can solve all of the problems faced by an individual, the particular components of a treatment programme must always form part of a well-rounded and carefully individualised strategy for rehabilitation.

ACKNOWLEDGEMENTS

We would like to thank Mr Sidney Locke, District Occupational Therapist, Crawley Hospital, for the use of parts of his Larvic Rehabilitation Lathe manual. Thanks are also due to Anne Goodrick-Meech, Senior Lecturer, Department of Occupational Therapy, Christ Church College, University of Kent, Canterbury, for updating the information in the lathe section.

USEFUL ADDRESSES

ACE (Aids to Communication in Education) Centre
Ormerod School
Waynflete Road
Headington
Oxford. OX3 8DD
0865 63508

BARD (British Database on Research into Aids for the Disabled), Handicapped Persons Research Unit
Newcastle Polytechnic, Coach Lane Campus
No.1 Coach Lane
Newcastle upon Tyne NE7 7XA
0632 665057

British Computer Society
Disability Specialist Group
Membership: Liam Madden, MBCS
Disabled Specialist Group
Department of Electrical Engineering
Imperial College
London SW7 2BT

CALL (Communication Aids for Language and Learning) Centre
University of Edinburgh
The Annex, 4 Buccleuch Place
Edinburgh EH8 LW9
031 667 1438

Centre for Special Needs Technology
Information Management Officer
Beechcroft, 14 The Gardens
Fentham Road
Erdington, Birmingham
B23 6AG
021 350 6188

IBM Support Centre for People with Disabilities
IBM Warwick
P O Box 31
Birmingham Road
Warwick CV34 5JL
Freephone: 0800 269545

National Occupational Therapy Special Interest Group in Microcomputers
c/o Mrs C. V. MacCaul
Keycol Psychiatric Day Hospital
Nr. Sittingbourne
Kent ME9 8NG

Nottingham Rehab (for MULE Exerciser)
Ludlow Hill Road
West Bridgford
Nottingham MG2 6HD
0602 234251

PC Independent Users Group
87 High Street
Tonbridge
Kent
NN9 1RX
0732 771512

RCEVH (Research Centre for the Education of the Visually Handicapped)
Birmingham University
Selly Wick House
59 Selly Wick Lane
Birmingham B29 7JE
021 471 1303

SEMERC's (Special Education MicroElectronics Resource Centre):

Bristol SEMERC
Faculty of Education
Bristol Polytechnic, Redland Hill
Bristol
BS6 6U2
0272 733141

Manchester SEMERC
Manchester College of Higher Education
Hathersage Road, Manchester
M13 OJA
061 225 9054

Newcastle SEMERC
Newcastle Polytechnic, Coach Lane Campus
No. 1 Coach Lane

Newcastle upon Tyne NE7 7XA
0632 665057

Redbridge SEMERC
Dane Centre
Melbourne Road
Ilford, Essex
1GI 4HT
081 478 6363

SEND
Special Educational Needs Database
On Prestel
SCET
74 Victoria Crescent Road,
Glasgow G12 9JN
041 334 9314

REFERENCES

ACE Centre. Switches and interfaces, 2nd edn. ACE Centre, Oxford

ACE Centre 1990 Electronic communication aids survey. ACE Centre, Oxford

Aggleton S 1987 Programming planning guidelines. National Occupational Therapy Special Interest Group in Microcomputers, London

Clark E N (ed) 1986 Microcomputers: clinical applications Slack, New Jersey, pp 7, 20

Colven D, Detheridge T 1990 A common terminology for switch controlled software. ACE Centre, Oxford

Creighton C 1985 Three frames of reference in work-related occupational therapy programs. The American Journal of Occupational Therapy 39(5): 331–334

Crofts F, Crofts J 1988 Biofeedback and the computer. British Journal of Occupational Therapy (February): 57–59

Cromwell F S 1986 Computer applications in occupational therapy. Haworth Press, New York

Data Protection Act 1984 HMSO, London

Dickey R, Shealey S H 1987 Using technology to control the environment. The American Journal of Occupational Therapy 41(11): 717–721

Green S 1989 Occupational therapy and information technology. Grass roots and tree tops. In: Information technology in health care — a handbook. Kluwer Publishing, Brentford

Hall M 1987 Unlocking information technology. The American Journal of Occupational Therapy 41(11): 722–724

Hope M H 1987 Micros for children with special needs. Souvenir Press, London

MacKenzie L M 1989 Introductory manual for occupational therapists using microcomputers in treatment. Tayside Health Board, Dundee

Newell A F 1985 Developing appropriate software. British Journal of Occupational Therapy (August): 242–243

Okoye R L 1989 Computer technology in occupational therapy. In: Hopkins H L, Smith H D (eds) 1989 Willard and Spackman's occupational therapy, 7th edn. J B Lippincott, Philadelphia

Ottenbacher K 1986 Technology and professional practice in occupational therapy: promise and perils of technology. Proceedings, 14th Federal Association of Occupational Therapists Conference, Brisbane, 204–211

Reed K L 1986 Tools of practice: heritage or baggage? The American Journal of Occupational Therapy 40(9): 597–605

Reid J (1990) Computers in occupational therapy. In: Occupational therapy in mental health. Churchill Livingstone, Edinburgh

Roberts C 1986a Focus on BBC computers. Proceedings, 14th Federal Association of Occupational Therapists Conference, Brisbane, 232–233

Roberts C 1986b The use of computers in occupational therapy at the Rehabilitation Unit, Odstock Hospital: a review. The British Journal of Occupational Therapy (May): 157–160

Rogers J C 1982 The spirit of independence: the evolution of a philosophy. The American Journal of Occupational Therapy 36(11): 710–715

Ross M 1987 Using microcomputers: a guide for occupational therapists. Paradigm Press, Perth

Rugg S 1986 A preliminary study of occupational therapy staff concerning the use of computers in their profession. British Journal of Occupational Therapy (October): 296–298

Saul K, Saul P 1986 Accessing remote databases using micro-computers. British Journal of Occupational Therapy (March): 76–78

Smart S, MacKenzie L, Richards D 1985 The design of viable software for use in occupational therapy. British Journal of Occupational Therapy (October): 296–298

Spicer M McG, McMillan S L 1987 Computers and occupational therapy. The American Journal of Occupational Therapy 41 (11): 726–732

Stoneman R 1985 The potential use of the microcomputer with patients suffering from cerebral vascular accident and head injury. British Journal of Occupational Therapy (June): 163–166

Szeto A Y J, Allen E J, Rumelhart M A 1987 Employability enhancement. American Rehabilitation 13: 8–29

Vanderheiden G C 1987 Service delivery mechanisms in rehabilitation technology. The American Journal of Occupational Therapy 41(11): 703–710

Weiss P 1990 The integration of computers into the occupational therapy department. The American Journal of Occupational Therapy 44(6): 527–534

West W L 1984 A reaffirmed philosophy and practice of occupational therapy for the 1980s. The American Journal of Occupational Therapy 38(1): 15–23

Wilson S L, McMillan T M 1986 Finding able minds in disabled bodies. Lancet 2: 1444–1446

Wright K 1990 OT Micro News (June): 2–8

FURTHER READING

ACE Centre 1989 Portable computers survey. ACE Centre, Oxford

Batt R C, Lounsbury A 1990 Teaching the patient with cognitive deficits to use a computer. The American Journal of Occupational Therapy 44(4): 364–367

Carter R 1989 The student's guide to information technology. Heineman, Oxford

Chorlton S 1986 National Occupational Therapy Special Interest Group in Microcomputers: 2nd annual conference. British Journal of Occupational Therapy (June): 191–194

Collin S M H 1988 Dictionary of computing. Peter Collins Publishing, Teddington

Disabled Living Foundation Information Service 1989 Computers and accessories for people with disabilities. ISD No 85/5 (revised July). Disabled Living Foundation, London

Ellison P 1971 The OB Help Arm. Nottingham Handcraft Company, Nottingham

Everson J M, Goodwyn R 1987 A comparison of the use of adaptive microswitches by students with cerebral palsy. The American Journal of Occupational Therapy 41(11): 739–744

Giles G M, Shore M 1989 The effectiveness of an electronic memory aid for a memory-impaired adult of normal intelligence. The American Journal of Occupational Therapy 43(6): 409–411

Gray C 1988 The importance of correct seating. Occasional paper. ACE Centre, Oxford

Johnson R, Garvie C 1985 The BBC microcomputer for therapy of intellectual impairment following acquired brain damage. British Journal of Occupational Therapy (February): 46–48

Kemball-Cook R 1990 Computer switches for the handicapped. How to buy them or make them yourself. National Occupational Therapy Special Interest Group in Microcomputers, London

Levy R 1988 Interface modalities of technical aids used by people with disability. The American Journal of Occupational Therapy 37(11): 761–765

Newman C, Sparrow A R, Hospod F E 1989 Two augmentative communication systems for speechless disabled patients. The American Journal of Occupational Therapy 43(8): 529–534

Nottingham Medical Equipment Company. NOMEQ operator's handbook — hydraulic table. NOMEQ, Redditch

Nottingham Medical Equipment Company. NOMEQ operator's handbook — Larvic lathe. NOMEQ, Redditch

Ridgway L, McKears S 1985 Computer help for disabled people. Souvenir Press, London

Saunders P 1984 Micros for handicapped users. Helena Press, Whitby

Skinner A D, Trachtman L H 1985 Brief or new: use of a computer program (PC coloring book) in cognitive rehabilitation. The American Journal of Occupational Therapy 39(7): 470–472

Smart S, Richards D 1986 The use of touch sensitive screens in rehabilitation therapy. British Journal of Occupational Therapy (October): 335–338

Thompson S B N, Hards B, Bate R 1986 Computer-assisted visual feedback for new hand and arm therapy apparatus. British Journal of Occupational Therapy (January): 19–21

Trevriranus J, Tannock R 1987 A scanning computer access system for children with severe physical disabilities. The American Journal of Occupational Therapy 41(11): 733–738

Turner, A (ed) 1987 The practice of occupational therapy, 2nd edn. Churchill Livingstone, Edinburgh

11

Orthotics

*Lorraine L. Pinnington and
Pauline Rowe*

INTRODUCTION

An orthosis is an externally applied device which is used to prevent deformity, support or protect a body segment and to assist in the restoration or improvement of function. In order to achieve these aims, it may be designed to assist or restrict movement of relevant body parts. Currently, the term 'orthosis' is used in preference to the term 'splint', and the study of their design, manufacture and use is known as 'orthotics'. At present, the nomenclature is a mixture of those terms which are based on the name of the designer or hospital of origin (eponyms) and those which indicate the area of the body over which the orthosis extends. Specific examples of these terms include the 'Capener' and an 'ankle-foot orthosis'. The latter category of terms are more useful because they provide some basic anatomical information and are potentially more internationally understood. However, in the past there was a tendency for orthoses to be given non-descriptive and arbitrary titles, such as a 'paddle' or 'cock-up splint'.

Whilst qualified orthotists undergo a specific course of training, other professionals, including occupational and physiotherapists, may be involved. Indeed, as occupational therapists are knowledgeable about many aspects of function, they are well qualified to consider the principles of orthotics in relation to the physical and practical demands of everyday life. Depending on the reasons for prescribing an orthosis, it may be 'static' or 'dynamic' (see p. 347) and designed for permanent or temporary use. Although occupational therapists are more usually concerned with the design and fabrication of temporary orthoses, they may also assist the orthotist in the manufacture of permanent ones. Certainly, whether the orthosis is temporary or permanent, she should participate in the initial assessment and the subsequent education of the individual regarding its use and potential benefit.

In the following sections of this chapter, emphasis will be placed on the principles of orthotics rather than providing detailed methodological instructions for the manufacture of selected orthoses. Since occupational therapists are predominantly involved in the provision of orthoses for the hand, many of the examples used here will be of that type. However, where appropriate, some principles will be illustrated by referring to orthoses for other parts of the body.

ASSESSMENT

An occupational therapist or medical practitioner may decide that an orthosis is required. Indeed, some operative procedures necessitate a specific orthotic regime and this should be discussed with the surgeon. Before embarking on the selection, design and fabrication of an orthosis a thorough and holistic assessment of the person must be carried out. The aim of the assessment is to determine the individual's personal and clinical needs and to ascertain which of these, if any, may be satisfied by supplying an orthosis. Although the assessment aims to gain information about many clinical, anatomical, personal and social factors, in practice the assessment may not be compartmentalised under these sub-headings.

Clinical and anatomical features

It is important to have clinical knowledge of the diagnosis and prognosis because these have implications for the aims of the orthosis and its design. Initially, information about the individual's medical history and current treatment can be gained from the case notes and through discussion with other personnel. If an orthosis is to become an effective and integral part of the person's total programme of treatment and rehabilitation, consideration must be given to any limiting or complementary factors which each regime imposes. Thus, if a priority of treatment is to provide active exercise to the dorsiflexors of the foot, it might be counter-productive to supply a static ankle–foot orthosis which passively supports the foot in dorsiflexion.

Although basic decisions about orthotic management can be made on the basis of the diagnosis, it is only by specific assessment of the individual that points of particular relevance may be focused upon and expanded.

A physical examination can supply important information about the current state of the individual and how the condition is affecting him. Since each person varies to some extent from the 'norm', it is often beneficial in uni-lateral conditions to compare the affected body part with the unaffected limb or side of the body. In this way, the therapist can determine what is the 'norm' for that person. Features which can be noted during this examination include:

- skin condition
- circulatory competence
- nail condition
- scars
- nodules
- oedema
- range of movement.

Skin condition

With regard to the skin, it is important to observe its colour, texture and integrity and to determine the extent of any sensory loss. The therapist will not only need to examine the skin covering the parts directly involved, but also those areas over which the orthosis will need to extend for purposes of leverage, pressure reduction and strapping. If an orthosis is supplied to a person with sensory impairment, it is particularly important to protect the person from warm materials whilst fabricating the orthosis. Furthermore, he must be instructed to check for early signs of pressure or skin irritation (see p. 349).

Oedema

Oedema is another factor which needs to be considered. Since oedema may be transient, regular fittings must be arranged to make adjustments. Comparison with the unaffected side can be of help in determining whether all the oedema has subsided. However, when comparing the upper limbs, one should allow for the possibility that slight differences may exist between the size of a dominant and non-dominant limb.

Range of movement

The alignment and range of active and passive movement at relevant joints should also be assessed. Range of movement may be limited by pain or by the underlying condition. On the other hand, if the joint ligaments are lax, movement may extend beyond its normal range. In addition, range of movement may be affected by soft tissue or boney deformity. Nevertheless, regardless of the cause or severity of the deformity, it may be necessary, in the initial stages, to accommodate it in the design of the orthosis. Ultimately, however, it is hoped that orthoses can assist in the reduction or correction of soft tissue deformities.

Personal and social factors

An integral part of the assessment is to ascertain the individual's requirements and priorities with regard to his personal, social and work-related pursuits. Clearly, this aspect of the assessment can only be carried out with the full and active co-operation of the person. Also, this involvement will help to ensure that the orthosis meets the needs of the person and facilitates his acceptance of it. Similarly, it is important that he understands the functions and limitations of the orthosis. If a person has unrealistic expectations of an orthosis, seeing it as an instant or miraculous cure, or conversely considers it as an encumbrance, then it is very unlikely that he will gain the full potential benefit from its use.

THE FUNCTIONS OF ORTHOSES

Ultimately, the aim of orthotics is to achieve an optimal anatomical position and physiological state, thereby maximising functional ability. The means by which these aims are attained may not only vary between individuals but also at different stages of treatment. Indeed, the wearing of an orthosis may, on occasions, impede or totally inhibit function, but will enable greater mobility following its precribed period of usage. During the initial assessment, specific aims and objectives will be identified, discussed and prioritised for each individual. Upon completion of the assessment, one or more orthoses can then be designed to meet the specific and often interdependent aims of treatment. In general, orthoses are provided to give external support or for the purposes of correction, protection and prevention. More specifically, these functional categories may include:

- pain relief, e.g. carpal tunnel syndrome
- facilitation of healing, e.g. ligament repair following whiplash injury
- prevention and correction of soft tissue deformity, e.g. burns
- maintenance of function in unaffected parts, e.g. support of wrist joint in rheumatoid arthritis
- maintenance of improvements achieved by other forms of treatment, e.g. passive stretching
- improvement or maintenance of joint alignment, e.g. prevention of ulnar deviation at metacarpophalangeal joints in rheumatoid arthritis

- assistance of weakened muscles, e.g. peripheral nerve lesion
- substitution for lost muscle power, e.g. peripheral nerve lesion
- protection of vulnerable anatomical structures, e.g. meningomyelocele cyst.

Position of rest

Sometimes, symptoms can be alleviated by providing rest to the affected body parts. Rest is most effectively achieved by supporting the body part in a correct, yet comfortable position. The resultant effects of rest can include the reduction of pain and inflammation, as in the inflammatory stage of rheumatoid arthritis, and the facilitation of healing as, for example, following a whiplash injury.

A position of rest is based on the natural position the part assumes with normal muscle balance between antagonist muscle groups. In the case of the hand, it is useful to base the position of rest on that assumed by the hand when it is resting passively palm upwards on a table (see Fig. 11.1). The wrist is in 10 to 20 degrees of extension and the distal and proximal interphalangeal and the metacarpophalangeal finger joints are slightly flexed. Whilst at rest the fingers adopt this flexed pattern because the flexor muscles are stronger than the extensors. When orthoses are constructed for the axial rather than appendicular regions, a prime objective is to achieve postural symmetry.

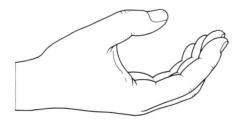

Fig. 11.1 Position of rest.

Position of function

On occasions, a body part can deteriorate as a result of impairment of neighbouring structures. If an orthosis supports an affected part in an appropriate position it can help to maintain function of structures at risk of this secondary involvement and thereby reduce the risk of deterioration of otherwise healthy tissues; for example, a position of some 20–30 degrees of wrist extension is necessary for full flexion of all the joints of the fingers and powerful prehension. Hence, a wrist extension orthosis has a direct and indirect effect upon upper limb function. Primarily, as stated earlier, it facilitates finger flexion and hand function, and secondarily, as a result of this increase in hand function, the more proximal joints of the upper limb are mobilised to enable a wide range of positioning of the hand.

According to Malick (1979), the position of function of the hand can generally be described as similar to that which it adopts when holding a ball (see Fig. 11.2). The wrist is in 20–30 degrees of extension, the thumb is abducted and opposed. The transverse arch at the level of the metacarpal heads is increased in curvature and the amount of flexion in the fingers is approximately 30 and 45 degrees at the metacarpophalangeal and proximal interphalangeal joints respectively.

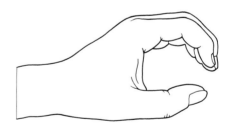

Fig. 11.2 Position of function.

Position of immobilisation

It may be necessary to immobilise a hand in order to allow healing to occur. Since this process may continue for a long period, it is important to maintain stretch on soft tissues to prevent contractures. An optimal position of immobilisation for the hand is illustrated in Figure 11.3. In this position, where the metacarpophalangeal joints are flexed to 90° and the proximal/distal interphalangeal joints are extended, the collateral ligaments are taut.

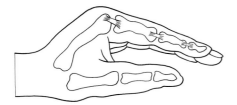

Fig. 11.3 Position of prolonged immobilisation (collateral ligaments of finger joints are taut).

Dynamic orthoses

Some orthoses have moving sections, secured to a static base. These 'dynamic', as opposed to 'static', orthoses can support structures in an optimal position by their static base and also assist or produce movement by their moving, i.e. dynamic, portions. Dynamic orthoses may have the additional aim of substituting for lost muscle power, be it a partial or total loss. They also provide balance and exercise for unaffected muscles, which help to maintain muscle condition and prevent contractures. In addition, the pumping action of muscle activity may help to reduce oedema. Furthermore, as dynamic orthoses encourage movement they help to prevent the formation of adhesions which would inhibit movement if left untreated.

The direction and size of the forces applied are paramount and must be mechanically and kinesiologically based. In general, 'dynamic' orthoses are more complex in design than 'static' orthoses, therefore it is advisable to develop expertise in the manufacture of static designs before progressing to dynamic ones. Although some basic points concerning the design of dynamic orthoses are given in the following section, more detailed guidelines can be obtained from such sources as Malick (1974) and Colditz (1983).

PRINCIPLES OF ORTHOTIC DESIGN

The general objective of the following discussion is to provide a theoretical framework and a check-list of criteria to assist in the design and fabrication of orthoses. As stated earlier, this approach has been adopted in preference to supplying descriptions of particular orthoses or details of their manufacture, because it was felt that this would be too restrictive and prescriptive. Furthermore, there are several specialist texts available which outline the orthotic management of specific conditions (see Malick & Meyer 1978, Fess & Philips 1987).

There are many anatomical, biomechanical and social factors which should be taken into consideration before designing an orthosis. In practice, these factors are often interrelated and dependent on each other. However, for the purposes of clarity, they will be discussed here under separate headings.

Biological and biomechanical principles

Whilst it is not intended to present a detailed coverage of the extensive and sometimes complex anatomical structures which an orthosis might encompass, reference will be made to the more salient anatomical and kinesiological features and some basic knowledge will be assumed. In particular, this section will focus on the surface anatomy of the body, methods of pressure reduction and management, and the protection of boney prominences.

Anatomical landmarks

The size and shape of an orthosis is partially determined by the body's anatomical structures and observable or palpable landmarks, such as boney prominences, joints and skin creases. These can provide a useful starting point when drawing a pattern or when trimming away excess material from a partially completed orthosis. Also, as these landmarks vary slightly from person to person in their size and exact location, correct fit and positioning will not be achieved unless they are taken into account when the orthosis is being shaped and moulded around the body part.

Thus an orthosis for the foot will be more comfortable if the material conforms to the curved plantar surface, which is created by the medial and lateral longitudinal and transverse arches.

Similarly, in the case of the hand, even when the palm is outstretched it is usually curved and slightly concave. These contours are formed by: the transverse palmar arches, the longitudinal arch, and the thenar and hypothenar eminences (see Fig. 11.4). Clearly, if an orthosis does not follow the contour of these curves, it is likely to cause pressure and discomfort. If an orthosis has been provided for functional purposes, care must be taken to avoid restricting movements which it aims to facilitate. Therefore, if a hand orthosis extended beyond the thenar or the transverse palmar creases (see Fig. 11.5) it would restrict movement at the carpometacarpal joint of the thumb and the metacarpophalangeal joints of the fingers and thereby impede the prehensile function of the hand. Furthermore, since the curvature of the palm normally varies during activity, orthoses should be moulded in an optimal position, thus allowing the splinted hand to be used for a variety of grips and functions.

In addition to being aware of the body's natural curves and skin creases, it is generally advisable to avoid boney prominences, or to accommodate them by following their contour (see p. 350). Boney prominences which usually require pre-cautionary action include: the ulnar styloid, the dorsum of the MCP joints and the lateral malleolus (see Fig. 11.6).

However, in some circumstances it is not possible to avoid a boney prominence because the

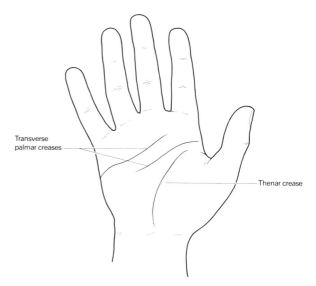

Fig. 11.5 Creases of the palm.

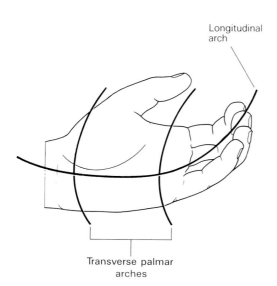

Fig. 11.4 Arches of the hand.

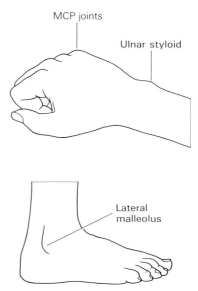

Fig. 11.6 Potential pressure points.

overall integrity and strength of the orthosis would be reduced if the material was cut back around the protrusion. Also, this would increase the pressure exerted over the skin which surrounds the boney prominence. This situation can occur when an ankle–foot orthosis, which encloses the calcaneum, is supplied to a person who is confined to bed and has vascular insufficiency. In these conditions, a pressure sore may develop over the weight-bearing heel. Whilst it might seem logical to cut a hole in the material which covers the heel, this may only transfer the problem, that is the pressure, to the skin which is beneath the circumference of the hole. A similar and classic problem can arise when a thermoplastic moulded seat insert is supplied to an immobile and underweight person. Here, the skin covering the ischial tuberosities is at risk and may deteriorate. This problem, is usually rectified by slightly tipping the moulded insert, rather than by excavating holes in the base of the seat.

Suggestions for reducing pressure at places of boney prominence will be considered further in the next section, where the general principles of pressure reduction and management are discussed.

Principles of pressure reduction and management

Since orthoses are often designed to rest or immobilise a limb, and to correct or reduce the progression of deformity, it is inevitable that some pressure will need to be exerted in order to overcome the effects of gravity and muscle contraction. Therefore, in order to avoid skin breakdown, reduction in vascular supply or nerve impingement, it is important that the degree of pressure exerted by an orthosis is carefully monitored and maintained at an optimal level. Furthermore, the negative consequences of applying pressure will be minimised, or perhaps totally avoided, if the pressure is evenly distributed over a large surface area. Nevertheless, a balance must be achieved between this reduction in pressure and the exposure of skin for sensory input, which is particularly important for hand function. Hence, when designing a palmar wrist extension orthosis, the forearm section usually extends along two thirds of its length to support and distribute the weight

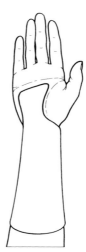

Fig. 11.7 Positioning of wrist extension orthosis in relation to palmar creases.

of the hand, but the distal section finishes at the transverse palmar and thenar creases, thus leaving the palmar surface of the hand exposed (see Fig. 11.7.). In the case of dynamic orthoses, the slings should be sufficiently wide to comfortably support the weight of the fingers. Similarly, if an orthosis is supplied to change the alignment of a body segment, pressure will be applied more safely if correction is achieved in several consecutive steps and only along one plane of movement at a time. Therefore, if a foot has adopted an equinovarus position, it is generally preferable to correct the varus deformity before attempting to correct plantar flexion.

In some circumstances, a deformity will only be reduced or corrected if pressure is simultaneously applied in diametrically opposed directions. This 'tri-point' principle can be illustrated by the swan-neck finger deformity, where the proximal interphalangeal (PIP) joint hyperextends and the distal interphalangeal (DIP) joint is flexed (Melvin 1989). Here, the finger can usually be corrected if pressure is simultaneously applied to the palmar surface of the PIP joint and the dorsum of the proximal and middle phalanges (see Fig. 11.8). The 'tri-point' principle of fixation could also be used to correct boutonnière finger deformity, knee hyperextension and spinal scoliosis.

When designing a 'dynamic' orthosis, although the principles which are listed above will apply to the static base, additional care will be needed to ensure that the dynamic components apply appropriate and controlled pressure. It is desirable to apply a constant force over a longer period of time rather than a stronger force for a shorter time span. The force should be sufficient to correct the abnormal segment, but not so strong as to totally inhibit the opposing movement. Generally, as Malick (1989) and Cannon et al (1985) point out, the force should be applied at right angles to the part being mobilised, an angle of pull less than 90 degrees tending to transfer forces into the joint and one of more than 90 degrees tending to distract it. The direction of the force applied must also correspond with lines of movement. This can be illustrated by considering the movement of the fingers. When they flex, they follow an oblique line which incorporates an element of adduction. As a result, flexed fingers point towards the scaphoid carpal bone (see Fig. 11.9).

Protection of boney prominences

It has already been noted that boney prominences may require extra protection from the effects of pressure, particularly if the person is unlikely to detect points of pressure himself because of impaired sensation or cognitive function. Pressure may be relieved from a boney prominence in at least two ways. First, if the area of skin which is proximal and distal (or medial and lateral) to the protrusion is padded, this will prevent the material from rubbing the skin (see Fig. 11.10). Alternatively, if the boney prominence is padded prior to moulding the orthosis, this will create sufficient space for the completed orthosis to be lined with a piece of soft material (see Fig. 11.11). However, if the orthosis is moulded over the prominence without padding in situ, then any subsequent attempts to line the orthosis would merely exacerbate the problem because the thickness of the lining material would increase the pressure that is exerted over the bone (see Fig. 11.12).

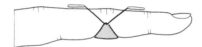

Fig. 11.8 Tri-point principle as applied to correct swan-neck deformity.

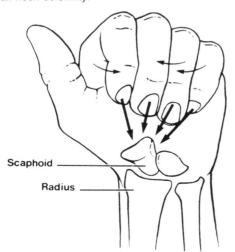

Fig. 11.9 Fingers' normal anatomical alignment in flexion is towards the scaphoid. (by permission of Cannon et al Manual of hand splinting, Churchill Livingstone, New York, 1985)

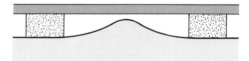

Fig. 11.10 Padding applied either side reduces pressure on prominence.

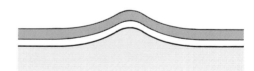

Fig. 11.11 Shape achieved when pre-padding is used in fabrication.

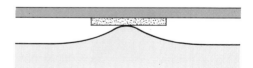

Fig. 11.12 Additional inner padding applied post fabrication merely increases pressure on prominence.

Social factors

So far, the focus of attention has been towards the anatomy of the body and the biomechanical principles of pressure reduction and management. Whilst these factors are important, it cannot be stressed enough that each orthosis should also be designed to accommodate the individual's needs and wishes.

In order to achieve this aim, the therapist should utilise the information which was gleaned during the initial assessment about the individual's personal, work and social circumstances, before designing and fabricating an orthosis. In addition, she should explain and discuss with the person the range of orthotic solutions which are available before reaching a mutually acceptable decision about the choice of orthotic design and material. However, it may on occasions be necessary to accept that the most medically suitable orthosis cannot be prescribed if it is practically unsuitable or cosmetically unacceptable to the individual; for example if the person lives alone he may not be physically capable of fitting and fastening a rigid or complex orthosis. In this situation, if it is not possible to arrange daily assistance, it may be necessary to select an alternative design or more pliable material.

If a person consents to surgery, he is also consenting to certain follow-up procedures, which may include an orthosis. Non-compliance with this regime may result in a poor outcome and this should be explained.

Cosmesis and comfort

Research and personal experience suggest that orthoses are frequently abandoned if they are unsightly or uncomfortable. In view of this, it is essential that every reasonable effort is made to improve the appearance and comfort of orthoses, regardless of whether they are supplied for temporary or permanent use.

The cosmetic appearance of an orthosis will be improved if:

- there are no unsightly pen marks — patterns should be inscribed by a sharp instrument rather than a pen

- there are no finger or nail prints
- the edges are neatly finished
- the orthosis can be cleaned
- the straps are neatly attached
- the orthosis is as unobtrusive as possible.

The comfort of an orthosis will be improved if:

- it is not unnecessarily heavy or warm
- it does not enclose the body segment in such a way that it pinches the skin or impedes circulation
- pressure is not exerted over a nerve which takes a superficial course
- pressure is not exerted over a boney prominence
- some air can circulate between the skin and orthotic material
- the edges and inside surface of the orthosis are smooth
- the straps are adjustable
- the straps are not placed over an area of sensitive skin nor over a boney prominence
- it is not unnecessarily complex and can therefore be fitted correctly and easily.

Whilst the aforementioned suggestions for improving the appearance and comfort of an orthosis are not exhaustive, it is hoped they will serve as a useful guide.

MATERIALS AND EQUIPMENT

Principles of material selection

Orthoses can be fabricated from a wide range of materials which have different properties. However, since the cost and availability of each material is likely to vary over time, these materials will not be individually described in detail.

In theory, a material should be selected on the basis of the therapist's clinical knowledge and understanding of the individual's personal needs. However, in reality, there are several economic and practical constraints which may limit the range of materials a department can utilise. Nevertheless, before addressing these limiting factors, attention will be drawn to the clinical features and orthotic objectives which should primarily guide the choice of material.

Clinical considerations

Clearly, there are a vast number of symptoms, or combination of symptoms, which may influence an occupational therapist's choice of material. Since it is impossible to list all of these clinical features, a sample of the more common and decisive factors will be discussed. These include:

- comfort
- risk of cross-infection
- respiratory function
- weight
- contractures
- skin condition.

In some cases, it is necessary to make frequent but small changes to the size or shape of an orthosis, for instance to accommodate fluctuating levels of oedema. Therefore, it is advisable to select a material which can be re-heated and adjusted as necessary, for example Orthoplast and Sansplint. If the area which needs alteration is small, then spot heating by the appropriate method may be used. This has the advantage of reducing the amount of time and discomfort the person is exposed to and is cost effective. On the other hand, if more extensive changes have occurred in the size or position of the body segment, as a result of weight loss or corrective serial splintage, it is usually preferable to make a replacement orthosis from new materials. In this situation, unless it is clinically detrimental, the less expensive materials, such as plaster of Paris or Hexcelite, would be useful. Furthermore, in order to minimise the risk of cross-infection, it is recommended that materials are not re-used, unless they are supplied to the same person and for the same body segment. When an orthosis is prescribed for a person with a respiratory disorder, it is prudent to avoid any material which produces dust or noxious fumes.

The importance of a material's strength and durability will vary according to the person's weight, whether the orthosis covers a weight-bearing surface and whether the orthosis has been supplied to resist the force of gravity or to correct a contracture.

It may be advisable to select a waterproof material, such as Orthoplast or Sansplint, if making a functional orthosis, as this would enable the person to continue with most routine domestic duties.

Although 'comfort' is a criterion which influences the choice of material selected for any orthosis, in some circumstances it is more important than others, for instance, if the skin is friable, as a result of injury or prolonged steroid therapy, the orthosis may only be tolerated if the material is relatively smooth, flexible and lightweight. In these circumstances, Plastazote may be an appropriate choice, as this provides cushioning and is relatively lightweight. Comfort may also be improved if the material is well perforated, thus allowing at least some air to reach the skin.

Economic and practical considerations

As noted earlier, there are several economic and practical factors which may limit the number of materials that a department can hold. If the department serves a population which rarely requires orthoses, it is not usually economically viable to hold a large or varied stock. Similarly, in these circumstances it would be unwise to order materials with a limited shelf-life. On the other hand, even if a department has a quick turnover, the manager may still decide to purchase one or two materials but in large quantities, thus enabling her to negotiate a discount with the supplier. Furthermore, it would not be practicable to stock those materials which are softened or mixed by expensive or specialist equipment unless they are used in sufficient quantities to justify the capital investment.

Finally, whilst it is inevitable that materials will be chosen on the basis of each therapist's personal preferences, experiences and training, every reasonable effort should be made to broaden and develop expertise wherever possible and to critically evaluate the materials that are available. In this way, it is hoped that the quality of practice will improve and that occupational therapists will be in a better position to provide suppliers with constructive comments and feedback.

Miscellaneous materials

In addition to holding a stock of orthotic materials, there are several small but essential items which are necessary for skin protection, material handling and strapping.

First, before moulding an orthosis, it is often necessary to protect the skin from the effects of heat by covering the body part with a length of cotton stockinette. Similarly, before using Hexcelite, water or lanolin should be applied to the person's skin in order to prevent the material from adhering to body hair. In addition, it is useful to hold a stock of soft, preferably self-adhesive lining materials. These may be attached to a complete orthosis to protect the skin from potentially abrasive areas, such as the inside surface of rivets.

Whilst most materials can be hand held when warmed to their working temperature, there are a few, such as Vitrathene and Plastazote reinforcer, which cannot be applied directly to the skin and can only be handled if gloves are worn. Also, these materials should be placed on a patch of cotton stockinette before heating to prevent the material from sticking to the oven shelf. However, most materials can be placed directly in the oven, provided the shelf has been lined with the waxy, brown, 'release paper', which is supplied by Smith and Nephew, between each sheet of Plastazote.

Several items may be required for strapping, including:

- leather
- velcro
- cotton webbing
- sheepskin
- plastic D-rings
- rivets
- glue.

Finally, in order to make 'dynamic' orthoses, a range of sundries will be needed:

- spring wire
- plastic tubing
- rubber bands
- metal dress hooks
- elastic, and
- leather

Equipment

The majority of orthotic materials require heating by means of hot water, an oven or steam before they can be moulded and applied to the body (or to a cast of the body). Two exceptions are plaster of Paris and Neofract. The former can be applied to the skin following submersion in cold or tepid water, whereas the latter involves mixing two tins of resin (see p. 354).

Although it is possible, if working in a community setting, to heat small pieces of low temperature thermoplastic material by pouring hot water into a bowl, it is safer to use an electric waterpan or 'Aquapan' which can be set to varying temperatures. Similarly, if purchasing an oven it is advisable to select a model which is fitted with a thermostat.

Some ovens also have a convector fan, which is particularly useful when heating large sheets of material as it helps to maintain an even temperature throughout the oven.

'Steam' and 'mixer' machines can be purchased from the respective suppliers of Fractomed and Neofract.

Miscellaneous equipment

In addition to the large pieces of equipment mentioned above, it may also be necessary to order a:

- heat gun
- glue gun
- soldering iron
- extractor fan
- plaster sink
- hole punch
- Stanley knife
- rolling pin
- spring wire jig
- pair of curved scissors
- tape measure

- rule
- plaster and wire cutters.

Although the purpose of this equipment is self-explanatory, it is necessary to mention the function of a portable wooden step and a wedge-shaped block. A wooden step can be used to support the foot of a seated person in dorsiflexion, thus leaving the therapist free to mould an ankle–foot orthosis. Similarly, a wedge can be used to support a person's forearm in supination, whilst the therapist applies material to the palmar surface of the limb.

Finally, an Allen key can be very useful for pushing two layers of material together and thus aiding adhesion.

PREPARATION

Before making an orthosis, there are several practicalities to which an occupational therapist should attend:

1. It is advisable to check that all necessary materials and equipment are to hand and in good working order.
2. Wherever possible, the person should be given an explanation of the manufacturing process and the opportunity to ask questions.
3. If it is felt that assistance will be required from another person at some point during the manufacture, this should be arranged in advance.
4. For the purposes of achieving optimal anatomical alignment, comfort and access, it is essential to check the positioning of the person.
5. The occupational therapist should be aware of her own body position; for example she should ensure that her hair does not brush against the person's face as she is working.

METHOD OF MANUFACTURE

Over the years many orthotic materials have been marketed and this range continues to increase as new ones are developed. Some of these materials are rendered malleable by a chemical reaction resulting from the combination of two or more components, and others by the external application of heat.

Such products as plaster of Paris and Neofract fall into the former category. In the case of plaster of Paris, water is added to the powdery gypsum which may be adherent to cotton material in slab or bandage form. An exothermic reaction occurs resulting in the formation of a new compound which, at first, is paste like and mouldable but then it solidifies and dries out to the state familiar to most people. Neofract again utilises a chemical reaction, this time between two components supplied in separate containers. To successfully combine these, specialist mixing equipment is needed along with adequate extraction and ventilation facilities. When thoroughly mixed the two components must then be poured into preformed stockinette moulds, rolled out to the desired size and then applied round the part and firmly held in position by an elastic bandage until the chemical reaction is complete and the compound material solidifies.

Many of those materials which require the external application of heat are thermoplastics, and an increasing number of these become malleable at temperatures low enough to allow them to be moulded directly onto the skin. From the three forms of dry, wet or steam heat, some thermoplastics can only be heated by one method whereas others can be heated by wet or dry heat, as summarised in Table 11.1.

Table 11.1 Methods of heating thermoplastics

Heating method	Materials
Steam	Fractomed
Water	Hexcelite, Aquaplast, Orfit, Coriform and Cellacast
Dry	Plastazote and Vitrathene
Water/dry	Orthoplast, Sansplint, Sansplint XR, Synergy, Polyform and Polyform lite

Each material has a different working temperature and some can be ruined by overheating. Also, some materials cannot be reheated. However, each supplier usually provides specific heating instructions for each product. Similarly, the particular properties of each material regarding degree of conformability, rigidity, stretch and shrinkage can be gleaned from the suppliers and of course through individual experience. Nevertheless, general useful tips for the handling of thermoplastics include the following.

• For those materials which in the raw state are very rigid, it may be helpful to use a Stanley knife or sharp scissors to cut out the approximate shape with as little wastage as possible. When cutting the material with scissors it is helpful to pull back one side of the material (see Fig. 11.13).

• The rough template of material can be partially heated, thus enabling an accurate shape to be cut, preferably using long, smooth scissor strokes.

• A chemical solvent such as Zoff or trichlorethylene can be used to remove surface grease or dust from the material, which increases its self-adherent properties. This may be useful, not only in fabricating the orthosis but also when utilising pieces of material to attach straps or dynamic components. In order

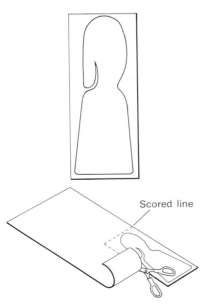

Fig. 11.13 Cutting an approximate template from cold materials.

for bonding to be effective, both surfaces must be dry.

• Talcum or plaster powder may be sprinkled on the surface of the material to reduce its self-adherent properties. This is useful when, during the manufacture of an orthosis, parts of the material come into close proximity and could inadvertently self-adhere.

• Spot heating by means of a heat gun, or by spooning water onto the material, can enable small adjustments to be made without the entire shape of the orthosis being affected.

• Do not rush. Even though some materials have a short working time it is often more than ample. If, until experience is gained, the working time is not sufficient, this may not cause a problem, since many materials can be reheated. Therefore, orthoses can be manufactured in several stages or modified to correct any faults. However, speed should be increased with practice and is usually desirable both for patient comfort and cost effectiveness.

• Some materials, for example Polyform and Sansplint XR, should be applied in a gravity-assisted position and handled as little as possible, to avoid stretching and unsightly finger marks. Less conformable materials, such as Orthoplast, can be held in situ by a crêpe bandage.

The basic outline, or pattern, of an orthosis can be achieved by one of three alternative methods, namely: individual measurement, standard template or pre-cut shape. Regardless of which method is used as a starting point, accurate adjustments and moulding are essential if the orthosis is to correctly fit the individual.

FINAL EXPLANATION AND INSTRUCTIONS

The success of an orthosis often depends on the quality of explanation and discussion that has occurred between the occupational therapist, medical practitioner, the person and, if necessary, his carers. This discussion should occur not only before and during the design and fabrication stages, but also prior to discharge. At this latter

Scored line

stage, any verbal explanation or instruction should, ideally, be reinforced by written notes. These should specify when, and for how long, the orthosis needs to be worn. Details about the cleaning, storage and maintenance of the orthosis should also be given. Although it is advisable to operate a system of 'follow-up', a written note of the therapist's name, address and telephone number should also be given. This will enable the person to contact the therapist as soon as he has any queries or experiences any difficulties with the fit of the orthosis. Finally, in order to avoid the potential risk of litigation, many departments now have a policy whereby clients are asked to sign a form stating that they have understood the instructions the therapist has given and that any alterations they make to the orthosis are done at their own risk.

CONCLUSION

This chapter provides an overview of the basic principles of material selection, orthotic design and fabrication. The approach is based on the premise that rigid solutions cannot be predicted for particular diagnostic groups because each case is unique: these concepts are illustrated in the following case example. It is argued throughout that orthotic management should be integrated with other regimens and based upon holistic assessment and review. The chapter serves as an introduction to orthotics, which the reader can supplement by further study, experience and research.

CASE EXAMPLE 11.1

Mrs Warmsley lives with her retired husband in a detached modern bungalow. The couple both enjoy travel and regularly visit their caravan in Wales. Mrs Warmsley is secretary of the local caravan club, but finds her hands and wrists tire when typing the minutes of meetings. Mrs Warmsley suffers from rheumatoid arthritis and experiences problems with general hand function. The arthritis particularly affects her left wrist which intermittently becomes inflamed and oedematous. However, even during a remission the joint is painful and unstable and her grip is weakened. She has received steroid therapy for several years, which has resulted in friable skin. Although an essential aspect of treatment includes support and rest of the wrist joint, Mrs Warmsley is keen to maintain independence and continue with her secretarial duties. In this instance, an 'off the shelf' elasticated orthosis, such as a 'Futura wrist extension orthosis', might encircle the wrist too tightly and would not fully accommodate fluctuating levels of oedema. Since this lady is retired and leads a sedentary lifestyle, more expensive hard-wearing materials, such as Orthoplast and Sansplint, are not necessary. Indeed, in view of her skin condition and pain, a softer more pliable and warm material such as Plastazote would be indicated. This could be strengthened with either Vitrathene or Plastazote reinforcer to give adequate wrist support. Finally, an enclosed design, with 'D' ring straps, would also help to ensure an accurate fit is maintained as the degree of oedema changes.

REFERENCES

Cannon N M et al 1985 Manual of hand splinting. Churchill Livingstone, New York, pp 6, 7

Colditz J C 1983 Low profile dynamic splinting of the hand. American Journal of Occupational Therapy 37(3): 182–188

Fess E E, Philips C A 1987 Hand splinting — principles and methods, 2nd edn. Mosby, Washington

Malick M H 1974 Manual on dynamic hand splinting with thermoplastic materials. Harmarville Rehabilitation Centre, Pittsburgh

Malick M H 1979 Manual on static hand splinting, 4th edn. Harmarville Rehabilitation Centre, Pittsburgh, vol 1, p 19

Malick M H 1989 Upper extremity orthotics. In: Hopkins H, Smith H (eds) Willard and Spackman's occupational therapy, 7th edn. Lippincott, Philadelphia

Malick M H, Meyer C M H 1978 Manual on the management of the quadriplegic upper extremity. Harmarville Rehabilitation Centre, Pittsburgh

Melvin J L 1989 Rheumatic disease in the adult and child: occupational therapy and rehabilitation, 3rd edn. F A Davis, Philadelphia, pp. 284, 562

FURTHER READING

Barr N R, Swan D 1988 The hand: principles and
techniques of splintmaking. Butterworths, London

Cannon N M et al 1986 Diagnosis and treatment manual for
physicians and therapists. The Hand Rehabilitation Center
of Indiana, Indianapolis

Cromwell F S, Bear-Lehman J (eds) 1988 Occupational
therapy in health care: hand rehabilitation in occupational
therapy. Howarth Press, New York, vol 4, numbers 3/4

Rose G K 1986 Orthotics, principles and practice.
Heinemann, London

Wynne-Parry C B 1981 Rehabilitation of the hand, 4th edn.
Butterworths, London

Part 3
Practice

We shall not cease from exploration
and the end of all our exploring
will be to arrive where we started
and to know the place for the first time.

T. S. Eliot *Four Quartets*

Introduction to the practice of occupational therapy

12

A basis for practice

Margaret Foster

INTRODUCTION

Occupational therapy is a rapidly developing profession which is currently consolidating its theoretical basis in order to provide a solid foundation for research and evaluation and to more clearly explain its philosophy to others.

For many years, occupational therapists have been using a variety of techniques in treatment and intervention, but only in recent years has there been a reappraisal of the value of individual methods and practices, the basis on which these have developed, and the ways in which they interlink within the various branches of occupational therapy.

Competence in any profession depends upon an understanding of the theory that underlies it. 'Theory', in this general sense, is that which provides a basis for practice. It encompasses philosophical viewpoints, paradigms, frames of reference, models, approaches, and particular *theories*. The occupational therapist needs to be conversant with these elements of theory as they have developed within her own profession, so that she has a clear understanding of the principles of her discipline and a sound basis from which to plan, implement, and justify her interventions.

While there are many texts available which present in-depth discussion of particular aspects of theory (see References and Further Reading), this chapter aims to provide an overview of the main aspects of occupational therapy theory which have application to the treatment of people with physical dysfunction.

The first sections of the chapter discuss the importance of theory to the profession of occupational therapy as a whole and to the individual therapist. Various terms used in the discussion of theory, such as 'paradigm', 'frame of reference', 'approach' and 'model', are defined. The interconnections between these areas of theory are then illustrated.

The next sections of the chapter turn to the application of theory to practice. First, specific theories that have had an important influence upon occupational therapy are discussed; these are the humanistic, occupations/activities, and psychosocial theories. The basic assumptions of each theory are outlined, and particular refinements on these theories as they have evolved within occupational therapy are described.

The remaining sections of the chapter are devoted to particular frames of reference that have had an important influence on the treatment of physical dysfunction, namely, the developmental, biomechanical, compensatory and learning frames of reference. The merits and limitations of each frame of reference are set out, and their relevance to today's changing practice is discussed.

THE IMPORTANCE OF THEORY

PROFESSIONAL RECOGNITION

Historically, there were only three true professions: the Church, law and medicine. In recent years, increasing emphasis has been placed on the terms 'profession' and 'professionalism' as more disciplines strive to attain status and recognition. Occupational therapy has been recognised as a profession since the 1930's.

To maintain and further its professional standing, occupational therapy must have a sound theoretical framework by which it can define itself and justify its activity. Like any profession, it must have a theoretical basis which is compatible with the social values of the community that it serves and which reflects the practices it employs (Yerxa 1979).

Before considering the nature and importance of this theoretical basis, we might first examine what qualities are essential to a 'profession' and to 'professionalism'.

What is a profession?

No one definition of what constitutes a profession exists, although various texts which outline the characteristics representative of a profession agree on a number of points. The following elements are generally considered to be fundamental to any profession:

- A unique body of knowledge which is pertinent to the practices and beliefs of the profession. Some knowledge may overlap with that of other professions, but the particular integration and utilisation of knowledge is unique to each profession.
- A sound theory base on which to explain the profession's philosophies and values. Many texts state that this theory base should be proven by investigation and research.
- Educational requirements in order to become a member of the profession; continuing education within the profession to maintain standards in the light of change.
- Autonomy in determining the rules of the profession and maintaining standards.
- Ethical responsibility to regulate the modes of behaviour of those within the profession and to protect the client.
- Professional commitment within the membership to adhere to the practices and beliefs of the profession and to further its development.

What is professionalism?

The Little Oxford Dictionary* defines professionalism as the 'qualities or typical features of

---

*The Little Oxford Dictionary of Current English, 1986.

professionals'. This definition extends the notion of professionalism beyond the possession of a knowledge base and cognitive skills to include the way in which the individual conducts himself and the competence with which he accepts the responsibilities of his profession. It encompasses the ways in which the person reflects the values of his profession in daily practice, and the responsibilities necessary to maintain competence. It includes the individual's fulfilment of professional obligations vis-á-vis consumers, his maintenance of professional standards and his specific role within the profession.

The British Association of Occupational Therapists' (1990) *Code of Ethics and Professional Conduct* defines the ways practitioners should meet professional obligations in relation to consumers in terms of responsibilities, relationships, professional integrity and standards of practice. Included within these are articles concerning professional demeanor, clinical competence, personal behaviour and professional development.

Implications for occupational therapy

It is therefore vital for occupational therapy to have a proven theory base if it is to continue to be recognised as a true profession. The study of theory should be an essential part of the education necessary to become a member of the profession.

Skill as a 'do-er' based on practice, repetition and experience reflects a technical level of competence. Professionalism, however, requires skill in *thinking*, in reflecting on previous experiences and linking these to theory and learning, and to the presenting problem, in order to ensure that the choice of 'doing' is the most appropriate for the particular situation.

A sound education in the theoretical principles of her profession enhances the ability of the therapist to confidently address issues, make considered decisions and defend outcomes. The ability to defend actions is a vital component in today's practice, in which there is an increased level of investigation and questioning. Litigation is occurring with greater frequency in many professional disciplines as clients challenge the results of practices.

A high standard of learning and of clinical reasoning enhances not only the standing of the individual but also the recognition of the profession as a whole. This may be reflected in academic credentials (diplomas, degrees or doctorates) but should also be evident in the ways in which members of the profession as a whole present themselves to others — the ways in which they demonstrate professionalism.

Members must be conversant with current theory and reflect their theories and beliefs positively in their practice. In order to maintain professionalism they should continue their own personal learning and development to ensure that their practice remains current, competent and ethical.

CLARITY OF PURPOSE

Theory is the lens through which we see reality more clearly. (Kielhofner 1985)

The history of occupational therapy demonstrates the consequences of basing a profession on a weak theory base. Lacking a solid theoretical framework, the profession was, particularly in the 1960s, diverted from its original purpose and allied itself more closely to theories from other professions which appeared to have a sounder proven knowledge base or which were particularly valued or fashionable at the time (see Ch. 2).

Since then, occupational therapists have begun both to question and to value their basic philosophy. Through the development of conceptual models, the analysis of approaches and the evaluation of practices, they have been able to justify the basis on which therapy intervention is founded and more clearly explain the aims and goals of practice to themselves and to others.

Without a theoretical framework a profession is like a ship afloat without a compass in a sea of change. It is at the mercy of the waves and tides of fashion, regularly changing course according to their ebb and flow, without ever reaching its proper destination. It is at risk of washing up on an unknown shore, where its crew will be likely to modify their behaviour to match the customs or culture of the natives and thereby gain acceptance.

Theory is the compass which guides the profession's progress, keeping its direction true whatever storms or changes in tides it encounters. Theory sets the course (the therapy process) and guides the passage (the intervention) to ensure that the ship reaches its chosen shore.

Theory provides a means by which our professional practice can be explained and clarified — for our own benefit and in response to others. It is a framework in which we can explain the philosophy of our practice, justify the value of interventions, and measure the efficacy of treatment.

The move to increase community-based services will place more occupational therapists in multidisciplinary situations where they will be working with colleagues from disciplines other than their own. Sound professional knowledge and expertise will therefore be essential to retain identity, educate others, and integrate occupational therapy practices into the multidisciplinary framework. The practitioner will need to be self-reliant within her discipline and demonstrate skills of independent thinking and clinical reasoning to meet people's needs and justify actions to others. In order to do this efficiently she will need a sound theoretical base to guide her judgements and develop practice expertise.

Theory is an integral part of competent professional practice. Mont and Ross remind us that 'there is nothing impractical about good theory . . . . Action divorced from theory is the random scurrying of a rat in a new maze. Good theory is the power to find the way to the goal with a minimum of lost motion and electric shock' (cited in Black & Champion 1976).

COMMON UNDERSTANDING

In a profession which has such a broad spectrum of practice it is essential to have a common understanding to retain professional identity within the membership and in the perception of the client.

During the 1960s and 1970s many occupational therapists moved into intensely specialised areas such as orthotics. Without a strong common theory base, specialised practitioners were at risk of losing sight of their true professional philosophy regarding the value of occupation and activity and the development of the self.

Lively debate and fierce argument surrounded this trend, which at times threatened to fragment the profession into individual specialisms, many of which were practice (doing) based, rather than philosophy (belief) based. The development of terminology, techniques and expertise specific to each area tended to isolate therapists from one another. How many therapists employed in areas of acute mental illness were able to freely share discussions about the goals of their practices with occupational therapists who had specialised in neurodevelopmental techniques?

Many occupational therapists were at risk of losing sight of the *occupational* nature of therapy, and of becoming divorced from others within their profession in their practices, values and roles. Frequently, this led to a closer alliance with the practices of another 'favoured' or influential profession within the work environment.

Such divergencies did nothing to enhance the understanding of the profession by patients, clients, other professionals and employers. When individuals received different treatments and advice from different therapists there was understandably some confusion, often followed by a loss of respect for the methods used or the information given.

How can such a situation be explained? Much was due to the emphasis on competence in 'doing' rather than on the value of knowing the *why* behind the 'doing', or on clarity regarding the philosophy and process of intervention. The development of theory based on holism and humanism and the organisation of problem-based intervention strategies has enabled therapists to more clearly understand and explain the projected aims and goals of their practices and thereby justify the variations in the methods used to achieve specific outcomes to meet individual requirements.

The occupational therapist has been recognised for the unique breadth of her practice, but only at the risk of being considered a 'Jack of all trades and master of none'. Mastery *in combination with* breadth will become increasingly important as treatment needs and the provision of health care change.

The clientele of occupational therapy has changed in recent years, and will change further in the future, to include more people with multiple pathology. This is occurring for various reasons, including:

- demographic changes, including an increase in the number of elderly people
- advances in surgical and survival techniques which enable people to survive longer following severe trauma and to live much longer with chronic medical conditions such as multiple sclerosis and cancer
- improved antenatal and neonatal care and diagnostic techniques which have enabled children with multiple handicaps to survive
- manpower demands which have led to simple orthopaedic conditions not being seen by occupational therapists in many areas because of the more pressing needs of those with chronic or more complex problems.

As a result of this shift in clientele, the narrow focus of earlier treatment techniques will be insufficient to meet people's needs. An increasing emphasis on a holistic understanding of the individual will be a spur to research into the merits of particular frames of reference and to investigation of how the many theories can be cohesively integrated to meet the complex needs of a changing clientele.

A BASIS FOR RESEARCH AND DEVELOPMENT

The interrelationship between theory and research in all areas of knowledge and development is well known. Theory forms the basis on which research is carried out, and research leads to the proving or disproving of theory.

The Little Oxford Dictionary defines research as 'careful search or enquiry into a subject to discover facts by study or investigation'. In the present climate of therapy, as the professions re-examine their practices in order to justify them to employers, managers and other professions, and with a view to meeting changing patterns of need, research and investigation is vital. Occupational therapists need to investigate the premises on which their interventions are founded and prove the efficacy of those interventions to others.

While many therapists, and others, intuitively recognise the benefits of various occupational therapy practices, there is currently a dearth of research by which the effectiveness of these has been measured or proven. Reliance on intuition and face validity does not provide a sound basis on which to assess the value of a given practice or to build further developments.

Many people view research as something done by others from which they are able to gain information. This is quite true as far as it goes. However, this view is often linked to a hesitancy to personally embark on research because it is perceived to be specialist, complex, highly intellectual, remote or even 'detached from the real world'.

In the past, occupational therapists have gained recognition as 'doers'. They have been active in devising and utilising methods to facilitate patients' and clients' abilities as doers and have been under pressure themselves to be doers as the number of people requiring their assistance has increased and the profession has expanded. This has inevitably been at the expense of time for research to qualify and quantify the results of the 'doing', or to promote new thinking.

Occupational therapists should all be involved in research in some aspect of their work, even if only to prove their own worth. This may be through the simplest form of evaluation of a particular practice or intervention, or through a more complex investigation of needs or modes of provision for future planning strategies. Research is also needed to develop more valid and reliable assessment instruments on which clinicians can confidently base their intervention strategies.

Investigation by Taylor and Mitchell (1990) reveals that many clinicians are not personally carrying out research because of the constraints of time, money, skills and caseload needs but are in favour of clinical research and keen to collaborate with experienced researchers and to learn from their findings. This collaboration could raise the level of clinicians' involvement in research and in so doing raise the level of their interest, expertise and satisfaction, which could further lead to the instigation of personal research investigations. Taylor and Mitchell conclude that 'the profession needs to draw on clinicans' interest in research and develop strategies for increasing their involvement and productivity through mutual and supportive experiences'.

Lyons (1985) states that therapists have acquired a 'modest, but respectable body of knowledge' which should be 'defined, researched and systematised so that it becomes evident, definable, defensible and saleable'. The expansion of our knowledge base is vital to the maintenance and promotion of our professional identity.

No profession can stand still if it is to retain its credibility, but change should not occur just for the sake of change. Whilst occupational therapy needs to keep pace with changing conditions, it should not lose sight of its original purpose.

Theory guides the attitudes and values of our profession. It forms the basis of our clinical reasoning (the questioning and determining of actions) and of our reflection on outcomes and the appropriateness of present practices. Theory based on sound reflection and proven findings makes a major contribution to the development of proactive thinking for future needs.

The history of the profession's divergence from its originating philosophy in the 60s and 70s, when developments occurred without the support of a strong, defined and proven theory base, provides further argument for research and planned development based on sound theory.

DEFINING TERMS

Frequently there are slight differences among health-care professionals in their understanding of theoretical terms. This may occur because some words are used differently from one profession to another. Additionally, the analysis of occupational therapy is a worldwide process and there are differences in the use and understanding of terms between nations and, depending on which source of information has been used, between individuals within one country. Therefore, definitions of terms as they are used in this text are given below.

PHILOSOPHY

A common use of the word 'philosophy' refers to a set of ultimate values, that is, a view of the meaning of life and of the significance of the world we live in. The philosophy of occupational therapy is based in the profession's view of what constitutes an acceptable or desirable quality of life. It determines the values, beliefs and practices of the profession, which are founded in what therapists consider is inherently good and provide a basis from which to approach theory and practice.

One of the earliest philosophies for the profession, put forward by Adolph Meyer in 1922, identified occupational therapy as 'an awakening to the fullest meaning of time as the biggest wonder and asset of our lives and the valuation of opportunity and performance as the greatest measure of time'. The philosophy of occupational therapy is discussed in greater depth in Chapter 1.

PARADIGMS

Kielhofner (1983) uses the word 'paradigm' to refer to 'an agreed body of theory explaining and rationalising professional unity and practice, that incorporates all the profession's concerns, concepts and expertise, and guides values and commitments'.

A paradigm imposes a shape upon a science. It derives from the values, principles and knowledge shared by members of a professional community, and determines the scope and boundaries of the profession, thus guiding practice, research and future development.

Paradigms are built by members of a profession. They are formulated to guide the development of theory and practice, and are eventually discarded as new findings and beliefs emerge to form a new paradigm. This is a natural process of development, which occurs in all areas of science. To take an historical example, after the explorations of Christopher Columbus and others the paradigm of a flat world was replaced by the paradigm of a round world. This shift in understanding further changed thinking and beliefs, and stimulated and guided new thinking and promoted other discoveries.

Paradigm developments have occurred in occupational therapy. The profession's initial paradigm was based on a view of man's need to be 'occupied'. This was replaced by a reductionist paradigm which emphasised body and mind mechanisms as discrete parts of a whole. The present paradigm combines elements from the previous two into a new whole reflecting occupational behaviour and performance. This paradigm has led to the development of new models, for example the human occupations model (Reed & Sanderson), the model of human occupation (Kielhofner) the activities health approach (Cynkin & Robinson) and new theories of occupational performance.

THEORIES

The Heinemann English Dictionary (1987) defines 'theory' as:

- 'a systematically organised group of general propositions used to analyse, predict or explain facts or events'
- 'the whole collection of ideas, methods and theorems associated with a study, e.g. "the number theory"'
- 'an explanation of the principles of a subject, such as art, as distinct from the practice of it'
- 'a conjecture or opinion — "that's your theory but I disagree."'

In the present text, 'theory' might be used in any of the first three senses listed above. Thus, 'a theory' is an organised and systematic set of principles by which phenomena can be predicted and explained; these principles may be more or less comprehensive, and may constitute a methodology. Theory as 'conjecture or opinion' is less relevant to our purposes, although it should be remembered that particular theories that are regarded as sound may have elements of conjecture within them; indeed, they may be found, in the light of later experience, to be untrue.

In the introductory sections of this chapter, 'theory' has been used in the third, general sense given above to refer to the discussion of the 'principles' of our profession as opposed to its 'practice'. It should be borne in mind, however, that just as our practice should be firmly grounded in theory, our theory should never be far removed from practice. A theory that is not readily applicable to and verified by practice may have to be revised or discarded.

The reader will also notice the slight shift in meaning that occurs when we move from the discussion of 'theory' in its widest sense (i.e. a type of discourse, as in: 'The subject of this chapter is occupational therapy theory') to the discussion of 'a theory' or 'theories' (e.g. Piaget's theory of intellectual development). Thus, within the philosophy and paradigm of occupational therapy *theory*, various particular *theories* come into play, some of which are unique to our profession, and some of which have been borrowed and adapted from other disciplines.

FRAMES OF REFERENCE

A frame of reference is an organised body of knowledge, principles and research findings which forms the conceptual basis of *a particular aspect* of practice. It is based on cognitive, perceptual, psychological and social considerations and is used to explain the relationship between theory and practice. Conte and Conte (1977) describe a frame of reference as 'the sum of cultural, personal and psychological biases that inherently reside in subjective man, and that serve to colour and interpret reality'.

Unlike a paradigm, which provides a *general* structure for thought, a frame of reference is related to a particular facet of practice. It is not, however, confined specifically to one method of intervention, but covers particular aspects of thinking which may form the basis of a number of techniques.

In day-to-day practice the occupational therapist uses her own personal frames of reference to guide her interventions and explain her actions. Occupational therapy models and techniques have evolved partly through experienced individuals using their personal frames of reference methodologically to develop principles for practice. They have built on their own values, theories, practice, knowledge, and research findings to develop techniques which may be used by many members of the profession.

Frames of reference are therefore important to the professional development of the individual therapist and of the discipline as a whole. They lead to the use of 'a standard set of facts to judge, control or direct some action or expression' (Reed & Sanderson 1983) and to clarity in the explanation, evaluation and evolution of professional theory.

As Mosey (1981) writes:

A frame of reference delineates a particular aspect of a profession and provides a central theme to which to refer for decisions regarding the appropriateness of the programme design and content . . . It influences the practitioner's choices and approach to treatment and thus gives unity, balance and direction to the treatment programme.

APPROACHES

Approaches are the *ways and means of 'doing'*, i.e. of implementing frames of reference. An approach consists of the rationale behind a specific technique and the way in which it is used in practice. An approach may be used singly or in combination with others to achieve an aim or goal. For example, the rehabilitative approach, which is based on the compensatory frame of reference — the belief that a problem can best be overcome by compensating for it rather than through learning or development to improve anatomical, physiological or psychological function — may be used exclusively to treat a permanent impairment. However, where the impairment is likely to be temporary the rehabilitative approach may only be used for a short time, to be phased out in favour of another approach as recovery commences.

An approach determines *how* an activity may be used. Within the rehabilitative approach the therapist will assist a keen gardener to devise ways in which he can continue his hobby, e.g. through the provision of adapted tools or through modifications to the garden design. Within the neurodevelopmental approach, the therapist will use gardening to promote sitting or standing posture, balance and bilaterality. Within a biomechanical approach, a heavy gardening activity such as digging may be used to improve muscle strength and activity tolerance in the lower limbs.

MODELS

According to the Oxford dictionary a model is 'a physical or symbolic representation of an object or idea', 'a simplified description of a system', or 'a representation used as a basis or design'.

Everyone is familiar with three-dimensional scale models which replicate in miniature a real *object*, such as a train. Some may also be familiar with simulation models, which aim to portray or simulate a *situation* or *place*.

A *conceptual* model has been described as 'an abstract representation of practice' (Hopkins & Smith 1988, p. 383). It presents *theories* or *ideas* in schematic form, e.g. through charts, plans, pictures or flow diagrams, often showing the interrelationships between the parts in the whole.

A conceptual model of professional practice represents the basic concepts or theories behind intervention in a diagram or chart form, delineating the framework for professional action. This will be based on professional values and beliefs and display the links between theory and practice. Such a model may be used to promote clearer understanding, to clarify the boundaries and roles of intervention, to determine assessments and practices and to deduce anticipated outcomes.

A professional practice model may apply to any area of the profession, providing a framework for a number of aspects of intervention in a variety of realms of practice and a diagrammatic tool for explaining complex theories.

LINKING TERMS

Frequently there is difficulty in linking together the terms defined above, particularly when there is no consistent interpretation of the terms between texts.

In the context of the present volume, the *paradigm* of occupational therapy will be considered as the basis of the fundamental principles of the profession. It is comprised of the concepts that therapists hold in common concerning the ways in which man uses and benefits from occupation, that is, from his involvement, interaction and activity in life. These concepts derive from and are supported by the profession's *philosophy* regarding the essential humanity of man and his participation with and in his environment.

Theories have developed from this paradigm (as well as from other areas of knowledge and learning) to reflect therapists' values and beliefs about the nature of occupation, the criteria for defining and achieving competence and the essence of humanism. These theories have further led to the development of a number of *frames of reference* with regard to how man learns, develops and performs within his environment. *Approaches* have been devised in order to apply the philosophies and theories within these frames of reference in clinical practice.

Within this hierarchy of professional thinking, *models* exist at two levels. Some models have been devised and drawn up to explain particular approaches in relation to frames of reference. Other models show the integration of frames of references with theories. Thus some models, such as the behavioural model, may be confined to a particular aspect or area of practice, while others, such as the model of human occupation, may be more broadly based, explaining the interrelation of a number of frames of reference in a theoretical whole.

THEORY IN PRACTICE

The practice of occupational therapy is eclectic in that it selectively draws upon various schools of thought in addressing a wide variety of needs. This eclecticism has permitted the use of a number of frames of reference, each of which may be used to determine particular techniques and approaches in practice. Inevitably, these frames of reference overlap and to some degree may be integrated with one another, but each is significantly different in

its underlying theories and beliefs. Humanistic, occupations/activities, and biopsychosocial theories support individual aspects of practice but also underpin wider frames of reference and are used concurrently with them to form the basis of many approaches to practice. In this way, *theories* and *frames of reference* complement one another.

THE HUMANISTIC THEORY

This is based in existential psychology which, founded on the theories of 'self-actualisation' and 'the self' as described by Maslow and Rogers, views the individual as a free and responsible agent capable of determining his own development.

In humanistic theory, man is considered as a whole being — a Gestalt — rather than a collection of parts. Humanism perceives man optimistically, believing that human nature is essentially 'good'. Such positive beliefs are reflected in the view that human beings have an innate drive to be creative, to love, to grow and to be productive.

Frame of reference

Humanistic beliefs are used as the basis for specific approaches, but are more widely applied to the ways in which the therapist respects the autonomy and individuality of her clients in whatever approach she adopts. The humanistic frame of reference is based in the recognition of the person's capacity for self-awareness and his right and freedom to choose his own actions. This is the opposite of the didactic authoritarianism which predominated in many professions' earlier practices — the 'professional knows best' syndrome.

Basic assumptions

- The person has the potential for awareness of personal needs, drives and goals and has the ability to change through opportunities and experiences
- The quality of intrapersonal and interpersonal relationships and rapport are important in the development of self-esteem

- The individual has the right to make choices and prioritise according to his personal perceptions of strengths and needs and the right to preserve or develop an internal locus of control
- The positive strengths and abilities of the individual to overcome difficulties, rather than his weaknesses, should be emphasised
- Merely 'being able to do' is not sufficient. Feelings of purposefulness, skill and achievement are vital components in self-actualisation and self-esteem.

Humanism in practice

Within the humanistic frame of reference, the therapist respects the individual as a partner in therapy. Partnership in assessment of needs and priorities and in the negotiation of realistic, purposeful opportunities is the basis on which the therapeutic relationship grows. The therapist's essential belief in individual self-determination is reflected in the ways in which she helps him to make informed choices from a range of suitable options without exerting control over his decisions.

Practices which reflect humanism

- self-rating assessments
- recognition of values, roles and beliefs
- non-directive counselling
- providing opportunities for expressive interactions
- providing opportunities for informed prioritising
- acceptance of opinions and choices.

THE OCCUPATIONS/ACTIVITIES THEORY

This, the earliest theoretical base for occupational therapy, was founded in the belief that occupation and activity are instrumental in achieving and maintaining health. Theories regarding the value of occupations and activities developed from studies by Meyer, Barton, Reilly and others, but have their beginnings in the view of the relation be-

tween activity and health that was taken by the Romans and ancient Greeks (see Ch. 2).

The basis of the use of this theory in occupational therapy is summed up in Mary Reilly's (1962) well-known statement: 'Man through the use of his own hands, as they are energised by mind and will, can influence the state of his own health'.

In recent years, many therapists have striven to clarify the differences in meaning between 'occupation' and 'activity' in order to more clearly explain the profession's philosophy. Occupation has been defined as:

- 'volitional goal directed behaviour aimed at the development of play, work and life skills for optimal time management' (Rogers 1984)
- 'The dominant activity of human beings that includes serious productive pursuits, and playful, creative and festive behaviours' (Kielhofner 1983)
- 'Man's goal directed use of time, energy, interests and attention' (American Occupational Therapy Association 1976)
- 'Those activities and tasks which engage a person's time, energy and resources and are composed of skills and values' (Reed & Sanderson 1980)
- 'An active doing process of a person engaged in goal directed, intrinsically gratifying and culturally appropriate activity' (Evans 1987).

The Little Oxford Dictionary defines 'activity' as a 'task or action' or 'being active'. Within the realm of occupational therapy, activity is said to be 'purposeful' when the value of its use is to 'achieve mastery and competence' in those activities which have significance to the person 'in terms of social, cultural and personal meanings that are describably real and symbolic' (Fidler & Fidler 1978).

In summary, activity is *doing*, whereas occupation is a state of *being*, most frequently achieved through active participation in activity.

While there has been some deviation from the occupations/activities theory, particularly while other ideas developed in the 1950s and 60s, the belief in the value of occupation has remained central to the profession, either overtly in the use of purposeful activities in therapy, or covertly in the belief that other forms of therapy intervention will lead to competence in occupational tasks. For example, biomechanical exercises to improve mobility can enhance the person's ability in daily living or work tasks, thus serving an 'occupational' end.

Recent analysis of occupations/activities theory has led to a fuller appreciation of 'occupation' and a broadening of the recognition of the purposefulness of activities. Modern models and approaches based on this theory have been able to organise knowledge of the stages and factors which lead to successful 'occupational performance' into sequential hierarchical patterns by showing the interrelationships between internal and external components more comprehensively. They have been able to integrate beliefs from other frames of reference to explain ways in which a broader range of activities may be used purposefully to achieve occupational goals.

Examples

The occupations/activities theory has been formulated and refined in various ways, as in:

- Clark's human development through occupation model
- Cynkin and Robinson's activities health approach
- Kielhofner's model of human occupation
- Reed and Sanderson's human occupations model
- Reilly's occupational behaviour model.

Basic assumptions

- Occupations/activities are vital components of balanced, normal, healthy living
- Occupations/activities can be used in a variety of ways to overcome dysfunction and promote health in body and mind
- The most positive outcomes are achieved through occupations/activities which are purposeful and goal directed, offering realistic challenges and achievable outcomes

- The greatest personal commitment is obtained when the activities chosen are relevant to the individual's life-style, roles, aspirations and needs within his environment and respond realistically to his present levels of function.

The model of human occupation (Fig. 12.1)

One of the most widely publicised current models within the occupations/activities theory is the model of human occupation. This was devised by Kielhofner, Burke and Igi, in the late 70s and early 80s and is still being developed and refined.

The model is based on the 'open system' theory, which perceives man as a cyclic system capable of change and development in response to experience. The open system has four facets:

- input: the receipt and taking in of information
- throughput: the internal ability to organise incoming information and formulate actions and responses
- output: the presentation or performance of the response as action in the environment
- feedback: the recognition or acknowledgement of the consequences of the actions or response.

This feedback is then accepted back into the system as new input to continue the cycle.

In simple terms, the open system is a means of explaining experiential learning, i.e. the ways by which man learns and develops within his environment. Through activity, man is able to interact with his environment (output) and from the responses he receives as input from his actions (feedback) he is able to make considered judgements (throughput) and objectively change his future actions (output).

The model of human occupation describes the structure of occupation within a hierarchy of three subsystems: volition, habituation and performance.

Volition is the highest subsystem and is composed of values, interests and beliefs about oneself. These are seen as the most influential factors in

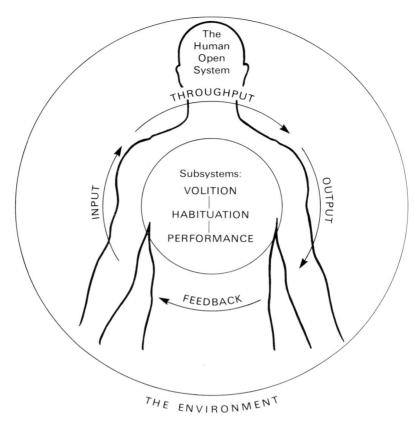

Fig. 12.1 Keilhofner's model of human occupation. (Adapted from Keilhofner 1985.)

determining priorities and goals and the driving forces which motivate the person to participate in activity.

The second subsystem is habituation, which is composed of personal habits and roles. These are linked to the driving forces of volition and are the basis of the person's perception of his roles, status and obligations, and of how these are organised in daily life.

The third subsystem is performance — the skills through which the person carries out various daily functions. These may be divided into process skills (for problem solving), interpersonal communicative skills and motor skills.

The three subsystems are seen to interact together, each providing input for the others.

The model of human occupation encompasses the physical, psychological and social aspects of performance and recognises the effects of the environment upon the individual. It can therefore be used in conjunction with a number of frames of reference to organise and structure investigative, analytical and intervention strategies. It can include within it a variety of therapeutic approaches in order to meet the particular volitional, habituational and performance requirements of the individual.

THE PSYCHOSOCIAL THEORY

This theory concentrates on the attainment of interpersonal and intrapersonal skills in the environment and was initially applied in relation to mental health. However, many of its principles are equally important in areas of physical or cognitive dysfunction in relation to social integration and role performance. The psychosocial theory may have application for those who have to make adjustments to living as the result of trauma affecting cognitive function (for example, following head injury) or for those who have a physical or perceptual dysfunction following disease or injury. Additionally, the initial acquisition of competent psychosocial performance may be limited or constrained through lack of opportunity or ability in the case of those who suffer congenital impairment.

Many practitioners, recognising the psychological and social implications of impairment, have incorporated aspects of the psychosocial theory into their frames of reference. These have been considered as factors to be included in planning holistic, humanistic intervention strategies, but have been combined with other areas within the frames of reference rather than being considered as a theory per se.

Mosey's psychosocial theory

The use of psychosocial theory in occupational therapy was expounded by Mosey in the 1970s and 80s. Mosey based her views on psychoanalytic and developmental theory, together with earlier occupational therapy theories. These included limitations identified in early habit training as used by Slagle, Fidler and Fidler's communication processes and Ayres' neurobehavioural orientation theory, together with her own previous theories of adaptive skills responses described in her *Recapitulation of Ontogenesis* (1966), a reflective summary of the stages of development of the individual.

Mosey's theories are based on the belief that individuals have an inherent need to explore the environment and that this need leads to a desire to be competent within that environment. The requirements to achieve competence are dependent on the nature of the society in which the individual functions and the social roles expected of and anticipated by him. The nature of the environ-

ment also has a significant effect on the process of learning.

Basic assumptions

- The process of social integration occurs through psychosocial learning regarding roles and role needs
- During illness the individual may lose skills but these can be relearned and regained
- Adaptation in each skill area occurs developmentally and is dependent on and related to adaptation in other skill areas
- Change (adaptation) occurs as a continuum from conscious learning and doing through non-conscious action to the adoption of unconscious habit as mastery develops
- Most adaptation occurs through practical interaction in a 'growth facilitating' environment which is realistic with regard to the area of need and provides opportunity to explore the skill area and receive feedback from it.

Mosey developed a biopsychosocial model in three main areas: analysis, development and acquisition. Within these areas she identified three frames of reference: the reconciliation of universal issues in the analytical aspect, the attainment of adaptive skills in the developmental aspect, and the adoption of roles in the acquisitional aspect. These may be described as follows:

Reconciliation of universal issue

This is 'concerned with the modification of intrapsychic content in such a manner that the individual is able to reconcile universal issues in a more adaptive manner' (Mosey 1966). Mosey identified eight 'universal issues': reality, trust, intimacy, adequacy, dependence/independence, sexuality, aggression and loss. She described change as occurring in four phases — communication, insight, assessment and working through. The individual is encouraged to become aware of his unconscious or unshared feelings, thoughts or beliefs about an aspect of one of the universal issues and to share or communicate them. These feelings are then explored and examined in order to promote insight. Following this, assessment occurs with a view to deciding whether to maintain the same beliefs or behaviours or to make changes in accordance with new insights. When the decision is to make a change, the individual will need support and help to work through any resulting anxieties or conflicts. Much of the process is facilitated through activities which promote transference, association and interpretation.

Adaptive skills

These form a 'developmental frame of reference addressed to those aspects of development considered to be crucial for adequate and satisfactory participation in a variety of social roles' (Mosey 1966). Adaptation occurs in seven main areas:

- perceptual/motor skill: the ability to recognise and make appropriate responses to sensory stimuli
- cognitive skill: the ability to process information and solve problems
- drive/object skill: the ability to manage and control personal drives in relation to current existing human and non-human objects
- dyadic interaction skill: the ability to engage and perform in a variety of one-to-one relationships
- group interaction skill: the ability to participate in a variety of group situations
- self-identity skill: the ability to recognise the self as an autonomous, competent, valued and developing being
- sexual identity skill: the ability to perceive one's sexual nature as 'good' and participate in long-term sexual relationships which are mutually pleasurable for those involved.

Mosey related these skills to stages of human development as described by Ayres, King and Llorens and identified ways through which an individual may be assisted to achieve such skills through learning in the environment.

Role acquisition (Fig. 12.2)

This is 'an acquisitional frame of reference addressed to those behaviours considered impor-

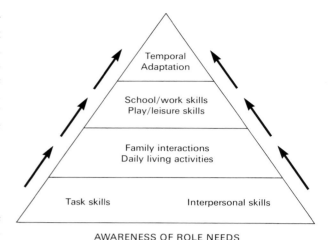

Fig. 12.2 Mosey's psychosocial theory: role acquisition (Mosey 1986).

tant for adequate participation in the major social roles' (Mosey 1986).

Acquisition of social roles is facilitated through group explorations which develop awareness and skills for successful interactions and performance within particular roles. The most basic skills for role acquisition are individual awareness of the needs of the role, competence in necessary personal tasks and interpersonal communicative skills. These are initially explored within the context of personal and family roles.

Social roles outside the family are developed through experiential group activities in which the task skills and interpersonal skills related to roles in school, at work and in social and leisure pursuits are explored. The culmination of role acquisition is 'temporal adaptation' — the ability of the person to recognise the appropriateness of each action or activity within a role, and to prioritise a number of tasks and needs realistically so that the requirements of different roles are adequately met.

Mosey's biopsychosocial model may be used in a number of ways in interventions for people with physical dysfunction. It may be used to address a particular aspect of intrapersonal or interpersonal dysfunction, or it may form a more general basis for determining approaches within a developmental or occupations/activities approach.

FRAMES OF REFERENCE RELATING TO PHYSICAL DYSFUNCTION

The approaches most frequently used in the last decade in Britain to overcome or compensate for physical dysfunction were the biomechanical, neurodevelopmental and rehabilitative approaches, which are based on the biomechanical, developmental and compensatory frames of reference. More recently, other approaches within the developmental frame of reference, such as the sensorimotor approach, have been used to promote particular aspects of function.

Occupational therapists also use other approaches and frames of reference in the field of physical dysfunction. For example, the cognitive approach, based on the learning frame of reference, may be used to identify the most effective way in which an activity might be carried out in order to promote learning in a particular aspect of living. In this approach, tests or assessments can be used to identify the ways in which a particular individual is best able to learn; for example, memory might be tested using verbal lists, pictures or demonstrations to determine what mnemonic techniques are most helpful for that individual, with a view to incorporating these into functional tasks.

THE DEVELOPMENTAL FRAME OF REFERENCE

This has had a significant influence upon occupational therapy practice since the 1940s; many approaches have been based on the theories of human development described by Piaget, Erikson, Freud and others.

Development occurs because of continuous interactions between nature (heredity, genetic factors and maturation) and nurture (the effects of experiences and the environment upon the individual). The development process affects the sensorimotor, cognitive, perceptual, personal and social domains of life. It can be attributed to: natural maturation; conscious interactions with the environment and external stimuli; the processes of learning; analysis, evaluation and making choices; and to uncontrolled occurrences which influence the individual.

Most frames of reference take into account some element of growth, progression and evolution but an understanding of human development is at the *core* of this frame of reference, dictating and guiding the stages of the approaches that derive from it.

Basic assumptions

- Dysfunction is due to incomplete, maladaptive or retarded behaviour. This may be the result of incomplete maturation, the inability to utilise input effectively or the paucity of stimuli
- The person has the potential for development
- Development occurs sequentially, each stage building on the previous one. Approaches relate closely to the stages of normal chronological human development
- Development occurs in sequential stages from the person's present level of capability. Missing or jumping stages is counterproductive
- Active co-operation rather than passive participation on behalf of the person involved facilitates greater development in most cases.

Examples

Some examples of developmental frames of reference which have influenced approaches to physical dysfunction are:

- Ayres' sensory integration model
- Rood's sensorimotor approach
- Llorens' developmental model
- Bobath and Bobath's neurodevelopmental approach
- Brunnstrom's movement therapy
- Voss, Ionta and Myers' proprioceptive neuromuscular facilitation approach.

Merits

- The developmental frame of reference uses theory to good effect by incorporating the normal processes of physiological and

psychological progression into intervention strategies
- The belief is one of optimism for each stage's completion and there is a defined progression
- The commencement point for intervention is flexible, reflecting the person's present state, and there is no definitive rate of progress. The programme is therefore adaptable to a variety of levels of need and rates of development.

Limitations

- Progress may appear slower than in some approaches as each stage should be achieved before moving on to the next
- The developmental frame of reference is inappropriate for deteriorating conditions
- Many individual approaches within this frame of reference require high levels of expertise which are fully developed only at a post-graduate level
- In order to attain maximum progress a coordinated, consistent approach is required from all members of the intervention team.

A sample approach

A widely used approach which is developmentally based is the neurodevelopmental approach as proposed by Karel and Bertha Bobath in the 1940s and 50s in the treatment of children with cerebral palsy. In recent years this has been extended and modified for the treatment of some adult neurological disorders, particularly hemiplegia as the result of cerebrovascular accident (CVA) or head injury.

This approach makes use of positions which inhibit abnormal postures and patterns of movement, but facilitate normal equilibrium, balance and righting reactions and encourage normal movement patterns. Its basic principles are derived from the neurological learning frame of reference and from theories of normal human development. The approach attempts to apply these principles to all aspects of activity throughout the day. It considers that the immature or damaged brain, because of the lack of opportunity to develop sophisticated balance control, or because of interruption or blocking of such patterns by trauma to pathways within the brain, gives rise to primitive or abnormal muscle tone and movement patterns. By inhibiting or suppressing these abnormal patterns, and then stimulating normal sensory, postural and motor patterns, the brain may be stimulated to develop normal patterns through alternative pathways. The neurodevelopmental approach is most successful if begun in very early life for the child with cerebral palsy, or as early as is practicable after a CVA or head injury.

The sequence of treatment follows the normal sequence of development of movement in children. Man is essentially symmetrical, and positioning and movement patterns aim to simulate and encourage bilaterality and symmetry whilst developing normal movement sequences. Alongside the development of motor patterns, stimulation of sensation and body awareness through touch and positioning is encouraged in order to assist the re-education of sensory pathways and to enhance the ability of the brain to interpret perceptual stimuli.

Integration of these principles within a programme of purposeful activities facilitates the development of sensorimotor control, which will then enable successful occupational performance. Concern has been expressed by some occupational therapists that the exclusive use of neurodevelopmental approaches in occupational therapy neglects such aspects as volition, motivation or occupational needs. For use in the occupational therapy framework, 'it is necessary to expand knowledge of the logical continuity beyond inhibition–facilitation techniques to activity, and to ways in which sensori-motor treatment principles can be applied during the performance of purposeful activity' (Pedretti 1985, p. 5).

THE BIOMECHANICAL (BODY/MACHINE) FRAME OF REFERENCE

This frame of reference has been the basis of many medical interventions throughout the century. It views the body as a functioning machine, made up of specific parts which may be damaged by disease or injury. This frame of reference is based in the desire to explain function scientifically and many of its basic premises formed the foundations on which exercise physiology, surgery and chemotherapy developed within the medical model. The body is seen as being made up of a combination of parts which join together to form a whole; however, the Gestalt (the sum of the whole being more than a combination of the parts) is not acknowledged. Treatment to overcome damage to a particular part results in the return of function. Therapeutic exercise or activity improves functional performance; this in turn leads to a sense of well-being, which promotes recovery.

Basic assumptions

- Successful human activity is based on physical mobility and strength
- Participation in activity involving repeated, specific, and graded tasks maintains and improves function
- Activity can be graded to meet particular demands progressively within a programme of intervention.

Approaches

Three slightly different biomechanical approaches were developed:

- Baldwin's reconstruction approach. (This was presented in 1918 and was one of the earliest documented 'physical' approaches)
- Taylor's orthopaedic approach (1934)
- Licht's kinetic approach (1957).

While each of these approaches have slightly different emphases, all are based in the biomechanical frame of reference, and thus in the physical field of practice. They are utilised in physiotherapy and in physical rehabilitation in occupational therapy to promote mobility, strength and activity tolerance (stamina). Their early popularity reflected the essentially scientific nature of medical development, particularly in the physical field.

Merits

- The biomechanical frame of reference makes good use of media and equipment to promote physical function
- It can be applied to a variety of creative and constructive activities
- It uses knowledge of activity analysis to good effect
- It has utilised increased knowledge of anatomical, physiological and kinaesthetic processes in man
- It has led to the development of specific techniques for measuring movement, strength and endurance.

Limitations

- The biomechanical frame of reference focuses on physical performance in the absence of volition or environmental influences. It is specifically based in physical activity with no reference to mental health or the psychological, social or emotional aspects of rehabilitation.
- It does not address the need for balance in activity in daily life. It emphasises lower levels for survival — mobility and physical function — but does not follow through to the higher levels of self-esteem and self-actualisation
- It is not applicable to conditions in which the central nervous system is impaired. The emphasis is on the promotion of physical mobility; therefore this frame of reference is not relevant to those with chronic or deteriorating conditions affecting mobility.
- There is a risk of didactic reductionism — the therapist controlling the programme and the person being a passive participant within a regime which does not necessarily reflect personal interests or promote an internal locus of control.

Current use

Biomechanical approaches were widely used in the 1960s but are less popular today, forming only a small part of the occupational therapist's treatment methodology. The mechanistic compartmentalisation of functional performance into physical actions contradicts the holism and humanism of occupational therapy's philosophy. Overcoming specific biomechanical dysfunction is only part of the management of the individual's total needs, mobility being only one part of function. However, since mobility *is* an important aspect of life, the principles of the biomechanical approach may form a part, if not the whole, of the therapeutic programme.

The changing nature of occupational therapy practice (which can be seen in the shift from hospital- to community-based work, and in the increase in the proportion of people with complex, chronic disabilities and neurological conditions) further limits the use of this approach. Increased awareness of the merits of broadly-based holism as opposed to specialisation may further reduce the importance of this frame of reference in the total intervention programme.

Many occupational therapists have already abandoned the exclusive use of many biomechanical practices, although certain measurement techniques and activity analyses are useful in particular aspects of treatment. Some features of the biomechanical frame of reference combined with other, less reductionist, approaches retain importance in specific areas of practice, particularly orthopaedics, sports medicine and the treatment of physical damage resulting from trauma. Other professions, including physical medicine, nursing and physiotherapy are adopting more humanistic, holistic philosophies, which may further contribute to the decline in popularity of the biomechanical frame of reference.

THE COMPENSATORY FRAME OF REFERENCE

This frame of reference is based in the belief that man is a functional animal and that his ability to function — by whatever method necessary — is essential to his well-being. It stresses the secondary benefit to be gained by improving performance in activity or occupation despite ongoing physical, cognitive, psychological or social disability. A number of different compensatory methods may be used to perform an activity. The successful completion of the activity, rather than a specific change in anatomical, physiological or psychological bodily processes, is the primary goal, for this is what will enable the person to succeed in society.

Compensation may be used to facilitate the performance of a variety of activities in daily life by the use of remaining abilities and strengths and of external compensatory aids, but does not directly contribute to changing the person's biological, physiological or psychological deficits. This is one of the oldest frames of reference for rehabilitation. It is not unique to occupational therapy, but is also used by physiotherapists, (for example, in the provision of walking sticks and frames), by orthotists and prosthetists, and to some degree by speech therapists when alternative communication equipment or techniques are recommended.

Basic assumptions

- Completion of daily role activities is a basic human need; the disabled individual can benefit by learning alternative methods for carrying out these activities
- People suffer short- and long-term dysfunction which cannot be immediately or significantly improved by other therapeutic methods, so there is a need for compensation for lost or limited abilities
- Residual capabilities can be supplemented by external aids to promote problem-solving
- The individual's involvement in choosing appropriate methods can be advantageous in promoting some general aspects of 'well-being'.

This frame of reference has been documented in occupational therapy primarily in terms of the rehabilitative approach (Trombly 1989).

Merits

- The compensatory frame of reference is a widely documented and widely used basis for therapy practice. Many therapists are familiar with it
- It is easy to explain and understand

- It makes good use of a problem-solving approach
- It can be used to meet immediate short-term needs or to compensate for long-term loss. It is therefore appropriate for acute needs, for example immediately following surgery, or for people with chronic or deteriorating disorders who are not likely to recover or improve
- A range of options is available, with considerable choice within them to meet a wide variety of needs
- There is no rigidly structured sequence of progression, so there can be flexibility to meet the particular needs of the individual.

Limitations

- Historically, this frame of reference has had a long association with the medical model, and so may be prone to reductionist or recipe-like thinking. The therapist may be tempted to 'prescribe' the 'best' method of compensating for a particular problem, rather than evaluate the range of options with the person concerned. A tendency, deriving from the medical model, to compartmentalise problems may fragment this potentially holistic approach into physical and psychological divisions.
- The recognition of permanence of loss of function may have negative connotations for the individual, who will then require considerable support.
- In choosing solutions the therapist may be at risk of succumbing to external pressures concerning the quickest or cheapest way of compensating, thereby denying personal choice. Compensation per se may be seen as a solution in cases where the use of other approaches and frames of reference may in fact promote or facilitate physical or psychological recovery or improvement.

The rehabilitative approach

This approach is most widely used to compensate for dysfunction in mobility, self-maintenance and domestic activities, but is also used in the pro-motion of work and leisure pursuits. It applies all the basic beliefs and practices of the compensatory frame of reference. Occupational therapists using this approach must recognise the individual's need to be actively consulted and involved in the choice of the most appropriate method of compensation; this involvement will help to motivate the person to accept and persevere with the chosen solution.

A therapeutic programme using the rehabilitative approach may include:

- The teaching of 'trick' movements, alternative techniques and the use of cognitive prompts
- The provision of prostheses or support orthoses
- The supply of adapted tools or equipment.
- The modification of the environment
- The provision of financial help
- The organisation of manual/social assistance.

The therapist using this approach must acknowledge the need for flexibility and adaptability in responding to a particular person's circumstances. It will obviously be advantageous in the majority of instances to consider the use of a 'trick' movement or technique, or of cognitive prompts, as these are constantly available to the person wherever he may be, and can be used to overcome a number of different problems. Support orthoses have similar value in potentially solving a variety of problems, provided they are worn consistently and correctly.

Adapted tools and equipment may have a wide application in some instances, but some equipment or tools may be specific to one particular task and may not be easily transferable or transportable. Environmental adaptations are often considered a more drastic measure, as they are more likely to overtly stigmatise the person with the problem and affect other members of the family; they are also more costly. An adaptation can usually be made to particular environments pertinent to the individual, e.g. home, work or school, but their rehabilitative value is limited to these locations. The implications of restricted freedom in the wider environment will still have to be addressed.

Financial benefits may be used rehabilitatively to purchase equipment or services to compensate for deficit; for example, a person who is unable to perform the full range of food preparation might buy an electric food mixer or microwave oven or make arrangements for prepared food delivery. Such financial benefits may enable the person to pursue personal preferences, depending upon the range of options available and the funding provided.

Arranging for helpers to assist with certain tasks will require the person to recognise his limitations and to decide that the tasks in question are essential to him, despite the loss of independence they entail. Increased dependence upon others may be viewed positively, by virtue of the social contact it brings. It also enables the person to conserve his energy for other personal priorities.

Obviously, as there is such a wide variety of options available in the rehabilitative approach, detailed assessment of functional capabilities and life-style needs is essential. From these findings the priorities and options for problem-solving should be discussed so that optimum solutions are found. These will depend on personal preferences and volition, the level, nature and probable duration of the dysfunction, and the social environment. Additionally, the person's potential to learn new skills and use equipment or other resources should be considered.

It may sometimes be necessary to explore a number of rehabilitative options before the optimal solution is hit upon. For the person with a progressive condition it will be necessary to re-evaluate the choice of options and methods used as the condition progresses, but this should be minimised by forward thinking and proactive planning.

THE LEARNING FRAME OF REFERENCE

This frame of reference, which is based on the work of educational psychologists and behaviourists such as Piaget, Bandura, Lorenz, Argyle, Hilgard, Thorndike and Skinner can be applied to the treatment of physical dysfunction. There is an element of learning in most aspects of therapy, but the theories of cognitive and conditioned learning are central to the beliefs of this frame of reference.

Basic assumptions

- The person has the capacity to learn through education
- The acquisition of positive skills and appropriate attitudes and behaviours will change the individual and promote well-being and social acceptance
- Behaviour is learned. 'Poor' or non-advantageous habits can be unlearned and replaced by lasting, helpful, 'good' habits through positive experiences and practice
- Learning occurs through different educational modes and may be basically cognitive or conditioned.

This frame of reference is used to support some of the approaches used within other frames of reference. It is a major influence in some aspects of practice, for example:

- social skills training
- assertiveness training
- anxiety/stress management
- joint protection and time management education
- behaviour modification.

CONCLUSION

Without a theory base a profession has no foundation and no planned direction. Without a theory base the professional will be ill equipped to assess the situations she is faced with and to respond to them in a realistic and organised manner.

Understanding the theory base of occupational therapy is a complex task, given the eclectic nature of today's practice, the diversity of individuals' needs and the current emphasis upon humanistic principles in therapy. Appreciation of the individual needs and drives of her clientele and an understanding of theory will assist the therapist in her professional reasoning and reflection.

The therapist herself is an individual with personal values and beliefs which may influence her choice of frames of reference. Recognition of these within the context of other frames of reference and the broader pattern of theory will enable her to more fully understand her own professional approach and that of others.

No profession stands alone; a sound theory base is necessary to identify the strengths and boundaries of a profession in the context of multi-professional health care provision.

No society stands still; theory is essential in guiding research and development in the profession, in order to meet the changing needs of individuals and ensure that the profession of occupational therapy remains up-to-date in its practices.

REFERENCES

American Occupational Therapy Association 1976 Occupational therapy: its definition and functions. American Journal of Occupational Therapy 20: 204

Black J A, Champion D J 1976 Methods and issues in social research. John Wiley, New York

British Association of Occupational Therapists 1990 Code of Ethics and Professional Conduct. British Journal of Occupational Therapy 53(4): 143–8.

Conte J, Conte W 1977 The association: the use of conceptual models in occupational therapy. American Journal of Occupational Therapy 31(4): 262–4

Evans K A 1987 Definition of occupation as the core concept of occupational therapy. American Journal of Occupational Therapy 41(10): 627–8

Fidler G, Fidler J 1978 Doing and becoming: purposeful action and self actualisation. American Journal of Occupational Therapy 32(5): 305–310

Kielhofner G 1983 Health through occupation. Theory and practice in occupational therapy. Davis, Philadelphia

Kielhofner G 1985 The model of human occupation. Williams & Wilkins, Baltimore

Licht S 1957 Kinetic occupational therapy. In: Dunton W R, Licht S Occupational therapy principles and practice. Thomas, Illinois

Llorens L A 1970 Facilitating growth and development. The promise of occupational therapy. American Journal of Occupational Therapy 24(1): 93–101

Lyons M 1985 Paradise lost! Paradise regained? Putting the promise of occupational therapy into practice. Australian Journal of Occupational Therapy 32(2): 45–53

Maslow A 1968 Toward a psychology of being. Van Nostrand, New York

Meyer A 1922 The philosophy of occupational therapy. Archives of Occupational Therapy. 1: 1–10

Mosey A C 1966 Recapitulation of ontogenesis: a theory for practice of occupational therapy. American Journal of Occupational Therapy 22: 426–432

Mosey A C 1981 Configuration of a profession. Raven Press, New York

Mosey A C 1986 Psychosocial components of occupational therapy. Raven Press, New York

Pedretti L W 1985 Occupational therapy: practice skills for physical dysfunction, 2nd edn. Mosby, St Louis

Piaget J 1950 Psychology of intelligence. Routledge & Kegan Paul, London

Reed K, Sanderson S R 1983 Concepts of occupational therapy. Williams & Wilkins, Baltimore

Reilly M 1962 Occupational therapy can be one of the great ideas of 20th century medicine. American Journal of Occupational Therapy 16: 1

Rogers C R 1967 On becoming a person. Constable, London

Rogers J C 1983 Eleanor Clarke Slagle Lecture. Clinical reasoning: the ethics, science and art. American Journal of Occupational Therapy 37(9): 601–616

Rogers J C 1984 The foundation: Why study human occupation? American Journal of Occupational Therapy 38: 47–49

Taylor E, Mitchell M 1990 Research attitudes and activities of occupational therapy clinicians. American Journal of Occupational Therapy 44(4): 350–355

Trombly C A 1989 Occupational therapy for physical dysfunction. Williams & Wilkins, Baltimore

Voss D E, Ionta M K, Myers B J 1985 Proprioceptive neuromuscular facilitation: patterns and techniques, 3rd edn. Harper & Row, New York

Yerxa E J 1979 The philosophical base of occupational therapy in 2001AD. American Occupational Therapy Association. Rockville, Maryland.

FURTHER READING

Ackerman W B, Lohnes P R 1981 Research methods for nurses. McGraw Hill, New York

Alexander L, French G, Graham G, King L, Timewell E 1985 Who needs a theory of occupational therapy? Do you? Australian Occupational Therapy Journal 32(3): 104–108

Allport G 1940 The psychologist's frame of reference. Psychology Bulletin 37(24)

Argyle M (ed) 1981 Social skills and health. Methuen, London

Argyle M 1978 Psychology of interpersonal behaviour. Penguin, Harmondsworth

Ayres A J 1973 Sensory integration and learning disorders. Western Psychological Service, Los Angeles

Baldwin B T 1919 Occupational Therapy. American Journal for Care of Cripples 8: 447–451

Bandura A L, Walters R H 1963 Social learning and personality development. Holt, Rinehart & Winston, New York

Bandura A L 1971 Social learning theory. General Learning Press, New York

Barnitt R 1990 Knowledge skills and attitudes. What happens to thinking? Proceedings of 10th World Federation of Occupational Therapists International Conference, Melbourne, Australia

Barris R, Kielhofner G, Watts H V 1983 Psychosocial occupational therapy. Ramsco, Maryland

Barton W E 1943 The challenge of occupational therapy. Occupational Therapy Rehabilitation 22: 262

Beck A T 1976 Cognitive therapy and emotional disorders. International University Press, New York

Berger R M, Patchner M A 1988 Planning for research. A guide for the helping professions. Sage, California

Black J A, Champion D J 1976 Methods and issues in social research. John Wiley, New York

Bobath B, Bobath K 1975 Motor development in the different types of cerebral palsy. Heinemann Medical, London

Bobath B 1978 Adult hemiplegia. Evaluation and treatment. Heinemann Medical, London

Bruce M A, Borg B 1987 Frames of reference in psychosocial occupational therapy. Slack, New Jersey

Brunnstrom S 1970 Movement therapy in hemiplegia. Harper & Row, New York

Calnan J 1984 Coping with research. Heinemann, London

Clark P N 1979 Human development through occupation: a philosophy and conceptual model for practice, part 2. American Journal of Occupational Therapy 33(9): 577–584

College of Occupational Therapists 1985 Research advice handbook for occupational therapists. COT, London

Corey G 1982 Theory and practice of counselling and psychotherapy, 2nd edn. Brooks/Cole, Monterey

Cracknell E 1984 Humanistic psychology. In: Willson M (ed) Occupational therapy in short term psychiatry. Churchill Livingstone, Edinburgh

Cynkin S, Robinson A M 1990 Occupational therapy and activities health: toward health through activities. Little, Brown, Boston

Eden S 1987 Ethnic groups. In: Bumphrey E (ed) Occupational therapy in the community. Woodhead Faulkener, London

Ellis M 1981 Why bother with research? British Journal of Occupational Therapy 44(4): 115–6

Erikson E 1950 Childhood and society. W W Norton, New York

Freud A 1965 Normality and pathology in childhood. Assessment and development. International Universities Press, New York

Hilgard E R, Atkinson C A, Atkinson R L 1975 Introduction to psychology. Harcourt Brace Jovanovich, New York

Hopkins H L, Smith H D (eds) 1988 Willard and Spackman's occupational therapy. Lippincott, Philadelphia

Kielhofner G, Burke J P, Igi C H 1980 The model of human occupation, parts 1–4. American Journal of Occupational Therapy 34(9–12): 572–581, 663–675, 731–737, 777–788

Levins M 1986 The psychodynamics of activity. British Journal of Occupational Therapy 49(3): 87–9

Mares P, Henley A, Baxter C 1985 Health care in multiracial Britain. National Education Council and National Extension College Trust, Cambridge

Mocellin G 1988 A perspective of the principles and practice of occupational therapy. British Journal of Occupational Therapy 51(1): 4–7

Parham D 1987 Toward professionalism: the reflective practitioner. American Journal of Occupational Therapy. 41(9): 555–560

Partridge C, Barnitt R 1986 Research guidelines. A handbook for therapists. Heinemann, London

Rood M S 1954 Neurophysiological reactions as a basis for physical therapy. Physical Therapy Review 34: 444–449

Royeen C B (ed) 1988 Research tradition in occupational therapy. Process, philosophy and status. Slack, New Jersey

Skinner B F 1938 The behaviour of organisms. Appleton-Century-Crofts, New York

Skinner B F 1968 The technology of teaching. Appleton-Century-Crofts, New York

Slagle E C 1988 Historical perspectives of occupational therapy. In: Hopkins H L, Smith H D (eds) Willard and Spackman's occupational therapy. Lippincott, Philadelphia

Taylor M 1934 The treatment of orthopaedic conditions. Canadian Journal of Occupational Therapy 2: 1–8

Thorndike E L 1932 The fundamentals of learning. Teachers College, Columbia University, New York

Wallis M A 1987 'Profession' and 'professionalism' and the emerging profession of occupational therapy, Part 1. British Journal of Occupational Therapy 50(8): 264–5

Willson M 1987 Occupational therapy in long term psychiatry, 2nd edn. Churchill Livingstone, Edinburgh

Young M 1984 Models of practice for occupational therapy. British Journal of Occupational Therapy 47(12): 381–2

13

Roles in daily life and professional practice

Sybil E. Johnson

INTRODUCTION

A role is a combination of attitudes and strategies which are used to maintain an individual's status and self-esteem. In other words, it is a part played or a function fulfilled by a person in particular circumstances. Nature enables animals to play many parts and to adapt to their environment. Man has throughout his history adopted many roles — hunter, fighter, farmer, wage-earner, and so on — in order to survive.

Life confers a variety of roles on every individual throughout his life cycle. Each of us is someone's son or daughter; many of us, as life progresses, become partners, parents, uncles or aunts, and grandparents. In addition to our familial roles we acquire others relating to work, interests and hobbies, beliefs and culture.

In order to maintain status and self-esteem in today's rapidly changing world, we enact different roles, in different places, with different codes of behaviour and appearance. We are profoundly influenced by these roles, which distinguish us as individuals and assign us a specific place in society. Our role at home may be that of loving parents whose every effort is concerned with family activities and with maintaining harmonious family relationships. Our work role will involve adhering to workplace rules and regulations and to a code of ethics, and may also entail adopting a particular way of dressing.

Roles are central to daily life. The occupational therapist needs to understand the relevance and importance of people's roles generally, including her own, and those of individuals in their particular family, culture and environment. The early sections of this chapter consider the roles people adopt through the normal stages of development from childhood to old age. The importance of maintaining 'role balance' is discussed, along with the difficulties that can arise when different roles conflict with one another and when accustomed roles are lost. Illness, disability or any other interruption to a person's routine life pattern will disrupt the roles he accepts as his norm. Enforced role changes — for example, from that of family provider to the 'sick role' — have to be dealt with and modified by the occupational therapist.

However, in the course of her work, the therapist herself must adopt and develop particular roles in response to varying circumstances. This chapter, therefore, outlines some of the roles occupational therapists perform in order to facilitate an individual's return, following illness or disability, to a balanced set of roles and behaviours. The therapist's roles may depend upon age, experience, expertise and status, and are influenced by the expectation that she will behave in a certain, acceptable manner, identified by her uniform, the work she undertakes, and the environment in which she functions.

In addition to the occupational therapist's clinical role, other roles will be enacted. These will vary with circumstance but will particularly relate to individuals referred to therapy and may include: facilitator, key worker, assessor, mentor, problem-solver, and teacher (Fig. 13.1). Several roles may be utilised simultaneously during a course of therapy with one individual and his family. At other times the emphasis will be on one specific role, for example, that of interviewer or listener.

The final sections of the chapter consider the roles played by the occupational therapist in relation to those enacted by other members of the multidisciplinary team. In particular, the use of a

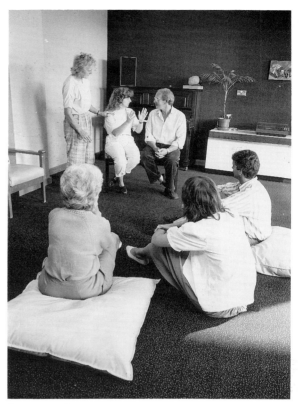

Fig. 13.1 Occupational therapists enact many roles, for example, that of teacher.

'key worker' is considered as a means of coordinating and facilitating the efforts of various professionals and of preventing 'role confusion' among colleagues as they work together in the interests of the disabled person.

THE DEVELOPMENT AND DISRUPTION OF ROLES THROUGHOUT LIFE

Development comprises an identifiable pattern of change in all people, from cradle to grave. During the various stages of human development individuals learn and master certain skills, building upon these as years pass, or putting them to one side if they are no longer required. During normal development from infancy through childhood and adolescence to adulthood an individual also develops or adopts certain roles (Table 13.1). This is a normal process and it is recognised that particular roles entailing specific types of behaviour are enacted by everyone in society. These roles will relate to status, to social convention, to culture and, in particular, to family life, in which people have roles as parent, child, sibling or partner. Society expects individuals to accept and conform to particular roles at different stages in their lives, for example, to the work role in adulthood.

If therapists endeavour to facilitate normal patterns of development in those with whom they work they need to understand how roles develop and change within and between life stages. This enables a therapist to modify her behaviour and professional role accordingly, thus assisting her to comprehend the multiple potential problems of the different life stages and the relationship of work, play, relaxation (Fig. 13.2), education, retirement and development itself with those stages.

Development of childhood roles

There are three periods of role development within childhood. The first, infant/toddler, is a period of very limited roles which begins with one of total dependency and develops into those of learner and player. It is only when the child approaches two years of age that he starts to adopt a family-member role, as he begins to recognise that he 'belongs' to a certain small group of people, which includes himself.

From the age of 2 until he is 5 or 6 his family-member role develops and he demonstrates this as

Table 13.1 Developmental stages and associated roles: a summary

Developmental stage	Associated roles
1. Infant	Total dependence — player, learner Family member role commences
2. Small child (pre-school)	Family member role increases Player role expands — experimentation with roles observed in others Friend role commences
3. Child (junior school age)	Increase in roles and experimentation Schoolchild Family member role continues to increase Friend role increasingly important Begins to perceive certain roles
4. Adolescent	Student Family member role subject to change over time Role experimentation — adulthood Friend role important — both sexes Worker — assumes equal importance with friend role Player — greater diversity
5. Adult	Partner, parent, homemaker Worker/breadwinner Leisure and friendship roles Social, organisational, cultural roles
6. Older person	Role continuity/gains — family, friends, work (paid or unpaid), leisure, education Role loss: bereavement, retirement, moving house

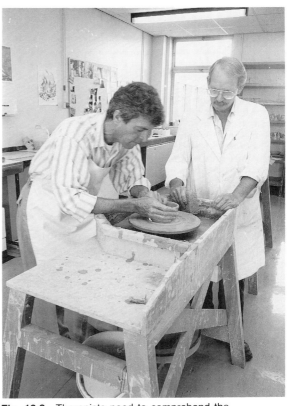

Fig. 13.2 Therapists need to comprehend the relationship between different life stages and work, play, relaxation, education, retirement and development itself. Recreational and creative outlets are vital ingredients for a balanced life-style.

he conforms increasingly to the demands of family life. His play role becomes more advanced and through this role in particular he first develops into the friend of another child of a similar age. He also experiments with other roles through play, copying his parents or other adults in, for example, work or home care roles.

During junior school years, i.e. when the child is from 5 or 6 to 11 years old, one observes a substantial increase in the roles he develops and with which he experiments. He becomes a schoolchild and this affects his other roles. Friendship within his peer group becomes increasingly important and may extend into membership of another group, for example, Cubs, Brownies and, later, Scouts and Guides. He increases his participation in home care activities and his access to additional role models becomes evident. At this stage he also begins to perceive certain roles and will act accordingly for example, by declaring 'I am a scout, this is my uniform and I have obtained these badges.'

Development of roles in adolescence

Adolescence is a period of transition from child to adult status. It is a time of experiment which aims to assist a young person to consolidate his identity, status and independence. He will still have student and family-member roles but he may also adopt a new worker role, particularly at weekends and during holidays, for example, by helping at a holiday play scheme or assisting in a local shop. This new worker role, along with the friendship role, is probably the most important. The adolescent may find, however, that he experiences role conflict for the first time, e.g. his student role may be at odds with his worker role. He may not be able to cope with others' expectations of his new roles initially, but as he grows and develops he will adopt new roles through negotiation with others or by conforming to the accepted norms of his society or culture.

Disruption of roles in childhood and adolescence

Children's and young people's roles relate primar-

ily to play, school, self-care, family life and peer interaction. The development of abnormal roles or the disruption or loss of normal ones commonly accompanies illness or disability, whether congenital or acquired. A severely handicapped child may not develop the concept of certain roles. For example, his immobility may prevent copying of adult work roles, and he may adopt a permanent 'sick role', particularly if his condition warrants lengthy stays in or numerous visits to hospital.

When a child's potential roles remain undeveloped, his parents' roles will be affected to a greater or lesser degree; for example, their caring role may increase, thereby interfering with or even excluding previous roles such as that of worker. Parents may place disproportionate importance on developmental milestones such as talking or walking but may overlook behaviours and subsequent roles related to play or peer interaction. A child may be overprotected or perceive himself as 'sick'. Roles relating to play and school may be severely disrupted and adjustment to possible roles may have to be sought; for example, the young person with muscular dystrophy will need to adjust and possibly relinquish certain roles as his abilities decrease.

Roles in adulthood

For the purposes of this discussion, let us consider adulthood as comprising the years between adolescence and normal retirement age, i.e. a span of approximately 40 years. Culturally and socially appointed and individually selected roles structure an individual's life. He will probably be a worker, parent and homemaker and will also enact other social or organisational roles dictated or influenced by leisure interests and/or friendships. Whatever roles he adopts will guide his performance; e.g. work roles will direct working day activity. Adopted roles will overlap and interrelate with daily routines, such as getting up and getting ready to go to work. The individual's roles and their relationship with his routines may be quite stable for long periods of time, peaking in middle adulthood when he has to divide his time among numerous roles. However, he may experience role conflict as he endeavours to meet the demands of family life, work and leisure.

Disruption of roles in adulthood

If an adult experiences physical limitations these will frequently interfere with his normal roles. If he is the family breadwinner and has an accident which results in permanent dysfunction it may not be possible for him to return to or maintain his former employment or work role. If, on the other hand, he attempts to resume that role he may have to modify his expectations, e.g. change employment. Role changes are exceedingly stressful both for the individual and his family. Conflicts may arise as a result of the differing expectations of family members, the individual believing he can achieve one level, the family another level of role performance.

Another significant role change in families concerns the parent/child relationship. The adult may begin caring for elderly parents, whilst his own children no longer need 'parenting'. This too may give rise to conflict, particularly concerning the nature of 'duty' and in which direction that duty lies.

Role loss in adults may mean reversion to lower-level roles — for example, to the role of 'dependant' — and can also result in loss of identity, decreased self-esteem and a sense of bereavement. The company director with advanced motor neurone disease will, for example, lose his high-status work role and may be forced to adopt less important roles within his family whilst attempting to salvage his self-esteem and to manage his grief.

The most significant effect of physical dysfunction on the adult is his enforced 'sick role', in which he may have a passive, dependent relationship with those caring for him, i.e. family, doctor, therapist, nurse. This role is wholly counterproductive. If the individual is to gain most benefit from his rehabilitation he has to take increasing responsibility for his own future and for his adaptation to temporary, permanent or progressive inabilities. In conjunction with his battle against the sick role he may have to contend with overprotection by his family, i.e. being treated as though he is more handicapped than his dysfunction dictates.

Frequently, his inability to participate in his previously accepted roles will result in confusion about his status and current roles, and will give rise to symptoms such as pain, fatigue or sensory loss not necessarily associated with his condition. In addition, the psychological effects of physical illness and disability may well disrupt his role performance, leading to imbalance or conflicting demands as he finds himself unable to meet the many obligations of several roles or attempts to achieve equally in all roles, for example, striving to be an active parent as well as a highly skilled worker.

Conversely, having too few roles will be more detrimental to the individual's mental health than the reverse position. Loss of roles affects individuals in different ways and their reaction to the loss often depends on which role they have to forgo. Hence, one person may suffer depression whilst others may succumb to stress-related illness, increased substance abuse or increased anxiety.

Roles of older people

People have less control over their roles as they grow older, and they need to adjust in order to maintain their identity and daily routines. Their roles are often extensive and may be associated with family, friends, voluntary work, alternative paid employment, education and leisure. Older people experience major role changes, primarily associated with retirement, moving house or the death of their partner. However, in order to maintain good health they need role continuity and role gains, that is to continue in certain pre-retirement roles and to replace roles they have lost, such as the work role.

Retirement for most people is a time of opportunity and enjoyment, of true relaxation and further learning. However, for some, adjustment is often more difficult. Changes to the individual's environment, for example an enforced change of home or the deaths of partners or close friends, over time cause repeated role loss to which the individual may respond by adopting negative roles. He may view himself as dependent, worthless or helpless, and as having no valued roles, at the same time as he has high expectations of himself, for example as a grandparent or as someone with much life experience to share.

Role balance

Role balance, i.e. a healthy distribution of 'work, rest and play', ensures that roles do not conflict or compete for an individual's time. Having different roles offers the individual rhythm, healthy change, time and energy for enacting the tasks associated with each (Fig. 13.2). Role balance is possible only when the individual has a sense of identity and purpose and the expectations and structure to guide and use his time in relation to paid or unpaid work, or home, his favourite pastime and visiting friends. Roles provide a means of directing him in the required behaviours and tasks expected within his cultural/social group and environment.

Role strain

At some time or other everyone suffers from role strain, i.e. being torn between two or more incompatible demands, for example, the need to study for an examination and the desire to spend the weekend with friends. Role imbalance can also be caused by role loss or by an initial lack of roles. Roles give the individual's life structure and direction; without them he has no identity or purpose and can become disorientated. Often, the loss of one role is followed by the adoption of another, e.g. as the student becomes a worker. In other circumstances (such as retirement or the death of a partner) roles may end more abruptly and it is then far more difficult to adopt new ones. Behaviour is more readily adapted to role loss if a person has other roles which can assume more importance, as in the case of a worker becoming a volunteer or returning to school.

Role change or loss

Role change or loss may be experienced by many potential recipients of occupational therapy and the therapist must ensure that her assessment and subsequent intervention cater for the unique needs of each individual, modifying and restoring roles appropriate for him, thus facilitating the return of purpose and direction in his life.

ROLES ADOPTED BY OCCUPATIONAL THERAPISTS

Roles, as described in the introduction above, are 'expected patterns of behaviour' associated with one's position in society. During the course of her duties an occupational therapist, of necessity, must adopt a very wide range of roles (Table 13.2). Commonly, she will enact the roles of assessor, information giver and receiver, educator, planner, interviewer and goal-setter. However, during specific interventions involving individuals or groups she may need to adopt still more diverse roles in order to assist people to overcome or come to terms with their difficulties. These roles may include advocate, counsellor, negotiator, mentor or carer.

An occupational therapist's key tool is her 'self', along with core skills, knowledge, attitudes and other attributes. It is often the approach and the role or roles adopted by the therapist which are the most significant factors in her intervention and an individual's progress. A therapist will continuously evaluate and modify her role(s) and adjust her expectations of the recipient of treatment. By increasing the degree of independence and autonomy offered, and by gradually reducing her support, she will pass responsibility to the individual.

Approaches and roles have to be selected with as much care as in any treatment medium. A range of factors must be considered, including the framework within which the therapist works, be this a multidisciplinary team utilising particular techniques, an occupational therapy team using a specific model or the environment in which the selected activity is to take place.

At this juncture it is probably useful to consider in a little more detail a number of the therapist's roles and their relationship to practice.

Table 13.2 Roles and the occupational therapist: a summary

Role	Function/purpose
Communicator/ interviewer	Giver/receiver of information Establishing working relationship Comprehension of individual and his perceived abilities/inabilities
Assessor	Identification of skills, problems, abilities Formation of baseline for intervention
Planner	Explorer of options in relation to needs Requires objectivity and realism
Negotiator	Influencing/exchanging ideas Mutual decision-making, agreeing on plans, resolving differences Motivating the individual
Adviser	Imparting information, knowledge, skills
Decision-maker	Selection/choice from range of options, increasing individual's ability to make own decisions
Role-model	Adopting roles to achieve empathy Modelling a desired set of behaviours.
Problem-solver	Identification of problem, options and resources to aid solution, choice of solution
Educator	Transfer of skills, knowledge, abilities to individual/carers
Goal-setter	Establishing aim(s) and planning strategies for achievement
Advocate	Understanding individual's needs/requirements and acting on his behalf
Counsellor	Listener, assistant, explorer of options/values/needs/solutions
Mentor	Counsellor, with knowledge and skills to guide, usually in relation to specific topics
Carer	Concern for individual within programme of intervention, providing media/techniques to meet his needs

Communicator

As communicator, information giver and receiver, the therapist adopts a role in which she aims to establish an appropriate working relationship with an individual. This is central to her assessment and to any subsequent intervention. It involves listening and observing, i.e. receiving as well as offering verbal, non-verbal and other information. Each therapist must develop listening skills if she is to begin to understand the individual with whom she is working, the problems he identifies as a priority, the interests which are most important to him, and his perception of his relationships with family members. Therapists are able to obtain a considerable volume of information from individuals and their carers if effective two-way communication is established.

Assessor

In her assessor role the therapist works with the individual to identify the skills he possesses and the functional difficulties he is experiencing. For example, physical dysfunction in a young adult poses many potential difficulties with his life roles. The therapist has to identify skills and abilities required for the roles which the young person values most highly. She must establish means of partial role participation, if full participation is impossible, and assist him to identify other or previously less important roles which he might adopt. Assessment establishes a baseline from which intervention to assist this individual can be planned and negotiated.

Planner

Planning entails exploring the options available to an individual, i.e. those which may enhance his overall function given his skills, needs, selected life-style and environment. This role requires the objectivity of the therapist, to which she will add her knowledge, skills and attitudes in order to assist the individual in clarifying the realities of his circumstances, his own and others' expectations, and the options that are open to him in the short and long term.

Negotiator

Negotiation is the process used to satisfy particular needs when another person controls what an individual requires. It is an attempt to influence others through an exchange of ideas or of something of material value. Making mutual decisions, resolving differences or agreeing upon plans can all be described as negotiation.

Occupational therapists aim to help individuals to assist themselves. The demotivated person may not wish to play an active part in his treatment programme, but if he is to progress and to build on his existing skills he has to begin to take charge of his own destiny. In these circumstances the therapist may resort to 'bargaining' with him or acting on his behalf for a specified period. She may provide opportunities for successful performance to reinforce baseline ability levels and promote a sense of achievement, and in so doing will need to discuss the options available to him.

Adviser

The occupational therapist possesses a wealth of information which can aid those with a wide range of problems. Intervention programmes usually include an element of advice-offering aimed to help each individual to resolve certain of his own difficulties. In these circumstances, the therapist can offer her support to the individual whilst he pursues advice given, or she can withdraw and allow him to proceed. However, she may ensure that she remains accessible so that the individual may return to discuss further options and advice. Essentially, however, she will wish him to adopt the role of information seeker, active participant, or advocate himself.

Decision-maker

Many people have previous roles removed when they become ill and one of these is the role of decision-maker who takes responsibility for himself. As a result, the person loses independence, has much lower self-esteem and adopts the role of 'sick person'. Initially the therapist may have to decide how firm she will be in encouraging the individual to undertake active tasks which may or may not be within his total capacity, i.e. which may cause him emotional stress or physical discomfort and, in turn, may affect his motivation and perseverance.

The therapist's continuing role as decision-maker in any intervention should decrease as the programme progresses. She should plan to allow the individual to make informed decisions based on information and choices which he comprehends. In some situations she may have to adopt the role she wishes the individual to accept so that she can evoke some response from him.

Role model

Role-modelling is a technique utilised by most therapists at one time or another. In role modelling the therapist adopts a particular role in order to empathise with an individual, to experience a set of circumstances from his viewpoint and to encourage him to behave in a particular way. This is especially important when the therapist is providing opportunities for an individual to develop behaviours and attitudes which are relevant in certain circumstances, for example, cooperating with a small group of people with a similar problem, when the therapist will assist the individual by modelling the required behaviour of courtesies, listening, verbal and non-verbal communication including posture.

Problem-solver

As problem-solving is a central element of all occupational therapy, the therapist must be skilled in identifying problems, considering options and resources for the resolution of those problems and implementing the selected alternatives. With the individual she may explore and work on his reintegration into previous routines and roles, assisting him to clarify and modify his expectations of the future. She may have to act, temporarily, 'in loco personae', i.e. in place of the individual, considering on his behalf the options and potential alternatives which best suit his lifestyle and level of motivation (see p. 51).

Other roles

Occupational therapists enact many other roles during the course of their work; these include researcher, enabler, facilitator, mentor, observer, educator/teacher, advocate, colleague, counsellor and carer. The role associated with being a therapist (Table 13.2) is in fact a combination of roles, adapted to individuals and their needs, and to the needs of professional colleagues or other team members. Roles adopted by the occupational therapist interrelate with the roles adopted by others; e.g. her role as enabler is a response to the 'sick person' role of the individual receiving treatment.

Role blurring

There are other important issues to consider regarding roles which relate rather more to team colleagues than they do to individuals receiving occupational therapy, although they have the potential to affect the latter. Role blurring, for example, is increasingly common and indicates that a number of professions, such as occupational therapy, nursing and social work, now share basic or specialist skills, e.g. communication or counselling. However, each team member also needs to understand the specific role, or core skills, of her fellow professionals. For example, the occupational therapist's core or specific skills relate to activity, its analysis and application in all areas of function — self-care, leisure, work and social relationships.

Role conflicts

Role conflicts do occur and a team needs opportunities to discuss individual roles and the skills that each member will utilise in her daily work. Each team member must comprehend her colleagues' skills and regular discussion and debate is needed in order to minimise potential misunderstandings, tension or arguments within the team.

Key workers

Many teams use a key worker. This person is allocated to a particular individual receiving team assistance in order to coordinate and organise his care. The key worker concept is used with increasing frequency in multidisciplinary teams. Her professional background will be secondary to the skills, abilities and motivation she demonstrates in assisting the individual.

The advantage of the key worker system, by which intervention is channelled through one person, is that work is not duplicated and communication between the team on the one hand and the individual and his carers on the other is enhanced. The specific skills of individual workers will be called upon when required, while communication and assistance of a more generalised nature is dealt with by one person who is in regular contact with the individual.

The advantage of working as a team is that several professionals, by virtue of their skilled roles and specialised training, can contribute a very wide range of perspectives to the treatment of an individual. Each profession has its own exclusive set of skills, and team members must identify and understand these if role confusion is to be avoided. Role confusion resulting from lack of comprehension of a each team member's professional and personal skills can cause inefficiency and lead to under-utilisation of particular professions.

CONCLUSION

Occupational therapists are interested in the individual's skills and the existing abilities and experiences he can utilise when performing everyday tasks which are important to him. The therapist also attaches importance to his attitudes and the concepts he has which affect his adoption and performance of particular roles. She must enable him, through the use of her own range of roles and through an understanding of others' feelings and perceptions about him, his behaviour and roles, to obtain a renewed perspective on his present circumstances. He may frequently need help to make positive progress along the dysfunction/function continuum, moving from helplessness, incompetence and inefficiency to exploration, competence and achievement.

REFERENCES

Bruce A B, Borg B 1987 Frames of reference in psychological occupational therapy. Slack, Thorofare, New Jersey

Finlay L 1988 Occupational therapy practice in psychiatry. Croom Helm, London

Hume C, Pullen I 1986 Rehabilitation in psychiatry — an introductory handbook. Churchill Livingstone, Edinburgh

Kielhofner G 1983 Health through occupation — theory and practice in occupational therapy. F A Davis, Philadelphia

Kielhofner G (ed) 1985 A model of human occupation: theory and application. Williams & Wilkins, Baltimore

Mosey A C 1986 Psychosocial components of occupational therapy. Raven Press, New York

Willson M 1983 Occupational therapy in long-term psychiatry. Churchill Livingstone, Edinburgh

Willson M 1984 Occupational therapy in short-term psychiatry. Churchill Livingstone, Edinburgh

FURTHER READING

Bee H L, Mitchell S K 1984 The developing person — a life span approach, 2nd edn. Harper & Row, New York

Bond J, Bond S 1986 Sociology and health care — an introduction for nurses and other health care professionals. Churchill Livingstone, Edinburgh

Gillis L 1980 Human behaviour in illness — psychology and interpersonal relationships, 3rd edn. Faber & Faber, London

Rose A M (ed) 1977 Human behaviour and social processes — an interactionist approach. Routledge & Kegan Paul, London

SECTION 2
Neurology

14

Introduction to neurology

Sybil E. Johnson

INTRODUCTION

The functions of the central and peripheral nervous systems are more complex and varied than those of any other system in the human body. When the nervous system functions normally it can be likened to a computer receiving and interpreting information from and transmitting messages to all other systems. Damage to any part of the system will cause dysfunction, which may affect all or some motor, sensory, intellectual and emotional functions.

People who have suffered damage to their central and/or peripheral nervous systems will respond in one of a number of ways. Some may recover all or a degree of their pre-morbid state spontaneously (e.g. in mild CVA); others may not recover from internal or external trauma without some form of intervention (e.g. in peripheral nerve lesion); those with progressive disorders will deteriorate over time in spite of treatment, as medical science has not yet discovered the means of preventing certain conditions (e.g. multiple sclerosis). Some cannot be replaced (e.g. spinal cord lesion), and although the impairment remains static, as in those people born with impairment, they may be able to gain varying degrees of improved function. Therefore, people with difficulties caused by neurological deficit require a variety of interventions to enable them and their families to live with the effects of their disorder and any subsequent disability.

This chapter offers the reader a concise introduction to the nervous system and to the conditions which impair its normal function, along with their causes, features, diagnosis and treatment. The conditions described are cerebral palsy, cerebrovascular accident (CVA), head injury, motor neurone disease, multiple sclerosis, muscular dystrophy, Parkinson's disease, peripheral nerve lesions and spinal cord lesions. These are included in this section for two main reasons. First, many of their features are similar and affect either upper or lower motor neurones or both. Second, it is useful to compare their respective treatments.

DEVELOPMENT OF THE NERVOUS SYSTEM

The nervous system is responsible for all motor, sensory, autonomic, intellectual and emotional functions and activity. Its development in size and intricacy is a complex process that extends from conception to maturity. Normal motor development begins with the presence of the neonatal reflexes, many of which gradually disappear over the first three or four months of life. As mature reflexes emerge these allow head control, posture and gross movements to develop, with eventual progression to the finely coordinated movements, perception and understanding required for complex activities such as driving a car. It is essential that occupational therapists understand the structure, development and normal function of the nervous system and how it enables a person to interact with his environment.

The relationship between normal development and the conditions described in the following chapters varies. Some conditions such as cerebral palsy impair development from birth; others, such as muscular dystrophy, affect development during early childhood. Normal development is not affected by disorders acquired after maturity, but specific damage to an adult's nervous system may impair normal function. For example, movement patterns affected by a CVA or head injury may require the sequential reestablishment of normal reflexes, muscle tone and head control; progressive conditions such as motor neurone disease and 'static' ones such as spinal lesions may necessitate simultaneous treatment for trunk control, sitting balance and so on.

THE CONDITIONS

This section outlines the causes, features, diagnosis and treatment of neurological and neuromuscular conditions.

Causes

The causes are many and varied and include trauma to the brain and other parts of the body, focal disturbances and chemical deficiences in the brain, genetic factors, and causes whose nature is unknown. Box 14.1 groups the nine conditions mentioned by *primary* cause and offers brief explanations where appropriate.

Features

The features of these disorders are also varied and numerous; it will perhaps be helpful to begin by summarising them under the three headings of 'input', 'interpretation' and 'output' (or control). Some conditions will present features from all three areas, whilst others will be confined to one.

Problems relating to input include:

- sensation loss: may affect perception of light touch, deep pressure, pain, temperature; can include anaesthesia, paraesthesia, neuralgia, hyperaesthesia
- proprioceptive deficits: change in or loss of joint or limb position sense
- visual difficulties: hemianopia, diplopia, blindness, nystagmus (can also hinder balance)
- hearing/balance deficits: deafness, tinnitus, vertigo
- taste: may be affected
- smell: may be affected.

Problems of interpretation:

- perception: difficulties with body image; astereognosis, figure/ground discrimination problems, visuo-spatial deficit, agnosia

Box 14.1 Neurological conditions grouped according to primary cause

Trauma	Focal disturbance	Genetic	Unknown
Cerebral palsy: before during and after birth, e.g. severe asphyxia, distortion of head during birth with tearing of tentorium	*Cerebrovascular accident*: focal disturbance of cerebral function; usually vascular in origin, i.e. cerebral infarction or haemorrhage	*Muscular dystrophy*: genetic, therefore familial and hereditary. Different types associated with different genes, e.g. Duchenne sex-linked recessive. Some spontaneous mutation	*Motor neurone Disease*: progessive degeneration of motor pathways
Head injury: direct trauma to head resulting in open or closed head injury			*Multiple sclerosis*: demyelination of nerves in central nervous system. Theories re cause: genetic predisposition and environmental factors
Peripheral nerve lesions: direct trauma to limb (may also be caused by infection, pressure etc.)			*Parkinson's disease*: cell degeneration in dopaminergic pathways of basal ganglia with consequent disturbance of neurotransmission systems. Theories related to idiopathic parkinsonism include environmental pollutants
Spinal cord lesion: direct trauma to spinal column and cord (may also be caused by infection, pressure etc.)			

- communication: receptive dysphasia
- cognition: see 'output', below
- insight: lack of insight impairs interpretation of numerous stimuli because the individual does not appreciate that he has a problem.

   Problems of output/control:

- muscle tone/control: spasticity, flaccidity, rigidity, ataxia, clonus, choreiform and athetoid movements, tremor (intention tremor or tremor at rest), fasciculation, tics, spasm, disturbance of mobility in terms of gait, balance, synergies

- reflex patterns: disturbed or absent
- disturbance of emotional control: lability, fear
- urinary/faecal control: retention, frequency, incontinence
- cognition: problems with memory, problem-solving, reasoning, organisational skills and learning
- behavioural control: aggression, agitation, depression, difficulty with personal relationships
- communication: expressive dysphasia, dysarthria, apraxia, problems with non-verbal communication.

Age groups

Figure 14.1 illustrates in chart form the age distribution of the nine conditions described in the following chapters. Neurological conditions can cause dysfunction from childhood into old age, and whilst one condition, i.e. cerebral palsy, is present from birth, others will be more prevalent in young adults or have a peak incidence during middle to late adult life.

Type of onset

Onset may be divided into two main types, insidious and sudden. An insidious onset is one in which relatively minor signs and symptoms appear in the early stages of a condition and increase in severity with time (usually over a period of years). The muscular dystrophies, Parkinson's disease, multiple sclerosis and motor neurone disease are in this category. Conditions whose onset is sudden, i.e. head injury, spinal cord lesion, CVA and peripheral nerve lesion, are usually caused by internal or external trauma. Cerebral palsy is somewhat different, being caused by brain injury at or around the time of birth, and relates to the 'sudden' category rather than the 'insidious' one.

Motor features

The motor features with which these conditions present vary, depending upon the site of the damage, i.e. whether it is an upper or a lower motor neurone lesion.

- *Upper motor neurone lesion.* The distribution of dysfunction is related to the anatomical site of the lesion. For instance, internal capsule damage is likely to cause a contralateral hemiplegia, with voluntary and more skilled movements most affected. Other disturbances may include raised muscle tone and spasticity, mild muscle-wasting due to long-term disuse, possible weakness of all muscle groups on the affected side, and perceptual and cognitive deficits.
- *Lower motor neurone lesion.* This results in the wasting of innervated muscles in an upper or lower limb(s) and/or trunk, weakness or paralysis, impaired cutaneous sensation and absent tendon reflexes.

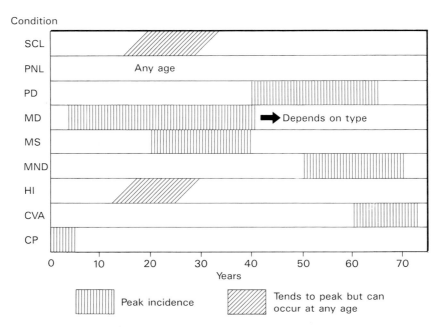

Fig. 14.1 Age groups affected by neurological conditions.

Table 14.1 summarises the differences between these two types of lesion, and Box 14.2 lists the conditions by lesion, i.e. upper, lower or mixed upper and lower.

Table 14.1   Upper and lower motor neurone lesions: contrasts

Changes to affected areas	Upper motor neurone	Lower motor neurone
Loss of power, paralysis	Present, but often incomplete; tends to affect entire limbs	Present and usually complete; affects muscle groups in limb(s) and trunk
Muscle tone	Spastic	Flaccid
Muscle wasting	Usually absent but disuse atrophy may occur	Usually severe
Sensation	Slight impairment only	Impairment more severe
Tendon reflexes	Present and exaggerated	Absent
Plantar reflex	Extensor response	Normal flexor response
Abdominal reflexes may be	Absent	Present

Box 14.2   Neurological conditions defined by lesion type

Upper motor neurone

Cerebral palsy
Cerebrovascular accident
Head injury*
Multiple sclerosis**
Parkinson's disease
Spinal cord lesion *above* L1

Lower motor neurone

Head injury:* if it has associated peripheral nerve lesion
Multiple sclerosis:** when plaques form at anterior root exit
Muscular dystrophy
Peripheral nerve lesions
Spinal cord lesion *below* L1

Mixed upper and lower motor neurone

Motor neurone disease

Sensory features

The extent of sensory loss ranges from no deficit at all to severe loss. The more severe and complex deficits are associated with upper motor neurone lesions, but milder deficits are not necessarily related to lower motor neurone lesions.

Muscular dystrophy and Parkinson's disease involve no sensory loss; motor neurone disease generally causes none, but in progressive bulbar palsy there is some loss of sensation on the posterior portion of the tongue.

Peripheral nerve and spinal cord lesions present with cutaneous sensory disturbance over the area supplied by the peripheral nerve below the lesion level. Additionally, people with peripheral nerve lesions may experience pain and the temperature and sweat control mechanisms of the person with a spinal cord lesion will also be affected.

Multiple sclerosis presents yet another picture of sensory disturbance with visual defects, in addition to numbness in the limbs or in the face. The most complex deficits present in CVAs, cerebral palsy and head injury caused by severe brain damage. Here, loss or impairment may include visual field disturbances, proprioceptive deficit, loss of sensation and hearing difficulties or loss. The pattern of sensory disturbance in these four conditions will never be identical in any two people because the area and extent of damage to nerves or the brain will vary.

Perceptual features

Only three of the conditions mentioned above commonly present with perceptual disorders: cerebral palsy, CVA and head injury. The ataxic type of cerebral palsy presents with difficulties in areas such as visuo-spatial relationships, whilst the other two conditions will give rise to deficits related to the lesion site usually within the right (non-dominant) hemisphere. Generally, both present with similar problems such as agnosia, spatial relationship disorder and apraxia.

Communication

All neurological conditions may affect a person's verbal and/or written communication. In some people, communication may not be affected in the early stages of some disorders but may deteriorate; in others, it is affected at onset.

Verbal communication in muscular dystrophy and in nerve and spinal cord lesions is unimpaired, except in instances of very high cervical cord lesions in which respiratory insufficiency affects speech. Written communication in these disorders will be affected to some extent, except in the case of people with paraplegia.

The remaining conditions all generally display both verbal and written communication dysfunction of varying degrees of severity, either from onset or with progressive deterioration. Cerebral palsy, CVA and head injury may present with one or more speech disorders, such as articulation difficulties or dysphasia. The ability to write will depend upon whether the dominant hand is affected. Depending on its type, motor neurone disease will affect communication in different ways. Thus, progressive bulbar palsy affects speech first, whilst progressive muscular atrophy and amyotrophic lateral sclerosis initially impair the ability to write. In the later stages all three types will result in impaired verbal and written communication. Multiple sclerosis impairs speech in the form of dysarthria and any degree of tremor results in difficulty in holding and controlling a pen. People with Parkinson's disease present differently. Their writing tends to be micrographic and tremulous, whilst their speech may be monosyllabic and low in volume.

Again, it is difficult to generalise; communication disorders in neurology will vary as much as the individuals who present with such deficits.

Cognitive function

Dysfunction of cognition may be present in four disorders. Children with cerebral palsy who also have learning difficulties will need assistance to overcome or manage their cognitive deficits. People with parkinsonism may have short-term memory dysfunction and difficulty interpreting facial expressions. People with CVA or head injury can present with the most severe cognitive deficits, including inattention, loss of concentration and memory and difficulty in learning new skills.

Intellect

There is no intellectual impairment in nerve or spinal cord lesions, motor neurone disease or multiple sclerosis, and intellectual function usually remains unaffected in muscular dystrophy. However, in the other four conditions intellectual impairment may be present. Cerebral palsy may be accompanied by learning difficulties. Parkinsonism slows down a person's mental processes and approximately one third of elderly people with the disease suffer from dementia which may be caused by other degenerative processes. Those who have suffered a CVA may show signs of impairment, depending on the lesion site. For people with head injuries, impairment may range from the mild to the extremely severe.

Continence

People with motor neurone disease, peripheral nerve lesions, muscular dystrophy and mild or moderate cerebral palsy remain continent. Those who have had a CVA may be incontinent initially. Likewise, those with head injuries may be incontinent in the early stages following their injury, but may return to continence. Incontinence is not usually a common feature in parkinsonism but occasionally it may be caused by constipation (pressure on the bladder by the bowel) or immobility, and frequency of micturition may cause episodes of incontinence for people with multiple sclerosis. The only people who suffer permanent continence problems are those with severe cerebral palsy or spinal injury, in which both urinary and faecal incontinence will require management regimes.

Emotional and psychological features

Inevitably, conditions which affect part of the nervous system give rise to a wide range of emotional and psychological problems. Depression, fear, anxiety, frustration, low motivation and self-esteem and emotional lability feature highly in most neurological disorders. Some are integral to the condition; emotional lability, for example, is typical in multiple sclerosis and in the weeks or months following a CVA. Depression is commonly experienced by people with parkinsonism, motor neurone disease and multiple sclerosis and by those who have suffered a CVA. Agitation and aggressive outbursts may occur in people with any neurological deficit. Whilst this is understandable when severe permanent disability is likely, in some cases the reaction seems disproportionate to the extent of the physical injury.

Nonetheless, whatever the condition and the emotional and psychological difficulties experienced by the individual, the immediate family and other carers may also have to cope with their own and their relatives' feelings and emotions.

Personal relationships

Disability, whatever its cause, affects the individual's personal relationships within his immediate and extended family, within his circle of friends and acquaintances and with people at work, school and elsewhere. Readers will find that subsequent chapters in this section include observations about a variety of relationships, roles within those relationships and the long-term effects that a person's disability may have on his roles as friend, sexual partner or parent.

Life expectancy

The diagnosis of a neurological disorder does not necessarily mean that a person's life span will be curtailed. Many people can expect a relatively normal life span following trauma or the onset of a disorder (such as those with a spinal cord lesion, cerebral palsy or parkinsonism), providing the condition is not complicated by other disorders. The other conditions present a different and more variable pattern. For example, 75% of people with multiple sclerosis have on average an expected life span of twenty-five to thirty years from the onset of their condition, but this is difficult to predict with any certainty. Of those who experience a CVA, approximately one third die within a short space of time, a further third survive with a severe disability and the remainder make a good recov-

ery. However, the cause of their CVA may be an ever-present reminder that their general health is impaired. Head injury presents a slightly different picture and life expectancy will depend on the severity of the original injury and resultant disability. Motor neurone disease and muscular dystrophy comprise different types within each condition. The three groups of symptoms in motor neurone disease can indicate whether a person's life may be curtailed drastically to a further three years or so, or whether he may look forward to approximately another fifteen years. Muscular dystrophy types also herald varying life expectancies. Children who develop the Duchenne type will only survive until their early twenties, whereas those with the other types may enjoy a relatively normal life span despite increasing disability.

A person's realisation that his life expectancy will be far less than he had anticipated whilst he was in good health is not necessarily a precursor of reactive depression and a loss of joie de vivre. Each person will have his own means of coping with these circumstances and it is important that all remaining years are filled with purpose.

Diagnosis

Prior to being treated any condition must be correctly diagnosed. In neurology this is not always a straightforward process and some diagnoses are made by a process of elimination as well as by the administration of specific tests. The taking of a history, and observation and discussion of symptoms and signs are important in all these disorders, particularly the degenerative ones, in which it is not always clear which condition is present. Spinal cord and peripheral nerve lesions, head injury and CVAs are relatively easy to diagnose almost immediately, using such procedures as reflex testing, observation of cutaneous sensory loss and of early deformity, X-ray and examination and sophisticated scanning systems. The diagnosis of cerebral palsy is usually straightforward but the possibility of other neuromuscular degenerative diseases has to be eliminated first. Duchenne-type muscular dystrophy is not apparent at birth and other types have an insidious onset at various life stages.

Therefore, in addition to taking a history and considering the signs and symptoms, the physician will rely on clinical observations as well as muscle biopsy and electromyography.

The diagnosis of multiple sclerosis has become more specific in recent years with visual and auditory evoked responses or potential testing. Evoked responses involve the artificial stimulation of pathways within the central nervous system in order to reveal disturbances of conduction. Visual evoked responses or potentials indicate whether or not delayed conduction from one eye compared to the other or to normal values indicates a lesion of the optic nerve. A similar technique is used to measure central conduction velocities in the auditory system. Testing of the cerebrospinal fluid for gammaglobulin may indicate abnormality in 50% of cases.

Electromyography in suspected motor neurone disease shows denervation with widespread fibrillation, and the sural nerve is usually biopsied to eliminate the possibility of other disease. Finally, the diagnosis of Parkinson's disease relies almost totally on the physician observing signs and symptoms and distinguishing them from other conditions which may present in a similar way in their early stages.

Treatment

The treatment offered to people with neurological conditions covers virtually the whole spectrum of available intervention, i.e. chemotherapy, surgery, nursing and rehabilitation. For certain conditions, treatment is relatively predictable. For instance, peripheral nerve and spinal cord lesions are treated with surgical repair and stabilisation of the injury site respectively, followed by the necessary rehabilitation. None of the other conditions' treatment is as clear-cut. Symptomatic treatment is utilised primarily for people with multiple sclerosis, motor neurone disease, cerebral palsy and muscular dystrophy; intervention may include chemotherapy, rehabilitation, and, in the case of muscular dystrophy, genetic counselling. Parkinsonism is treated with chemotherapy and rehabilitation with the correct balance of drugs being central to the whole rehabilitative process. CVA and head injury intervention will depend very much on the causes of the damage and its severity. The causal factor in CVA such as subarachnoid haemorrhage, may need treatment (particularly in younger people), as will any resulting impairments, but on the whole treatment is conservative, i.e. consisting of chemotherapy, nursing and rehabilitation. The range of severity of head injury presents widely varying pictures. A mild injury may require only advice and observation, whereas a severe injury will require life-saving treatment initially, followed by nursing care and rehabilitation over a number of years.

In addition to offering standard medical, surgical, nursing and rehabilitative procedures, the intervention provided by multidisciplinary teams working with people with neurological deficits has to be innovative in order to enable each person to attain his optimum health and ability levels.

PRINCIPLES OF OCCUPATIONAL THERAPY

A degree of spontaneous recovery in the nervous system following trauma is much more common than one might imagine. The continuing development of medical science offers new ideas about the recuperative powers of brain tissue, and the potential benefits of reeducating alternative areas of the brain to adapt to new functions are being explored. However, the effects of damage to the nervous system can result in major dysfunction in a person's physical, psychological, social and emotional life, particularly if the cause and resultant symptoms can only be alleviated to a minor extent.

People with neurological conditions need occupational therapy from an early stage; for example, the brain-injured person needs kinetic, tactile and aural stimulation; those who have had a CVA benefit from intervention as soon as any life-threatening episode has passed; and those with progressive disorders require assistance as soon as a diagnosis is suspected or confirmed. Each person's need for intervention will vary according to his condition, its progressive or non-progressive nature, and his personality, age, strength of character, attitude, insight and life-style.

The principles underlying the practice of occupational therapy in the treatment of neurological conditions are identical to those used in any other area of intervention. However, neurological conditions do present unique problems and challenges. The therapist will modify her pattern of intervention accordingly, while working within the framework of the occupational therapy process (see Ch. 4). This 'systems' approach of referral, information seeking, assessment, objective-setting, planning, implementing, monitoring and evaluating forms the basis of intervention regardless of the specific models, approaches and techniques utilised.

Assessment of people presenting with neurological dysfunction is continuous throughout the period of intervention. The types of assessment administered may vary according to each person's presenting problems, condition, life-style, past, present and anticipated future roles and those activities which they consider most important. In order to identify areas of function and dysfunction, specific assessment using functional activities and/or standardised tests may encompass cognitive function, physical abilities, sensory deficits, interpersonal skills and psychological and emotional states.

Treatment goals will be directed towards optimising existing and potential abilities and skills and minimising dysfunction, assisting individuals to adjust to their circumstances and recommending environmental adaptations. Intervention, wherever it occurs, will emphasise the home and family environment and relationships, concentrating on activities identified as priorities by the person and his family, helping them to come to terms with functional abilities, residual dysfunction or deterioration. Occupational therapy should also aim to help people to strike a balance in their lives, by enabling them to make informed choices about daily activities. (For instance, should a person struggle to dress himself each morning or should he accept appropriate help so that he can retain his energy and enthusiasm for school, work or hobbies?) This is particularly important for people whose condition is progressive, for they need to learn to monitor and evaluate their own functional status on a continual basis, enabling them to seek assistance as needed over a period of years rather than weeks or months.

The occupational therapist's monitoring, evaluation and review of an individual's function and/or dysfunction varies considerably in neurology. Following the initial, intensive period of assessment and treatment the person may be discharged from the therapist's active caseload. However, most people will either be offered a review date for a reassessment and discussion of their function and any further problems or will be advised to contact their therapist when particular activities become more difficult. The pattern whereby the therapist's input is followed by a period without active intervention and then by more input may continue for the duration of a person's life, particularly for those who have progressive conditions.

APPROACHES USED IN OCCUPATIONAL THERAPY

The occupational therapist will utilise many approaches to treatment within neurology — developmental, neurodevelopmental, sensory-integrative, humanistic, rehabilitative, cognitive, behavioural and psychotherapeutic. The approaches she uses with one person will depend upon his needs, problems and life-style and in practice she may utilise several approaches simultaneously.

Initially, the therapist tends to use one approach or to apply particular aspects of complementary approaches, particularly if the individual has sustained brain damage. For instance, the head-injured person with hemiplegia may be treated neurodevelopmentally initially, possibly in combination with humanistic and behavioural approaches. As the person's function improves and he has to consider independence in his own home, the therapist's emphasis may shift towards rehabilitative or modified neurodevelopmental principles to facilitate his independence.

The approaches used with progressive disorders are less clear-cut, but tend towards the rehabilitative, humanistic and psychotherapeutic, given that the individual's function over a long period will be of paramount importance to him and that very specific use of some approaches will not be conducive to achievement.

In the longer term, the therapist will use a single approach or a mixture of approaches best suited to the needs of each person, modifying her intervention as required whether it is short-term and intensive or occurs at intervals over many years.

CONCLUSION

Most of the conditions described in the following chapters have a long-term effect on the person and his family and impinge on all aspects of their lives. Therefore, the occupational therapist, along with the individual, his carers and her team colleagues must plan and implement intervention which is realistic, takes account of people's wishes as well as their needs and offers each person choice. Whilst the tasks of daily living may be important, the psychological and spiritual well-being of an entire family are integral to any therapy programme. It is a relatively straightforward matter to facilitate physical adjustment to disability, but therapists also need to use their considerable skills to assist families to adjust and to learn how to live with and manage disability and any subsequent handicaps utilising, if they so wish, the range of statutory and non-statutory services available to them.

FURTHER READING

Bannister R 1985 Brain's clinical neurology, 6th edn. Oxford University Press, Oxford

Downie P A 1986 Cash's textbook of neurology for physiotherapists, 4th edn. Faber & Faber, London

Hildick-Smith M 1985 Neurological problems in the elderly. Baillière Tindall, London

Houston J C, Joiner C L, Trounce J R 1985 A short textbook of medicine, 8th edn. Hodder & Stoughton, Sevenoaks, Kent

Matthews W B 1982 Diseases of the nervous system, 4th edn. Blackwell Scientific Publications, Oxford

Cerebral palsy

Jenny Wilsdon

INTRODUCTION

Cerebral palsy (CP) is a non-progressive disorder resulting from a variety of causes. It is mainly a dysfunction of tone, posture and movement secondary to brain abnormality or damage and may also be associated with additional handicaps. Onset occurs before brain growth and development are complete, that is, from conception to the second birthday. The incidence of CP is approximately two per 1000 live births.

Although the disorder is lifelong, that is, it cannot be cured, it is not unchanging. Movement patterns may change during development, maturation and/or intervention. This chapter, therefore, explores the important contribution that the occupational therapist can make in assisting the individual affected by CP to achieve a maximum level of independent function in all areas of living.

The chapter begins by reviewing the main characteristics of CP, including its causes, diagnosis, and types, together with the problems associated with the condition and their prognosis. Essential to an appreciation of the obstacles posed by CP, however, is an understanding of the normal patterns of development which it delays or preempts; accordingly, these patterns are discussed next. The role of the occupational therapist in treating CP is then described in broad terms, and general principles of practice are set out.

Next, the chapter turns to more specific aspects of occupational therapy intervention in CP; these include early intervention; the facilitation of correct posture; training, advice and support in self-care tasks; the assessment and development of hand and gross motor function; and support in overcoming mobility, communication, perceptual and behavioural problems. Attention is also given to the use of orthoses in CP and to possible adaptations to the school, home and work environment that will aid the person with CP to meet his full potential. Finally, the importance of the advice and support that the occupational therapist is able to offer to family members and carers is emphasised.

CHARACTERISTICS OF CEREBRAL PALSY

AETIOLOGY

A number of factors have been identified as predictors of increased risk of CP. These include:

- maternal intellectual impairment
- fetal malformations
- birth weight of less than 2100 g
- delayed first cry (after two minutes)
- neonatal seizures
- respiratory distress syndrome.

The vast majority of those affected by CP have an unknown or prenatal aetiology. Known causes may be classified as follows:

- prenatal (conception to birth)
  — genetic disorders
  — maternal disorders
  — primary fetal abnormalities
  — infections, cerebral infarcts (CP a secondary effect)
- perinatal (during the birth process)
  — birth trauma to normal fetus
  — prenatally caused CP leading to abnormal birth process

- neonatal (0 to 28 days)
  — infections
  — acute metabolic disorders
  — blood group incompatibility
- postnatal (1 to 24 months)
  — cerebral infections
  — head injury: accidental, non-accidental
  — CNS infections
  — haemorrhage: subdural, intraventricular.

DIAGNOSIS

This is usually straightforward for the overall disorder but some neuromuscular degenerative diseases, such as Wernig-Hoffmann disease (acute infantile spinal muscular atrophy) mimic the features of CP and must be eliminated from the diagnosis.

CLASSIFICATION

The disorder may be described as a delay and/or deviance, that is, as a delay in reaching normal developmental milestones and/or a deviance from the normal sequence or pattern of development. The precise nature of the disorder is determined by the location of damage within the brain, as follows:

Spastic

The clinical features of spastic CP are those associated with damage to the cerebral cortex and corresponding pyramidal tracts. Motor problems include paucity of movement, increased resistance to passive movement, muscle spasm, clonus, exaggerated deep tendon reflexes and absence of change in muscle tone associated with a change in posture, for example, moving from a supine to a sitting position. Although the sensory and proprioceptive nerve endings are intact, within the brain the perception and interpretation of stimuli may be affected; therefore, sensation may be abnormal, decreased or increased.

Subgroups identify the distribution within the body:

- hemiplegia: involvement of an upper limb

and a lower limb on the same side of the body
- diplegia: involvement of both lower limbs to a greater degree than the upper limbs
- quadriplegia: involvement of all four limbs equally or upper involvement greater than lower.

Dyskinetic

In this type, abnormalities in motor coordination affect the body as a whole. This is associated with damage to the basal ganglia and extrapyramidal tracts. Subgroups are as follows:

- athetosis: irregular writhing movements exaggerated by active movement and disappearing or decreasing during sleep. There is variable muscle tone from low tone (floppiness) to high tone (stiffness). Athetosis is often associated with chorea (jerky, excess movement), in which case it is termed *choreoathetosis*.
- dystonia: the adoption of bizarre, purposeless posturing of the extremities or the body as a whole. Muscle tone is variable.
- hypotonia: a lack of or decrease in muscle tone coupled with a lack of resistance to passive movement. The deep tendon reflexes may be diminished or increased. This may be the initial presentation of motor dysfunction of a child with CP and changes in tone may evolve.

Ataxic

In this form of CP the cerebellum is the site of damage. Features include primary incoordination and lack of balance. An intention tremor appears on active movement.

Mixed

Those who display more than one type of CP as described above are said to have mixed CP.

Figure 15.1 indicates the distribution of CP types; Table 15.1 lists their presenting characteristics.

1. Spastic — combined	66%
a. hemiplegia	30%
b. diplegia	16%
c. quadriplegia	20%
2. Dyskinetic	21%
3. Ataxic	3%
4. Mixed	10%

Fig. 15.1 Distribution of types of cerebral palsy.

ASSOCIATED HANDICAPS

The majority of people with CP have one or more of the following associated handicaps:

- Learning disabilities and intellectual impairment. IQ scores of less than 70 are recognised in over one half of individuals with CP. Severe intellectual impairment with an IQ score of 50 or less is seen in one third. Dyskinetic types generally score higher than spastic types. Amongst spastic types those with quadriplegia most often fall within the severely intellectually impaired group.
- Epilepsy. Epileptic fits of various types accompany CP in about one third of all cases. Most commonly occurring in the first two years, and sometimes appearing later, they may or may not continue throughout life. Again, the highest incidence is with the spastic types and the lowest with dyskinetic CP.
- Visual defects. One third have visual problems of varying degrees of severity; these include blindness (often cortical), homonymous hemianopia (usually with hemiplegic CP), refractive errors and strabismus.
- Hearing defects affect 10% of those with CP. Not all such defects are primary, however; conductive hearing loss, for example, is often secondary to frequent middle ear infections. High tone deafness often accompanies athetoid CP.
- Speech and language problems are present in 50% of cases of CP. Dysarthria is the most frequent with athetoid CP, dysfluency and dysrhythmia with ataxic CP and receptive and expressive dysphasias with spastic CP.

Table 15.1 Presenting characteristics of cerebral palsy

	Spastic quadriplegia	Spastic diplegia	Spastic hemiplegia	Athetosis	Ataxia
Muscle tone	Increased tone, difficulty in relaxing			Variable; early, often floppy	Reduced tone
Passive movement	Resisted, tone increased			Either compliant or very resistive	Compliant
Active movement	Slow, stiff, abnormal patterns			Difficulty inhibiting other movements; writhing, jerky movements	Often quick and uncoordinated
Distribution	All body involvement, upper limbs > lower limbs	Lower limbs > upper limbs	Ipsilateral upper & lower limb	All body involvement	All body involvement
Head/neck	Turning poor, possible neck extension	Unaffected	Unaffected	Extension	Tremor
Trunk	Stiff, limited rotation; later, scoliosis	Weakness, limited rotation	Later, if leg shortened or hip retracted, lateral spinal curve	Extension, poor rotation	Adopted postures are usually normal but movements grossly uncoordinated, combined with an intention tremor
Shoulders	Retraction, adduction	Mild retraction	Retraction, adduction	Marked medial rotation	
Elbows/wrists	Flexion	Mild Flexion	Flexion	Extension/flexion	
Forearms	Pronation	Possible pronation	Pronation	Marked pronation	
Hands	Fisting, thumb adduction	Possible fisting	Fisting, thumb adducted	Hyperextension of fingers	
Hips	Extension, adduction; later, windswept deformity	Strong adduction and medial rotation	Possible retraction with adduction	Extension	Possible hypermobility of the joints
Knees	Extension	Extension, later flexion	Extension	Extension	
Feet	Plantar flexion	Plantar flexion	Plantar flexion	Plantar flexion	
Walking pattern	Not usually achieved	Delay, on toes with hips & knees flexed, thighs adducted, often scissored	On toes with leg thrown out to side on swing-through	May not be achieved. Otherwise, erratic, jerky, uncoordinated. Arms and legs flail	Wide base, staggering, falling gait
Speech/feeding	Tongue thrust, jaw clamping, swallowing & breathing difficulties all hinder feeding; speech very poor if achieved	Not usually affected, may be delayed	Facial involvement is unusual	Facial grimacing. Swallowing & breathing difficult. Speech irregular, slurred & difficult to understand. Tongue & palate involvement	Speech may be staccato and monotonous

• Other problems frequently associated with CP are disorders of perception, emotion, behaviour and sleep.

PROGNOSIS

The eventual outcome will depend upon the type of CP, its severity and its associated handicaps (see Table 15.2). Those with mild CP, those with a significantly higher IQ and those who pass through mainstream education are most likely to achieve full independence and competitive employment. Those with a significant physical handicap and those with intellectual impairment are most likely to achieve partial independence and to be employed within sheltered employment. In cases where a severe physical disability is combined with intellectual impairment independence is unlikely to be achieved. These are general prognoses, of course, and other factors — i.e. family support, general health, regular education, vocational training, and, most importantly, the motivation of the individual — will affect the degree of independence attained.

NORMAL DEVELOPMENT

Prior to discussing the role of occupational therapy in the treatment of cerebral palsy it is necessary to consider normal development. Although the knowledge of developmental milestones (see Ch. 3) is a basic prerequisite of intervention, of greater importance is the knowledge of how development occurs, i.e. the sequence and pattern of development and learning.

MOTOR CONTROL

The development of motor control over any part of the body follows a sequence from instability to stability and, finally, mobility. In the development of head control, for example, this sequence might be described as follows:

• instability: initially, a child lying prone can lift his head only momentarily; the movement will be jerky and unreliable
• stability: after practice the movement becomes controlled and reliable
• mobility: eventually, the child is able not only to lift his head at will but to turn his head in the direction of a visual or auditory stimulus, for example, a toy or his mother's voice.

The development of motor control also occurs in a fixed 'direction', so to speak; that is, it takes place in sequences which can be described as:

• cephalo-caudal
• proximal-distal
• medial-lateral.

Table 15.2 Use of terminology — mild, moderate and severe cerebral palsy

	Mild	Moderate	Severe
Type	Spastic hemiplegia Spastic diplegia Athetosis Ataxia	Spastic hemiplegia Spastic diplegia Athetosis Ataxia	Spastic quadriplegia Athetosis
Function	Independent living	Supported living	Totally dependent
Mobility	Independent walking, possibly with aids	Self-propelled wheelchair, very unsteady walking or crawling	Push-chair
Hand function	Unlimited	Limited	Non-purposeful
Intelligence	> 70	70–50	< 50
Speech	Sentences	Phrases, single words	No recognisable words
Education	Mainstream	Mainstream with support	Special education facilities
Work	Full employment	Sheltered or supported employment	Unemployment

These developmental patterns may be illustrated as follows:

- Cephalo-caudal. Motor control moves down the body from the head to the pelvis. As in the above example, the baby gains control of his head and then gains voluntary control of his pectoral girdle and upper trunk. This is shown in a prone position as he raises himself up onto his forearms to see more of his surroundings. By progressing to the use of extended elbows he gains control of his lower trunk. This enables him to rotate and flex his trunk; for example, when he sits on his mother's lap with his pelvis supported he is able to turn and bend towards her or to objects which attract him. Finally, when pelvic control is achieved he is able to sit on the floor unsupported, and to turn and bend to one side and back again without losing his balance (Figs 15.2, 15.3).

- Proximal-distal control develops at the same time as cephalo-caudal control. As the baby, lying prone, learns to prop himself up onto his forearms he gains control of his shoulder girdle, the proximal part of his upper limb. The elbow joint moves through the stages of instability, stability and controlled movement as the baby progresses to the use of extended arms. He can transfer his weight through to one side and leave the other arm free to reach for

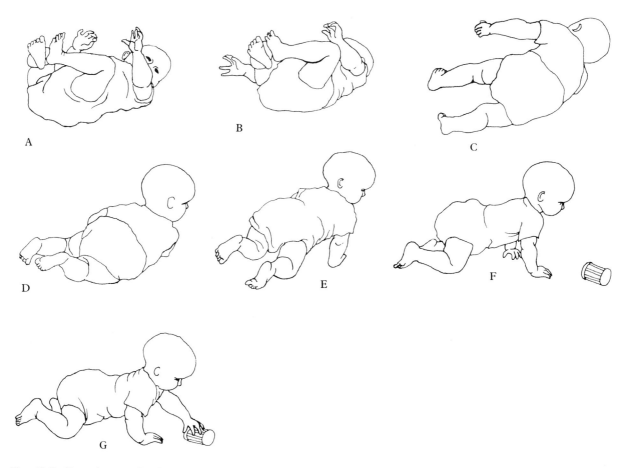

Fig. 15.2 Normal motor development: rolling from supine to prone position and up into crawl position (head leading). (Drawings by Sarah Denvir reproduced from Griffiths M, Clegg M 1988 *Cerebral Palsy: Problems and Practice*, Souvenir Press [Educational & Academic], London, by kind permission of the publisher.)

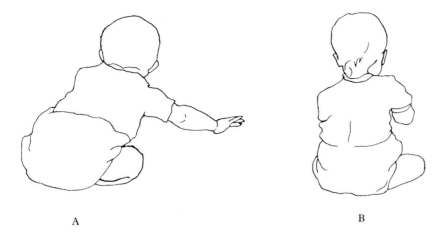

A   B

Fig. 15.3 Normal motor development: pushing up from the crawl position into unsupported sitting (head leading). (Drawings by Sarah Denvir reproduced from Griffiths M, Clegg M 1988 *Cerebral Palsy: Problems and Practice*, Souvenir Press [Educational & Academic], London, by kind permission of the publisher.)

his toys. The proximal-distal sequence is also followed in the legs from pelvic and hip control in crawling, to knee control in standing and ankle and foot control in walking (Fig. 15.4).

● Medial-lateral. This sequence applies to the hands and feet; control progresses from the medial to the lateral arch in the foot, and from the little and ring fingers through the middle finger to the index finger and thumb of the hand. Ulnar grasp is achieved before a refined pincer grasp.

ACQUISITION OF SKILLS

The acquisition of each new skill or activity occurs in three phases:

- trial and error
- consolidation
- acquisition.

● Trial and error. At this stage a new skill is emerging. It may lead directly from a previously acquired skill (for example, as walking follows from standing) or it may be accidental or spontaneous (for example, discovering that pulling at a sock will make it come off the foot).

● Consolidation. Once the correct movement or effect has been achieved it is repeated until it

has been perfected.

● Acquisition. Here the skill or activity is executed in an easy and relaxed manner and can be used for play and pleasure and as a basis for new skills.

Thus, in the trial and error phase of walking, the child takes a tentative step forwards, usually lifting his leg too high or taking too long a step, and falls. In the consolidation phase, he manages three or four steps and enjoys practising but will revert to the previously acquired skill of crawling for speed and pleasure. In the acquisition phase, walking becomes the preferred method of locomotion.

It must be recognised that the acquisition of various skills is interrelated. Being able to feed oneself depends upon motor skills (head control, trunk control, hand function, hand/eye coordination), intellectual ability (understanding what food is and what it is for) and perceptual skills (knowing where one's mouth is and where one's hand is in relation to mouth and food). If one is asked to feed oneself, the understanding of language is also a prerequisite.

The knowledge of normal development is not only important for the therapist working with children, but provides the basic theory behind the neurodevelopmental or neurosequential approach

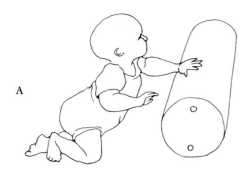

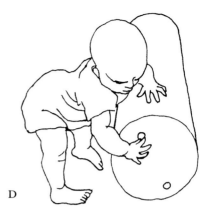

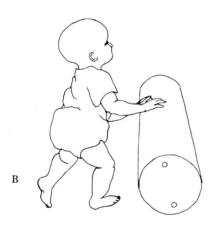

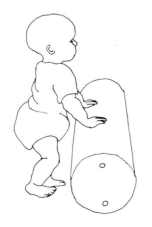

Fig. 15.4 Normal motor development: moving from the crawl position into standing and cruising position (head leading). (Drawings by Sarah Denvir reproduced from Griffiths M, and Clegg M 1988 *Cerebral Palsy: Problems and Practice*, Souvenir Press [Educational & Academic], London, by kind permission of the publisher.)

used by many therapists for the treatment of both childhood and adult disorders.

THE ROLE OF THE OCCUPATIONAL THERAPIST

The person with CP may be referred to the occupational therapist at any time during his development from infancy to adulthood. If the diagnosis of CP is made at or soon after birth, intervention will probably commence whilst the baby is in the special care baby unit (SCBU). Diagnosis might not be made, however, until it is evident that certain developmental milestones such as rolling over, sitting and standing have not been reached within normal limits. This is most likely to occur with the milder forms of CP. On rare occasions, a child or adolescent who has 'slipped through the net', moved to a new area or arrived from another country will be referred to the occupational therapist for the first time. Most persons with CP will receive advice and support from an occupational therapist throughout their lives, sometimes in the foreground as new problems arise, often in the background as the person adapts to his handicap and life-style. In the early years, intervention is usually frequent and intensive, gradually tapering off as the child moves through school age into adolescence and adulthood. As an adult, the person with CP may call upon the services of the occupational therapist as life changes occur — for example, a new job, new home, marriage and children. The holistic approach taken by the occupational therapist will involve her not only with the individual but also with his family (mother, father, siblings, grandparents), teachers, employers and partner.

Intervention cannot be rigidly subdivided into early, middle and late stages of treatment, as the form it takes will be determined largely by the severity of the CP, the personality of the individual and the support he receives from others. Some people with severe CP will require the multisensory input of early intervention throughout their lives; others will attain independence in many areas as their chronological age allows.

Assessment

The aim of the occupational therapist's assessment is to identify the individual's abilities and problems as a basis for setting objectives and planning her intervention. Assessment will consist of the following components:

Observation

The therapist will observe how the person achieves or tries to achieve certain goals; his understanding of various tasks; his level of concentration and motivation; his functional ability; the time taken to perform tasks, and the sequence of achievement. Observation of how the mother or carer handles and responds to the individual can be very instructive. For example, if the mother carries the person with total support, as one would a baby of one or two months, this would suggest that the individual lacks gross motor control. Similarly, the level of language used by the mother may indicate the level of intellectual function. The occupational therapist should provide a number of toys, activities and situations which give the individual the opportunity to demonstrate his various abilities.

Information

This can be gathered from the individual, his family and from other professionals.

Handling

The occupational therapist must handle the person in order to assess muscle tone, joint range of movement, sensitivity to touch and positional change and responsiveness to facilitation of movement.

Formal assessment

This becomes more appropriate as intervention progresses. It may take the form of a standardised perceptual battery, a formal functional assessment or a developmental checklist.

Aims

Specific aims, objectives and intervention programmes will depend upon the individual's prognosis, that is, upon the type and severity of his CP, his intellectual ability and his expected rate of progress. General aims are:

- to facilitate the normal developmental process, through direct contact, adaptations to the environment, provision of equipment, education, counselling, encouragement and support of the individual and family
- to provide opportunity for exploration, play, learning and maturation
- to enable the individual to achieve his maximum level of functional independence.

PRINCIPLES OF PRACTICE

A number of approaches to practice are used by the occupational therapist when treating the person with CP, the main ones being:

- behavioural
- biomechanical (see Ch. 11)
- neurodevelopmental.

Behavioural principles are the foundation for the treatment of problems of a psychological and/or emotional nature. They are employed to elicit changes in, or adaptations to, behaviours in response to specific stimuli.

Biomechanical principles emphasise range, strength and tolerance of movement as necessary components of a person's ability to perform functional life tasks. These principles may be employed during the later treatment stages of a person with mild CP who has achieved some voluntary muscle control.

Neurodevelopmental principles lie behind a number of treatment approaches utilised by the therapist with the person with CP. The most commonly used are briefly described below:

- Bobath approach. This emphasises the experience of normal posture and movement through the inhibition of abnormal postural reflexes, tones and patterns and the facilitation of normal balance and equilibrium reactions, thereby encouraging normal movement patterns.
- Peto approach (conductive education). This aims at the attainment of functional or task-orientated goals through group activity, using repetition, rhythm and vocalisation.
- Ayres approach (sensory integration). This attempts to develop and coordinate multisensory input and motor output with sensory feedback, utilising planned and controlled sensory input to elicit an adaptive response.
- Rood approach. This emphasises the normalisation of tone and desired muscular responses through the application of specific sensory stimulation. It aims to facilitate progress through the developmental sequence of sensorimotor control (for example, rocking on all fours before crawling). All movements used in treatment must be purposeful. The principles of repetition are applied to strengthen and consolidate normal movement patterns of stability and mobility.

The therapist, in her problem-solving or pragmatic approach to treatment, will employ these principles and approaches according to the person's needs and her own experience. Generally, a mixture of the above is used, providing an eclectic approach to treatment. Often one approach will predominate, but emphasis will change in accordance with individual needs.

EARLY INTERVENTION

The occupational therapist may be involved with a moderately or severely affected baby during the neonatal period and the first contact may take place in the special care baby unit (SCBU). The initial aim will be to support and advise the parents; this will be the aim not only of the occupational therapist but of all the members of the multidisciplinary team involved in the SCBU.

The arrival of a new baby is a time of great change for any family, particularly if he is the first baby. The baby will have been looked forward to for a number of months. If there has been a history of miscarriage or difficulty in conceiving, the baby will be especially precious. The relationship between the parents will have changed and will continue to change as they adjust to the baby's arrival and their relationships with him. The news that their baby has problems which will affect his development (the diagnosis of CP may not be initially apparent) will be devastating. The parents will experience shock, disbelief, anger and guilt. They will have to pass through the grieving process and mourn for their lost normal baby before they can accept their handicapped baby.

During this period the therapist's role is to support the parents; in doing so she must work closely with the other team members. The mother/baby and father/baby bonds are vitally important at this stage; therefore, the occupational therapist should encourage the parents to actively participate in all treatment programmes.

Parents are anxious and unsure when handling and caring for their new baby and a handicapped baby brings additional worries; therefore, advice and encouragement are of paramount importance. Advice on handling and stimulating the baby should be coupled with encouragement and praise to help the parents become more confident. A 'normal' baby has no voluntary motor control and requires total support of head and trunk, whilst his arms and legs usually adopt the flexed posture and so look after themselves. The baby with CP, however, may be floppy or stiff and is therefore more difficult to hold and care for. Floppy arms and legs need to be remembered and supported. Arms and legs which are stiff make nappy changing and dressing difficult. Slow, smooth movements are required as quick, jerky movements will increase the spasticity. Parents will need to be taught how to decrease the spasticity, for example by flexing the baby's hips and knees before attempting to abduct the thighs at nappy change.

Babies develop spontaneously, that is, without apparent intervention, in many areas. Vision and hearing gain voluntary control as a baby learns to turn his head to look and listen in response to a variety of auditory and visual stimuli. A baby with CP will need help in this regard however; because he is unable to turn his head, stimulation must be brought to him. A SCBU is full of sights and sounds but not those which normally surround a developing baby. If the baby requires this specialist medical support for more than a few days, multisensory stimulation must commence before he goes home. The parents should be encouraged to bring in items from home, particularly all the usual baby paraphernalia, which is preferable to that used by the hospital. His mother's choice of soap and talc, for example, will enable the baby to know his own smell. As the parents wash and clean their baby and massage lotion onto his body they will quickly learn how to handle him, forge bonds with him, and build their own confidence. As they cuddle him he will learn their personal smells and recognise them apart from the professionals who also handle him.

Toys to stimulate the senses are also important. Musical and squeaky toys encourage location of sounds and bright or reflective toys stimulate vision. Communication is vital and parents should be encouraged to talk to their baby and to tell him what they are doing to him. A baby with spastic CP will relax and anticipate movement if he is spoken to and stroked before handling; if he is touched or picked up unexpectedly, he will jump and stiffen. Talking to a handicapped baby is often difficult, as he may not respond. Parents may become discouraged. The occupational therapist can provide support and encouragement by setting an example. The way in which she handles, stimulates and communicates with the baby is often the model which parents imitate and adopt.

POSITIONING

Positioning is used in the treatment of CP to prevent contractures and deformity, to facilitate movement, and to enable function. A given position may further any or all of these aims. The basic positions used are lying (supine, prone, side), sitting (floor, side, chair), and standing. Most positions can be supported with one's own body (i.e. with the mother's, therapist's or teacher's body), with everyday furniture and objects, or with specialised furniture and equipment.

Lying

Supine

The supine position is the least used, as stimulation to the back of the head may trigger a full extension pattern and it is difficult to use the upper limbs against gravity. However, this position can be used to stretch those in a total flexion pattern or when encouraging eye contact and early communication skills in the young or severely affected person. Supine lying can be supported as follows:

- own body: babies and small children can be positioned on an adult's lap (Fig. 15.5A, B)
- everyday: for use with people of any age; the adult can position herself astride the person on the floor (Fig. 15.5C)
- special: for the moderately or severely affected person wedges made from foam or wood with harnesses and supports (Fig. 15.5D, E) can be used.

Prone

This position is used to prevent flexion contractures of the lower limbs, encourage head control and enable upper limb function. It can be assisted as follows:

- own body: lying supine (on the floor, bed or sofa) the adult can position a baby or small child on her chest. The adult supports the

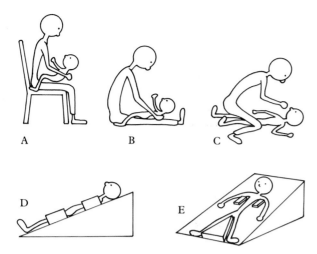

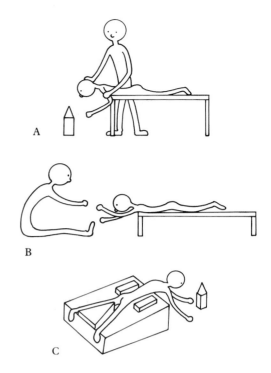

Fig. 15.5 Positioning: supine lying.

Fig. 15.6 Positioning: prone lying.

baby's head; a slight bouncing movement will stimulate the neck extensors and allow some weight to be taken by the baby. This position is particularly successful with floppy babies. With the adult standing, the person with CP can be positioned at right angles, e.g. on a plinth, facilitating both head control and upper limb function (Fig. 15.6A).

- everyday: the person can be supported in the prone position using a bed, sofa, cushions from the sofa or pillows (Fig. 15.6B).
- special: a wedge made form foam or wood with harnesses and supports will hold a person securely in the prone position (Figs 15.6C, 15.7).

Side-lying

This position provides total body support, including the head; facilitates shoulder protraction and brings hands into the midline; enables upper limb function (lower arm is in midline with gravity eliminated and upper arm is brought to midline, assisted by gravity); and inhibits spastic posturing of the lower limbs. It is particularly beneficial for the person who experiences difficulty in maintaining a symmetrical posture prone or supine. In itself, side-lying is not a supportive position; therefore, support must be provided, especially to

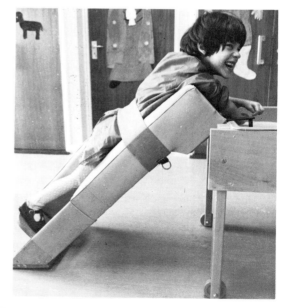

Fig. 15.7 Positioning: prone board enabling hand function.

the head, trunk and the uppermost lower limb. Side-lying can be facilitated as follows:

- own body: this position is tiring for the adult so should only be used for short periods of time. The baby or small child is positioned in side-lying on the floor, protected by a rug or foam mattress. The adult is positioned on all fours astride the child, with one arm supporting the head and spine and the other facilitating play, one leg behind the child to support the lower back and under leg, and the other between the child's legs to position and support the uppermost leg (Fig. 15.8A).
- everyday: as above, but the position can be used with a person of any age. Support is provided by foam blocks, cushions or pillows.
- special: side-lying boards are available in many forms from various manufacturers and custom-made boards can also be fashioned from heavy density foam or orthotic materials such as Plastazote and Hexcelite. The boards should be adjustable, if possible, so that alternate sides can be used (Fig. 15.8B).

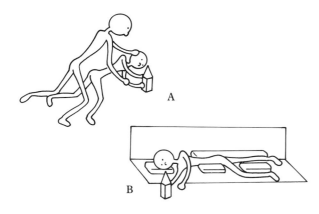

Fig. 15.8 Positioning: side lying.

Sitting

The main aim of the sitting position is to enable function, for example: learning — play, reading, writing; personal tasks — eating, toileting, dressing, applying make-up, shaving; communication — looking, listening, talking; leisure activities — games and hobbies, watching television.

The sitting position provides a stable base from which head, upper trunk and upper limb movement is made easier. The two main types of sitting are floor sitting and chair sitting.

Floor sitting

'W' sitting (Fig. 15.9A) and 'tailor' sitting (Fig. 15.9B) should be discouraged, as both encourage backward pelvic tilt (sacral sitting) and flexion contractures of the lower limbs. Floor sitting can be further subdivided into long-legged sitting and side sitting.

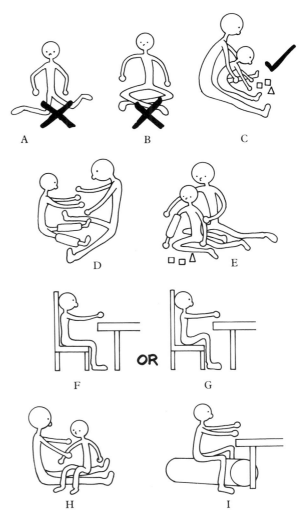

Fig. 15.9 Positioning: sitting.

Long-legged sitting provides stretch to the hamstrings and Achilles tendon with hip abduction and lateral rotation and enables hand function by bringing the hands into the midline assisted by gravity. This position can be supported as follows:

- own body: the adult sits on the floor with legs astride; the person with CP sits in the same direction, close to the adult's body, thus obtaining support for the trunk and pelvis. The legs can be supported in extension and lateral rotation by the hands (if not needed for the head and arms), leg gaiters (see p. 434) or by the adult's legs. With the adult's arms free, upper limb function can be assisted (Fig. 15.9C).
- everyday: the person may require trunk support to the rear, so sitting with his back to a wall, corner or sofa will help. Leg extension supported by gaiters will leave the adult free to face the individual for play, eye-contact and communication (Fig. 15.9D).
- special: various floor sitters are available, with or without trays or tables, harnesses, head supports and pommels (to encourage abduction and lateral rotation at the hips) (Fig. 15.10).

Side sitting: although an asymmetrical posture, this is used to provide a position in which weight-bearing through one upper limb is encouraged whilst the other limb is kept free for function. It is particularly useful for those with spastic hemiplegia. Side sitting can be supported by:

- own body: a person can be supported by an adult sitting behind in a similar position, providing support for and weight through the shoulder and elbow joints. An arm gaiter may be utilised to hold the elbow in extension (Fig. 15.9E).

Chair sitting

The correct posture is one in which the head is upright, the spinal curves supported, the person's weight distributed evenly through the buttocks and thighs, the knees at 90° and the feet plantigrade. Some people may require their hips and

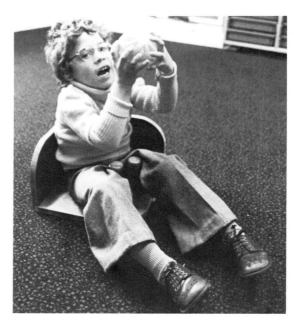

Fig. 15.10 Positioning: corner floor sitter; supported sitting to enable hand function.

knees to be more flexed in order to inhibit spastic posturing (Fig. 15.9F,G). Support can take the following forms:

- own body: a small child can be supported in the sitting position on an adult's thighs. This is especially useful for undressing and dressing (Fig. 15.9H).
- everyday: baby chairs, high chairs, kiddy chairs, dining chairs, pushchairs and armchairs can all be successfully utilised by most individuals. The addition of cushions, foot stools or tables will often suffice in maintaining a good sitting position.
- special: the severely affected person often requires more support in the sitting position, either to prevent deformity or to enable function. Many variations are available; therefore, assessment, selection and fitting are of vital importance. For people with tightness of the hip adductors, an astride or bolster chair may be the most suitable (Fig. 15.9I). Extra support can be provided using foam wedges, harnesses or moulded inserts. A chair should not only foster a good

position but should also be appropriate for the function required, for example watching television, eating, going to the shops.

Standing

Standing positions should encourage an upright posture (enabling perception of height and distance), prevent flexion contractures, ensure weight-bearing through the hip joints (essential for bony joint development), and facilitate stability of the knee and ankle joints prior to independent standing and walking. The following support can be provided:

- own body and everyday: whilst the child stands at a sofa, chair or table the adult supports his hips and knees in extension (Fig. 15.11). This is particularly useful for those with spastic diplegia who can use their upper limbs but require support for their lower limbs. Gaiters can be used to hold the knees in extension, thereby freeing the adult's hands to facilitate function in the upper limbs for those with more severe CP.

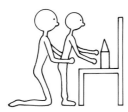

Fig. 15.11 Positioning: standing.

- special: prone standers, flexistands and standing frames are available, providing a wide range of positions and support (Fig. 15.12).

Relative positioning

The position adopted by the individual and adult relative to each other has important implications. The ideal positions are:

- face to face, as this promotes symmetry and eye contact

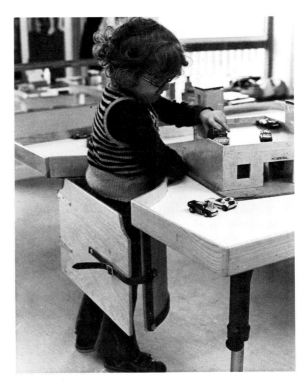

Fig. 15.12 Positioning: special equipment to enable standing (The Amesbury Quadra table).

- one behind the other, which removes distraction and enables the adult use of her own movement patterns when facilitating movement, as in feeding and dressing.

Looking upwards may stimulate the total extension pattern (Fig. 15.13A); in this case relative positions must be taken such that eye contact is on a downward gradient from the individual to the adult (Fig. 15.13B). Positioning oneself to the side of a person with CP encourages asymmetrical posturing, as it forces him to turn, stimulating the asymmetrical tonic neck reflex and making swallowing, chewing and vocalisation extremely difficult.

PERSONAL SKILLS

The overall aim of treatment is independence of function, and this should be achieved with those who have mild CP. People with moderate CP may

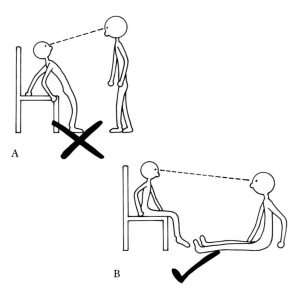

A

B

Fig. 15.13 Relative positioning.

be expected to gain a degree of independence in most areas, either with the help of aids to function or with the support of their carers. For those with severe forms of CP, the aim is to minimise the time and effort required by the carer in performing these functions for the individual.

Toileting

Problem areas include:

- sitting on the potty/toilet
- getting onto and off the toilet
- wiping
- bladder and bowel control
- toilet training
- removing and replacing clothing
- menstruation.

Sitting on the potty/toilet

Various toilet aids are available. Whether these are used in the short or long term will depend upon the individual's degree of success in acquiring head and trunk control and balance. The young child may be secure on a potty which has a large base with back and side supports. The standard

Watford potty chair has a higher back and sides with a removable front bar which prevents the child falling forwards. If the person is thin and bony, and thus finds the toilet aperture too large and uncomfortable, an insert with or without sides will help. Special toilet chairs which are either attached to the lavatory pan or slide over the pan are suitable for more severely affected people. These chairs have various accessories, for example head and trunk supports, harnesses and footrests, which can be added and adjusted to suit the individual.

Getting onto and off the toilet

Appropriately sited handrails will assist the person who is unsteady but otherwise independent and a step or platform around the base of the toilet will help if the toilet is too high. The dependent older child or adult may be too heavy to transfer onto the toilet, especially if the area is small, and in such circumstances a commode in the bathroom or bedroom will make toilet times easier.

Wiping

This is always an awkward task, requiring good hand function, balance and body perception. If tearing paper from a roll is difficult, a flat-pack of single sheets or wet-wipes may be easier. Wiping aids are available but these are often not suitable for a person with CP; an automatic washer or bidet can give the individual total independence.

Bladder and bowel control

People with severe CP are unlikely to achieve full control or to be able to make their needs known. If bowel habits are regular, routine toileting using the previously described aids can help the carer. Shop-bought terry or disposable nappies are adequate for the young incontinent child, but the older child and adult will need special pads, pants or larger nappies. The type of protection will depend upon the individual's needs and the availability of supplies from the local continence service. The help of the continence adviser should be sought.

Toilet training

The occupational therapist is unlikely to be directly involved with the routine of toilet training but she can assist by ensuring that the physical aspects of toileting, as described above, are appropriate for the individual.

Removing and replacing clothing

Mastering this aspect of toileting is of vital importance in giving the person with mild CP confidence and independence in using the toilet at school, work and in social settings. Clothing should be loose and limited to a few layers. It should have elasticated waistbands, which are easier to manage than belts, buttons and zips. Adapted clothing using Velcro fastenings is especially suitable for those in wheelchairs.

Menstruation

Menarche is always a time of change for the individual and the family. The severely affected child may or may not reach menarche at the usual time; occasionally, there is precocious puberty but often it is delayed. The parents are often unprepared; they may regard their dependent daughter as a child and menstruation may come as a shock. Menstruation may exacerbate certain problems, such as epilepsy, and so medication may be used to restrict the cycle. If the girl is doubly incontinent more frequent changing of pads will suffice. The girl with moderate or mild CP may wish to choose her own type of feminine hygiene (either pads or tampons) and advice, practice and, possibly, aids will be required. Some women who are wheelchair dependent, especially those with athetosis, find that pads are hot and do not stay in position, and therefore prefer the security of tampons. They may require special aids for insertion or removal or may depend on a carer.

Bathing

Bathing is a time for cleansing, relaxation and play. The pros and cons of bath versus shower change throughout the person's development and stages of independence. In the early stages bathing is preferable, as it gives an opportunity for play in the relaxing medium of warm water. Those who are severely affected may find that purposeful movement is made easier by the natural buoyancy of the water. Later, these benefits may be outweighed if a shower proves to offer personal independence or to be easier to use with a person who is severely handicapped. Safety is the main concern of any method of bathing. In the early stages, the lifting of a baby or child into and out of the bath will not present problems; however, the maintenance of a safe position will be more difficult. A bath mat may be sufficient to prevent a child slipping in the bath. A simple bath aid fashioned from a washing-up bowl (Fig. 15.14) will provide support in the sitting position and similar suction-based seats are available from baby shops. The more severely affected child with poor head and trunk control, or a continually writhing child, will require more support; this can be provided by a variety of special bath aids or inserts. As the severely affected person becomes heavier and larger a shallow bath insert, lifting bath seat or hoist may be necessary; alternatively, a shower stall which accommodates a special chair may be more suitable. Selection will depend upon the individual, his carer and family and the space

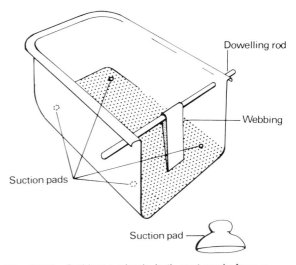

Labels: Dowelling rod, Webbing, Suction pads, Suction pad

Fig. 15.14 Bathing: a simple bath seat made from a washing-up bowl to maintain the sitting position.

available. Hair washing within the bath is easier with a shower attachment and 'halo' face protector. A wide selection of bath aids (e.g. rails, bath boards, seats, special baths) may provide the moderately or mildly affected person with bathtime independence.

Shaving is easier and safer using an electric rather than wet razor. Toothbrushes with padded handles, electric toothbrushes and pump-action toothpaste dispensers may aid independent teeth cleaning, but individual, custom-made aids may be required. Shaving, brushing teeth, putting on make-up, brushing or drying hair and so on will be easier to perform when seated on a chair or stool in the bathroom.

Feeding

Potential problems include:

- chewing, swallowing, mouth closure
- taking food from spoon
- maintaining a satisfactory posture
- taking food from plate to mouth
- picking up food with hand, spoon, fork
- cutting up food
- controlling liquids.

Babies and toddlers are dependent upon others for their feeding needs; in this respect children with CP are no different. However, some will remain dependent throughout their lives and others will need intensive intervention in order to achieve independence. Most forms of CP affect the face, tongue and palate muscles, causing the first two types of problems on the above list. These difficulties are dealt with primarily by the speech therapist. The occupational therapist must be conversant with the speech therapist's approach so that feeding programmes and interventions are complementary.

Posture

The positions adopted by the individual and his helper are very important. If the helper sits to one side the person must turn, thereby losing his symmetrical posture and possibly stimulating the asymmetrical tonic neck reflex. It is also very dif-

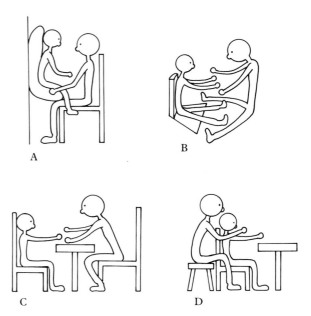

Fig. 15.15   Positions for feeding.

ficult to swallow with the head turned. Ideally, the helper should be directly in front, in order to maintain the person's position, facilitate mouth closure and chewing, and prevent teeth clamping. A small child can be positioned on the helper's lap with his back against a wall or corner (using a pillow for comfort) (Fig. 15.15A). A table can be positioned to one side to hold food and tissues. The older child or adult can be positioned in a floor sitter or suitable chair (see p. 420) with a narrow table between him and the helper (Fig. 15.15B,C). A grab bar fitted to the table, for the person to hold with one hand whilst eating with the other, will facilitate symmetry.

Taking food from plate to mouth

The table should be positioned at axilla height and close to the chest so that the distance from the plate to the mouth is reduced. This position allows the person to keep his elbows on the table, thus affording stability and reducing intention tremor. If the person needs assistance with this manoeuvre the helper should sit directly behind him so that she can use her own natural feeding pattern (Fig. 15.15D).

Picking up food

Hand control is essential and should be practised away from mealtimes (see p. 428). Appropriate foods should be provided for finger feeding; whole carrots, sausages, chips, salad items, biscuits, bananas and apple quarters, for example, are easier to grasp than smaller or chopped-up foods. Cutlery handles can be padded or adapted for attachment to the hand. Stodgy foods such as mashed potatoes, Weetabix and milk puddings stick to the spoon and thus can be used early in the feeding programme. Some people find stabbing food with a fork easier than scooping with a spoon. Dishes can be stabilised on the table with a non-slip mat or damp dish-cloth; alternatively, special suction-based dishes can be used. Plates with special lips, high sides or a plate-guard will stop the food sliding off the plate. Feeding aids should be provided with discrimination and discarded as independence is achieved.

Cutting food

While it is appropriate for a small child to have his food cut up for him, the older child and adult will want to be independent. Special cutlery, such as the combined fork/knife or rocker knife may be suitable. If such items are unacceptable away from home, the person should be encouraged to take packed lunches to work or school and to select foods from restaurant menus which do not require cutting.

Controlling liquids

Problems with controlling the lips and tongue often lead to liquids dribbling back out of the mouth. In the early stages, thickened liquids such as soups, custards and thick milkshakes can help the person to gain control. The difficulty may be in controlling the flow of liquids (i.e., tipping too much into the mouth); this can be eliminated by using a straw or a cup with a lid, or by putting only a small amount of liquid into the cup. Both hands can be used with a double-handled cup, thus promoting symmetry and better control.

People with an intention tremor often find a cup with a weighted bottom easier to use.

Mealtimes are an important social occasion in which the person with CP should be included, even if he is not actually fed at this time. This enables him to take part in family discussions and provides an ideal opportunity to learn social skills and mealtime etiquette.

The occupational therapist can provide the more independent person with opportunities to acquire skills related to mealtimes, for example food preparation, cooking, laying the table, nutrition and shopping. This can be started with the young child by using 'make-believe' play such as dolls' tea parties, setting up a shop, cooking in a Wendy House, or making dinner with Play-Doh; these activities also provide practice in gross motor control, hand function, perception, communication and social skills.

Sleeping

Problems associated with sleeping include:

- too much sleep
- too little sleep, disturbed sleep patterns, hyperactivity
- waking during the night, possibly having fits
- restlessness, falling out of bed
- inability to move or turn over in bed
- adopting abnormal postures.

Too much sleep

Often associated with severe forms of CP, this problem is sometimes found in the child who is described as 'very good' or 'no bother at all'. If the child sleeps for long periods during the day, opportunities for exploration, learning and play are severely limited and motivation may be very low. The aim is to provide frequent stimulation to discourage unwanted sleep. Waking periods should be gradually increased and a regular routine of sleep and wakefulness established. A programme of multisensory stimulation and varied activities of short duration supervised by a number of people and in different environments should be implemented.

Too little sleep

A person who does not sleep through the night should be provided with a very active day, with physical activity as well as mental stimulation. Naps should be avoided and a wind-down routine before bedtime (e.g. taking a warm bath, having a milky drink and listening to a bedtime story) will help to establish a healthy sleep pattern. If these measures fail to induce a full night's sleep other action will be required, given that parents or carers need to 'recharge their batteries' overnight. Sedatives may be prescribed, but these may affect alertness the following day. Arranging for a night-sitter or periods of respite care with a link family may be more appropriate.

Waking

Some people with CP are wakened during the night by cramps, spasms or fits. The new listening devices which plug into the household electrical circuit are an ideal way to alert parents or carers to the individual's distress.

Restlessness

For any child, outgrowing the security of a cot and learning to sleep in a bed can be a difficult process. The person with CP may have particular problems with physical security, and it may be easier to achieve the process in stages, for example by placing the mattress directly onto the floor, then onto the divan base and, finally, fitting the legs. Placing the bed in a corner, against the walls and using two or three 'baby-shop' bedsides should safely contain most individuals. Those with greater problems may need a sleeping harness attached under the mattress or an 'all-in-one' bottom sheet and duvet cover, which functions as a large sleeping bag attached to the bed.

Inability to move

If a person is unable to change position during sleep, stiffness, cramps, spasms and pressure sores can develop. It is impractical to expect the parents or carer to get up frequently during the night to reposition the individual. Turning beds, or mattresses which automatically and regularly change the areas of pressure may be necessary. Sheepskins and polystyrene bead filled mattresses also help to prevent pressure sores.

Abnormal postures

During sleep a person with CP may adopt positions which encourage deformity or contractures. Night splintage (see p. 434), foam wedges and bean-bags, in various combinations, can be used to support limbs or the whole body in a more satisfactory position.

Dressing

Problems with dressing may be of a physical, psychological or perceptual nature:

- physical: difficulty in controlling the limbs, maintaining balance, and holding gaze on the task to hand
- psychological: poor motivation, concentration, understanding, memory
- perceptual: apraxia, inaccurate body image, difficulty with sequencing and with understanding position in space and orientation of self and clothing.

The person with severe CP will be dependent upon someone else to dress and undress; therefore, the aims of intervention will be to teach the helper useful techniques and to advise on clothing which makes dressing and undressing easier and quicker. Positioning the individual on the floor, bed or specially fitted work surface is safer than using one's lap, a chair or a wheelchair. Techniques to inhibit spastic postures will facilitate the movement of limbs into and out of clothing. Clothing should be loose, free from unnecessary fastenings and limited to a few layers.

Physical

A good sitting position (see p. 419) is essential to trunk control and balance; it also facilitates head control, thus enabling the person to look at what he is doing.

Psychological

Problems in this area require the activity to be analysed (see Ch. 6) and the broken-down task to be taught using the backward chaining technique (Box 15.1). This method enables the therapist to monitor very small achievements rather than the whole task, which may not show any progress. These small but important improvements also motivate and encourage the individual to continue. If motivation is a problem the activity should be made more interesting and/or rewarding. With children and those with low intellectual ability the ideal motivator is that of dressing up either in adults' clothes (to be like Mummy or Daddy) or in costumes. Undressing can be rewarded by playing in the splash pool or body painting.

Box 15.1 Example of the backward chaining technique

Task: **Breakdown:**	Pulling off a sock Sock off from toes Sock off from forefoot Sock off from heel Sock off from ankle Sock off from leg (complete task)
Reward:	Verbal praise, clapping
Prompts:	Verbal — 'sock off' Gestural — demonstration of action Physical — hands over hands to assist
Session one:	Therapist tells individual what is to take place. She gives the individual a physical prompt to remove the sock as far as the toes. If the individual completes the task without prompts, reward is given and progress can be made to the next stage. If the task is not completed, verbal, gestural or physical prompts are used until the task is completed.

Perceptual

Various activities can be used to help the person to grasp the dressing/undressing process. Large

dolls can be used at first to show the differences between front and back — face/tummy/knees/feet versus no-face/back/bottom/no-feet; the child can then begin to apply this understanding to his own body. Dolls can be used to demonstrate which items of clothing cover which parts of the body. Dressing dolls can also provide practice in manipulating different fastenings (Fig. 15.16).

Tactile experience — proprioception and sensation — is very important; it will assist the child's understanding to actually *feel* the resistance when tugging down trousers and getting them caught over his bottom or to 'lose' his feet and try to 'find' them again.

The understanding of body parts, clothing and of the position of the body in space are all essential prerequisites of dressing. A person will be unable to respond to the instruction 'put your arm into the sleeve' if he does not know what his arm is,

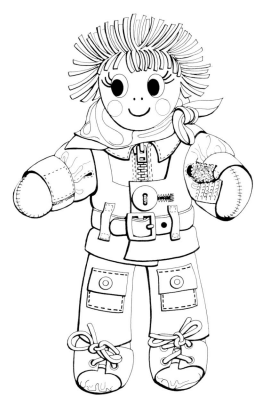

Fig. 15.16 Dressing practice: a doll whose clothes supply a variety of fastenings.

where it is or what a sleeve is. Activities may include: chanting body rhymes (e.g. 'Head and shoulders, knees and toes'); making a necklace of large beads and putting it on over the head; putting rubber quoits or rings up and down the arms and legs; standing in a hoola-hoop and pulling it up to the waist and up and over the head. Mirrors are useful for checking front and back, assessing neatness and motivating the person as his appearance changes. If problems persist into adolescence and adulthood, different motivators will be required, such as dressing up to go out, changing for hydrotherapy or swimming, and putting on clothes more suitable for a different, enjoyable activity.

HAND FUNCTION

Hand function is not assessed in isolation but as a later stage of upper limb development (see p. 412), since shoulder and elbow stability and mobility are required before hand control can be attained. Hand function is also assessed as an integral part of overall function and as such indicates intervention needs.

It is vital that, in working toward improvement in hand function, the sequences of normal development (see p. 411) be understood and respected. For example, the therapist must bear in mind that a stable trunk position (see p. 419) is a prerequisite for upper limb control. Similarly, activities to encourage shoulder control should not require the person to have either elbow or hand control. Hand painting, for example, in which the therapist applies the paint to the person's hand and large sweeping movements are made over a large piece of paper, avoids the frustration that will inevitably follow the person's attempts to make finer movements of which he is still incapable. Results will be easily achieved, providing positive feedback. When shoulder stability has been attained, activities to encourage elbow control can commence. Weight-bearing through the elbow joint (see p. 420) will promote joint stability. Dipping the hand into foods and taking the hand from plate to mouth will encourage controlled mobility of the elbow. When shoulder and elbow control have been achieved, work on hand func-

tion can commence. Picking up hand-size toys (2″ cubes, cars, balls, cups) and dropping them into a bucket will promote gross grasp and release. Controlled placing and releasing of grasp can be practised by putting pegs into holes, wooden men into boats, animals into pens, shapes into posting boxes and cars into garages. Activities for the control of forearm supination and pronation include pouring sand or water from cup to cup, drinking from a cup and using screwing rods.

Unlike the gross or full hand grasp, the tripod and pincer grips require finger differentiation; that is, in these grips not all fingers perform the same function. In the tripod grip the thumb, index and middle fingers are flexed to pick up or hold the object, whilst the ring and little fingers are slightly extended and abducted to provide balance for the hand. Constructional toys, building blocks and board games utilise this grip. The pincer grip is similar, but only the thumb and index finger are used for grasp whilst the other three fingers balance the hand. This is the most accurate and finely controlled grip and is used for picking up very small objects and performing complex bimanual tasks (e.g. threading beads). Final differentiation of the fingers allows one finger to be used alone, as in pointing, or pressing a switch. When individual hand control is achieved differentiation of each hand is possible; that is, one hand is able to perform one action whilst the other performs a different one. (For example, when drawing a line with a ruler or drawing round a template, one hand controls the pencil whilst the other positions and steadies the ruler or template.) Some people with CP, particularly those with hemiplegia, may never achieve hand differentiation; associated or mirroring movements of the more severely affected hand continue to occur and restrict hand function. Activities which encourage hand skills are limited only by the imaginations of the child and therapist; examples include using Play-Doh to make food for tea parties, making roads in the sandpit, or washing dolly's clothes and pegging them out. Remedial games and activities (see Ch. 10) such as pottery, cookery and woodwork are more suitable for the adolescent and adult with CP and hand function problems.

These are the basic stages of arm and hand control; the therapist should remember that the degree of upper limb control will affect the ability to perform other functions such as dressing, feeding, putting on make-up and shaving. A person who is only at the stage of shoulder and elbow stability has insufficient hand control to use cutlery; therefore, he should be expected to finger feed or to require aids.

Orthoses may be necessary to prevent or correct upper limb deformities or to facilitate function (see p. 434).

GROSS MOTOR FUNCTION

Gross motor control, coordination and balance are essentially the province of the physiotherapist; however, the occupational therapist providing treatment for CP should bear in mind that all skills are interdependent. She should not only be aware of the individual's level of attainment in these areas but should also incorporate the physiotherapist's treatment principles within her own intervention.

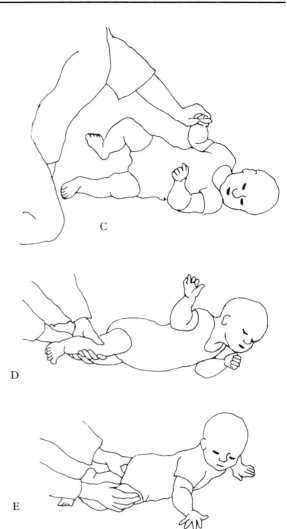

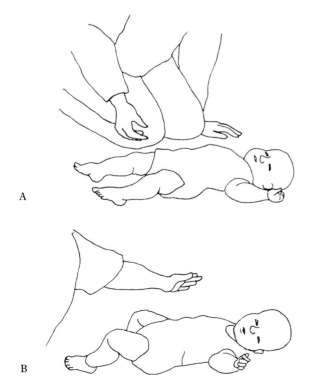

Fig. 15.17 The child with spastic diplegia moving from supine to prone position. Compare with Fig. 15.2A–E. (Drawings by Sarah Denvir reproduced from M. Griffiths and M. Clegg, *Cerebral Palsy: Problems and Practice*, Souvenir Press [Educational & Academic] Ltd, London, 1988, by kind permission of the publisher.)

The importance of gross motor function is evident in, for example, the young child with spastic diplegia who when lying on his back is unable to bring his hands into the midline to play (Fig. 15.17A). He needs to roll over onto his stomach to free his hands but even when his head is turned he is unable to roll over (Fig. 15.17B). The therapist will need to facilitate this manoeuvre either from the upper limb (Fig. 15.17C) or the lower limb (Fig. 15.17D), so that when lying prone the child has his hands free for play (Fig. 15.17E).

The child with athetosis is able to roll over but the movement pattern is uncontrolled and abnormal, taking much effort and often ending in frustration (as he ends up, for example, even further away from the toy he was trying to reach) (Fig. 15.18). It may be a long time before he is able to sit unsupported and therefore use his hands for play; the therapist can support this position whilst facilitating or encouraging hand function (Fig. 15.19).

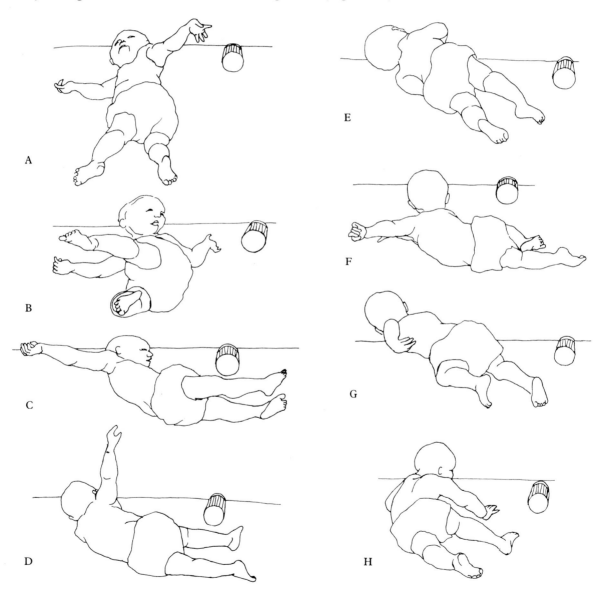

A

B

C

D

E

F

G

H

Fig. 15.18 The child with athetosis rolling over towards a toy. Compare with Fig. 15.2A–G. (Drawings by Sarah Denvir reproduced from M. Griffiths and M. Clegg, *Cerebral Palsy: Problems and Practice*, Souvenir Press [Educational & Academic] Ltd, London, 1988, by kind permission of the publisher.)

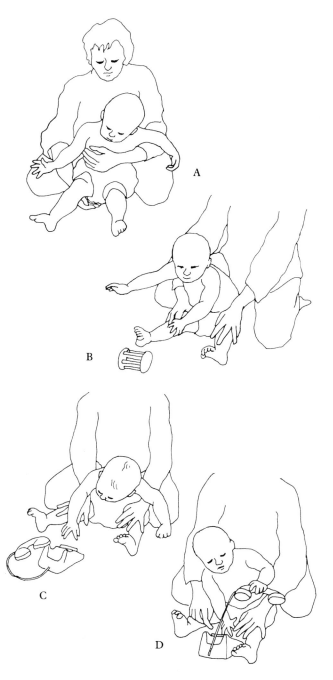

Fig. 15.19 The therapist supporting the child with athetosis in the sitting position to enable hand function. (Drawings by Sarah Denvir reproduced from M. Griffiths and M. Clegg, *Cerebral Palsy: Problems and Practice*, Souvenir Press [Educational & Academic] Ltd, London, 1988 by kind permission of the publisher.)

MOBILITY

Locomotion

The person with severe CP will be dependent upon wheelchairs and someone to propel them. The needs of the person and his family require careful assessment before wheelchair selection is made (see Ch. 9). Two chairs are often required: a buggy type for short journeys and outings with the family and a more supportive chair for everyday use. Many accessories are available to customise the basic chair for individual needs; these include head and trunk supports, harnesses, pommels, footstraps and moulded inserts. It is important to teach the family how to use the wheelchair correctly and safely, especially when an array of accessories has been provided. Wheelchairs will need to be modified or replaced as the person grows or his needs change. The person with moderate CP may use a wheelchair continuously or intermittently for long distances outside the home or for travelling around the school or college campus. The options are a self-propelled or electrically powered wheelchair or a tricycle (this can be foot or hand propelled with or without battery facility). Brightly coloured wheelchairs and tricycles are available which are often more acceptable and aesthetically pleasing; decorating in keeping with the latest craze in stickers can personalise them. Proficiency tests can be arranged to teach usage and maintenance for the individual, parents and teachers. Moderately and mildly affected children and adults may use a variety of walking aids: rollators, tripods, crutches and sticks, together with orthoses and/or special footwear, can enable independent locomotion.

Transport

It is accepted that travelling by car is safer with the use of seat-belts and car seats. These precautions are especially important for the person who has poor balance and saving reactions and limited control over his movements. The occupational therapist can advise parents on an appropriate car seat and, should more support be required, provide extra padding and/or harnesses. There are special car seats for the adult or larger child who requires more support than that provided by normal car seat-belts. If the person is transported to school or to a training centre by bus or taxi, provision should be made to ensure safety using either a seat or a harness. It may be easier and safer to transport the person in his wheelchair; some vehicles can be supplied or adapted to provide this facility. If the person is eligible for the Mobility Allowance a car may be purchased through the Motability Scheme. Under certain conditions the age at which a person can learn to drive a motor vehicle is reduced from 17 years to 16 years. Cars can be adapted to overcome a number of problems and special driving centres have been established around the country which provide assessment and instruction. Some individuals are unable to cope with either the speed or intricacies of driving standard vehicles but may achieve independence using a battery-driven car or scooter. Independence in transport can greatly enhance the quality of life for the person with CP, enabling him to work where he chooses and participate in a variety of social and leisure activities.

COMMUNICATION

The assessment and treatment of specific communication problems is provided by the speech therapist. However, the occupational therapist needs to be aware of these problems and their implications if she is to effectively communicate with the person affected by CP. She must be familiar with the speech therapist's approach so that intervention is complementary rather than antagonistic. Problems may occur in the reception, interpretation and/or expression of language. When working with a person who has attention or hearing problems the therapist should provide an environment that is quiet and distraction-free, and interaction should, preferably, take place on a one-to-one rather than a group basis. The therapist should position herself directly in front of and on the same eye level as the person. If he has problems with language interpretation, instructions should be accompanied by gesture or demonstration to provide visual as well as auditory input. Those with expressive problems should not be rushed, but given time and encouragement to

speak. The occupational therapist must use language commensurate with the developmental level of the person with CP; for example, if he is at the stage of two- or three-word phrases the therapist's instructions should be concise. Thus, in dressing, the instruction should be 'arm in' accompanied by gesture, not 'please put your arm into this sleeve'. The individual and speech therapist may be using an alternative means of communication, for example Makaton or Blissymbolics, and the occupational therapist must be familiar with the system and able to use it appropriately. A person with severe CP may require an electronic means of communication; the occupational therapist will be involved with the speech- and physiotherapist in assessing for a suitable aid (see p. 433).

PERCEPTION

Problems with perception may be subsequent to any form of brain damage or injury. Therefore people affected by CP are liable to show disorders of perception (see also Chs 16, 17). The assessment of such problems in CP differs from that of persons who suffer brain damage later in life in that standard assessment batteries are usually inappropriate; since the person with CP will need intervention before he is developmentally able to complete the required tasks, the therapist must depend upon observation and inference. For example, problems with body image may manifest themselves when a child is unable to cross a room without bumping into the furniture. This in itself presents difficulties as the cause may involve vision per se or figure/ground discrimination. The therapist should create various play opportunities which will help to identify the specific perceptual problem. As the treatment of perceptual problems is started early with the person affected by CP, the therapist can utilise many of the childhood games and activities which would be inappropriate for an adult. Nursery rhymes such as 'this little piggy', 'round and round the garden', 'eye, nose, cheeky, cheeky, chin', as well as body and face painting and games such as 'Simon says', all help to establish body image. Miniature assault courses providing obstacles to crawl under, over, through and around help to establish figure/ground discrimination and position in space. Perceptual problems will influence all areas of function, including personal skills, hand function, mobility, homecraft and education, and must be considered when planning intervention in any area.

MICROCOMPUTERS

The use of the microcomputer has grown rapidly over the last few years in the workplace, in education and in the home. Children and adults alike have found them invaluable as tools and as playthings and occupational therapists use computers for assessment, treatment and administration. The microcomputer has opened many doors for the person with CP — literally, by means of environmental control systems, and metaphorically, as communication aids. The occupational therapist may advise the person with CP on the suitability of a system, the position in which to use the computer and the means of access to the computer. A number of devices are available for access; these include pointers attached to headbands, mercury switches, light-sensitive switches, suck and blow devices, touch-sensitive pads, joysticks, mice, and concept keyboards. The occupational therapist, working with an electronics engineer, can usually design and construct special individual access devices if the above switches fail to meet the needs of the person with CP. In this way even the most severely physically handicapped person can be accommodated (see p. 434).

BEHAVIOUR

The person with severe or moderate CP may exhibit the following behaviours:

* self-stimulation or self-mutilation: rocking, head-banging, eye-gouging, teeth-grinding, hand-biting, masturbation
* aggression towards others
* screaming, breath-holding.

Management and behaviour modification programmes are usually directed by a clinical or educational psychologist but must be agreed to and implemented by parents, therapists and teaching staff so that the approach is consistent.

Preventive or protective measures may be necessary but must be accompanied by a programme to change or modify unwanted behaviours. For example, if hand-biting is a problem splints may prevent the hands from getting to the mouth (see p. 434) but this behaviour is often replaced by mouth-biting or head-banging. The person with mild CP may exhibit behaviours associated with a handicapped person trying to compete with peers; these include attention-seeking and immature behaviours, temper tantrums and over-dependency. Parents and teachers will need advice, reassurance and support through these episodes. If problems persist, referral to the psychology service will be appropriate.

ORTHOSES

Orthoses can be used as part of the problem-solving component of the occupational therapy process. The orthoses shown in Table 15.3 are suggested solutions to given problems. The exact method of their application and the materials used will depend upon:

* the precise problem
* the affected person
* the equipment available
* the knowledge and experience of the therapist
* financial considerations.

The occupational therapist may try a variety of designs and materials until a suitable solution is found. Some orthoses can be made and/or supplied by the surgical appliances department. These are usually permanent, heavy-duty, and more expensive. Fixed postural deformities require the utilisation of serial orthoses, that is, orthoses which are reshaped at regular intervals until a satisfactory position is achieved. (This goal may be impossible to reach, in which case the aim will be to prevent further deformity.) The following sequence of aims would be followed in correcting a flexed wrist/hand deformity:

1. Realignment, that is, correction of any deviation from the midline
2. Bringing the flexed wrist into the neutral position

Table 15.3 Orthoses for persons with cerebral palsy

Problem	Aim	Orthosis	Material	Other treatment	CP type
Head banging: intentional — self-stimulation/ mutilation; accidental — falls from fits or incoordination	To protect the face and head	Helmet (A)	Plastazote, leather, skate-boarder's crash helmet	Psychologist, behaviour modification	Severe intellectual impairment
				Physiotherapy, balance, gross motor coordination	All types
Mouth open: continual drooling, difficulty with feeding, speech	To facilitate mouth closure	Chin cup attached by elastic to lightweight head bands (B)	Canvas and elastic webbing, chin-cup — thermoplastic	Speech therapy, voluntary control	Athetosis
Access to computer required, only head control possible	To facilitate computer access	Helmet as above, attach pointing stick, mercury switch, light control			Athetosis, spastic quadriplegia
Tightly fisted hand, passively correctable	To maintain functional hand position (C)	Mitten-shaped paddle, supporting full palmar surface of forearm, wrist, hand, fingers and thumb. Serial orthosis (D)	Thermoplastics	Physiotherapy, passive stretching	Spastic hemiplegia, quadriplegia, baby in SCBU, older child or adult
Fixed flexion deformity of wrist & hand — pressure sores likely	To achieve a satisfactory position or to prevent further deformity			Surgery — tendon lengthening	
Fixed flexion deformity of elbow		Serial orthosis, full-length arm cylinder	POP, fibreglass casting tape		All types
Inability to maintain elbow extension	To support elbow in extension for weight-bearing (see p. 420)	Full-length arm cylinder, wrap-around arm gaiter (E)	Reinforced Plastazote, canvas with steel staves		
Hand function marred by inability to actively abduct thumb	To facilitate thumb abduction to enable controlled grasp and release	Working or active orthosis to dorsal aspect of hand and base of thumb	Thermoplastics	Physiotherapy, towards voluntary control of movement	Athetosis, spastic diplegia, hemiplegia
Hand function marred by inability to actively extend wrist	To facilitate wrist extension to enable hand function	Wrist cock-up orthosis	Thermoplastics, off-the-shelf canvas, Plastazote		
Intention tremor restricts hand function	To reduce tremor to enable function, writing, feeding, shaving, putting on make-up	Weighted wrist band	Close-woven cloth holding lead shot in compartments		Ataxia
Hand-biting, self-mutilation/ stimulation	To prevent hand to mouth movement but allow finger function	Arm cylinder with adjustable hinge at elbow	Thermoplastics; hinges: various	Psychologist, behaviour modification	Severe intellectual impairment
Poor trunk control

Asymmetrical trunk posture | To enable an upright, symmetrical posture in chair, wheelchair, free floor sitting (see p. 419) | Adjustable corset with shoulder straps, possibly with groin strap (E) | Hexcelite, Plastazote, thermoplastics, canvas, leather | Physiotherapy, muscle strengthening and control | All types |

Table 15.3 (con't)

Problem	Aim	Orthosis	Material	Other treatment	CP type
Difficulty with nappy change, dressing, walking caused by tight hip adductors	To achieve a satisfactory position or to prevent further deformity	Leg cylinders with adjustable abduction bar (G)	Plastazote thermoplastics	Physiotherapy, passive stretching. Surgery, adductor tenotomy	Spastic quadriplegia diplegia
Fixed knee flexion deformity		Serial orthosis, full-length leg cylinders	POP, fibreglass casting tape	Surgery, hamstring tendon lengthening	
Inability to maintain knee extension	To support knee in extension for standing, long-legged sitting, (see p. 420)	Full-length leg cylinder, wrap-around gaiter	Reinforced Plastazote, canvas with steel staves	Physiotherapy — voluntary control	All types
Fixed plantar flexion; deformity of ankle/foot	To bring foot to plantigrade position	Serial orthosis — as below	POP, fibreglass casting tape	Physiotherapy — passive stretching surgery-tendon (achilles) lengthening	Spastic quadriplegia, diplegia, hemiplegia, athetosis
Toe walking, dynamic plantar flexion (in standing, foot is plantigrade but walking increases spasticity, therefore foot is pulled into plantar flexion)	To hold foot 90° plus of dorsiflexion to facilitate heel strike	From above calf bulk to extend past toes, cut-out over heel to encourage proprioceptive feedback (H)		Physiotherapy — correct gait pattern	Spastic diplegia, hemiplegia

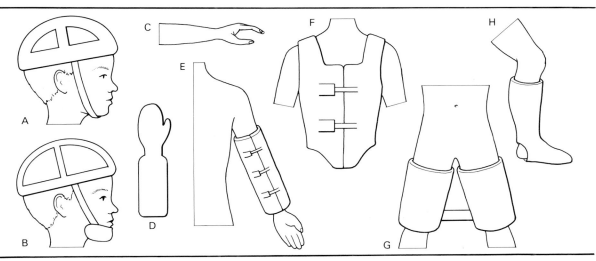

3. Bringing the flexed metacarpophalangeal joints of the fingers into the neutral position
4. Extending and abducting the thumb.

If all of these aims are achieved, then the wrist can be brought into slight extension.

EDUCATION

Historically, children with a physical and/or mental handicap were educated within special schools, that is, away from mainstream education. However, over the past few years changes within the education system have altered the situation of those with learning disabilities (encompassing all handicaps). The Warnock Report (1978) highlighted the need for those with learning disabilities to be integrated within the mainstream education system. The Education Act 1981 and the subsequent Education Reform Act 1988 instigated the Statementing procedure for those with 'Special Educational Needs'. This was followed by the inclusion of all children within the National Curriculum (with allowable exemptions). These changes have affected the occupational therapist in both the assessment and the treatment of children with CP. The occupational therapist may be requested to report on the occupational therapy needs of the child as part of Medical Needs within the Statement of Special Education Needs. Reassessment and review of needs is carried out annually, or at shorter intervals if there is a change in the child's needs.

Formerly, when handicapped children were educated in special schools, treatment was carried out with a large number of children on one site, often by a therapist who worked solely within the school. Now children with CP attend school throughout an authority's area, often with only one child in each school. Consequently, the child may not have the intensity of treatment previously available in special schools. Therapists face practical difficulties in visiting all the schools. They may also be reluctant to take a child out of class, thereby making him appear special or causing him to fall behind with his work; after school, however, the child is often too tired for therapeutic activity. One solution is to run intensive therapy groups during the school holidays with children of similar skills and problems. These can be organised like well-structured play schemes, with input from the occupational, physio- and speech therapists. Help with managing a number of children may be forthcoming from teachers who want to understand more about these children, from adolescents as part of their community service, and from parents. These therapy groups provide an opportunity for full reassessment, evaluation and review of intervention. Holidays are also an ideal time for home visits to check on equipment and the home

environment and to liaise with the family, who are often forgotten when a child attends school.

Integration

The occupational therapist will be involved in preparing and supporting the child before he starts school or when he changes schools. She will need to visit the school well in advance to assess and advise on the environment, i.e. on access, stairs, lifts, ramps and the equipment needed for the child to participate in all parts of the National Curriculum. Preparation and support for teachers and peers is also vital.

Personal skills

The child will not want to stand out from his peers; therefore, great emphasis must be placed on achieving independence before integration. He should be able to take himself to the toilet and manage by himself (adaptations may be necessary), to feed himself (a packed lunch may be suitable if he has difficulty with cutlery), to serve himself if hot meals are supplied and to dress and undress for PE and playtime. The therapist should also give consideration to the following:

- Positioning/seating: a good position at desks, tables and workbenches is essential to enable function in the classroom, laboratory, workshop (metal and woodwork) and kitchen
- Mobility: around the classroom, all of the above rooms, from the classroom to the playground and around the playground and school campus
- Hand function: intervention may be required to enable the child to participate in all activities, from early skills, e.g. using scissors, pasting, to the later skills used in fine arts, science experiments and vocational activities
- Gross motor control: practice in balance and coordination will facilitate participation in games, drama, movement to music, crafts and kitchen activities
- Handwriting: this may require specific intervention or, if it is too great a problem and delays the child's learning, the provision

of an alternative, such as a typewriter or word processor

- Perceptual problems: these may affect many areas of learning and will need constant monitoring and intervention as difficulties arise.

Liaison

Exchange of information between the therapist and the classroom teacher is of vital importance. The therapist should discuss her aims with the teacher and describe how they might be achieved. Often the teacher will be able to incorporate some of these objectives within her curriculum for the class as a whole. If the teacher finds a task with which the child is experiencing difficulty, for example drawing lines with a ruler, the occupational therapist can give the child a short, intensive programme either at school or at home, out of sight of his peers, so that he does not fall behind. Problems should not be pessimistically anticipated, as often a child, especially one who has initiative and perseverance, will overcome problems in his own way; this gives the therapist an ideal opportunity to learn methods of overcoming difficulties to use with other children.

HOME SKILLS

The person with moderate CP is expected to be partially independent. He is unlikely to live alone but will need to perform some household tasks himself. Basic home skills should form part of the occupational therapy programme for the adolescent. These should include: making a hot drink, getting a snack meal, cleaning and tidying his room, answering the telephone and, possibly, visiting the local shops. Those with less severe dysfunction who are expected to live independently should be able to manage all home skills, from cooking, cleaning, laundry, budgeting and nutrition to opening a bank account and selecting suitable accommodation and furnishing. The occupational therapist should ensure that all aspects are assessed and that information, advice, and intervention is supplied as necessary. Aids and equipment may be required to achieve independence.

Home environment

The baby or young child with CP is unlikely to require major alterations to the home environment, but as he grows older and heavier and his needs change the accommodation may become unsuitable. As the effects of CP are lifelong, it is possible to anticipate some future needs. The person with severe or moderate CP will be safer, easier to care for (or more independent) in ground-floor accommodation. This may be in an unmodified bungalow, a purpose-built bungalow or a ground-floor extension. Accommodation should have access and manoeuvrability suitable for a wheelchair, a bathroom and bedroom with suitable adaptations and an area for leisure or play. Any alterations to the home should be considered well in advance and discussed with the family so that changes are acceptable and as unobtrusive as possible. The person with mild CP may be able to become completely independent only in a 'user-friendly' environment; he will need the occupational therapist's assistance in arranging his home to best advantage.

EMPLOYMENT

The person with mild CP should be able to manage full employment, although he may require assistance in choosing suitable work and help with adapting the work environment. The occupational therapist will need to liaise with the person and his employer and with the special services available for people with disabilities in employment. The Youth Employment Officer will liaise with the school careers officer in providing vocational guidance and information on job and educational opportunities. He or she can be contacted through the local Careers Office. Those who wish to continue their education or to enrol in vocational training colleges will find provision for people with disabilities at many centres of further and higher education; individual prospectuses will give details. There are also a number of residential colleges around the country which offer special facilities for the more physically handicapped person as well as various vocational training and further education courses. The Disablement

Resettlement Officer (DRO), based at Job Centres, can help the person to find suitable employment and can offer support to the employed. He or she may refer the person to a Training College specialising in the assessment and training of people with disabilities. The Disablement Advisory Service helps with access and alteration to the worksite and the installation of special equipment such as ramps, toilets, lifts and occupational aids. The Rehabilitation Engineering Movement Advisory Panels (REMAP) can advise on the design and supply of special items of equipment which will help individuals to overcome specific problems at work.

The person with moderate CP is more likely to need sheltered or supported employment. Workshops vary from open employment to those provided by the social services or non-statutory sector. The previously mentioned services may also offer information, advice and support.

The person with severe CP will usually transfer from school to a local authority training centre offering sheltered work with continuing education in personal, independent living and social skills. Special Needs Units attached to training centres offer placement for people with severe physical and mental handicaps, with input from therapists so that intervention programmes are continued. The Spastics Society run industrial units around the country, some with residential hostel accommodation, specifically for people with CP; referral is made directly to the Spastics Society.

ADVICE AND SUPPORT

The long-term effects of CP on the family depend upon their attitude to handicap and to the affected individual. Some parents are unable to come to terms with or accept their handicapped child. For some, who feel unable to cope in the long term, the only answer is adoption. Often adoption takes place early in the child's life; the therapist will be involved throughout this process with both the foster or adoptive parents and the original family. Other parents accept the child as a member of the family but refuse to believe the diagnosis or recognise its implications. Another difficulty occurs when one parent accepts the child and the other

does not; relationships between the parents and between the parents and child are affected and the therapist should be aware of the effects on the child in particular. Such difficulties may remain unresolved, resulting in divorce or in one parent immersing himself in work whilst the other's life revolves around the handicapped person.

The majority of parents of children affected with CP accept them as individuals and encourage independence. However, the transition from childhood to adolescence and adolescence to adulthood will be no less problematic than in any other family. As life changes occur the person with CP may lack self-confidence and become frustrated or bewildered. These emotions are not exclusive to people with CP, but the presence of a disability may make these feelings occur more frequently or more strongly. The emergence of self-identity and the development of social and sexual relationships are trying processes in which the occupational therapist can offer advice and support. Parents, siblings, grandparents and partners need to understand all aspects of the individual's handicap, problems and treatment programme if they are to help and support the person. Their main role, however, is that of family member — mother, father, brother, sister, and so on.

The occupational therapist can also provide advice about holidays and social and leisure activities and can make referrals to other agencies such as social security, the Spastics Society, local support groups and counselling services.

CONCLUSION

Cerebral palsy is a lifelong disorder which affects many areas of function. It is not, however, an unchanging condition and the occupational therapist can play a major role in facilitating improvement. She must work closely with the affected person, his family and with other professionals; she must be prepared to offer advice, support, education and intervention in widely ranging areas of function. The occupational therapist is instrumental in enabling the person with CP to become 'his own person' and to achieve his full potential.

USEFUL ADDRESS

Information and advice can be obtained from:

The Spastics Society
12 Park Crescent
London W1N 4EQ

FURTHER READING

Abercrombie M L J 1964 Perceptual and visuomotor disorders in cerebral palsy. Heinemann Medical, London

Anderson E M, Clarke L, Spain B 1982 Disability in adolescence. Methuen, London

Caston D 1981 Easy to make aids for your handicapped child. Souvenir Press, London

Department of Education and Science 1978 Special educational needs: report of the committee of enquiry into the education of children and young people (Warnock Report). HMSO, London

DiMario F J, Sladky J T 1989 The cerebral palsy patient: neurologic disorders affecting the lower extremity. 6 (4): 761–790

Eckersley P, Clegg M, Robinson P 1986 The 1981 education act: guidelines for physiotherapists and other paediatric professionals. Chartered Society of Physiotherapy, London

Finnie N R 1977 Handling the young cerebral palsy child at home. Heinemann, London

Gordon N, McKinlay I 1980 Helping clumsy children. Churchill Livingstone, Edinburgh

Griffiths M, Clegg M 1988 Cerebral palsy: problems and practice. Souvenir Press, London

Griffiths M, Russell P 1985 Working together with handicapped children. Souvenir Press, London

Hegarty S, Pocklington K 1981 Educating pupils with special needs in ordinary schools. NFER Nelson, Windsor

Hewitt S 1970 The family and the handicapped child. Allen & Unwin, London

Illingworth R S 1983 The development of the infant and young child: normal and abnormal. Churchill Livingstone, Edinburgh

Klein M D 1982 Pre-writing skills. Communication Skills Builders, Tucson, Arizona (In UK: Winslow Press)

Klein M D 1983 Pre-dressing skills. Communication Skills Builders, Tucson, Arizona (In UK: Winslow Press)

Klein M D 1987 Pre-scissor skills. Communication Skills Builders, Tucson, Arizona (In UK: Winslow Press)

Kogan K L, Tyler N, Turner P 1974 The process of interpersonal adaptation between mothers and their cerebral palsied children. Developmental Medicine and Child Neurology 16: 518–527

Levitt S 1984 Paediatric developmental therapy. Blackwell, Oxford

Nolan M, Tucker I G 1988 The hearing impaired child and the family. Souvenir Press, London

Routledge L 1978 Only child's play. Heinemann Medical, London

Russell P 1984 The wheelchair child. Souvenir Press, London

Scrutton D 1984 Management of the motor disorders of children with cerebral palsy. Spastics International Medical Publications, Oxford

Sheridan M D 1975 Children's developmental progress — from birth to five years. NFER Publishing, Windsor

Simeonsson R J, McHale S M 1981 Review: research on handicapped children: sibling relationships. Child Care Health and Development 7: 153–171

Ward D E 1984 Positioning the handicapped child for function. Phoenix Press, St Louis, MO

Wedell K 1973 Learning and perceptuo-motor disabilities in children. Wiley, London

16

Cerebrovascular accident

Sue Hirst and Ruth Larder

INTRODUCTION

This chapter discusses the particular challenges faced by the occupational therapist in helping individuals who have suffered a cerebrovascular accident (CVA) or stroke.

The first section of the chapter defines CVA and describes its incidence, prognosis and causation. A very brief introduction to neuroanatomy is provided, with a view to explaining the neurological damage that can result from CVA. Characteristics of normal movement and posture are also outlined, together with the possible effects of CVA on motor control. The chapter then turns to other clinical effects of CVA, such as sensory deficit, spasticity, emotional disturbance, speech disorders, and perceptual dysfunction.

Next, the chapter describes in detail the specific role taken by the occupational therapist in facilitating rehabilitation following CVA, beginning with her assessment of the impact that the CVA has had upon the individual's motor, sensory, perceptual, and cognitive function, and upon his ability to resume his former level of activity and independence. Likely aims of the rehabilitation programme are set out, along with practical suggestions for treatment in such areas as the prevention of deformity, reduction of spasticity, enhancement of independence in personal and home care, management of perceptual problems, and resettlement at home and work.

Finally, specific physical problems that may present obstacles to rehabilitation are briefly described; these are the 'pusher' syndrome, shoulder and ankle problems, and multiple diagnoses.

Although a problem-solving, rehabilitative approach is emphasised throughout the chapter, the therapist is urged to tailor her treatment programmes to the needs and potential of each individual. The presenting problems of CVA are many and varied, and no one approach can offer solutions to them all. Therefore, the therapist must be flexible in her interventions, always keeping the individual's own priorities firmly in mind, and ensuring that her treatment complements that provided by the other members of the multidisciplinary team.

CHARACTERISTICS OF CVA

'A cerebrovascular accident is a rapidly developed clinical sign of a focal disturbance of cerebral function of presumed vascular origin and of more than 24 hours duration' (WHO 1986).

Excluded from this definition are episodes which resolve spontaneously within 24 hours. These, termed transient ischaemic attacks (TIAs), may precede a completed stroke; a predisposing medical condition such as hypertension may be present.

Stroke syndromes of slow, insidious onset are more likely to be due to another cause, such as a cerebral tumour; in such cases a full medical history is vital in order to establish an accurate diagnosis.

INCIDENCE AND PROGNOSIS

The incidence of strokes is about 1.8–2.0 per 1000 of population per annum. About 70% of all strokes occur in people over 70 years of age. Approximately 80% show some useful recovery and are able to return home (Rankia 1957); 60% of the total number regain independence in activities of daily living (ADL) and 30% are able to resume normal activities. The risk of mortality increases with age and the presence of associated conditions such as heart disease.

AETIOLOGY

Ischaemia

Occlusion of one of the major cerebral blood vessels (middle, posterior, anterior) or of one of their smaller branches is the most common cause of CVA; 70–75% of all strokes are attributable to occlusion.

Atherosclerosis

Intracranial arteries which have degenerative atherosclerotic changes may become occluded if platelets adhere to the damaged endothelial lining, forming a thrombus. The tissue beyond the occlusion is consequently deprived of blood which carries oxygen, and so becomes infarcted. The function normally performed by that area of the brain is lost or reduced, depending on the severity of the lesion. This type of CVA is most common in elderly people.

Embolus/thrombus

A stroke may also be caused by an embolus, a part of a thrombus which breaks away and is carried by the circulatory system into the smaller vessels of the brain, where it becomes lodged, thus depriving distal brain tissue of its vital blood supply. Particularly susceptible to this type of occlusion are people with cardiac disease in which emboli arise from the left atrium or ventricle and cause problems in the middle cerebral arteries in particular.

Haemorrhage

A smaller percentage of strokes is caused by cerebral haemorrhage and may occur at any age due to a rupture of abnormal blood vessels. In elderly people, hypertension, particularly in combination with arterial degeneration, may result in the rupture of small intracranial arteries. Sites prone to this are the internal capsule, pons, thalamus and cerebellum.

In younger people the presence of aneurysms or, more rarely, arteriovenous malformations (angiomas) may lead to cerebral haemorrhage; the Circle of Willis is a particularly susceptible site.

Pathology

In the case of haemorrhage, as with occlusive strokes, the area of the brain normally supplied by the ruptured vessel will be deprived of its oxygen supply. Additionally, function will be reduced in the area of the brain into which the blood has leaked. This area, however, may regain function if the blood is reabsorbed or the resulting haematoma surgically evacuated.

NEUROANATOMY

The following is a brief introduction to the neurological consequences of CVA. The reader is advised to consult appropriate texts of neuroanatomy and physiology for more detailed information.

Blood supply to the brain

The brain obtains its blood supply from two main pairs of arteries: the internal carotid and the vertebral arteries. These, together with other arteries, form the Circle of Willis (Fig. 16.1).

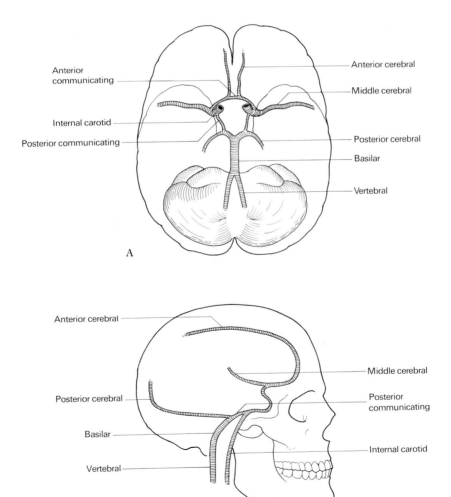

Fig. 16.1 The Circle of Willis: (A) basal view and (B) lateral view.

The Circle of Willis can act as a safeguard, allowing blood to flow to an infarcted area via an alternative route if a vessel is occluded, but where there is severe degenerative arterial change this may not be possible.

Nerve pathways

Sensory nerves

Sensory information from the trunk and limbs is conveyed via sensory nerve fibres in the peripheral nerves to their cell bodies in the dorsal root ganglia. Central collateral processes arise from these cells and pass from the dorsal roots into the spinal cord. From here, different types of sensory information are conveyed to the sensory cortex via separate pathways (Fig. 16.2).

Nerve fibres conveying information about *light*, *touch*, *vibration* and *joint position* travel up the ipsilateral side of the spinal cord (i.e. the same side on which they entered) along the dorsal columns to the brain stem dorsal column nuclei. There, they synapse with secondary neurones, which send nerve fibres to the opposite side to ascend to the thalamus in the medial lemniscus. From there, tertiary neurones send nerve fibres to the sensory cortex of the central hemisphere on that side.

Fibres carrying information about *pain* and *temperature* pass their impulses to second sensory neurones, which then cross to the opposite (contralateral) side of the cord. These then travel up to the thalamus in the spinothalamic tract, where they synapse with other neurones to convey the impulse to the sensory cortex in the parietal lobe.

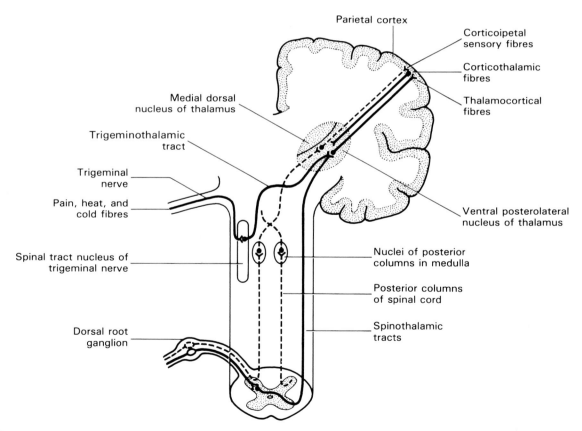

Fig. 16.2 Ascending sensory pathways in the brain and spinal cord. (Reproduced by kind permission of the publisher from Walton J N 1985 Brain's diseases of the nervous system, 9th edn. Oxford University Press, Oxford.)

Motor nerves

Weakness on one side of the body occurs as a result of injury to upper motor neurones in the opposite side of the brain. The motor nerve fibres, axons or pyramidal tracts arise from the motor cortex on one side of the brain, passing down through the internal capsule (see p. 445) to the medulla, where about 90% cross to the opposite side to form the lateral corticospinal tracts. They then continue down the spinal cord to the appropriate level, where they synapse with a second (lower motor) neurone. This passes out as a peripheral motor nerve fibre in a mixed peripheral nerve to skeletal muscle on that side of the body (Fig. 16.3).

The deficits resulting from CVA will depend on which area of the motor cortex is affected. The cells which control the movement of the legs originate on the superior aspect of the hemisphere, while those concerned with facial movements are on the inferior aspect, as can be seen in Figure 16.4.

Optic nerves

Some of the optic tract fibres cross at the optic chiasma, while others do not. The area of any

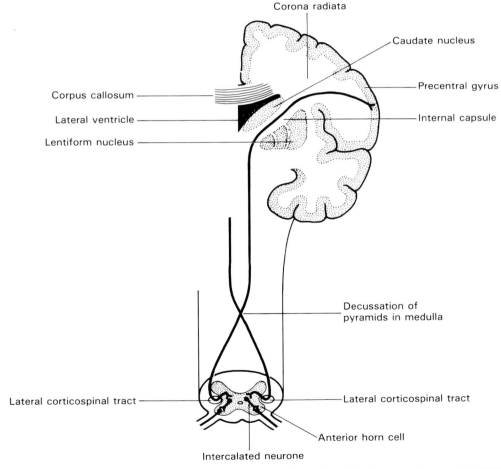

Fig. 16.3 Descending motor pathways in the brain and spinal cord. (Reproduced by kind permission of the publisher from Walton J N 1985 Brain's diseases of the nervous system, 9th edn. Oxford University Press, Oxford.)

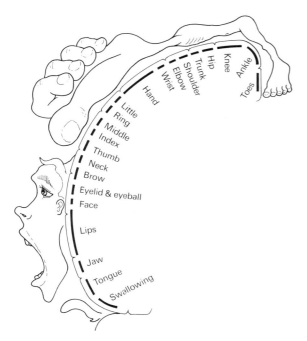

Fig. 16.4 The motor homunculus showing the representation of body in the motor area of the brain.

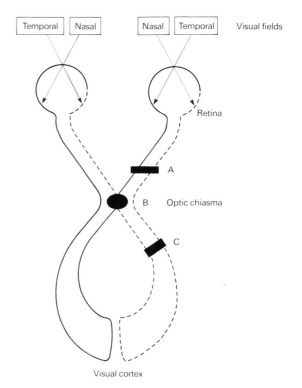

Fig. 16.5 Visual pathways and lesion sites. Lesions at site A result in total blindness in one eye; at B–bitemporal hemianopia; at C–homonymous hemianopia.

visual field deficit will depend on the site of the lesion. In CVAs the most common lesion produces homonymous hemianopia with loss of vision in half of each eye on the same side as the lesion. However, as the back of the eyeball receives information from the opposite side of the environment, the net effect is to be unable to see information presented on the opposite side to that of the lesion (Fig. 16.5).

Facial sensation

Sensory fibres in the trigeminal (5th cranial) nerve serving the face enter the spinal nucleus of the trigeminal nerve, where they synapse with secondary neurones. Their axons cross the midline to ascend on the opposite side in the trigemino-thalamic tract to the thalamus. There, they synapse with neurones which send axons to the sensory cortex of the cerebral hemisphere on that side (see Fig. 16.2).

It can be seen, therefore, that the central pathways for both sensory and motor function cross over, so that a lesion in one hemisphere of the brain results in disability on the opposite side of the body.

Location of lesions

Internal capsule

The internal capsule within the hemispheres is the site where bundles of motor nerves, sensory nerves and the fibres of the optic tract pass in close proximity to one another. Lesions in this region may cause loss of motor ability and sensory appreciation as well as hemianopia.

Cerebellar and brain stem CVAs

The pyramidal system works in conjunction with the extrapyramidal system to produce smooth movements. The extrapyramidal system (which consists of fibres from the premotor area, the basal ganglia and the brain stem) and the cerebellum are jointly responsible for coordinating the smooth contraction and relaxation of muscle groups and the maintenance of posture and body equilibrium. Lesions in these areas result in impairment of posture and righting reflexes and loss of control of voluntary movement, with intention tremor if the person attempts to move his affected limb (ataxia). Ataxia may involve one or more limbs: it can be unilateral or bilateral and may involve the trunk, causing unsteadiness when standing and walking (truncal ataxia).

Vertigo and vomiting may occur at the onset of a brain stem stroke and are common with obstruction of the posterior inferior cerebellar artery. Nystagmus (jerking of the eyes during voluntary eye movements) and disturbance of coordination of simultaneous eye movement (conjugate gaze) can also occur.

If the nuclei and nerve tracts controlling extraocular movements are affected, strabismus (squint) or diplopia (double vision) may be present. With lesions low in the brain stem (e.g. in the medulla), the lower cranial nerve nuclei and axons may be affected, giving rise to bulbar palsy with dysphagia (difficulty swallowing), dysarthria (slurred speech) and difficulty with coughing. This should be distinguished from pseudobulbar palsy, which has similar symptoms, but is due to bilateral upper motor neurone lesions within the motor cortex.

NORMAL MOVEMENT

The therapist needs a thorough understanding of normal movement in order to treat the motor and sensory manifestations of stroke as described above. Normal movement occurs automatically; for example, the individual does not generally have to think consciously about moving from a sitting to a standing position. However, individuals move in patterns which may vary slightly according to various factors such as build, personality, habits and pain.

In order to move normally, the central postural control mechanism is needed, accompanied by normal sensation, tone, balance, righting and equilibrium reactions and reciprocal innervation.

Patterns of movement

When an individual moves deliberately he chooses how to do so by selecting the movement and controlling it; he does not move in gross motor patterns but in refined, highly selective patterns of movements.

Sensation

Everyone is aware of pain, temperature, pressure and proprioception. All these are integrated from the periphery and transmitted to the centre, providing feedback to facilitate normal movement. Sensation is also necessary for the maintenance of balance.

Normal tone

This provides a background for normal movement. Normal tone allows freedom of movement without conscious thought. Tone needs to be sufficiently high to support the body and to enable it to move against gravity but not so high that it impedes movement. Automatic adjustment, for example moving from a sitting to a standing position, relies on normal tone — without it the body cannot support itself and the person falls over.

Balance, equilibrium and righting reactions

During everyday activity the body's tone and posture adjust automatically to take account of the effects of gravity and to maintain balance. The body needs to be maintained in equilibrium while supporting surfaces move (as when one rides on a bus), or are uneven (as when one walks over rough terrain).

Reciprocal innervation

Reciprocal innervation facilitates the graded interplay of agonist and antagonist muscles so that selective movement is possible. Co-contraction, i.e. the simultaneous contraction of flexors and extensors, ensures stability of a joint to allow it to be used functionally.

KEY POINTS AND POSTURAL SETS

Key points are points of control within the body where changes in postural tone occur to allow normal movement.

The central key point (CKP) can be represented as a circular band taking in the lower part of the sternum and T6–7; the proximal key points are the two shoulders and the pelvis.

Postural sets are positions or postures of symmetry or alignment of key points from which normal movement occurs. They allow the individual to move with or against gravity, and to perform purposeful, selective movement. Abnormal patterns start to develop if the individual is unable to maintain or regain alignment of the key points in a given postural set.

Postural sets include supported and unsupported sitting, standing, prone lying and supine lying. In each set there will be a particular influence of tone.

Sitting

In sitting the individual has a large base of support and thus requires less muscle tone to maintain his posture against gravity.

In supported sitting the CKP lies behind the peripheral key points. Here, the overall influence of tone is toward flexion, whereas in unsupported sitting a person will use active extension of the pelvis, lumbar spine and CKP to negate the effects of gravity.

Standing

In standing a person is relatively unstable in that his base of support is very small and his centre of gravity is distant from that base. Normally, a higher level of postural tone is needed to support oneself against gravity, with the main tendency being toward extension. However, there is some selective flexion, as the shoulders will normally fall forwards.

Prone and supine lying

These two sets are not often used during occupational therapy but it is still important to understand their influence on tone. In prone lying the position of the CKP in relation to the others dictates an overall flexor pattern, whereas in a supine position the CKP is in front of the others, resulting in an overall extensor pattern. The most usual time to adopt one of these positions is during sleep and by using a variety of positions the development of overall flexion or extension can be avoided.

CLINICAL FEATURES OF CVA

The effects of a CVA can be extremely diverse. Some observable changes in posture and tone have already been outlined. Other relatively common problems are considered below (Fig. 16.6).

Sensory disturbance

The maintenance of posture and normal movement requires the efficient transfer of information between the sensory and motor systems. Disturbances in vision and proprioception, for example, will affect the quality of information received from the sensory system; this then impairs the quality of the motor system's reactions, i.e. movement.

The senses are utilised in the learning and relearning process; therefore, a person with major sensory deficits — for example, total lack of sensation in the hemiplegic side — often rehabilitates more slowly and with less success than another whose senses are intact.

If perceptual problems are present in conjunction with sensory deficit, the risk of injury will be greater; for example, if a left inattention exists with a total sensory loss, the person will be at great risk from burns or scalds when working in the kitchen. In order to prevent unnecessary injury the individual needs to understand the potential danger in such circumstances. He will need to learn and develop compensatory techniques, which may include visual, tactile or auditory cues, such

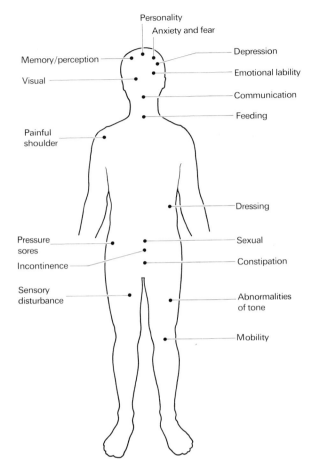

Fig. 16.6 Areas that can be affected by a CVA.

as using his unaffected hand to test the temperature of water.

Abnormal patterns of movement

A hemiplegic person may present with abnormal patterns of movement, or synergies, due to abnormal tone, sensory deficit, and loss of balance, equilibrium and righting reactions. Flexor or extensor synergies can be seen in the upper or lower limb, depending on the activity being performed. For example, when bringing food from the plate to the mouth a flexor synergy may be seen in the upper limb. As the shoulder moves into abduction this results in mass flexion of the upper limb.

Abnormal muscle tone

A paralysis (plegia) or weakness on the side of the body contralateral to the lesion is usually the most observable result of a stroke; the face, neck and trunk muscles can be involved as well as the limbs. Muscle tone alters following a stroke. Hypotonus (reduced tone) is usually present immediately after the episode and presents with limp, flaccid limbs and a reduction or absence of resistance to muscle movement. Although hypotonus may persist, it is usually followed by hypertonus (increased tone). This can present in typical patterns of spasticity as resistance to passive movement increases. If the individual tries to move whilst exhibiting increased tone he may be unable to produce selective movement, demonstrating abnormal patterns of movement instead; for example, his upper limb may become flexed due to the pull of the spastic muscle groups.

Typical patterns of spasticity

Neck

The neck is flexed toward the hemiplegic side and rotated slightly towards the unaffected side so that the face is turned towards that side (Fig. 16.7).

Upper limb

The scapula is retracted, the shoulder girdle depressed and the humerus adducted and internally rotated. The elbow is usually flexed and the forearm pronated, although in some cases supination may occur. The wrist is flexed, with some ulnar deviation, and the fingers and thumb are flexed and adducted.

Trunk

The trunk is flexed laterally to the hemiplegic side.

Lower limb

The pelvis is retracted and the hip extended, adducted and internally rotated. The knee is extended and the foot plantar-flexed and inverted with the toes flexed and adducted.

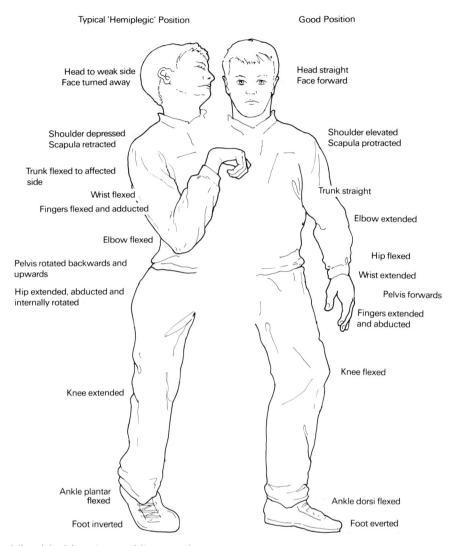

Typical 'Hemiplegic' Position

Good Position

Head to weak side
Face turned away

Head straight
Face forward

Shoulder depressed
Scapula retracted

Shoulder elevated
Scapula protracted

Trunk flexed to affected side

Wrist flexed

Fingers flexed and adducted

Elbow flexed

Pelvis rotated backwards and upwards

Hip extended, abducted and internally rotated

Trunk straight

Elbow extended

Hip flexed

Wrist extended

Pelvis forwards

Fingers extended and abducted

Knee extended

Knee flexed

Ankle plantar flexed

Foot inverted

Ankle dorsi flexed

Foot everted

Fig. 16.7 Typical 'hemiplegic' posture and its correction.

Associated reactions

Associated reactions have been described by Walshe (1923) as 'released postural reactions in muscles deprived of voluntary control'.

These reactions may occur when a person attempts too difficult a task or is anxious or upset. When carrying out a task, for example dressing the unaffected side, associated reactions may be seen in the affected arm and leg. The individual can be taught to inhibit these reactions, for example by placing the clothes in a position that encourages extension rather than flexion; alternatively, he can be taught how to overcome the reactions once they have occurred.

Emotional disturbances

Many people become emotionally labile following a CVA, exhibiting uncharacteristic emotion, for example crying or laughing at inappropriate times.

This is often distressing and embarrassing for the individual and his relatives, who may not understand that these changes in behaviour occur as a result of the CVA.

However, true mood changes do occur and may include depression — a result of the person's understanding of his changed situation. Frustration and aggression may also present, particularly if the individual has communication difficulties. Additionally, he may be anxious and apathetic.

Different approaches need to be used in dealing with people who exhibit emotional lability and true mood changes. In the former case, a simple explanation that this is occurring as a direct result of the stroke may be sufficient to reduce the individual's and his relatives' distress and embarrassment. The person may also benefit from being given reassurance and the opportunity to express his emotion and cope with it in his own way.

In the latter case, true mood changes may have a more permanent effect on motivation and performance, hampering rehabilitation in the long term. In these circumstances it may be necessary for the therapist to work with a clinical psychologist to implement strategies to enable the person to overcome his difficulties.

If the individual becomes depressed, cognitive processes may also be slowed, impairing reasoning and the retention of new information. This will further detract from the success of a treatment programme.

If possible, any negative emotions should be channelled into productive activity; for example, kneading dough and baking bread could benefit someone who is exhibiting frustration and aggression by providing both an outlet for emotion and a satisfying end product.

Activities should be selected in cooperation with the individual to ensure maximum motivation and, therefore, maximum therapeutic value.

Speech and language disorders

Speech and language disorders normally occur in people who have a lesion in the dominant hemisphere (usually the left).

Dysarthria

This occurs when the muscles involved in speech are weak or paralysed; speech becomes slurred, although there is no language deficit.

Dysphasia

This may be divided into expressive and receptive dysphasia.

Expressive dysphasia, which is caused by a lesion in Broca's area, is the inability to express oneself through speech even though comprehension of the spoken word may be intact. A person who is expressively dysphasic may be able to sing or speak on an automatic basis; for example, singing hymns, counting or reciting days of the week may be possible.

Receptive dysphasia occurs as a result of a lesion in Wernicke's area and is the inability to comprehend the spoken word, although on first acquaintance an individual may appear to understand speech on a superficial level. This may be due to him picking up nonverbal cues such as facial expressions or gestures.

A combination of expressive and receptive dysphasia is termed *global aphasia*.

Visual disturbances

The most common visual disturbance is homonymous hemianopia resulting from trauma to the optic tract or visual cortex in the occipital lobe. This is a visual field defect in which the person is unable to see half of the visual field while looking straight ahead. The same side of the visual field is lost for each eye; this is commonly the same side as the hemiplegia. It may be peripheral, sparing central vision, or it may 'split' or divide the central field of vision. In some people vision may be lost in only one quadrant, giving rise to quadrantanopia (Fig. 16.8).

Functional difficulties associated with visual disturbance are often related to safety in the kitchen, negotiating stairs and crossing roads.

Perceptual deficits

Perception is 'the ability to interpret sensory mess-

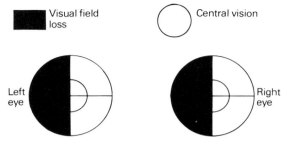

A Left homonymous hemianopia splitting central vision

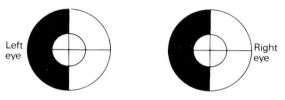

B Left homonymous hemianopia sparing central vision

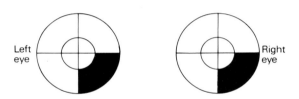

C Right lower quadrantanopia sparing central vision

Fig. 16.8 Homonymous hemianopia.

ages from the internal and external environment such that the sensation has meaning' (Zoltan et al 1986).

Following a CVA certain perceptual deficits may be present, their type and extent depending upon the site of the lesion. Perceptual dysfunction occurs when the sensory end organ is intact but the area within the cortex concerned with interpretation of the stimuli received by that organ is damaged.

The main categories of perceptual disturbance are outlined briefly below; again, the reader is encouraged to gain a deeper understanding from specialised texts.

Agnosia

A person is unable to recognise familiar objects using a given sense although the corresponding sense organ is undamaged. For example, a person with visual agnosia may fail to recognise personal objects such as hairbrushes or combs using sight but may identify them correctly through touch. If a person has problems with agnosia he may put himself at risk from injury, for example by inadvertently putting a knife in his mouth.

Spatial relationship disorders

- *Figure/ground*. The individual has difficulty differentiating foreground from background. He may have difficulty finding his matching shoe in a wardrobe.
- *Position in space*. The person has difficulty orientating himself or objects within the surroundings; for example, he may look on top of the bed when told his shoes are under the bed.
- *Form constancy*. The individual may have difficulty recognising everyday objects when they are seen from an unusual angle, in unusual positions or are of different sizes but similar in design, for example a hairbrush and a toothbrush.
- *Depth/distance perception*. The person may misjudge depth and distance and so have difficulty when negotiating stairs or trying to fill a cup.

Apraxia

This is a loss of ability to perform a previously learned movement although the individual retains the motor power, sensation and coordination essential to the action. It may take several forms and it is common for two or more forms to coexist. Apraxia might be demonstrated by a person who, wanting to make tea, is able to take the kettle to the tap but cannot understand how to get the water into the kettle.

Body image/body scheme disorders

Body image is the mental representation of one's body that expresses one's feelings and thoughts whereas body scheme is the postural model of the body's physical structure.

Included in body image and body scheme disorders are unilateral neglect/inattention and failure of right/left discrimination.

Unilateral neglect/inattention is the inability to respond appropriately and consistently to stimuli from one side of the body. This is common following right hemisphere strokes. An individual may bump into objects on one side or may only eat the food on one side of his plate.

When right/left discrimination is affected the concepts of right and left are no longer understood and the individual is unable to identify the right and left sides of his body.

THE ROLE OF THE OCCUPATIONAL THERAPIST

The occupational therapist works alongside the individual who has suffered a CVA and his carers, as part of the multidisciplinary team. Her work will complement that of other members of the team in enabling the individual to achieve his personal goals and maximise his independence.

At various stages of the rehabilitation programme the therapist's role will change considerably in accordance with the findings of continuous assessment; for example, in the early stages of treatment good positioning may be the most important aim, whereas safety in the kitchen may take priority later on.

ASSESSMENT

Assessment forms an integral part of intervention and is a component of each treatment session.

Due to the complexity of the information required to form an accurate assessment it may not be possible to build a full picture of the individual's abilities and problems in one session. He may become easily exhausted; therefore, alternative sources of information such as medical notes and the observations of nurses and relatives should be used to complement the information gained from the person himself. A full and accurate assessment needs to be done before priorities for the treatment programme are established. This assessment should include information about the person's previous level of health, independence and life-style, as these will affect the outlook for rehabilitation.

The therapist's knowledge of the individual's current abilities will not only form a baseline for treatment but will also help to boost the person's morale and maintain his level of motivation.

When assessing a person's problems it is essential to determine not only what these are, but also why they have arisen, so that their specific causes can be addressed. For example, the person may be unable to dress independently due to a loss of postural control, a faulty body scheme or problems with sequencing; equally, he may be apraxic or lacking in motivation to complete the task. The cause of the problem should be considered on a personal basis so that treatment can be planned to meet the individual's needs.

Specific areas of assessment are outlined below.

Initial observation

Through observation the therapist can amass a great deal of information about the individual's condition. Working from the head to the foot, she should consider the following for example:

- head/face
  - facial expression
  - any asymmetry
  - visual inattention to one side
  - mouth drop and drooling
  - position of the head
  - muscle tone of face and neck
- trunk
  - asymmetry in posture, noting any flexion and rotation
  - muscle tone
  - weight distribution
- upper limb
  - position and awareness of limbs
  - muscle tone
- lower limbs
  - position and awareness of limbs

— muscle tone
— weight distribution
• feet
— any inversion.

Loss of postural tone

This may be observed whilst the individual attempts to maintain his posture, for example when sitting. He may tend to fall to one side, being unable to correct himself or prevent himself falling. If he can maintain a stable posture he may be unable to change it (e.g. to move from lying to sitting or sitting to standing).

Range and quality of movement

The range and quality of movement can be measured or assessed functionally, that is, in activities such as feeding or transferring. Such activities will indicate the individual's abilities in static and dynamic sitting balance and his upper limb range of movement. They will also demonstrate whether movement patterns are normal or synergistic, and whether they occur without associated reactions, notably flexion in the affected upper limb and extension in the lower limb.

Sensation

Testing for touch and temperature sensation, stereognosis and proprioception is necessary, as deficit has been shown to have a major bearing on functional ability.

• *Touch*: light touch sensation can be tested by lightly touching the person's skin, working proximally to distally; results may be recorded in diagram form.
• *Temperature* can be tested using two test tubes, one containing warm water and the other containing cold water.
• *Stereognosis*: the individual's ability to recognise objects by touch can be tested by asking him to name objects felt but not seen, e.g. items placed inside a cloth bag. If communication is a problem an object out of sight can be matched from a selection that can be seen (see also p. 581).

• *Proprioceptive loss*: the therapist can test for this by moving the affected limb into a position while the person has his eyes closed. He then has to copy the position with his unaffected limb.

Visual problems

The therapist can test for hemianopia by standing behind the individual and moving an object from the lateral field of his vision towards the centre, first from one side, then from the other. The person should indicate when he can first see the object. A simple diagram can be used to chart visual field loss.

Functional activities may also be used to indicate visual field loss; for example, the therapist can ascertain at what position the person can see his knife or soap. Hemianopia is often associated with neglect of the affected side.

Speech and language disorders

Ineffective communication is a major cause of frustration and depression, sometimes resulting in reduced motivation and slower rehabilitation.

As these areas will be more comprehensively assessed by a speech therapist, liaison is essential to ensure that the most effective means of communication is used by each member of the team. An accurate assessment of the individual's receptive abilities may indicate that visual cues are a more appropriate means of communication than verbal cues. This type of information is particularly important when helping him to learn new skills or relearn former ones, such as peeling a potato using a spike board.

Perceptual dysfunction

Standardised assessments for perceptual dysfunction can be used to identify the extent of specific problems that the individual may mask during normal activities. Examples of these are the Chessington Occupational Therapy Neurological Assessment Battery (COTNAB) and the Rivermead Perceptual Assessment Battery (RPA).

These are standardised and validated tests. Standardisation ensures that the assessor does not affect the outcome of the test, whilst validation ensures that the test actually assesses the area it is designed to assess.

Other, non-standardised tests are available as assessment tools. These include scanning sheets, sequencing cards and body image jigsaws. Functional assessments may also indicate a range of perceptual difficulties; for example, an analysis of someone making a drink may show that he has difficulties in such areas as figure/ground differentiation, shape and object recognition and sequencing.

Cognitive function

Standardised tests which aid the assessment of cognitive function include the Rivermead Behavioural Memory Test and the Clifton Assessment Procedures for the Elderly (CAPE).

In assessing particular aspects of cognitive function it is important to take account of a number of specific factors which may influence the individual's performance. These include consideration of any senses that may be relevant to a task; for example, elderly people can experience visual or auditory deficits which may give a false impression of their abilities. If they fail to hear a kettle whistling and consequently let it boil dry, they may be considered unsafe or forgetful, when in fact their hearing may be the problem.

A suitable environment for testing is essential. Potential distractions such as extraneous noise or other people nearby should be avoided, thereby enhancing the individual's ability to concentrate.

Activities of interest to the individual may give a more accurate indication of his cognitive abilities, as lack of interest can result in inattention and poor motivation.

Functional assessment

It is important to assess and record a person's level of independence in ADL as this will often form the baseline of treatment. Only skills relevant to the individual need to be considered. For example, if an elderly lady did not cook her meals prior to her stroke, then assessment in this area is of little value. Continual assessment will indicate areas of improvement as well as areas in which the individual may need support in the longer term.

In addressing functional problems the cause of the difficulty needs to be ascertained. For example, if the individual is unable to wash his face it may be because he cannot cross the midline, has an inattention, has extensive loss of postural control or lacks understanding or motivation.

Home assessment

If the individual is being treated at home, problems can be addressed as they arise. If, however, the person is being treated in hospital a home assessment may be necessary to ensure that the transition from hospital to home is as smooth and trouble-free as possible.

Assessment in a person's home environment is described in Chapter 7, but four areas which may be of particular importance for those who have had a CVA are briefly summarised below:

- *Access*. If the person is unable to manage the access with any mobility aids, e.g. a wheelchair or walking frame, then adaptations such as a ramp, half steps or rails may be indicated.
- *Doors and corridors*. The width of these may hamper mobility around the house if the individual is dependent on a wheelchair or walking frame. Widening the doors may be possible and thresholds may need to be removed.
- *Stairs*. Problems ascending or descending may indicate the need for a second banister and two walking aids, one of which can be situated upstairs, the other downstairs. More major adaptations may include a stairlift or through-floor lift as an alternative to bringing a bed downstairs.
- *Transfers*. If the individual is having difficulty with any transfers then the height of the furniture may need to be adjusted to make standing easier; for example, a raised seat and rail could be used in the toilet.

It may prove impossible to adapt existing accommodation to suit the needs of the individual. Rehousing to more suitable premises may be a possible alternative but this may have far-reaching effects on the person and his family. The convenience of more suitable accommodation needs to be weighed against the disadvantages of being removed from familiar surroundings and from local support networks. It may also be more difficult for relatives and carers to visit the individual in a new location and provide the necessary levels of support.

APPROACHES TO TREATMENT

A wide variety of approaches are available to the therapist treating individuals who have suffered a stroke. These include the Rood, Brunnstrom, Bobath, Proprioceptive Neuromuscular Facilitation, Conductive Education and Rehabilitation approaches. Each has its own particular emphasis and for this reason it is essential that people from different disciplines agree on a broad base of treatment. This will ensure that the individual being treated is approached in a consistent manner by all concerned. For example, if one team member is aiming to inhibit associated reactions, others should take this into account in the course of their own interventions.

The merits of each approach need to be considered in conjunction with the aims of the individual. This may result in the adoption of a number of components from several approaches; for example, the principles of a neurodevelopmental approach could be applied to an adapted rehabilitative technique to ensure that the latter does not permit any undue increase in tone. As no single approach will solve all individuals' problems, the therapist will need to gain a good working knowledge of a wide range of approaches.

AIMS OF TREATMENT

Although the individual may present with a number of problems which can be treated separately, the therapist should maintain a holistic outlook, as it is the *combination* of the individual's problems which prevents him from being independent. For example, resolving body scheme problems may not make someone independent in dressing if he also has problems sequencing the activity.

After assessment a treatment programme should be formulated, taking into account the individual's particular needs and priorities.

Some broad aims of treatment may include the following:

- prevention of deformity
- maintenance of full range of movement
- reduction of spasticity and promotion of normal movement
- maximisation of personal independence
- maximisation of independence in domestic activities
- exploration of coping mechanisms for psychological problems
- management of perceptual problems
- resettlement within the family
- reestablishment of work and leisure roles.

Preventing deformity

Good positioning is essential in both the early hypotonic stage and the later hypertonic stage of muscle tone. The individual needs to be encouraged to take responsibility for his own positioning as early as possible. Education for relatives should also be provided. The individual should be taught to recognise increase in tone, what causes it and how he can reduce it himself. Good positioning should be constantly reinforced by all members of the multidisciplinary team so that it is maintained for as great a part of the day as possible.

Positioning should aim to break up any abnormal patterns and inhibit increased tone such as flexor pattern in the upper limb with retraction of the scapula, and extensor pattern in the lower limb, again with retraction of the hip.

Lying

The positions illustrated in Figure 16.9 will inhibit increased tone.

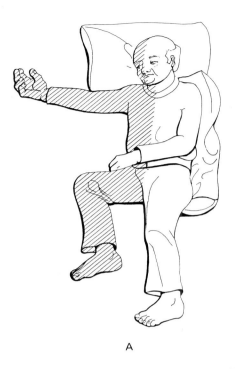 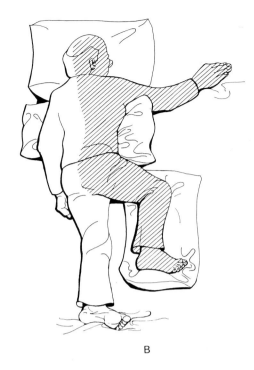

A   B

Fig. 16.9 Positioning while lying down. (A) Supine. (B) Prone.

Sitting

When sitting at a table to carry out an activity such as eating with the unaffected hand, the individual should place the affected upper limb/forearm and hand in a position within the visual field (Fig. 16.10).

Maintaining range of movement

Unless a full range of movement is maintained in all joints, good functional movement may not be possible, or may at least be painful, once motor recovery occurs. It is therefore important for the occupational therapist to complement the work of physiotherapy and ensure that the individual puts each affected joint through its full range of movement regularly. For example, in dressing practice a good range of upper limb movement can be achieved.

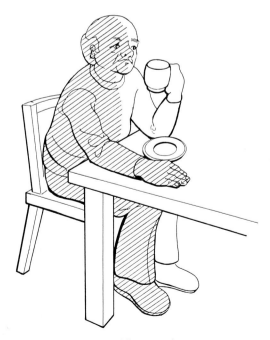

Fig. 16.10 Positioning while seated.

Reducing spasticity and promotion of normal movement

An individual would gain maximum benefit from being treated by an occupational therapist immediately following a session in physiotherapy. This arrangement would ensure that the occupational therapist was able to concentrate on functional activities rather than first having to spend valuable time reducing any abnormal tone.

During treatment the overall influence of tone on any working position needs to be considered in relation to the person's needs. For example, with someone who has low tone and a largely flexed posture, work in a standing position, if possible, would facilitate an increase in tone with an overall extensor pattern (although there should be some natural flexion around the central key points). With such an individual work in a sitting position is likely to have less effect on low tone, and to further encourage flexor tendencies. The position adopted for work is therefore important, in both gaining and maintaining normal tone.

The effect of work in a given postural set should be monitored throughout treatment. In the above example, work in standing may be indicated at the beginning of a session, but if left in standing for too long, the person's tone may increase excessively. This would affect his ability to perform normal movements. Alterations of the postural set would avoid this.

Treatment media which cause stress, anxiety or over-exertion will result in both spasticity and associated reactions and so would best be avoided.

Depending on the severity of the stroke, work on trunk movement may be needed. Activities performed in a sitting position which encourage lumbar extension and even weight distribution include remedial games on an elevated board and darts. Such activities can be adapted to encourage side flexion and rotation by being placed in varying positions. Throughout the treatment, attention should be given to the affected limbs to ensure that they are well positioned, e.g. that the foot is flat on the floor in a neutral position.

In a standing position, weight transfers practised first with feet parallel and later with one foot in front of the other will promote good standing and walking patterns. Walking technique can be re-emphasised while the individual is participating in ADL or in other therapeutic activities in the occupational therapy department.

Maximising personal independence

Building on the previous aims of good positioning and normal movement patterns, independence in ADL needs to be achieved — provided that this is a priority for the individual. It may be that he prefers to direct his energies into activities which give him pleasure and improve his quality of life, leaving more routine tasks to carers. In this case, it is essential to ensure that carers are taught the easiest and safest way to assist with and/or complete any task.

Turning in bed

As the ability to turn over is a prerequisite to being able to get out of bed, rolling in bed should be practised (Fig. 16.11).

Sitting up

This is usually easier if the individual turns himself onto his affected side first. Then his unaffected arm can be brought forward across his body to push up on the bed. He should move his legs off the side of the bed prior to pushing up.

Transferring

Transferring to the affected side will encourage weight-bearing through the affected leg, thus helping to prepare the individual for standing. Transferring to the unaffected side should also be practised, as it may be necessary in some situations, for example in getting on or off the toilet. It may also be safer for some elderly people and help to increase their confidence in their ability to transfer. Assistance with transfers may be reduced gradually as the individual improves; for example, the therapist in Figure 16.12 could reduce her control of the affected knee as active control is gained.

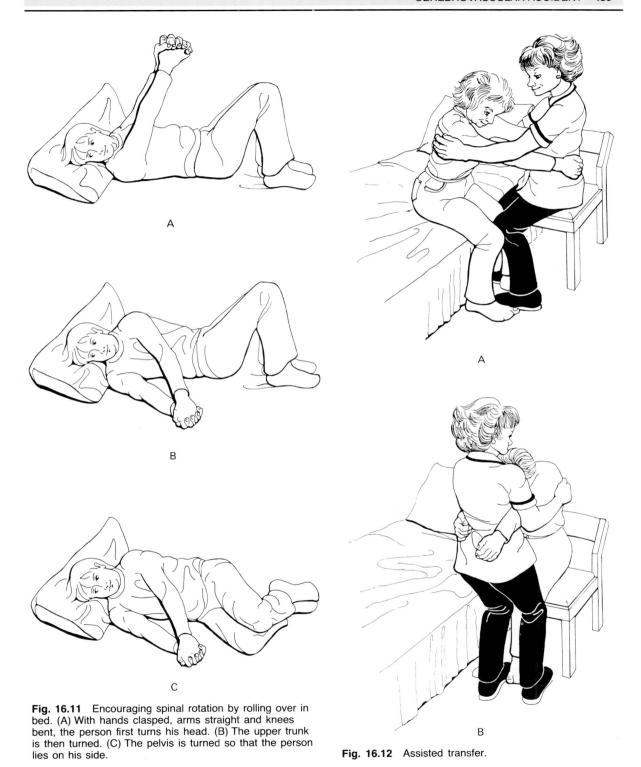

Fig. 16.11 Encouraging spinal rotation by rolling over in bed. (A) With hands clasped, arms straight and knees bent, the person first turns his head. (B) The upper trunk is then turned. (C) The pelvis is turned so that the person lies on his side.

Fig. 16.12 Assisted transfer.

Eating and drinking

This may be a problem due to functional difficulty, swallowing difficulties, and perceptual and/or visual problems. Again, a problem-solving approach should be adopted. The exact nature of the problem should be identified and treatment planned accordingly. The assistance of other professionals should be sought as appropriate. For example, a speech therapist can help with swallowing difficulties and a dietician can ensure a balanced intake of sufficient calories for those who are able to tolerate only small amounts of food. A dietician may also be able to advise about foods which will assist the individual to maintain his fluid intake; for example, if he is unable to control fluids within his mouth, thickeners such as Carobel could be used.

When the person is eating the position of his head, arm and hand in relation to his food is important. This means that suitable seating arrangements are essential; for example, if an individual is to use his wheelchair at mealtimes then domestic armrests may be needed so that he can place the chair up close to the table; or, if he has an unstable upper limb the height of the table may be important so that he can rest his elbow and use it as a pivot, so stabilising his arm.

Equipment such as large-handled cutlery may be useful if grip is affected; cutlery such as Dynafork or Splayd which compensates for reduced or absent return of movement may be used in the long term. Straws can be used to encourage good lip closure in the early stages.

Personal hygiene

Personal hygiene is important in the maintenance of self-esteem and dignity, and an individual may prefer to struggle to complete his basic hygiene routine rather than rely on help from others. Potential problem areas include shaving, where lack of sensation may lead to the individual cutting himself with a hand razor. This could be overcome by using an electric razor. Teeth cleaning can be made easier by using toothpaste in a pump dispenser rather than struggling with a tube and cap.

Washing and bathing practice can be used as treatment media as well as a means to independence. They are useful in providing sensory stimulation and in addressing perceptual problems such as poor right/left discrimination.

It may be easier for the person to wash in bed initially and as recovery occurs to progress to sitting and finally standing at a wash-basin, as this is a more natural position for this activity.

Bathing

Safety is particularly important in the bathroom and elderly people may already have problems which make it difficult to get in and out of the bath. Bathrooms are often small and access to the bath may be awkward. These factors need to be taken into account when considering whether the individual would be safer bathing or strip-washing.

If it is impossible for the individual to get in and out of the bath in his usual way, equipment may be needed to ensure his safety; for example, a non-slip mat, a bath board and seat or a Mangar/Aquajack bath aid could be used. Grab rails may also be useful. A shower with level access may provide a suitable alternative to a bath for people who are ambulant or wheelchair dependent.

Useful items in the bathroom may include a long-handled sponge or brush to reach inaccessible places, a soap mitten to maintain control of the soap and eliminate the need to soap a flannel or sponge; and a suction nailbrush to aid cleaning of the nails on the unaffected hand.

The bathing method selected should suit the needs of both the carer and the individual; for example, a hoist may be necessary to safeguard the carer from back injury.

Dressing (Fig. 16.13)

Dressing is often a problem; this may be due to loss of balance, movement or sensation, perceptual problems, or reduced concentration and energy. The reason underlying the problem needs to be ascertained so that dressing procedures can be developed to meet the individual's needs. For example, if the individual has functional movement of his left upper limb but normally tends to

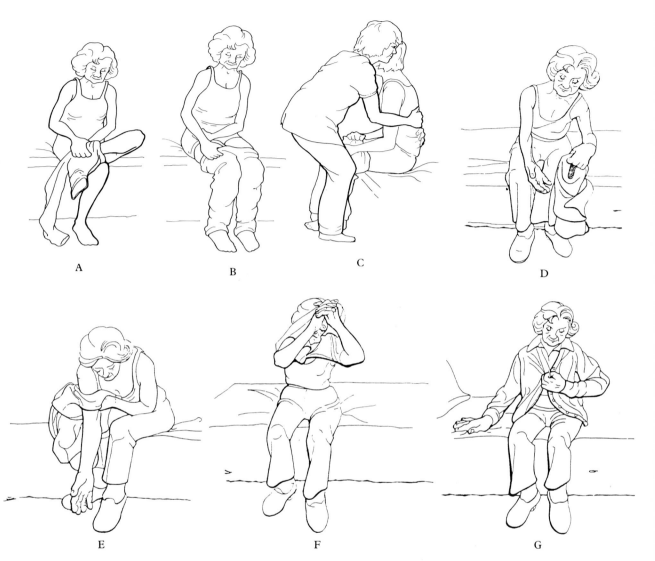

Fig. 16.13 Dressing to encourage functional movement while inhibiting patterns of spasticity. (A) Dress affected leg first by crossing it over the unaffected one. (B) Uncross legs to dress unaffected limb. (C) Assisted stand to pull up trousers. (D) For top garments extend arm, protract scapula and rest hand between knees. (E) Lean forward and extend arm through sleeve using gravity. (F) Clasp hands and lock thumbs under neck part; push garment over head by externally rotating shoulders. (G) Weight bear through affected arm while fastening garment with unaffected one.

ignore it, placing his clothes on his left-hand side may encourage use of the neglected arm.

Joint treatment sessions with a physiotherapist will facilitate good posture and balance, and assist in the maintenance of normal tone. Positions and movements least likely to trigger primitive reflexes and associated reactions should be used. Move-

ment patterns which go directly against typical spastic patterns can be encouraged. In Figure 16.13E, for example, the extended arm, assisted by gravity, is pushed through the sleeve, whereas pulling the sleeve of a garment up over the affected arm whilst in flexion may cause increased spasticity in the limb.

Practical dressing problems may need to be considered in the later stages if return of function is not forthcoming. Equipment which may improve independence if leaning forwards is a problem includes long-handled shoehorns, elasticated shoelaces and stocking/sock aids. Button hooks, Velcro or buttons on elastic may make fastenings easier.

Independence in dressing may not be a priority for the individual if he tires easily or has a great deal of difficulty in completing the task. In such a case it may be more appropriate to consider the carer's needs and provide education on easier methods to help the person. For example, the carer may need to learn how to pull up her relative's trousers while holding him in a standing position.

Maximising independence in the home

It may be important to maximise independence in domestic activities if this is a priority for the individual. His previous role may have included responsibility for most domestic activities but following a CVA this may change of necessity or choice. Alternatively, the individual may take a greater part in home life, relinquishing previous responsibilities that he can no longer manage. The therapist's attention to such tasks as housecleaning, shopping, meal preparation, laundry, budgeting and gardening should reflect the individual's abilities, needs and priorities.

Work on particular skills should be appropriate to the individual and be carried out with a full knowledge of the person's residential circumstances, including the type, design and organisation of his home and how much help there is available from the family and/or outside agencies.

The therapist can assist the person to reestablish a routine, to regain confidence in his abilities, and to build up stamina to cope with a full day. She may be able to help him improve particular physical skills and/or recommend appropriate labour-saving expedients such as using a food mixer, cleaning the floor with a long-handled mop, or hiring a window cleaner. Safety in the kitchen will be particularly important. Previously used methods may now be impossible and new ones may need to be practised and adopted, for example holding a kettle in a different way, using a bread and butter board or sitting down to iron. Specific tasks may need to be broken down into simple stages at first and upgraded as the individual becomes more able and confident.

Where the individual is a member of a family unit the therapist may help the family to organise itself so that each member has responsibility for particular tasks such as bed-making, gardening and shopping, ensuring that the disabled member still has a role yet is not overburdened.

Managing perceptual problems

Having assessed the extent of perceptual deficits the therapist must devise a programme that addresses these. Treatment can be carried out using functional tasks and/or through transfer of techniques whereby abilities gained in one situation may be carried over to other tasks; for example treatment for visual field deficit involving exercises such as circling a particular letter on a scanning sheet would be designed to carry over and improve the individual's visual field in a functional activity. Transfer of training techniques does have limitations, particularly for people who are disorientated, depressed, unmotivated or who present with receptive dysphasia. It may be difficult to explain the purpose and relevance of an obscure task, whereas the aims and benefit of a functional activity will be more readily apparent; for example relearning to sequence an activity through the use of picture cards may be less effective than actual practice in the activity.

Suggestions for treatment of perceptual problems are given below, but more in-depth knowledge can be gained from consulting specialised texts. In providing treatment in this area, the therapist should bear in mind that the individual may be left with residual deficits for which he will need to learn compensatory techniques in the long term.

Agnosia

Recognition can be encouraged by repetition, matching objects, reinforcing correct answers and by using other senses; for example, photographs of familiar objects can encourage the individual to memorise their names.

Spatial disorders

Suitably graded activities can help the individual to recover his grasp of spatial relations; for example, if he has figure/ground problems he will more easily be able to select an appropriate item from a drawer containing two or three items than from a full drawer. Such tasks can then be gradually upgraded to a more normal level of stimulus.

Perception of form constancy may be improved by presenting the individual with the same object in various positions and sizes and then asking him to identify it. Alternatively, specific computer programmes may be employed.

Apraxia

Although apraxia is often difficult to treat the following guidelines may be of help:

- Break down the activity into individual components, teaching each component to the person and gradually reassembling them to form the complete task
- Encourage graded practice of difficult tasks
- Guide limbs through the specific movements required, gradually withdrawing support as the person learns the task
- The person may find it easier to carry out a task if he sees it demonstrated by the therapist first, rather than relying solely on verbal instructions
- When demonstrating, the therapist should sit alongside the person, not opposite, as this could cause confusion with regard to spatial orientation
- Encourage the person to learn to perform the task in a specific sequence, as this may make it easier to remember.

Unilateral neglect

In all situations the individual should be encouraged to take account of stimuli from his affected side. This can be encouraged by suitable positioning of his bed or chair within the environment to ensure that some stimulation comes from both sides.

Resettlement

For the person who remains at home following his CVA, treated and supported by his general practitioner and other community-based personnel, all assessment and treatment will take place at home. This can reduce trauma for both the individual and his carer, and precludes the need for resettlement within the family. The return home after a hospital stay may be fraught with difficulties as the individual and his family suddenly realise the extent of his disability and recognise that previous active roles and full participation in family life are now impeded.

In order to alleviate potential difficulties it is appropriate for likely role changes to be anticipated prior to discharge, thus avoiding some of the stresses change may cause. This may involve the negotiation of role changes within the family; for instance, a man may agree to accept responsibility for the home whilst his wife goes out to work.

Whether the individual has been admitted to hospital or cared for at home following his CVA it is important to identify any environmental changes necessary to facilitate his return to optimum function. Chapter 9 describes various home modifications, many of which may assist the person who has had a stroke. Once any adaptations have been installed, additional support such as home help, community nursing or voluntary services may be arranged. If this takes place whilst the individual is in hospital he may be able to take weekend leave from the ward in preparation for his return home. Short periods at home are most valuable as they enable the family to reinforce skills learned in hospital and to prepare for the future. If the services suggested above are already provided during this period the trial will be more realistic and may indicate any further, unexpected areas of need.

Consultation with other members of the multidisciplinary team is essential to ensure that appropriate follow-up, such as treatment in a day hospital or outpatient clinic, is provided.

A local stroke club may provide a social outlet and support for the family, enabling them to discuss particular situations and problems with people in similar circumstances.

Work

If the individual was working prior to his stroke, detailed discussion with him and liaison with his employer, if appropriate, will be necessary in order to ascertain whether he can return to his job or to another post in the same company, or whether alternative options need consideration.

The therapist will need to identify aptitudes and skills retained, impaired or lost and relate these to work requirements. Assessment should also indicate possible solutions for difficulties in such areas as timekeeping, communication, manual dexterity and standing tolerance.

Each person's future employment will depend on his potential level of function and the flexibility of his employer and of the work of the company. If his former job is still a feasible option a gradual return to full-time work may be negotiated. If alternative work with the same employer is agreed upon, the individual will need preparation for this change.

If neither of these options is realistic, and if the individual wishes and is able to return to paid employment, the Disablement Resettlement Officer (DRO) should become involved. The DRO, with his knowledge of employment training and retraining, of specialist assessment and training centres, of the possibilities for adapting work environments, and of modifying equipment or providing equipment to facilitate work, will be able to offer objective advice and help.

The impact of unemployment on people of working age has far-reaching financial, social and psychological consequences. The individual's loss of his former employment role is likely to increase his feelings of frustration and helplessness. The development of new roles may help to compensate for this loss; for example, the person may find he is able to take over the preparation of meals, thus freeing his carer for tasks he can no longer com-

plete. This would help to contribute to his sense of worth and 'belonging' within the family unit.

Leisure

A person's interests and hobbies may offer important stimulation and motivation during treatment and may even be an essential starting-point for rehabilitation if he is depressed or anxious. The introduction of a familiar activity early in the treatment programme may encourage participation and help to build a good rapport between the therapist and the individual. This can then be built on as aims of treatment are established in keeping with the individual's own priorities.

Leisure activities may also need to be actively encouraged, as most people suffering a CVA will be of retirement age or unable to return to work due to the severity of the stroke and subsequent dysfunction. Activities which can be pursued together with family and friends will be important in maintaining the person as part of his normal social unit.

The purposeful use of leisure time offers relaxation and utilises existing skills and knowledge. It ensures that days are balanced in terms of self-care, work and relaxation. Some leisure activities such as reading or listening to music may be carried out in the usual manner. Others may need to be adapted in response to specific needs; for example, if the person is now unable to drive he may need assistance to identify the best alternative transport which will allow him to visit his grandchildren. If previous interests can no longer be pursued due to physical, cognitive, perceptual or psychological barriers, it may be necessary to introduce a range of activities more suited to the person's abilities.

It may be, however, that a particular individual has no hobbies or interests in life other than sitting at home and watching television. Such established patterns may be difficult to break and the question must arise as to whether it is appropriate to try.

PHYSICAL PROBLEMS WHICH CAN HINDER REHABILITATION

Following a stroke some people experience a number of problems in addition to the ones identified above which can affect levels of independence in the long term.

Pusher syndrome

This is the name given to a group of symptoms with which some people present. It is characterised by the following problems:

- In all positions the person pushes towards the hemiplegic side with his unaffected side.
- He resists any passive correction of his posture by 'fixing' with his unaffected side.
- His head is usually pulled towards the unaffected side while he is sitting.
- When he sits in a wheelchair his trunk will be flexed and shortened on the unaffected side with his head turned to the same side. His unaffected arm grasps the side of the chair and he will push himself over to the affected side. He will also push against the back of the chair, with the result that his bottom slides forward in the chair.
- When he sits unsupported his trunk will be flexed and shortened on the unaffected side while the affected side is elongated. His head will be turned to the unaffected side with the weight on the affected side.
- When standing he will push towards his affected side and often shuffle his unaffected foot sideways to allow him to push more. He takes little weight through the affected limb.
- When transferring weight to the unaffected side he will resist and express fear of falling.
- When transferring he pushes excessively with his unaffected side, which causes him to move backwards, over to the hemiplegic side.
- When rolling onto his unaffected side he will again resist.
- The 'pusher' often has sensory impairment and perceptual problems, such as neglect of the affected side, dyspraxia, hemianopia and body image problems.

Management

- Fear and anxiety will increase pushing; therefore, it is important to reduce these at every opportunity. For example, dressing practice could be carried out initially in a chair rather than sitting on the bed.
- Wheelchair footplates should be positioned so that the individual's hips and knees are flexed to 90°.
- A pelvic strap can be used while the person is sitting to prevent him from sliding his bottom forwards and pushing back against the chair.
- The 'pusher' should not be encouraged to self-propel in a wheelchair or to pull himself up into a standing position using the furniture, as this can reinforce the pushing syndrome.
- Transfers to the unaffected side will usually decrease tone.

Shoulder problems

Subluxed shoulder

The main feature of the shoulder joint is mobility rather than stability, making a great range of movement possible. As a result the shoulder is easily traumatised and malalignment is common. In subluxation the shoulder girdle drops, the scapula is depressed and retracted, and the humerus slips downwards. Treatment should involve correct positioning at all times to help prevent this. Maintenance of a full, pain-free range of movement is also necessary.

Activities designed to stimulate normal tone in the muscles around the shoulder joint should be encouraged; these might include baking, with the individual seated on a plinth.

Painful shoulder

A painful shoulder can occur early or late after a CVA but can be avoided with good management. The individual will often complain of pain in a specific site initially, with the pain gradually becoming more generalised if the cause is not addressed.

Actions which contribute to a painful shoulder are ones in which the scapula and humerus do not move in a synchronised manner. This causes soft tissue structure to be squeezed between the acromion and head of humerus, as when the upper limb is lifted by the wrist without movement of the scapula being facilitated. In addition, failure to externally rotate the humerus when the limb is abducted may cause pain in the greater tuberosity as it encroaches on the other bony structures in the joint.

Management to prevent a painful shoulder developing involves good positioning and a programme to maintain full range of movement. Once a painful shoulder has developed, the trunk and shoulder should be adequately mobilised before any activity is carried out. If this is not undertaken, further damage to the structures around the shoulder joint will result, thus increasing pain.

It may be necessary, therefore, to see the person immediately following physiotherapy sessions. Activities designed to gradually increase the range of movement with the arms supported, for example pushing dominoes into position with a bilateral grip, are useful initially.

Ankle problems

Normal walking requires some degree of active dorsiflexion of the ankle and toes. Extensor spasticity interferes with dorsiflexion and some people have excessive plantarflexion of the toes in standing and walking. This may cause instability if not treated and lead to injury to the ankle.

Decreased sensation can also cause difficulties at the ankle joint, as the person will not be aware of the degree of pressure being put on his foot. Good early positioning is important and the individual should be encouraged to be aware of his foot when sitting or transferring. Carers should also be taught the importance of correcting the position of his feet.

Bandaging of the ankle will encourage dorsiflexion. A crepe bandage can be applied over the shoe to hold the foot in dorsiflexion and to help prevent supination. An ankle-foot orthosis can be used on a more permanent basis than bandaging, keeping the foot in dorsiflexion. Liaison with the physiotherapist regarding the ordering of an ankle-foot orthosis may be necessary. Tubigrip can be placed over the person's shoe to enable the foot to slide along the floor. This is particularly useful in the early stages of walking, when there is insufficient hip, knee and ankle control.

Multiple diagnosis

Elderly people in particular are likely to have had other problems, conditions or deficits before they suffered their stroke. Such problems might be a cardiac condition, arthritis, diabetes and associated problems, Parkinson's disease, amputation or poor vision and hearing.

When treating people with multiple diagnoses it is necessary to first identify their previous level of independence, i.e. personal and domestic ADL, range of movement, tolerance level, ability to mobilise, motivation, attitudes, support received before the CVA and general life-style.

Following very comprehensive assessment, a treatment programme must be planned that takes the severity of the other conditions into account and sets goals that the person can realistically achieve.

CONCLUSION

The flow chart given in Figure 16.14 provides a summary of the treatment process employed by the occupational therapist when working with individuals who have suffered a CVA. The therapist must bear in mind throughout her intervention, however, that since the problems precipitated by CVA are extremely varied in kind and degree, no one therapeutic approach will solve every problem that her clients encounter. It is her responsibility to find the particular combination of approaches and techniques that will best assist the individual to improve his quality of life and regain an optimum level of activity and independence. As CVA has a potential impact on all areas of the individual's life and function, the contribution of occupational therapy to his rehabilitation is likely to be wide-ranging, and to offer the therapist many challenges and rewards.

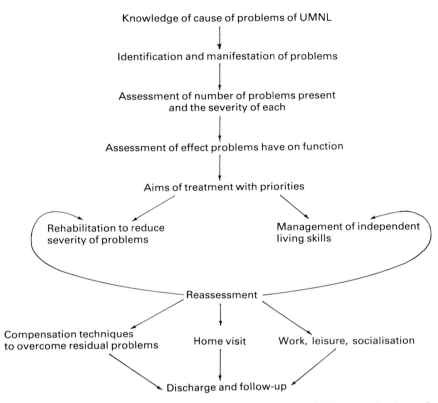

Fig. 16.14 The occupational therapist's treatment of a person who has had a CVA summarised as a flow chart.

REFERENCES

Rankia J 1957 Cerebral vascular accidents in patients over the age of 60. Scottish Medical Journal 2: 200–215

Davies P M 1985 Steps to follow — a guide to the treatment of adult hemiplegia based on the concept of K & B Bobath. Springer-Verlag, Berlin

Zoltan B, Siev E, Freishtat B 1986 Perceptual and cognitive dysfunction in the adult stroke patient. Slack, New Jersey

FURTHER READING

Bobath B 1978 Adult hemiplegia: evaluation and treatment. Heinemann, London

Cotton E, Kinmans R 1983 Conductive education for adult hemiplegia. Churchill Livingstone, Edinburgh

Eggers O 1983 Occupational therapy in the treatment of adult hemiplegia. Heinemann, London

Lindsay K W, Bone I, Callander R 1986 Neurology and neurosurgery illustrated. Churchill Livingstone, Edinburgh

Pedretti L W 1980 Occupational therapy — practice skills for physical dysfunction. Mosby, St Louis

Ross J S, Wilson K J W 1981 Foundation of anatomy and physiology. Churchill Livingstone, Edinburgh

17

Head injury

Steve McWilliams

INTRODUCTION

Head injury may be defined as damage to living brain tissue caused by an external mechanical force. It is usually characterised by a period of altered consciousness, amnesia or coma that can be very brief (lasting minutes) or exceedingly long (lasting months/indefinitely). The consequences of the resulting tissue damage can be so diverse and affect such a variety of physical, cognitive, behavioural and psychosocial abilities that no two head injuries are ever alike. Apart from the actual extent of the tissue damage, personality, insight and motivation are all important in terms of influencing the ability of the individual to make a good recovery. Age is also significant, as the younger person may have a more adaptable brain. On the other hand, however, he may have a less responsible personality and therefore be less amenable to the hard work involved in recovery.

It is because no two cases of head injury are alike that this chapter does not aim to set out a fixed treatment programme for the occupational therapist to implement. Rather, the most important features of head injury are described, followed by general principles and strategies that the therapist can adapt to the case at hand.

The chapter begins with a description of the primary and secondary forms of brain damage resulting from head injury, along with their typical complications and early sequelae. The course of recovery to be expected after head injuries ranging in severity from 'mild' to 'very severe' is also outlined. Focusing on moderate and severe cases, the chapter then describes the consequences of injury for physical, cognitive and psychosocial function. The discussion then turns to the role of the occupational therapist in assisting head-injured people toward an optimum recovery, taking in turn the acute, post-acute and late stages of treatment and considering the rehabilitation aims and strategies appropriate to each phase. The specific physical, cognitive and psychosocial problems that the individual is likely to encounter in each phase are described.

Throughout the chapter, the implications of the individual's head injury for his family and friends is stressed, along with the need for the occupational therapist to encourage those close to the individual to become actively involved in the rehabilitation process.

PATHOLOGY

In cases of head injury it is often difficult to locate the exact site of the lesion, as damage may be diffuse, and trauma to one part of the head may cause damage in a more remote part of the brain. For instance, a blood vessel damaged at the site of the trauma may disrupt the blood supply to another area of the brain, thus affecting the function of that area; e.g., if the anterior cerebral artery is damaged this will disrupt the blood supply to the motor cortex, thus leading to paralysis of the opposite leg.

Head injuries can be classified under two main headings:

1. *Open head injury*. The coverings of the brain are ruptured, for example by a bullet wound. Relatively localised areas of the brain tend to be damaged, resulting in fairly discrete and predictable disabilities.

2. *Closed head injury*. The skull may be fractured but the coverings of the brain remain intact, as, for example, when the head collides with another object such as the windscreen of a car. In contrast to open head injuries, closed head injuries tend to cause more diffuse tissue damage, resulting in a mosaic of disabilities that are more generalised and highly variable. The generalised, and often subtle, nature of the disabilities arising from closed head injuries are often difficult to clearly identify and conceptualise.

PRIMARY AND SECONDARY DAMAGE

There are primary and secondary processes by which brain damage occurs.

Primary damage

The primary forces occurring in head injury are compression, tension and shear (twisting). These forces produce both diffuse and somewhat localised damage.

Contusion

This describes the damage caused, for example, by the head striking the windscreen of a car. The brain, which is floating in and cushioned by cerebrospinal fluid, smashes into the skull as the head hits the windscreen. This compression at the site of the impact tears and bruises nerve fibres and is termed a contusion. Certain areas of the skull, most notably the base of the frontal and temporal lobes, have bony ridges which enhance the likelihood of contusion at these sites. As the compression wave travels through the brain, further damage occurs. In addition, because the brain is a jelly-like mass and is surrounded by fluid, it will often 'rebound' from its initial impact and be driven against the opposite side of the skull. This is referred to as the *coup/contrecoup phenomenon*, i.e. blow/counter-blow (Fig. 17.1).

Shearing injuries

These can cause diffuse damage and occur when the brain rotates severely within the cranial vault. The brain is anchored at its base by the spinal cord and the cranial nerves and its upper aspects are

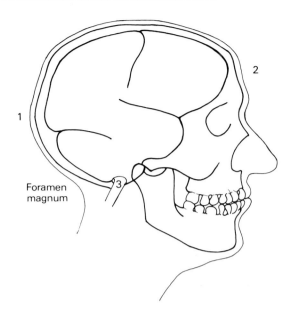

Fig. 17.1 Contrecoup lesion. As the head is thrust forward, damage may occur (1) in the occipital area (2) in the frontal area (3) at the base of the brain.

supported by a bath of cerebrospinal fluid. Thus, if the head is rotating at the time of impact, the skull will stop its rotation while the brain within does not, at least not until its anchor of nerve tissue has been severely stretched. This shearing, twisting action is not limited to the base of the brain but continues upwards to higher levels with a decreasing force. The billions of thread-like nerves are stretched to such an extent that they either snap altogether or are at least temporarily dysfunctional. Of those nerves that are merely stretched, some will recover function, while others will degenerate and pull apart like the more seriously stretched and snapped nerves.

Tension

Tension or stress on nerve fibres occurs as the brain moves within the head as a result of the forces applied to it. Stretched fibres may be stretched and damaged or snap and degenerate.

Secondary damage

In cases of primary damage, secondary mechan-

isms commonly come into play, resulting in further damage. Haemorrhage, for example, prevents oxygen and other nutrients from reaching their target tissues which may result in damage or necrosis of these tissues and also damages brain tissue as the pooled mass of blood compresses and displaces nerve fibres. Intracranial pressure may rise as the brain swells due to increased fluid retention and increased blood flow. This may cause the brain tissue to herniate through the foramen magnum.

FRACTURES OF THE SKULL

- Simple fracture — the skull is fractured but the skin is intact
- Compound fracture — the skin is also broken
- Comminuted fracture — the skull is broken into several pieces
- Depressed fracture — the fractured bone is driven inwards. This will require surgery to elevate the depressed bone, although this may not be urgent if there is no evidence of intracranial haemorrhage or cerebral compression.

The seriousness of a fracture will depend on its type and location. Simple fractures require little attention but compound fractures bring the danger of bacterial meningitis, although the risk is greatly reduced by the administration of antibiotics. Damage to the underlying brain is the main complication.

COMPLICATIONS REQUIRING SURGERY

The following complications may occur with or without fractures of the skull:

Subdural haematoma

This is a serious and common complication. Only slight trauma may be sufficient to cause rupture of blood vessels between the dura mater and arachnoid mater. The bleeding causes a haematoma, an accumulation of blood within the tissues that clots to form a solid swelling, which will in time produce cerebral compression and cause the person to become drowsy and to complain of headache. Eventually his level of responsiveness will deteriorate. Subdural haematoma may develop rapidly (acute subdural haematoma) or slowly; this is the chief reason why the head-injured person should be kept under observation for at least 24 hours. Acute subdural haematoma should be suspected if the individual no longer responds to painful stimuli. Computerised tomography (CT) scanning will show the location of the haematoma and surgery will be required to evacuate it.

Extradural haematoma

This most commonly occurs in the frontoparietal region when the middle meningeal artery is torn, for example by fractured bone, causing bleeding between the skull and the dura mater. The ensuing haematoma usually collects quickly and as it grows the person becomes increasingly drowsy and restless. There will be dilation of the pupil on the side of the haematoma with increasing paralysis of the opposite side of the body. The CT scan will show a shift in the midline position of the brain. Surgery should be immediate to evacuate the haematoma and stop the bleeding.

Intracerebral haemorrhage

This usually occurs soon after injury when there is continuous bleeding into the brain substance, but it is not very common. The person will show a reduced level of responsiveness. The site of the haemorrhage can be determined by physical signs in relevant parts of the body; for example, a middle cerebral haemorrhage in the dominant hemisphere may produce dysphasia. A burr hole is made over the site and the dura opened so that the haematoma can be removed.

ASSESSING THE SEVERITY OF HEAD INJURY

Fortunately it is possible to determine, at least in general terms, the severity of a given injury soon after the initial insult. The Glasgow Coma Scale (GCS) rates three key responses: eye-opening

ability, motor responsiveness and verbal responsiveness. With a scale ranging from 3 to 15, a Glasgow score of 8 or below indicates true coma, i.e. one in which there is no eye-opening even in response to painful stimuli, no movement in response to simple commands and no comprehensible words uttered. People whose comas last more than 6 hours are considered to be severely injured, whilst those lasting from 1 to 6 hours are moderately injured and those whose period of unconsciousness is less than 1 hour are considered to be mildly injured.

Another recognised yardstick for assessment of the severity of head injury is the duration of post-traumatic amnesia (PTA). PTA is defined as the time interval between the injury and the reinstatement of continuous day-to-day memory. However, it should be noted that this is *not* the same as the interval between the injury and the first remembered event after the injury. A moderate injury is one causing PTA of less than 24 hours, a severe injury one causing a PTA of 24 hours or more (Table 17.1).

Table 17.1 Classification of head injury. (Adapted from Medical Disability Society (1988) The Management of Traumatic Brain Injury.)

	Period of unconsciousness	Post-traumatic amnesia
Minor:	15 minutes or less	
Moderate:	More than 15 minutes but less than 6 hours	less than 24 hours
Severe:	6 hours or more	24 hours or more
Very severe:	48 hours or more	7 days or more

EARLY SEQUELAE

The outcome of recovery after head injury depends to a considerable extent on the treatment given at the site of the accident. Immediate intervention consists of keeping the airway clear and preventing further blood loss from other injuries. Speed is essential so that the person can receive any necessary surgery as soon as possible. If he has had a head injury severe enough to cause concussion he should either be admitted for obser-

The person needs to be observed for 24 to 48 hours and brought back to hospital IMMEDIATELY if he:
1. Becomes increasingly sleepy
2. Becomes unconscious
3. Complains of INCREASINGLY severe headaches
4. Complains of blurred or double vision
5. Vomits repeatedly
6. Has a fit

Fig. 17.2 Observations.

vation, or relatives should be instructed to monitor him for the first 24 to 48 hours and report the development of any untoward signs (Fig. 17.2).

The severity of the effects of head injury will also depend on other injuries incurred at the time of the accident, such as burns, fractures or internal injuries. These need to be treated in conjunction with the problems produced by the head injury itself; this combination of problems may well produce far more serious consequences than head injury alone.

Management at this stage involves good nursing care of the unconscious patient. Observation is essential so that complications such as subdural haematoma are recognised as early as possible. Treatment is designed to prevent complications as far as possible, as these may prevent or limit recovery.

Damage to respiratory organs

This may result from obstruction of the airway, either through the accumulation of secretions, blood or vomit, or through fractures of adjacent bones compressing the airway. This obviously calls for immediate treatment and an airway has to be passed. The person may need frequent suction to clear the airway. If he does not regain cough and swallowing reflexes after 24 hours a tracheostomy will be performed to facilitate suction and ventilation. A ventilator may be needed in cases of severe respiratory insufficiency.

When treating people with respiratory problems, the occupational therapist should understand the use of resuscitators and be aware of environmental factors, such as a dry atmosphere, which may aggravate the individual's condition.

Skin

Because skin is prone to breakdown it is essential that all potentially vulnerable pressure areas are cared for. The immobile person may quickly develop sores, particularly if he is incontinent or restless, as he may rub the skin off prominent areas such as the ankles. Sores will delay recovery and lead to infection.

Atrophy

Atrophy, i.e. wasting of muscles, and *contractures* must be avoided. The individual's limbs should be put through a full range of passive movements regularly by the physiotherapist. Night orthoses may be required to prevent deformity. Treatment can be difficult if there is disturbed muscle tone or decerebrate rigidity and in those who are grossly disturbed. *Myositis ossificans*, i.e. calcification and bone formation in muscles and around joints, is common in those with head injury.

Other fractures

Other fractures may occur at the time of the accident. It may not always be possible to treat these in the normal way, particularly if the patient is very disturbed, i.e. skin traction on lower limb fractures. The disturbed patient may not understand why his leg is restricted and so try to dismantle the traction rendering it ineffective.

Peripheral nerve injuries

These may occur due to the vulnerable position of, for example, the ulnar, median, sciatic and lateral popliteal nerves. Injury to these nerves may cause weakness in the muscles they supply and loss of sensation over the relevant area of skin. These injuries must be checked for after consciousness has returned, as they may be missed during the acute life-saving stage.

Incontinence

This problem is common in the early stages and the individual may need to be catheterised to control incontinence and to reduce the possibility of sores. There is always a risk that catheterisation will cause infection of the urinary tract and it should therefore be discontinued as soon as possible. Bladder training should be instigated and the person asked to pass urine at regular timed intervals day and night. This requires a great deal of work and coordination on the part of all staff concerned in order to be successful.

Visual impairment

This may occur due to damage to any part of the visual pathways (Fig. 17.3). In addition to *hemianopia*, i.e. loss of half the field of vision, there may be impairment of either the upper or lower fields of vision, or of any of the visual quadrants. There may be *diplopia*, i.e. double vision, or *nystagmus*, i.e. inability to coordinate the movements of the eyes. Both diplopia and nystagmus may be treated by covering one eye with a patch so that the visual input is reduced. The patch must cover each eye alternately so that one does not become lazier than the other. It is extremely important for the occupational therapist to understand the visual problems that people may present so that these are not mistaken as symptoms of other dysfunctions. Some visual difficulties may persist and become long-term, for example hemianopia due to permanent damage to the posterior aspect of the optic tract.

Epilepsy

This occurs in a large number of those who are head injured. Damaged brain tissue may leave a scar which can act as an irritant and a focus for electrical discharge, thus leading to fits. Fits are particularly likely after damage to the fronto-parietal or temporal lobes. They may occur at any time after injury and therefore all head-injured people are routinely prescribed anticonvulsants for at least two years post injury.

The occupational therapist should be competent in the procedures for keeping the airway clear and preventing the individual from injuring himself during a fit. He should be observed during a fit and these observations should then be reported to the ward sister or doctor concerned. Treatment should avoid potentially dangerous situations and activities, for example, using power tools.

Fits can be very distressing for both the individual and his relatives, who should be given the opportunity to talk about their worries.

Post-concussional syndrome

This is more commonly noted after minor injuries. The individual complains of headaches, intolerance of noise and irritability. He may have some impairment of memory, be unable to concentrate and complain of inability to work. He may suffer from insomnia. This usually clears up fairly quickly but in some cases it persists and is known as chronic brain syndrome.

COURSE OF RECOVERY

The course of recovery from a head injury is dependent upon the severity of the initial insult. Typical recovery patterns are outlined below for injuries ranging in severity from 'mild' to 'very severe'.

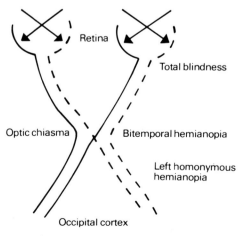

Fig. 17.3 Common lesions of the visual pathway.

Mild injuries

People experiencing mild injuries, i.e. having no or at most a brief loss of consciousness, may receive no medical attention, or only brief hospitalisation for routine tests and observation. Neurological examinations are usually normal and even though some nausea, dizziness and headache may be present, it is often assumed that no permanent, structural damage has occurred. Despite this assumption, many people who have suffered mild injuries are unable to resume and maintain their pre-injury performance level and continue to experience the symptoms of post-concussional syndrome, i.e. dizziness, impaired concentration, fatigability, depression, irritability, headache, insomnia, defective memory and restlessness. These symptoms may interfere with all aspects of daily living, including work, home life and social relationships. Unfortunately most people affected by post-concussional syndrome do not understand what is happening to them. Many of the problems they experience are subtle and difficult to recognise, both for the injured person and for those around him. These mild mental impairments can often lead to feelings of incompetence, frustration and guilt for the individual. He appears to be normal but family and friends may be critical and unable to understand why he fails to resume pre-injury responsibilities. It is not uncommon for him to return to work, fail to perform adequately and then lose his job. After failing at one or two subsequent jobs it becomes apparent that some real problems do exist. It is often at this point that professional advice and rehabilitation is sought.

Moderate injuries

Moderate head injury is characterised by a period of unconsciousness of between 1 and 24 hours. These people will be hospitalised and receive some degree of rehabilitation. Whilst there is much variability in the amount of physical, cognitive and psychosocial disability resulting from a moderate head injury, it is usually at least 6 to 12 months before return to work is contemplated or achieved, although significant numbers may not be able to return even at this stage.

Severe injuries

People with a coma lasting more than 24 hours are said to be severely injured. Such people tend to have more severe physical deficits because of damage to the brain stem. After acute medical care they should receive a protracted period of rehabilitation both as an inpatient and, where facilities exist, as an outpatient, or in the community. Rehabilitation may last several years and focus on improving levels of self-care and independence, as well as on meeting vocational needs, generally at a much later date. Those able to return to work generally do so in a much reduced capacity and many severely injured people may only be able to work in sheltered employment. They often remain dependent on their families and/or social service agencies for care or at least regular supervision and support.

Very severe injuries

These people have coma lasting weeks or months, after which the persistent vegetative state emerges. In this coma-like state they have sleep/wake cycles, in which they allow themselves to be fed but usually do not speak, follow commands or indicate any ability to understand what is said to them. If this state persists very long after coma has ended, it is unlikely that any real improvements will ever be made.

CLINICAL FEATURES

The clinical features resulting from head injury are as varied as the physical, cognitive and psychosocial functions that the brain itself supports. The focus in this section is on the relatively common features resulting from moderate and severe injuries.

Physical deficits

- *Paralysis* may involve all limbs. Muscle tone may be lost, reduced or increased as a result of damage to higher centres of the brain responsible for the regulation of muscle tone and the integration of muscular reflexes. The initial loss of tone, i.e. hypotonus or flaccidity, is usually replaced by an increase in tone, i.e. hypertonus or spasticity. Where higher centres are damaged reflex activity will predominate.

• *Ataxia* implies disturbance of muscular contraction and tone leading to an inability to coordinate movements. Ataxia is caused by damage to the cerebellum, which regulates muscle contraction and joint position, thus affecting and controlling balance. Muscle power, however, is not usually affected. Damage to the cerebellum will lead to incoordination of movement with inaccuracies in speed, timing and direction. Loss of sensation and of proprioception, i.e. the ability to feel the position of joints and limbs in space, will considerably exacerbate the situation and the person will try to compensate through vision.

• *Extrapyramidal tremor* is due to damage to the extrapyramidal system, in particular to the basal ganglia, and manifests itself by continued tremor, caused by fluctuating tone in opposing muscle groups.

• *Disturbances of equilibrium and righting reactions* are caused when the centres of the brain concerned with these mechanisms are damaged, resulting in the inability to place and maintain the body in the required position against gravity. Postural adjustments to maintain balance are upset.

• *Sensory disturbance* may be caused by damage to the sensory area of the cerebral cortex and posterior column tracts in the brain, causing lack of appreciation or distortion of sensation. There may be disturbances in tactile discrimination (pain, temperature, texture) and/or proprioception.

There may also be disturbances in the functions of the other special senses as a result of damage to the central processing centres of the brain rather than to the sensory organs (e.g. eyes, ears) per se, although these may also be damaged. There can thus be disturbances in visual, auditory, gustatory and olfactory perception.

• *Disturbances in speech* may occur while language comprehension remains intact. Two common deficits are:

— *Dysarthria* — difficulty in articulation of speech due to injury to the motor speech nerves

— *Apraxia* — impairment of articulatory programming in the cortex.

It must be stressed that these are purely motor problems and are not caused by impairment of the cognitive processes of interpretation and understanding of written and spoken language.

Cognitive deficits

• *Attention and concentration* difficulties may manifest themselves as an inability to filter out irrelevant background stimuli. The person responds to the most salient stimulus even though it may not be the most relevant and thus he is very distractable.

• *Memory and learning* deficits are very common. Invariably, head-injured people do not remember events around the time of the injury and for a variable period immediately before it; this is known as *retrograde traumatic amnesia*. Memory for these events is very unlikely to ever return. Memory for events prior to the injury may be disturbed although deeply ingrained material generally remains intact. Perhaps most significant is the difficulty most head-injured people face in their ability to learn and remember new material.

• *Perceptual deficits* occur when there is a disruption in the process of organisation and interpretation of incoming stimuli leading to an inappropriate response. Such deficits may include spatial relationship problems, body-image disorders and an inability to recognise familiar objects.

• *Language deficits* imply a disruption of linguistic competence and performance in contrast to speech deficits, which are purely motor. *Dysphasia* is the most common and can be (1) expressive, i.e. a difficulty in expressing language either verbally or in writing, (2) receptive, i.e. a difficulty in understanding spoken and/or written language, or (3) a combination of the two.

Psychosocial deficits

In the early stages of recovery from head injury, the person may exhibit behavioural disturbances and poor psychosocial function. Such disturbances may include emotional lability, aggressive outbursts, disorientation, impulsiveness and agitation. Typically there is an improvement in psychosocial functioning, although irritability, impulsiveness, poor frustration tolerance, denial, anxiety and depression may persist. It is arguable whether such symptoms are a direct result of brain damage or a psychological reaction to the situation in which the person finds himself.

THE ROLE OF THE OCCUPATIONAL THERAPIST

The common clinical features following head injury outlined above might be conceived as 'micro-deficits'. Micro-deficits such as ataxia, poor concentration and memory problems may combine in innumerable ways to form larger patterns of dysfunction or 'macro-deficits'. For example, a partial paralysis would certainly impede independent living activities, but when a paralysis is combined with a memory or attention difficulty an entirely different picture emerges. Such macro-deficits produced by particular combinations of micro-deficits can produce substantial handicaps in any of the following areas: activities of daily living (ADL), social involvements, educational/vocational activities and family relationships. Rehabilitation for the head-injured person must focus on both the micro-deficit level and, perhaps more importantly, on the more holistic macro-deficit level.

PRINCIPLES OF TREATMENT

1. Therapeutic intervention should commence as early after injury as is feasible.
2. Treatment should be provided in a holistic manner. The person should not be regarded as someone with a collection of particular deficits but rather as a whole person whose multiple needs require an integrated response.
3. Since the occupational therapist works as a member of a team, treatment approaches should be well coordinated with the other team members and treatments should complement one another.
4. Therapy should focus on micro-deficits and macro-deficits simultaneously. Whilst it is important to try to rectify specific problems such as concentration/attention difficulties within the treatment setting, it is equally important, if not more so, to focus on the person's functional abilities, for example daily living skills. Therefore, attempts to overcome a cognitive problem should be made on both 'fronts' simultaneously.

THE OCCUPATIONAL THERAPY PROCESS

The following points should be considered by the occupational therapist when assessing and planning treatment at any stage after head injury. Refer also to Chapter 4 for more detailed information.

Gathering information

1. About the individual. It is important to know as much about the individual as possible before setting overall aims and planning treatment. Relatives, friends, employers and teachers, for example, are all sources of information.

Information should be requested regarding family circumstances: for example, names, ages, relationships, educational/work background, hobbies and interests, personality, likes and dislikes.

2. About the injury. It is also necessary to understand the individual's condition in detail in order to establish a baseline from which to plan treatment. Medical notes, doctors, nurses and other professionals are important sources of information.

Information is needed regarding: date of injury; circumstances of injury, i.e. driver, pedestrian, industrial accident, assault; extent and location of damage, i.e. open or closed injury, temporal or frontal damage; any other injuries; any other relevant previous illness/disability.

Assessment

Assessment of the head-injured person may need to take place over several sessions as the individual's concentration span may be greatly reduced and he may tire easily. The environment in which he is assessed is also important. It should be quiet, well lit, comfortable and free from distractions. The person should be seated and relaxed.

Assessment should be through both observation of and interaction with the individual. Careful notes should be taken to record all responses, including duration, strength, quality and consistency of response.

As well as functional capabilities, areas to be assessed may include physical ability, cognitive function and behaviour. In the early stages of recovery it may not be realistic to attempt formal assessment; however, information about the person's abilities can be gleaned through careful observation. The therapist should observe his position and posture, motor control, eye and head movements, communication ability and response to commands.

For those people who are more alert or who are at a later stage of recovery it may be relevant to use more standardised assessment procedures such as the Rivermead Behavioural Memory Test (RBMT) (Wilson et al 1985) and the Chessington Occupational Therapy Neurological Assessment Battery (COTNAB) (Tyerman et al 1986). The RBMT is an assessment of functional memory in areas where the head-injured person is likely to encounter problems, e.g. remembering names, recognising faces, remembering an appointment. The COTNAB assesses four broad functional areas, i.e. visual perception, constructional ability, sensory-motor ability and ability to follow instructions. Both these assessments are valuable tools in obtaining a baseline from which to plan and evaluate treatment.

Treatment planning and evaluation

The following points should be considered in treatment planning.

- Different types of injuries produce different patterns of disabilities and rates of recovery. Therefore, the knowledge of the type of injury will help determine treatment priorities.
- Treatment should be directed towards improving functional abilities and social skills.
- Targets for therapy should be established on the basis of short- and long-term goals. Short-term goals can be considered as priorities for treatment and usually comprise some aspect of disability or behaviour which, if not improved, will become a major obstacle preventing rehabilitation in other areas.
- Continuous evaluation and modification of treatment is essential.

Progression of treatment

Rehabilitation of the head-injured person is a continuous and prolonged process and can be divided into three phases. The first is the acute phase, which takes place in the hospital, generally in the intensive care unit or neurosurgical ward. The second is the post-acute inpatient rehabilitation phase which may take place in a specialised ward or inpatient rehabilitation centre where available. The third phase is the long-term follow-up care shared by outpatient facilities and the community.

As the person progresses through these phases, treatment goals will probably change in accordance with progress. Initially, long-term goals may be quite unforeseeable, as the early short-term goals, such as encouraging the individual to swallow or to participate minimally in an activity, are very basic. Later the long-term goals may be to enable him to be as independent as possible with a view to returning home, so that the short-term goals at this stage would be, for example, to aim for balance and coordination and for independence in relevant ADL. Later still, the long-term goals may be to return the person to some form of employment, in which case the short-term goals would be to develop relevant skills such as speed, manual dexterity or accuracy.

TREATMENT IN THE ACUTE PHASE

The occupational therapist has an important part to play even in the very early stages of recovery from head injury, when treatment would take place on the ward (Garner 1990).

Aims of treatment

- Increase the level of awareness by using controlled stimulation.
- Promote orientation and reduce confusion.
- Prevent deformity and promote good positioning and posture.
- Facilitate family involvement in rehabilitation and offer support.

Stimulation and activity promote recovery of the injured brain. Deliberate and therapeutic stimulation is the beginning of the process of restoring the integrative action of the nervous system. The individual should be encouraged to respond appropriately to direct stimulation and environmental influences. All five senses should be stimulated in order to promote recovery but the therapist must be careful not to over-stimulate or flood the system, which will lead to either withdrawal or agitation. Any interaction with the person must be accompanied by slow, clear and precise words of explanation, orientation and encouragement.

- Tactile stimulation can be used with contrasting stimuli — heat/cold, roughness/smoothness, hardness/softness, deep pressure/light touch — on various parts of the body to encourage tactile discrimination and appropriate responses.
- Auditory stimulation involving familiar sounds such as voices, music or animal calls can be used to stimulate him, allowing periods of rest.
- Visual stimulation involves having familiar objects such as photographs and personal belongings within the person's visual field. It is better to have isolated objects in strategic places where they can be utilised specifically rather than to have a collection of things together.
- The senses of taste and smell should not be forgotten. The familiar smells of perfumes, polish, foods, and so on, can be used in stimulation.

Before attempting gustatory stimulation using bitter, sweet, salty and sour sensations, it must be ensured that the individual has an effective swallow and gag reflex.

As suggested above, the occupational therapist should encourage orientation by giving clear and precise explanations as to what is happening. Orientation can be further encouraged by keeping familiar objects near the individual, having a clock and calendar in view, and by facilitating as normal a wake/rest routine as possible.

The occurrence of a head injury in one family member has a devastating effect on the others, who in the early stages will feel bewildered and helpless and will need much support, guidance and encouragement. They should be encouraged to participate in rehabilitation. The individual often responds more positively to a relative, and as it is often the relatives who will be responsible for continued care and support in the community, they need education and the opportunity to share their fears and anxieties. It often helps them to share their feelings with others who have experienced similar circumstances, and the national head injuries association, Headway, may be of value to them.

TREATMENT IN THE POST-ACUTE PHASE

Once the individual has begun to recover consciousness and his condition has stabilised, the intensive and prolonged programme of rehabilitation begins.

Aims of treatment

- Facilitate normal movement patterns and inhibit abnormal reflex activity
- Increase independence in ADL
- Facilitate adaptation to perceptual deficits
- Promote strategies for managing memory and overcoming learning difficulties
- Facilitate socially acceptable behaviour and social competence
- Ensure appropriate community resettlement.

These aims of treatment are obviously very broad and by no means exhaustive. The complexity of deficits following head injury necessitates individualised treatment planning and it is perhaps better to consider how the occupational therapist can assist with some of the most common problems.

Paralysis

When paralysis is present it is essential to maintain range of movement of the joints and to prevent contractures. It is also important to ensure that affected parts are not neglected: the individual should be encouraged to take responsibility for them. This can be facilitated by using bilateral activities and by ensuring that the affected parts are always within the person's visual field (Eggers 1983); for example, the affected arm should be positioned on the table in front of him at meal times (Fig. 17.4). Further activities should encourage weight-bearing in order to stimulate the

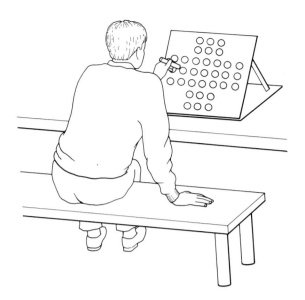

Fig. 17.5 Activities involving weight-bearing help to stimulate proprioceptors and reduce spasticity.

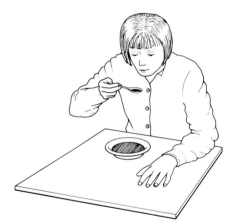

Fig. 17.4 The left (affected) arm is brought forward into a spasticity inhibiting position.

proprioceptors and should aim towards stability of the affected joints. For example, with the affected arm positioned on a chair or plinth at his side, the person can then be encouraged to cross the midline with the unaffected hand in playing solitaire, using a guillotine or printing. The therapist may need to support the elbow in the weight-bearing position (Fig. 17.5).

Spasticity

Treatment of spasticity should aim at normalisation of muscle tone and the inhibition of spastic patterns (Bobath 1978). Good positioning of the body is vital in inhibiting spasticity and forms a firm base from which normal movement can be facilitated. It must be remembered that normal movement cannot be superimposed on patterns of spasticity and, therefore, before any attempt to facilitate movement is made, the spastic pattern must be broken down, working proximally to distally, that is, from the centre of the spasticity outwards. Several factors will encourage spasticity and should therefore be avoided, such as increased effort or working against resistance, fear, anxiety and pain.

Activities which encourage trunk rotation and weight transfer will help to reduce spasticity in the trunk muscles and to increase stability and balance (Fig. 17.6). Also, activities which encourage the person to lean forward can lay the groundwork for the ability to stand from sitting (Eggers 1983). Activities such as printing, basic woodwork and remedial games can all be used to facilitate both these movement patterns (Fig. 17.7).

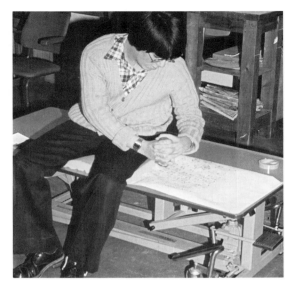

Fig. 17.6 Bilateral stamping to practise trunk rotation. The patient sits on a low plinth with his feet flat on the floor and turns from the ink pad on one side to the paper on the other side.

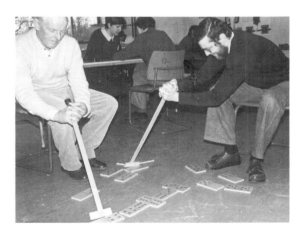

Fig. 17.7 Floor dominoes used to increase balance through leaning forward and to encourage bilateral arm activity.

For more detailed information on the treatment of spasticity, refer to Chapter 16.

Ataxia

The treatment of people with ataxia is problematic. Adding weights to body parts can help control the tremor during activity but this does not decrease the ataxia. However, weights should be used with caution because they may cause muscle bulk to increase.

There are strategies which can be used to compensate to some extent for lack of coordination. For example, if activities such as preparing food can be carried out in a sitting position then the person does not need to think about controlling ataxia in his lower limbs but can concentrate on his upper limbs. Likewise, if hand activities such as eating can be carried out with elbows resting on the table, he only has to control movement from the elbow instead of from the shoulder.

People with ataxia often find it difficult to slow down their speed of activity. They try to work at their previously normal speed, which is now impossible. They should be given opportunities to learn to work within their present ability. 'Placing' activities, such as draughts or noughts and crosses, using wooden blocks which must be lifted from one place to another, provide good initial training, allowing the person to work at the required slow pace and control the tremor between each move. With improvement the size of pieces can be reduced and the precision and speed increased (Fig. 17.8).

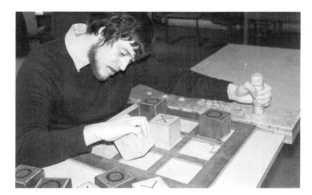

Fig. 17.8 Noughts and crosses used to treat ataxia. The spastic left arm is brought forward into a spastic inhibitory position while the right arm is used for gross co-ordinating movements.

Sensory disturbance

Sensory disturbance may lead to neglect and disuse of the affected part of the body and, due to diminished or absent sensory feedback, puts the individual at risk of injuries such as burns, cuts and pressure sores. Therapy may help him to distinguish different temperatures, textures and shapes, and may also encourage him to use vision as an aid to avoiding potentially hazardous situations. ADL such as dressing, washing and shaving may all be made more difficult by tactile disturbances but also by proprioceptive loss. In such cases the therapist should encourage compensatory strategies to facilitate independence. When abnormal proprioception is present the individual should be encouraged to move his affected joints using his unaffected arm. Purposeful activities involving the affected joints aided by an unaffected part, such as bilateral draughts, printing or sanding, should be incorporated into treatment. Adding different weights, incorporating changes in direction, giving resistance to movement and weight-bearing through the affected limb will all provide stimulation for the proprioceptors.

Perceptual problems

Perception is the process of organising, interpreting, storing and responding to information received from one or more sensory organs (Zolton 1986). Perception is required in order to make sense of, and interact with, the environment. Disorders of perception can occur following head injury and may impair function and cause confusion, agitation, bizarre and meaningless behaviour or apathy. As the damage in head injury is often diffuse, perceptual problems may not be as clearly defined as in other forms of brain damage, for example that caused by cerebrovascular accidents. The reader should refer to Chapter 16 for more detailed information on specific perceptual deficits and their treatment.

There are two main approaches to the treatment of perceptual disorders. The first is the *transfer of training* approach whereby the individual practises particular perceptual tasks with the intention of generalising to functional activities. For example, if a person has a unilateral neglect which is causing problems with dressing, he might practise assembling jigsaws of body parts and perform activities involving scanning to the neglected side; the intention is, by improving awareness of the affected side, to increase independence in dressing. While the evidence in support of this approach is scarce, it is beneficial in highlighting to the individual that there is a problem which needs to be addressed.

The second approach to treating perceptual problems is a purely functional one, whereby a person with a dressing problem would undertake repeated practice aiming to increase his independence.

It may be difficult to identify particular perceptual problems in those who have sustained head injuries, as these may combine with other deficits to form functional problems; for example, it may appear that the individual who has a problem in finding his way around the ward, rehabilitation centre or hospital has a spatial awareness deficit or topographical disorientation, i.e. a route-finding difficulty. However, this may not be the case as the problem may be the result of general confusion and disorientation or a memory difficulty, or a combination of these. Such difficulties are best tackled in a functional manner by ensuring that rooms are well signposted and by practising particular routes. These people often function better in familiar surroundings such as their own homes.

Memory

There may be several reasons why a person is unable to use his memory successfully. He may not be paying enough attention to the task and so not absorb the information; or he may not be storing the information; or he may be unable to retrieve that which is stored (Wilson 1987).

Loss of memory can be aggravated by hospital routine, as the person tends to be told what to do, and when and where to go, so that he need not think for himself. Even though the head-injured person's memory problem may persist, there are many ways in which the occupational therapist can help him increase his independence. In planning treatment, however, the therapist should bear in mind that there is no evidence to suggest that practice on memory games, such as Kim's game, generalises to improvement of memory in all aspects of function.

Management of memory deficits may include

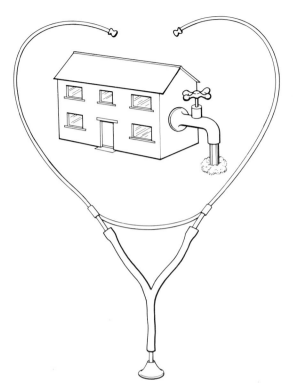

Fig. 17.9 A typical visual image which might be used to remember the name of Dr Waterhouse.

use of both internal and external aids. The use of internal aids might include forming a visual image associated with a name to be remembered (Fig. 17.9), learning rhymes or stories in order to remember and recall information, and devising first-letter mnemonics. External aids include diaries, notebooks, calendars and lists (Wilson & Moffatt 1984).

Difficulties may arise in teaching the person to use memory aids in that he may not acknowledge that he has a deficit, may not wish to use memory aids, or may forget to use them. The therapist must be persistent, and encourage him to incorporate memory prompts into his daily routine — for example, looking at his diary of the day's events at a particular time of day, in a particular place.

Personality/behavioural changes

Both personality and behavioural changes are common after head injury. An individual's personality consists of a complex combination of the idiosyncratic characteristics which make up his distinctive character. Following head injury any such characteristics may change and such symptoms as lability of mood, inability to control emotions, apathy and euphoria are common. Likewise, behavioural traits such as aggression, sexual disinhibition and other attention-seeking behaviours are common. It is arguable whether such changes are a direct result of brain damage or secondary to it in the respect that they may be born out of frustration. Whatever the cause it is possible to control behaviour in the right circumstances by using behaviour modification techniques (Fussey & Giles 1988).

Behavioural techniques can be utilised to extinguish unwanted behaviour or shape existing behaviour into a more socially acceptable pattern, and are based on the principle that if desired behaviour is rewarded then the use of that behaviour will be encouraged. They need to be very carefully structured and well coordinated for them to be successful. The following points should be borne in mind:

- A common response must be adopted by the whole team, including family and friends.
- The reasons for therapy must be clearly understood by all concerned, including the individual.
- Targets should be set as low as possible and raised gradually. If the individual does not achieve success initially he will become discouraged and perhaps cease to cooperate.
- Rewards for desired behaviour must be given as soon as possible after the behaviour has occurred.

Rewards should be appropriate for the particular person. Material rewards may be more acceptable in the early stages, but later they should be replaced by social rewards. A points system may be more suitable: i.e., points can be awarded for achieving the target or deducted for unacceptable behaviour; they can then be exchanged for rewards when a set target has been reached. Whatever form of reward is chosen, it must be easily controlled within the intervention setting.

Every care must be taken by all members of the team that the programme is strictly adhered to and the individual is not manipulating events.

LATE STAGE TREATMENT

Unfortunately it is often the case that once the head-injured person is sufficiently mobile and orientated to return home, he is discharged from hospital with little support and follow-up. At this stage his problems are often only just beginning. Both the individual and his family feel abandoned, experiencing increasing social isolation. For the head-injured person, rehabilitation may well be required over many years if he is to maximise his potential for recovery and adjustment; in this late stage of treatment, the occupational therapist has an important part to play.

Aims of treatment

- Continue to address specific 'micro' deficits
- Maximise level of social re-integration
- Maximise independent living skills
- Facilitate strategies to assist with new learning
- Resettle into work where possible
- Offer continued family support

Again, these are broad aims. Late stage rehabilitation should aim to equip the person with the skills needed to live in the least restrictive environment possible. This may involve work in a diversity of areas, ranging from meal planning, shopping and cooking to community orientation and the effective use of community resources. The occupational therapist can also help in retraining social skills and competences. Rehabilitation within the community entails the development of a programme by the different professionals involved, supplemented where necessary and possible by other carers. These other carers will include the family as important key workers who need to be trained and helped to cope with the stresses of long-term rehabilitation.

Community-based rehabilitation enables the team to capitalise on the available resources to be found in the area, such as training colleges, schools and adult training schemes. The community ap-proach allows the individual to remain a part of the community whilst the last stages of rehabilitation are completed and thus there is less chance of the individual and his family becoming socially isolated.

WORK (OR NON-WORK) RESETTLEMENT

At some point the individual will reach a stage where no further dramatic improvement is likely. There are many possible alternatives to be considered when this stage is reached. The individual's physical, cognitive, emotional and social abilities need to be considered before he and his family are counselled on his future prospects.

There are those who recover sufficiently to return to their previous employment, although this may mean gradual re-integration; it may take a significant length of time for them to achieve previous competency levels.

Most employers are very supportive and may be able to find work in a lesser capacity for those who are unable to return to their previous jobs, although it may be difficult for individuals to accept a change in status.

When work assessment and/or retraining is necessary the Disablement Resettlement Officer (DRO) should be involved. The DRO may refer the individual to an Employment Rehabilitation Centre (ERC) for assessment of his capabilities to return to his previous job or, if his pre-injury employment is no longer feasible, for assessment of his other skills and aptitudes.

It is unfortunate, however, that a significant number of severely head-injured people may not be able to return to employment or at best only return to sheltered employment, which in itself is a very limited provision. Although employment opportunities are limited in the United Kingdom there is a great deal of interest in an American scheme which has yielded encouraging reports of success of work resettlement of the head injured population. The scheme uses a 'job coach', i.e. a person who gives on-the-job training and support to the individual until he has mastered the job and then gradually reduces the amount of support offered.

Even if open or sheltered employment is not an

option, it should be remembered that there may be training/educational opportunities available. Employment training courses, colleges for people with disabilities and special needs departments of tertiary colleges are all worth consideration and investigation.

It should also be stressed that it is rarely the person's physical disabilities which prevent a return to employment; rather, cognitive and behavioural problems more commonly prevent successful reintegration.

HELPING THE FAMILY

Despite the efforts of therapists working in the few specialist head-injury rehabilitation centres and in more general rehabilitation settings, most head injured people suffer a protracted period of recovery and adjustment and often some degree of residual disability. The burden of care often falls to the immediate family.

Family members have to face problems resulting from a combination of primary neurological damage and secondary psychological repercussions as the person struggles to meet social demands for which he is no longer adequately equipped. Common primary changes include lack of insight, egocentricity, hyperactivity, impulsiveness and lack of emotional control; secondary changes, including reduced self-esteem, loss of self-assurance and confusion, are thought to emerge from repeated failures and frustrations.

Families often struggle to provide for as many of their relative's needs as possible and, despite their resourcefulness, warrant continued professional support and guidance.

CONCLUSION

The consequences of head injury are multi-faceted and complex. They may include physical, cognitive, behavioural, emotional and psychosocial disabilities. Each case is different; accordingly, this chapter has not attempted to offer a 'recipe' for rehabilitation. Rather, it has provided a broad outline of some of the most salient features of head injury and suggested aspects of rehabilitation in which the occupational therapist has an essential role, whilst stressing the importance of individualised treatment. Each head-injured person presents with a unique combination of problems which offer a challenge to rehabilitation services to cater creatively for his very special needs.

REFERENCES AND FURTHER READING

Bannister R 1972 Brain revised. In: Clinical neurology, 4th edn. Oxford University Press, Oxford
Bickerstaff E R 1978 Neurology, 3rd edn. Hodder and Stoughton, London
Bobath B 1978 Adult hemiplegia: evaluation and treatment, 2nd edn. Heinemann Medical, London
Clark-Wilson J, Giles G M 1990 Occupational therapy for the brain injured adult. Chapman and Hall, London
Evans C D 1981 Rehabilitation after severe head injury. Churchill Livingstone, Edinburgh
Eggers O 1983 Occupational therapy in the treatment of adult hemiplegia. Heinemann, London
Fussey I, Giles G M 1988 Rehabilitation of the severely brain damaged adult. Croom Helm, London
Garner R 1990 Acute head injury. Chapman and Hall, London
Hayward R 1980 Management of acute head injuries. Blackwell, Oxford
Medical Disability Society 1988 The management of traumatic brain injury. A Working Party Report of the Medical Disability Society.
Tyerman R, Tyerman A, Howard P, Hadfield C 1986 The Chessington Occupational Therapy Neurological Assessment Battery. Nottingham Rehabilitation, Nottingham
Wilson B A 1987 Rehabilitation of memory. Guildford Press, New York
Wilson B A, Cockburn J, Baddley A 1985 The Rivermead Behavioural Memory Test. Thames Valley Test Company, London
Wilson B A, Moffatt N 1984 Clinical management of memory problems. Croom Helm, London
Wood R L I, Eames P G 1989 Models of brain injury rehabilitation. Croom Helm, London
Zolton B, Giev E, Freishtat B 1986 Perceptual and cognitive dysfunction in the adult stroke patient, 2nd edn. Slack, New Jersey

18

Motor neurone disease

Helen E. Stoneley

INTRODUCTION

Motor Neurone Disease (MND) is a chronic fatal degenerative disease of the central nervous system. It is characterised by a selective loss of lower motor neurones from the pons, medulla and spinal cord together with loss of upper motor neurones from precentral gyri of the brain (Jones & Ramaiah 1986). The process of degeneration is remarkably selective, leaving intelligence, special senses, cerebellar, sensory and autonomic function intact. The aetiology of the disease is unknown, although various theories of causation have been investigated, including toxic poisoning by lead or mercury, viral infection and autoimmune diseases, without any positive results (Trombly 1989). The onset of the disease is usually after the age of 40, although occasionally it may appear in younger people (Table 18.1).

Table 18.1 Incidence of MND

Type	Age	Male:female	Prognosis
Progressive muscular atrophy	under 50	5:1	5–10 years
Amyotrophic lateral sclerosis	over 55	3:2	2–5 years
Progressive bulbar palsy	over 60	2:3	1–2 years

This chapter begins with a description of the clinical features of the three types of motor neurone disease, followed by its diagnosis and medication. The role of the occupational therapist is then discussed in detail in two sections: (1) during the early stages of treatment and (2) during the later stages. The following areas in which the occupational therapist is likely to intervene are covered: psychological and emotional factors, personal care, home management, general mobility, housing, communication, employment, leisure and finance. The chapter concludes with a section on the carers and families of the individual and discusses the role of the occupational therapist in providing support for them when the individual is dying and during bereavement.

CLINICAL FEATURES

There are three main types of motor neurone disease.

1. Progressive muscular atrophy. This is characterised by progressive lower motor neurone disease weakness and the wasting of muscles. It presents as asymmetrical wasting and weakness of the small muscles of the hands. The age at onset is usually under 50 years with more males than females being affected in a ratio of 5:1. The prognosis is 5 to 10 years.

2. Amyotrophic lateral sclerosis. This is the commonest form of MND. It is a combination of both upper and lower motor neurone weakness without muscle wasting. The age of onset is usually over 55 with more males than females being affected in a ratio of 3:2. The prognosis is 2 to 5 years.

3. Progressive bulbar palsy. This is characterised by a lower motor neurone lesion resulting in weakness in the musculature supplied by the cranial nerves controlling speech and swallowing. This affects mainly the elderly and is slightly more common in women. The prognosis is 1 to 2 years. Table 18.2 summarises the three types.

Initially it may be possible to differentiate

Table 18.2 Clinical features of MND

Type	Motor neurones	Muscle
Progressive muscular atrophy	lower	weakness, wasting, fasciculation of any limb or trunk muscles, small hand muscles involved
Amyotrophic lateral sclerosis	upper & lower	weakness without wasting, spasticity rigidity
Progressive bulbar palsy	lower	weakness, wasting & fasciculation of lower facial muscles

between the three types but in the final stages there are likely to be signs of both upper and lower motor neurone involvement. The initial symptoms are most frequently focal or segmental weakness of the hands, lower extremities or shoulders which may include symptoms of muscle weakness with atrophy, cramping and fasciculation. The degeneration then widens to include a number of motor cells, and widespread paralysis affects a large part of the body (Jones & Ramaiah 1986).

Diagnosis

There is not a specific test which is used to determine whether a person has MND, but the combination of upper and/or lower motor neurone involvement with no sensory abnormalities and with changes in the reflexes are sufficient to confirm diagnosis. Other tests are often carried out routinely to eliminate any other cause of the symptoms (Cochrane 1987).

Medication

There is no specific treatment available and therefore the only drugs which are prescribed are for the relief of symptoms, for example:

- painful cramps
- spasms
- excessive saliva
- infections. (Cochrane 1987)

OCCUPATIONAL THERAPY

As MND is an incurable and progressive disorder the occupational therapist's role is one of providing assistance and support for the duration of the illness. It is important that a good relationship is formed between the therapist and the family to ensure that contact can be maintained at regular intervals in order that the highest levels of physical, personal and social function are achieved.

Aims of treatment

It is vital to have individual aims and goals for each person at each stage of the condition and therefore the following are offered as a broad guideline only:

- To assess and maintain the person's optimum level of independence.
- To advise in relation to his life-style and environment and support the person and his family.
- To plan for their future needs and wishes.

EARLY STAGES OF TREATMENT

At this stage the individual shows signs of muscle imbalance, increased muscle fatigue caused by excessive energy expenditure, and decreased mobility and function. The presenting features may be:

- foot drop causing mobility problems
- difficulty in speaking, causing communication dysfunction
- severe weakness in the hands, causing difficulties with activities of daily living.

The individual is often undergoing tests to identify the cause of his loss of function, the time between the initial symptoms and a firm diagnosis differing from person to person. The way individuals react to the diagnosis will often depend upon their previous knowledge of the condition, its subsequent disabling effects and the reaction of their relatives. However, the reaction is often determined by the way in which the information

is presented to them and by whom. When a terminal diagnosis has been given, most people will be shocked and will take some time to adjust. Some hospitals now provide a counselling service for people who have a terminal diagnosis and a number of consultants will, where this service is not available, advise the families to contact the Motor Neurone Disease Association.

Assessment

The initial assessment must be extremely comprehensive and thorough as this will not only provide the therapist with a measure of the person's needs at any stage of the condition, but will also offer an indication of its course. At a later stage it will indicate its rapidity and therefore assist her to plan realistically for the future with the individual and his carers. It is important to establish at an early stage exactly what information the family members have been given about the condition, whether the full implications of MND are understood and their feelings and attitude to this information.

Goals

Realistic goals which will meet the family's needs, assist them to cope with daily and weekly variations and are appropriate to their way of life and environment must be discussed and established. The goals will need regular review and evaluation as further difficulties arise.

INTERVENTION AREAS

Psychological and emotional factors

Individuals react in innumerable ways when told they have motor neurone disease. Feelings of disbelief, commonly followed by anger directed at those closest to him will be displayed as the person grieves for a future which is curtailed. Each family will cope with these feelings in different ways and the therapist can assist them by listening, discussing worries and steering them towards as positive an outlook as possible for the future.

Meeting future needs and deciding how and

when these can be achieved should, ideally, take place in an objective and positive manner. The therapist will be able to judge when that time has arrived whilst supporting the carers as the recipients of anger and the individual as someone who may also be confused, depressed and full of misgivings.

Plans for the future need to be clarified. These plans include the practicalities of daily life, but they must also cater for a much wider range of human needs. The latter will relate to the individual's past, present and potential future lifestyle and encompass the roles he has enacted within the family, for example breadwinner, homemaker, parent. Equally important is the way in which he has and will continue to structure his daily life knowing that his condition will eventually severely impair his familiar routines. The therapist should aim to ensure that his and the family's motivation is enhanced by whatever means are acceptable, for example by the person maintaining a hobby or interest that involves all or key family members.

In reality, plans may frequently be blocked, particularly by the individual. Often he may wish to seek a second opinion regarding his diagnosis or pursue alternative therapies such as acupuncture or herbal remedies, and it is important that the person is psychologically and emotionally supported in these endeavours, providing there is no danger to his health.

Carers should receive as much support as the individual, as their feelings and needs are often overlooked. Time must be allowed for discussion of their needs and concerns, even if this takes place away from the family home and their partner.

The psychological and emotional issues underlying MND must be dealt with in tandem with the physical needs of the family. The occupational therapist's counselling and supportive skills are usually very much appreciated by the family and these complement the practical advice and help she offers. If the family members also wish for moral support and counselling from someone else, they can be put in touch with the Motor Neurone Disease Association.

Personal care

As weakness, particularly when it affects the small muscles of the hand, can be a presenting feature of MND, it is important to ensure that early assistance and advice are given, not only to resolve any initial problems but also to assist the person to plan for his future. Therefore it is necessary to establish realistic priorities with him, i.e. does he want to use his abilities/energies on personal activities of daily living or hobbies? It is important to remember that resolutions to problems should include:

● changes in method or technique where applicable
● assistance offered by carers when and where appropriate
● equipment provision as necessary.

Dressing/undressing

Clothing which is roomy, easy to put on, warm, lightweight, easy to launder and comfortable is advisable. Either fastenings should be in an easily accessible position and should be larger than usual, or garments should have no fastenings as they are easier to manage. Both the individual's and carer's needs should be considered, and ease of management may, over a period of time, indicate a change of style if this is acceptable.

Eating and drinking

The loss of function in the small muscles of the hands can make these tasks difficult. The use of large-handled lightweight cutlery may help the person maintain independence. Drinks will keep warm for longer periods in lightweight insulated beakers which are also easier to lift to the mouth. It may be necessary to introduce a two-handed beaker or a straw when the mobility of the upper limb becomes seriously impaired.

The therapist and family also need to review, regularly, the position in which the individual eats and drinks. It may help, for example, if he supports his weak upper limbs by resting both or one elbow on the table when he drinks; a dining chair with arms may offer him more stability and reassurance, enabling him to concentrate on his meal rather than his balance and general position.

Washing

It is important to give basic advice in the early stages to ensure that independence can be maintained, and therefore advice, for example on sitting at the basin to wash, may be all that is required.

Bathing

This is unlikely to be a major problem at this stage, but certain items of equipment, for example a non-slip mat and grab rail, may be required to provide extra support and reassurance.

Care of teeth

For the sake of the person's self esteem it is important that he cleans his own teeth. Adaptations to the handles of toothbrushes can be provided to help him and basic advice given on possible changes to equipment, for example replacement of a conventional toothbrush with a battery controlled one.

Toileting

The provision of rails or a high seat may be all that is required at this stage if the person is experiencing weakness in the lower limbs. The therapist must check the position of the flushing mechanism on the toilet and toilet roll holder to ensure that both are accessible.

Grooming

It is important to ensure that equipment with small diameter handles, for example shaving items, combs, brushes and make-up applicators, is enlarged if the small muscles of the hands are affected.

Home management

Assistance and advice in home care, including the garden, the person's hobbies and any pets, should be given as appropriate to the individual, his traditional family roles and his continuing wishes and needs.

Home maintenance, do-it-yourself jobs and car maintenance are usually the province of the man in a household, though increasingly partners tackle such tasks together. As motor neurone disease progresses, the individual and family may well have to accept more assistance from decorators, builders and others, particularly if family members are unable to help.

For someone who has always been proud of his skills this is exceedingly difficult to cope with and he will need to be consulted and involved in tasks as much as possible and supported through his feelings of increasing helplessness.

Gardening

Where possible it is important to support the continuation of this interest, and therefore early advice on suitably adapted garden equipment may be of assistance. It is essential to stress the importance of the person not becoming overtired and therefore ensuring that rests are taken at frequent intervals, and that sitting to undertake tasks may be advisable. A number of items of adapted garden tools are available, for example long handled shears, and careful consideration will need to be given to the individual's needs.

Other hobbies

These can be many and varied and include anything from car maintenance to embroidery. In most cases it will be possible for the person to continue with his hobby to some extent initially. If his key interest was sport it may be possible to continue as a spectator in order to maintain contact and interest. In some instances it may not be possible to continue either actively or as a spectator, in which case advice as to alternative activities which can be undertaken is important.

Catering and housekeeping for the family

If appropriate it is important to encourage the individual to remain in control of this for as long as possible, and advice from the therapist in the early stages can often make this possible. As muscle fatigue can be a problem to the person with MND he must be encouraged to do as much as possible without overtiring himself. The therapist should therefore give advice about activities which can be carried out using alternative methods or from a seated position, for example preparing vegetables and washing up. She should discuss the planning of these activities, how they might be easier to complete or who could help, to ensure that they are 'timetabled' to the person's liking. Some minor alterations in the positioning of certain items and/or to the kitchen itself may be necessary to allow him to maintain his involvement and control. The use of labour-saving devices such as food processors, pre-cooked meals, freezers and microwave ovens may also assist.

Cleaning and laundering

Carrying out small amounts of washing and cleaning and having frequent breaks will help the person initially, as will use of the appropriate equipment. It is, however, important to plan for the future and therefore it may help him to consider sending large items of washing to a laundry and arranging for help with the cleaning.

Shopping and deliveries

Initially, the person may only require help to transport the shopping. However, it is important to consider his long-term needs and investigate which shops, if any, offer a delivery service as this can help him to remain independent for as long as possible.

General mobility

Mobility

Where the initial symptoms affect the lower limbs, mobility indoors and outside will need to be con-

sidered. Wherever possible both the occupational therapist and physiotherapist should undertake the assessment and advise accordingly. They should suggest the most suitable means of mobility, recommend any mobility equipment required, and advise on its maintenance. Initially walking sticks and crutches may provide the necessary support, but later a walking frame may be required for indoors and a wheelchair for outdoor use.

It is always important to introduce the use of a wheelchair with care as both the individual and the carer may resist its provision, feeling it marks a drastic change in the person's condition.

Transport

At this stage it may be possible for the person to continue to drive. However, it is advisable to ensure that he informs both his insurers and the Driver and Vehicle Licensing Centre of the nature of his disability. At some stage he will be eligible for an 'orange badge'. This is a scheme which is available for both drivers and passengers. The badge, which is issued by the local authority, permits longer parking in restricted areas, but eligibility will be dependent on the person's level of disability. Additional information about this scheme is contained in Chapter 9.

Housing

If weakness presents in the lower limbs, the person may have already started to consider his future needs. The solution to his problems may be quite simple or complex depending on his present home environment. He may only require the provision of rails in the bathroom or the doors to be widened if he lives in a bungalow. Alternatively he may need a lift or the provision of ground-floor facilities if the property is two storey.

It is extremely important to start discussing the person's future needs at this stage as building work can take many months. Moving house may be contemplated by the family but this should only be considered as a realistic solution in the light of the person's prognosis.

It is essential to advise on the type of properties which may be suitable, for example:

- the building should have no steps
- the access to rooms should have ample manoeuvring space
- the kitchen and bathroom should have sufficient room to turn a wheelchair.

It is also important to ensure that the family have considered their long-term needs. Moving to be nearer family and friends who can offer support and assistance in the later stages may mean that the family lose the support network of the local community. These considerations need to be discussed and thought through before any decisions are made.

Communication

The initial problems in communication which may be displayed are a change in tone and an inability to use expressive speech. The person may talk in a monosyllabic tone. Much help and support can be gained by an early referral to the speech therapist who will be able to make a thorough assessment of the person's dysfunction and monitor his deterioration, as well as giving advice on any exercises which may assist at this stage of the illness.

Writing

Where the small muscles of the hands are affected it may be difficult for the person to write and therefore advice will be required on equipment which may assist in overcoming this problem. Initially this may be adaptations to writing utensils but in paid employment typewriters or computers may be involved.

Telephone

It is important to ensure that the person's independence is maintained, both whilst he is in employment and whilst at home, for as long as possible. There are a number of different types of telephones available and British Telecom offer advice on their range. These vary from those which can alter the volume of the voice and therefore can work for someone who has reduced voice strength, to those which can dial preset numbers. In the later stages, because of a multitude of symptoms, an environmental control system may be considered.

Orthotics

The individual may require orthoses at various stages of the disease. In the initial stage the most frequently used orthosis will be one which will allow functional positioning of the hand and support for the ankle and foot in order to assist in transfers, for example spring-assisted wrist and finger orthoses and ankle–foot orthoses to assist in standing, walking and transfers.

Employment

If it is at all possible for the person to continue to work this must be encouraged. His ability to continue working will depend on the type of job he has and his period of service with his workplace. Some employers are willing to retain an employee with the company for as long as they can and will make necessary adjustments to the type of work he is able to do. Alterations may be required to enable him to have access to the building or to toilet facilities. The Department of Employment's disablement resettlement officer is able to authorise grants for alterations for disabled people in open employment and will provide any special equipment to enable them to do their job.

Transport to and from the workplace is a factor which needs to be addressed along with mobility within the workplace.

Eventually an individual will decide, preferably with the employer, that he is no longer able to continue to work. This will be an extremely emotional time, even if he has reached this conclusion himself. The therapist's involvement at this stage and her knowledge of the individual and the family will enable her to offer the appropriate support and advice.

Finances

These will vary, depending on each individual's circumstances. It is, however, necessary to ensure that each person, and his carer, are receiving the appropriate benefits and are directed to the appropriate agency for advice, for example the Department of Social Security.

LATER STAGES OF TREATMENT

The later stages are characterised by progressive muscle weakness and deterioration of mobility. It is important that the person maintains his independence for as long as possible, particularly in performing tasks important to him. In order to do so the carer will have to continue to be involved in all the decisions which are being made. In addition, carers need continuing support and advice concerning when and when not to assist and how to help.

Assessment

Due to the pattern of deterioration in MND, general assessment is ongoing. However, specific assessment of particular functional or emotional areas will be completed as the need is foreseen or arises.

INTERVENTION AREAS

Personal care

Dressing

As the ability to dress independently decreases, the therapist will need to deal with each presenting problem in the way which is most appropriate and acceptable to the person and his carers. Once dressing independently becomes impossible, the carer should be shown the easiest way to support, dress and make the person comfortable.

Eating/drinking

Independence in eating and drinking should be prolonged for as long as possible because of the importance of maintaining the person's self-esteem and belief in his own abilities. Additionally, the experience of being fed by someone else, no matter how careful and caring she maybe, is unpleasant. The use of adapted cutlery (Fig. 18.1) and mobile

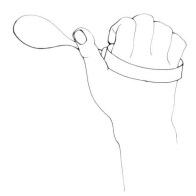

Fig. 18.1 Adapted cutlery may help an individual with poor grip to continue to feed himself.

arm supports can prolong this capacity, providing plates, dishes and beakers are appropriately placed.

Individuals with progressive bulbar palsy symptoms will also have the added problems of swallowing and choking. In these instances advice on dietary changes is necessary and a dietician's assistance will ensure that a suitable, well-balanced diet is maintained. Control of saliva is impaired by poor head control; i.e. the person's head falls forward and makes it difficult for him to swallow, and therefore positioning and supporting of the head must be considered. When swallowing becomes a problem the diet should be varied and tasty and include foods which are smooth and firm in texture, i.e. of a 'puree' consistency.

Swallowing difficulties are often accompanied by choking and this causes distress. Meals should therefore be taken in small quantities and at frequent intervals, as this will prevent exacerbation of the problems and overtiring due to effort. It is also important to ensure that the fluid intake remains high, as reducing this will only cause more problems, for example constipation and dehydration.

Bathing and toileting

Whilst the provision of bathing and toileting equipment can be a short-term solution to the problems arising, there are few properties which can easily accommodate a wheelchair in the bathroom and therefore alterations often have to be undertaken to provide internal access to a toilet and, where possible, washing facilities.

Washing/bathing/showering

The majority of individuals wish to remain independent. It is therefore important to consider whether there are areas where this independence can be maintained.

Washing at the basin. In the majority of cases, if access can be given to hot water, soap and a towel, the individual can usually manage to wash his own hands and face. This does not necessarily mean that he requires access to the basin: it can be done if a bowl is brought to his bed.

Bath. In a number of cases it may be possible to continue to use the bath by using a hoist. This can be a floor-fixed hoist using a rigid seat, a mobile hoist using slings as long as there is sufficient clearance under the bath, or an electric tracking hoist. There are also a number of specially designed baths which incorporate seats or hoists which may be useful. (See Chapter 9, Hoists.)

Shower. If there is sufficient space to provide washing facilities then initially a wheel-in-shower allows the person more independence, although it can be more difficult for a carer to assist.

The wheel-in-shower can be created by means of a special acrylic shower base which provides level access for a self-propelling shower chair. If structural alterations are being carried out it may be possible to provide a non-slip floor covering which is drained by means of a gradual slope towards a drainage hole, thus making the whole floor a 'wet' area. A number of different types of shower chairs are available; the most suitable would probably be one which was self-propelling with an adjustable/reclining back rest with detachable arms and foot rests.

Strip washing/blanket baths. If upper limb weakness is present then independent washing is likely to be very difficult. Initially it may be possible for the person to maintain independence by working out a routine so that different areas of the body are washed on different days.

Bath attendant. Eventually independent bathing will be impossible. To assist both the carer and the individual, help may be obtained from the community nursing service.

Toileting. The course of MND may prohibit any of the more sophisticated means of toileting assistance, in which case carers need advice and support in techniques to help them cope physically and psychologically with their relative's very personal needs. Upper limb involvement often dictates domestic alterations which include the provision of a special toilet to facilitate cleaning the perineum and allow the person to preserve his independence. Examples of this type of toilet are the Closomat toilet and the Medic Loo. These may be of benefit to those with a longer life span.

In some cases it will no longer be possible to gain access to the toilet and the provision of a commode, particularly for use at night, must be considered. It should:

- be stable
- be the same height as the wheelchair seat
- have detachable arms
- be suitable for wheelchair transfers.

During the day a suitable urinal can reduce the number of visits to the toilet.

Incontinence. This is not normally a problem associated with MND. However, towards the end of the illness, there may be some degree of incontinence caused by infection or constipation. The assistance of the local continence adviser should be sought as she will be able to advise on and provide suitable products such as pads or sheets.

Menstruation. For women still menstruating, their cycle may cause problems of management. Self-adhesive pads are the easiest to manage, but, for those wishing to continue using tampons, a number of special inserters can be obtained. It is usually best to avoid belts and hooks as these are the most difficult to manage.

Care of teeth. It is important that the individual's teeth are regularly brushed, either by himself or the carer. Alterations can be made to the toothbrush to enlarge or shape the handle or provide a long-reaching angled handle or strap fastening to help him maintain his independence.

Home management

The individual's ability to take an active role in running the home will steadily decrease, although he may still wish to retain control over some activities, such as deciding on or participating in the decision about family menus. It may be necessary to explore the possibility of external help from the social services department or privately paid help to assist in running the home. However, it is essential to allow him to continue to contribute for as long as possible, with support, for the sake of his self esteem.

General mobility

Transfers

It is important to ensure that the transfers which are carried out are as easy as possible. This can be achieved by ensuring that the heights, where possible, are the same, that all surfaces are stable and that brakes are applied on the wheelchair.

Beds

Initially the person may encounter increasing difficulty in getting into and out of a low bed, and this may be resolved by raising the bed. Some people who have MND find that their sleep is disturbed by painful limb cramps, spasms and anxiety. Initially they will be able to adjust their position themselves without disturbing their carer. However, when the person is no longer able to adjust his position without help, it may be necessary to consider the provision of an alternative bed.

There are a number of beds available which all have different features. The provision of an electrically operated bed allows the person to adjust his head and feet positions at the touch of a button. A number of these beds also have a height adjustment mechanism. This can be extremely beneficial for the carer as it obviates the need for her to bend to assist in activities of daily living as it can be adjusted to the right height for all transfers.

When the therapist is assessing for one of these beds it is necessary to consider whether any hoisting equipment will be required in the future as not all beds have sufficient clearance underneath to facilitate this.

It may be necessary for the therapist to advise on a change of bedding from blankets to duvet, the latter being lighter, warmer and therefore easier to manage.

Chairs

A comfortable high chair is essential in order to facilitate the person's comfort and independence for as long as possible, and wherever possible his own chair should be raised. If a replacement chair is being considered, this should take account of his long-term needs and should ideally have:

- an adjustable position
- a mechanically lifting seat
- support for his legs and feet when he is sitting.

Mobility

The person's walking ability will now have decreased and he will almost certainly require a wheelchair for outdoor use and possibly for indoor use. This is often a very traumatic time for him and his family, and the issue of a wheelchair may be strongly resisted. The therapist must be sensitive to the feelings of the family members and must identify their reasons for resistance in order to help them to adjust to the idea.

The initial wheelchair assessment is very important. Both the individual and his surroundings must be considered and the carer's needs ascertained. The therapist will then be able to determine the most suitable chair for the person's current needs and for any subsequent changes in his requirements. An outdoor lightweight folding wheelchair may be provided initially, as this facilitates overall mobility including transportation by car. For indoor use a Glideabout may be useful, particularly where there is insufficient space for a standard wheelchair without home alterations.

Lack of upper limb strength means that a self-propelling chair may be unsuitable, and therefore consideration should be given to the provision of an electrically-powered chair. Assessment for mobile arm supports should be undertaken as these will facilitate the person's upper limb function.

If he spends long periods of time sitting in his wheelchair, care of his pressure areas is vital, and a pressure-relieving cushion (the type depending on the chair and the needs of the individual) must be provided.

Transport

Transfer into and out of a car and storage of the wheelchair are likely to be the main problems in transporting the individual. Therefore, family members need training in safe and efficient methods of transfer if this is appropriate. If this is not feasible one of the car hoists currently available may assist them; for example an hydraulically operated hoist with tracking can be fitted to the car roof allowing the person to be transferred from the wheelchair to the car seat by means of a sling. One such type is the Burville car hoist. Some of the mobile hoists can be used for this purpose. However, it is often difficult to transport a mobile hoist and a wheelchair in the car for use at the end of the journey.

Hoists

Transfers will become more difficult as the condition progresses. A mobile hoist may help, but the decision of 'which hoist' will have to be based upon the needs of the individual, the needs of the carer and the available space within his home. In a small number of cases electrically operated hoists, ceiling fixed or run on a gantry, may be provided. The contraindications attached to the supply of these hoists are:

- time for installation
- cost
- lack of flexibility once the hoist has been fixed in position.

(See Hoists in Ch. 9.)

Housing

As previously mentioned, the therapist and family need to continuously monitor and identify whether any structural alterations are required to the property. The rapidly deteriorating nature of the individual's condition dictates very advanced forward planning so that alterations are completed as they are needed. However, it is important that all concerned are aware of the length of time the alterations will take and understand the procedures which have to be followed for grant approval, building regulations and planning permission if these are required. The types of alteration which can be considered will vary considerably depending on the individual's needs, the family's needs and the type and tenure of the property. If possible, the work should be kept to a minimum in order to cause the least amount of disruption to the household whilst giving the maximum benefit.

The doctor in charge of the person's care should be consulted before any major plans are drawn up, as specific information concerning the individual's general health and his prognosis can assist the therapist in planning realistically for the individual's future needs.

Access

Access to the property must be reviewed as the person's condition deteriorates. Initially he may be able to manage a small step, but once he is confined to a wheelchair it is important that suitable ramps are provided. In some instances the position of the step prohibits the installation of a conventional ramp and it is therefore necessary to consider a step lift which can cover raises of 700 mm to 1800 mm.

Stairlifts

Stairlifts can provide access to the upstairs bedroom and bathroom. It is important to consider the future course of the disease and ensure that the lift permits wheelchair transfers at the top and bottom of the stairs and provides a supportive seat and a seat belt. Ideally a lift which will carry a wheelchair is preferable, but unfortunately these types will only fit a small number of staircases. It is important to ensure that there is sufficient space for the wheelchair to manoeuvre around upstairs, and door widths must be checked and altered, if necessary and if possible, to facilitate this.

Through-floor lifts

These provide another option. In these cases it is necessary to be aware of the Local Authority guidelines for the installation of lifts as some authorities have strict regulations requiring through-floor lifts to be enclosed at first floor level. The fire officer will be very familiar with these regulations and may well need to see and approve any plans for building alterations, to ensure that there is sufficient time for the disabled person to evacuate the building in the event of fire. The guidelines for lift installation are under constant review and can vary from area to area.

Communication

At this stage the person's problems are likely to be fairly severe, particularly if he has progressive bulbar palsy. His ability to communicate using voluntary speech will now be quite limited, and it is likely that only his carers will be able to understand him. If the speech therapist is not already involved then her help can be invaluable at this stage, both to the individual and the carer. She can offer advice about techniques as well as provide simple, yet effective aids to communication, for example word and picture charts, communication charts, boards and cards.

Environmental control systems

The individual may well benefit from such a system as it can assist him in communication as well as give him some measure of independence. The systems are available through the Department of Health following an assessment and recommendation by a Regional Assessor. The two main systems, POSSUM and SEC, can be used to dial a telephone number, receive calls and operate an alarm, speaker lock and electrical equipment, for example a lamp, radio and television. The control mechanism which is installed is chosen to suit the abilities of the individual, for example it might be a touch pad or a 'suck blow' tube. If a complete environmental control system cannot be provided, social services may supply equipment such as intercoms or speaker locks to help the person overcome his particular difficulties.

Leisure

Once the person is no longer working he should, wherever possible, be encouraged to continue with his hobbies or interests, particularly if these provide some social contact. It may be possible for him to use some of the skills which he had previously used whilst in employment. If he cannot maintain previous interests it may be necessary to consider alternatives which offer a positive and rewarding use of time. Ideally, they should stimulate him mentally, ensure some degree of social contact, involve one or more of the family and offer non-participatory involvement, for example listening to music instead of playing, watching sport instead of participating.

CARERS/FAMILIES

The responsibility of caring often falls on the family members; this may be a shared responsibility or involve just one individual. Often the main carer is the partner and her needs must be assessed alongside those of the individual. She is as much the professional 'responsibility' of the therapist as the person himself. In some instances it will not be possible to satisfy the needs of both and in these situations it is necessary to negotiate a solution which is acceptable to both.

The carer may feel isolated and may need support, either from others who are in a caring role or from other carers of people who are suffering from MND. She may require the therapist's help to put her in touch with the appropriate organisations.

Respite care

One of the frequent, main concerns of carers is what would happen if they were suddenly unable to continue to care for any period of time because of, for example, sudden illness. They need reassurance and an opportunity to consider the possible options/solutions. These may include hospital or hospice admission or a support network of other carers.

The carer will not be able to continue to care without a break. She may take one day off a week whilst her relative attends day care, or the care may be shared with a hospital or hospice so that the individual has a number of weeks at home followed by a number of weeks in the hospital or hospice. This can often be difficult to organise because of the pressure on beds, and it can also be difficult to persuade the family members that the break is required, as they will often continue to visit daily instead of using the break to relax. However, even if they have a 'psychological' need to visit, they are relieved of physical caring for a time.

This time is particularly difficult for the relatives when they are aware of a short prognosis or where there are communication problems and the relatives are acting as interpreters. Because of these problems the carers often feel guilty about taking a break from caring, and the support of those who are in a similar position and their therapist can prove invaluable and reassuring.

Dying

At some stage the individual and family need to discuss whether he wishes to die at home, and before any decision is taken they may wish to clarify how death may occur, for example from respiratory infections.

If he is nursed at home, then support will be made available from specialist nurses dealing with terminally ill people in the community. The occupational therapist should also maintain personal contact during these final weeks and days in order to support the whole family emotionally and psychologically. She may not be offering specific practical help at this stage but this is immaterial. The presence of someone the family knows and trusts and who will listen, is of vital importance to them.

Bereavement

After the individual has died, the carer may wish to see the therapist to talk about the final stage and to deal with the return of any equipment. It is often beneficial for carers to talk to the staff who have been involved with the care as they find the void left by the death of their partner/relative difficult to come to terms with initially and they may need a brief period of support and counselling from an appropriate and acceptable person.

MOTOR NEURONE DISEASE ASSOCIATION

The Motor Neurone Disease Association is a registered charity which was formed in 1979. Its aim is to bring together all those people who are concerned with MND in any way, whether they are professionals or families and sufferers.

It is a voluntary organisation and its funds are directed towards two main areas:

1. The support of research projects into the disease and its management
2. The provision of patient care.

The head office is in Northampton where information is available about the work of the MND Association. The Association produces extensive information in the form of leaflets, both for use by professionals and the general public. The Association employs a number of regional care advisers who are available to the sufferers, their families and the professionals.

The Association is also able to loan equipment where it is not available locally, and is able to offer financial help to those in need. Members of the Association receive a quarterly newsletter with up-to-date information on local and national events.

Motor Neurone Disease Association
38, Hazelwood Road
Northampton NN1 1LN

CONCLUSION

Work with people with MND is always challenging because of the rapidly deteriorating nature of the disease. It allows the therapist the opportunity to work closely with an individual and his family, using all her skills to assist them to adapt to the continuous change whilst maintaining the life-style they choose to lead.

REFERENCES

Cochrane G M 1987 The management of motor neurone disease. Churchill Livingstone, Edinburgh

Jones D L, Ramaiah R S 1986 Distribution of motor neurone disease. Patients in occupational therapy departments. The British Journal of Occupational Therapy 49(8): 260–262

Trombly C A 1989 Occupational therapy for physical dysfunction, 3rd edn. Williams and Wilkins, Baltimore

FURTHER READING

B.S 5776 Specification for powered stairlifts

B.S 5900 Specification for powered home lifts

Cochrane G M 1989 Motor neurone disease. British Journal of Hospital Medicine Vol 41

Mathews W B 1982 Diseases of the nervous system, 4th edn. Blackwell Scientific Publications, Oxford

Wilkinson I M S 1988 Essential neurology. Blackwell Scientific Publications, Oxford

19

Multiple sclerosis

Jenny Goulter

INTRODUCTION

Multiple sclerosis is the most common of the demyelinating diseases. Incidence of the condition, however, varies widely in different geographical areas; for example it is very low in the tropics but high in the temperate zones of both the northern and southern hemispheres. In Britain it affects 1 in 2000 of the population.

This chapter begins by describing the pathology, aetiology and clinical features of the disease, as well as the course, diagnosis, treatment and prognosis. The overall aims of intervention by the occupational therapist during the initial interview and in the areas of personal independence, home management and general mobility are then described. Much practical information is provided to guide the occupational therapist in these areas. The chapter concludes with a discussion of the general housing needs of a person with multiple sclerosis during the course of the disease. The importance of providing information about the support services at the appropriate time is stressed and addresses of some of the most useful associations are provided.

PATHOLOGY

Multiple sclerosis (MS), or disseminated sclerosis

as it used to be called, is the most common progressive disease affecting the central nervous system. The disease affects the white matter in the brain and spinal cord leading to progressive weakness and disability. During the course of the condition demyelination occurs, which is the destruction of the myelin sheath (protective covering of the nerves) in patches both in the brain and spinal cord. These patches become sclerotic, can vary in size, and occur irregularly through the brain and spinal cord. They become shrunken in appearance resulting in the conductivity being seriously affected.

AETIOLOGY

The cause of multiple sclerosis is still unknown despite many theories and intensive research. Theories such as an infection, autoimmune reaction, diet, climate, life-style, circulatory disturbance causing temporary or permanent ischaemia in the affected areas, have all been suggested but none proven.

Hereditary factors have also been inferred and again, although not proven, there seems to be an increase in familial incidence.

COURSE

The disease is characterised by remissions and relapses. During a remission, temporary or prolonged improvement may occur. There is never a set pattern between one remission and another and there is no way of foreseeing when a relapse will occur. No two cases ever present the same pattern but some factors, such as trauma, surgery, influenza, pregnancy and stress, are known to precipitate a relapse.

DIAGNOSIS

The disease is usually diagnosed in young adults between 20 and 40 years of age and is slightly more common in women than in men. Occasionally it may be diagnosed later in life but this is often in hindsight, on examination of a person's past medical history.

CLINICAL FEATURES

The clinical features from the onset will vary from one individual to another. There may only be an isolated symptom or a combination of several, for example nystagmus and paraesthesia. The initial onset may only last for a short period of time and be followed by a remission. However, as the condition progresses, the following disturbances will become apparent, depending on the areas of the brain and central nervous system affected.

Visual

Involvement of the optic nerve may give rise to blurred vision, severe pain and tenderness of either one or both eyes. Diplopia (double vision) and nystagmus (oscillatory eye movement) or ptosis (drooping of the eyelid) may be present. In some severe onsets, blindness in one or both eyes has been known to occur on a temporary basis.

Motor and sensory

General weakness and 'clumsiness' in one or both lower limbs in the early stages are common, indicated, for example, by toes catching on irregularities in the ground causing tripping. This may also be associated with a feeling of heaviness. Paraesthesia gives rise to numbness and tingling in the extremities. Ataxia (muscular incoordination) and hypotonus (diminished muscle tone) will be present if the cerebellum is affected; and with pyramidal involvement, spasticity leading to flexor spasm and contracture and exaggerated reflexes will occur.

Bladder and bowel

Frequency, urgency and incontinence of urine cause particular concern to the individual. Retention of urine and constipation may also occur.

Sexual problems

Partial or complete impotence may occur. Lack of sensation and lack of vaginal lubrication will also cause distress, as well as incontinence.

Psychological/emotional

Euphoria, when it occurs, is quite significant. Depression is often present due to the emotional reaction to the diagnosis, and in some cases can become severe enough to require specific treatment.

Communication impairment

Slurred speech is not uncommon and will occur if the bulbar area of the brain is affected. The speech may become slow and deliberate with emphasis on each syllable.

A common picture of multiple sclerosis is one of a variety of symptoms, such as an ataxic gait, intention tremor, incoordination and loss of dexterity. The person will become weak and easily fatigued, and as the condition progresses he will become increasingly dependent on others.

TREATMENT

As the cause of multiple sclerosis is still unknown there is no curative treatment available, so it is a matter of management of the condition rather than treatment *per se*. The use of corticotrophin (Acthar Gel) and tetrocosactrin (Synacthen Depot) can shorten the acute episodes but does not prevent relapses. The spasticity may be treated with baclofen (Liorasal) or dantrolene sodium (Dantrium).

Individuals with multiple sclerosis have a low level of essential fatty acids so a diet of unsaturated fats is recommended, for example corn oil or Naudicelte capsules (sunflower seed oil) or gluten-free diets.

Physiotherapy is essential in helping the individual to maintain balance and mobility skills. Occupational therapy is also essential for the maintenance of mobility, personal independence, social and leisure interests. District nurses, social workers and speech therapists play an important role in the overall management of the individual.

PROGNOSIS

People with multiple sclerosis may live for two to three decades with the disease, but eventually extreme weakness, ataxia and loss of movement render them totally wheelchair or bed bound. The cause of death is usually as a result of intercurrent infection.

THE ROLE OF THE OCCUPATIONAL THERAPIST

As multiple sclerosis is a progressive disease, the role of the occupational therapist will be one of paramount importance, both in the early stages following diagnosis and in the long term, giving assistance and support, not only to the individual, but also to the immediate family members and other carers. The importance of building a good working relationship from the outset cannot be overemphasised as it will enable the occupational therapist to work with the individual in order to find ways of overcoming difficulties, to encourage him to lead as normal a life as possible — physically, mentally and socially — despite increasing disability.

Following an initial assessment the therapist should aim to solve any immediate problems, i.e. those of particular concern to the individual. Further contact will depend on the course of the condition but should be maintained on a regular basis.

It is essential that the therapist works closely with other members of the team at all times to ensure that an overall coordinated approach is both made and maintained. For instance, the community occupational therapist must work alongside the treatment team in the hospital where the person may be admitted periodically for a re-assessment of chemotherapy or intensive rehabilitation. The therapist must be aware of all the relevant resources available.

These resources may include:

- appropriate financial benefits such as mobility and attendance allowances
- help at work through the Disablement Resettlement Officer
- appropriate support networks, for example home help, meals on wheels and voluntary organisations.

OVERALL AIMS OF INTERVENTION

As the cause of MS is unknown, it is difficult to discuss treatment as such, but the general management of the condition and the intervention by the occupational therapist should aim to:

- assess and maintain the person's maximum level of personal independence at all times
- advise and support both the individual, family and/or carers
- maintain and restore where possible the person's maximum physical, mental and social capacity

- enable the person to maintain his dignity despite increasing disability
- advise and assist the person regarding employment
- advise with caring for the home and family
- introduce other resources at appropriate times (see Fig. 19.1 Chart of resource needs).

THE INITIAL INTERVIEW

The initial interview between the therapist and the individual will be of extreme importance as the relationship will probably continue over many years. It is imperative, therefore, that the occu-

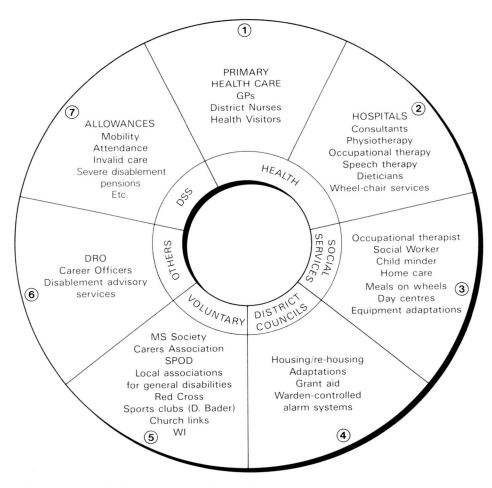

Fig. 19.1 Likely resource needs for people with multiple sclerosis.

pational therapist does not rush the interview but gives the person sufficient time to discuss problems, fears and anxieties. The therapist must be a good listener as this will enable her to gain a clear picture of the immediate family set-up, home and work circumstances, if appropriate, and social networks and interests.

It is important that the therapist discovers the individual's attitude to his disability and what, if anything, he knows of the condition.

In the early stages, the person may not have been informed of the diagnosis, as the results of tests are awaited or because his doctor has decided not to tell him. If, however, he is aware of the diagnosis, he may still be going through the grieving process. The pace at which the therapist can begin to work through problems will depend upon the ability of the individual to discuss issues. It is important, however, that he and his family are helped towards adopting a realistic attitude to the future.

PERSONAL INDEPENDENCE

It is likely that personal independence will begin to be affected from the onset of the condition due to incoordination, loss of sensation and general weakness. Early advice and assistance will be needed to enable the person to tackle difficulties, not only as they arise, but also in preparation for future problem-solving. Problems can often be solved by using alternative methods of approach, labour-saving techniques and, as a last resort, equipment which will assist independent living.

Dressing

Clothes which are light in weight, loose fitting, have 'give' and are strong enough to withstand pulling and stretching are advisable. Consideration should be given to the number of layers of clothing a person needs for warmth and how this will affect ease of dressing and undressing. Clothes which are easy to launder are also advisable.

It is not practical for anyone to buy a complete new wardrobe of clothes at a particular time, so advice in the early stages should help the individual to overcome dressing problems without too much anxiety. Fastenings at the front are easier to manage and the use of Velcro, large buttons and large zip pullers will help compensate for poor coordination. Nowadays, clothes which have been designed especially with the disabled person in mind are available and the therapist should seek out these outlets or help the family to locate them.

As the condition progresses and the person begins to experience problems with bladder control, protective clothing such as pants and pads may be needed. The choice of clothing will play an important part in helping the individual maintain continence. Weakness and incoordination will make it difficult for him to remove pants and trousers quickly. Wrap-round skirts and slacks or trousers with elasticated waist-bands can be pulled down more easily.

For a man, an extra long fly will help if a urinary bottle is used and, in the later stages when he has to be catheterised, an opening in the inner leg seam of his trousers will allow a leg bag to be emptied quickly and easily.

Eating and drinking

Incoordination, tremor and loss of sensation make eating and drinking difficult tasks and they can become an embarrassment for the individual. Adapted utensils can be used in the following ways:

- Cutlery with built-up grips or hand straps will help those with poor grip.
- Specially designed built-up plates, for example, will prevent food being pushed off the plate.
- The use of non-slip mats will help to stabilise plates and dishes.
- The introduction of weighted bracelets will help the individual to overcome the difficulties of tremor.
- Insulated mugs, with double hand grips, that protect the hands from burns and keep drinks hot, will help to compensate for both loss of sensation and tremor.
- In the later stages, flexy straws will obviate the need for the individual to hold a cup or mug.

Personal Hygiene

Washing/grooming

In the early stages, from general weakness alone, the individual may have to adopt a sitting position when carrying out washing and grooming activities. Alternative methods of using soap, such as soap dispensers, soap on a rope, a flannel mitt or a liquid soap dispenser may help the individual to overcome limited grasp. A long-handled bath brush and sponge will allow the user to reach his lower limbs, feet and back more easily.

Cleaning teeth may also pose a problem for the individual due to tremor and limited grasp, and this may be overcome by using an electric tooth-brush, toothpaste dispenser and/or water pik.

Shaving can become difficult due to poor grip and incoordination. Wet shaving may be made easier with a loop-handle grip fixed to a razor. Electric and battery-operated razors are not always a suitable remedy as they are heavier to hold. A razor holder, or strapping in conjunction with the elbow being supported, may be helpful.

Hair care problems may be overcome with the use of a long-handled comb or brush. A change in hair style which is both easy to manage and falls into place could be suggested. A shower spray, either over a bath or attached to basin taps, will help with the management of hair washing.

Make-up application may be more of a problem due to the finer movements required to hold and control items such as lip-sticks, mascara and eye shadow. Again, enlarged handles may help, but often a change, for example from a foundation powder to an all-in-one liquid base, may be a more effective way of overcoming such difficulties.

Use of the toilet

Initially, the person may only experience difficulty in using the toilet when rising from the seat. Thus it is important that the height of the toilet is correct for the individual; if a change in technique is not possible, the correct toilet height and possible installation and positioning of grab rails may be sufficient to help the person overcome any difficulties. As the condition progresses, the use of a commode on wheels, for example the Mayfair

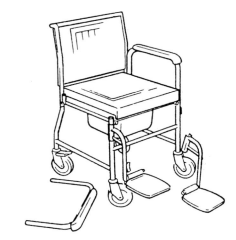

Fig. 19.2 The Mayfair commode.

(Fig. 19.2) which can be pushed over the toilet, may help to eliminate the need for some transfers. A reacher for toilet paper can extend the reach. Where grip and coordination are poor, single sheet toilet paper is a good alternative.

When the condition reaches a stage where transfers are becoming a more obvious problem, the therapist will need to consider:

- the general layout of the toilet and bathroom and the space which will be needed for wheelchair use
- alternative means of transfer, i.e. with assistance
- the possible installation of an overhead hoist or use of a mobile hoist.

Bathing/showering

General weakness, lack of coordination and fatigue will make it increasingly difficult for the individual to get in and out of the bath. However, the use of a combination of bathboard, seat, non-slip mat and well-positioned grab rails may be all that is required. If he gets too tired, strip washing whilst sitting may be advisable. When taking a bath, it is important that the therapist advises the individual not to have too hot a bath as heat will weaken and fatigue him and, therefore, exaggerate the difficulties of getting out. As balance and coor-

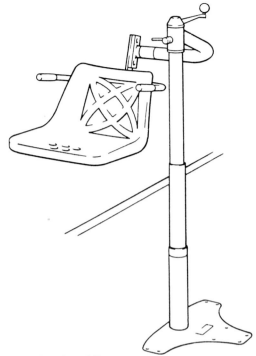

Fig. 19.3 The Auto Lift.

dination deteriorate, more complex equipment may need to be considered, such as a Mangar bath aid, Auto Lift (Fig. 19.3) or hoist.

Showering may well be an acceptable alternative and, if this is the case, a specially designed shower tray for a wheeled shower chair would need to be considered. A thermostatically controlled shower unit will be imperative as loss of sensation could lead to scalding.

HOME MANAGEMENT

All aspects of general home management will need discussion, including household cleaning, food preparation, cooking and shopping, and general mobility around the home environment.

It is important that the normal role of the individual should be maintained as far as possible as the psychological and emotional effects of role loss will have a detrimental effect on well-being and performance; for instance, if a housewife is unable to continue her usual routine in the preparation of

family meals and depends on her husband, she will feel inadequate and that she is becoming a burden to her family. The general problems of fatigue will be in evidence with all daily routines so it is important that the therapist advises and encourages each person to plan his days, allowing time for activity and rest alternately.

Food preparation/cooking

As far as possible all food preparation should be undertaken sitting down. This will help the individual to overcome problems of balance and fatigue. Various alternatives regarding the position of work surfaces, layouts of kitchens, aids to independence and labour-saving techniques will need to be considered in conjunction with all family members who use the kitchen and its facilities. Safety aspects in the kitchen must be highlighted at all times. The large number of available labour-saving items and kitchen aids makes it impossible to mention them all, but a few well-chosen pieces such as a stable vegetable slicer/peeler, electric tin opener and a spread board (Fig. 19.4) may be sufficient. The therapist can advise on labour-saving and safe techniques, such as using a chip basket in a saucepan for boiling vegetables to make draining easier and eliminate the risks of burning from the boiling water.

The general layout of the kitchen must be considered to ensure safety for the individual. It may

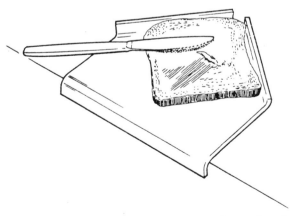

Fig. 19.4 A spread board, illustrating buttering a slice of bread.

not always be possible to achieve an ideal layout as this will depend largely on the space available and finances. However, problems of mobility around the kitchen and moving articles from one area to another can be solved with the use of a trolley. Suitable and accessible cupboards and shelving and their proximity to working surfaces may need attention. If visual disturbances are present, ways of identifying the contents of storage jars, for instance, will need to be considered.

The individual's lack of coordination and loss of sensation may make cooking difficult. Saucepans which are light and have wooden handles may be an answer, and guards to cookers and special control knobs, such as those advised by both the Gas and Electricity Boards, may be appropriate.

Frozen meals may be an acceptable alternative for some people, combined with the use of a microwave oven. Other electrical appliances, such as food processors and drink dispensers, may not only be labour saving but also help the individual keep his independence for a longer period of time. Floor surfaces should be, as far as possible, of a non-slip variety as spills will be dangerous. If or when the individual is wheelchair bound, the layout of the kitchen will need to take into account the height of work surfaces. It is usually prudent to have an area suitable for wheelchair use as well as one suitable for other members of the family.

Cleaning

As mentioned above, it is important for the therapist to help the individual decide how to tackle household tasks and plan the day or week in order to avoid fatigue. She may recommend that he continues with lighter tasks but that heavier tasks are managed by other family members or by a home help.

Laundry

Most households these days have a washing machine; nevertheless it is advisable to split the weekly washing and ironing so that a little can be undertaken at a time rather than all at once. If a washing machine is not available, the home help may be able to undertake this by visits to the laundrette. Some social service departments provide a separate laundry service, primarily for people who are incontinent. Ironing should be carried out in a seated position and, as previously mentioned, when buying new clothes in is advisable to buy those which need minimum ironing. Likewise, sheets which are crease resistant are invaluable.

Shopping

General weekly shopping may gradually be taken over by other members of the family or carers, but it is important that this is not done too rapidly to the extent that the individual acquires a sense of uselessness. Supermarkets with wheelchair access make it feasible for the person with multiple sclerosis to continue to participate. Other retail outlets are becoming more aware of the need to provide facilities for wheelchair users and the therapist should be aware of these to encourage the individual to continue with smaller and more personal shopping for as long as possible.

Transport

Transport will become more of a problem as the condition progresses. Various methods of transport may be appropriate, depending on the locality: for example, if the home is within easy reach of local shops, the person may be able to cope with an outdoor electric chair and be able to undertake some shopping. There are national schemes to facilitate easy transport, such as the car badge scheme, mobility allowance and motability. Where local schemes such as Dial a Ride, Dial a Bus and parking concessions exist, the therapist should advise accordingly. The National Key Scheme for public toilets also needs a mention as any anxiety the individual may have over toileting when going out can be easily overcome with this facility.

GENERAL MOBILITY/MOBILITY AIDS

In the early stages, the use of simple walking aids may be required. Whilst the individual is still ambulant, the normal heel–toe gait should be maintained and good posture encouraged. Walking should be encouraged for as long as possible but, whereas it may still be safe to walk in the home, the use of a wheelchair outdoors may be appropriate to avoid fatigue and the risk of falling on uneven surfaces.

The timing of the introduction of a wheelchair is crucial, not only in terms of safety but also from the psychological point of view. Very often people with multiple sclerosis see the introduction of a wheelchair as depressing. However, if the approach is both tactful and well timed, with the benefits of using a wheelchair stressed, it may be easier for the person to accept: for example, the use of a wheelchair will enable him to continue to carry out activities he enjoys such as outings, general shopping and holidays.

Other areas of general mobility which need to be assessed will include the heights and accessibility of bed, chair and toilet. The length of time the person will be able to maintain his independence in these areas may be increased with a technique change or the provision of bed-raisers, high chairs, appropriately positioned grab rails and raised toilet seats. Once a wheelchair is introduced, the heights must ideally be the same as the wheelchair seat to facilitate transfers. General instructions for safe, assisted transfers whilst the person is still weight-bearing will need to be given to his carers. As general weakness, lack of coordination and non weight-bearing occur, the need for mechanical assistance from a wheelchair to all areas may become necessary.

SOCIAL INTERACTION

It is important from the onset that the individual and his family are encouraged to maintain social contacts of all kinds for as long as possible. Problems of mobility and incoordination, speech impairments and difficulties with bladder control make it difficult for him to anticipate his ability to 'carry on as normal'. The therapist will need to give him help and guidance to overcome these problems and allay his fears in order to avoid isolation; for example, a toileting programme may be worked out to ensure a regular routine. The continence adviser will be able to give expert advice to the individual.

Leisure activities

Special interests and leisure activities will become increasingly important as the condition progresses. If the individual is unable to continue to work, he will have more time to fill. This will be particularly important for the person who may not be able to continue in the role of bread-winner. Activities which can involve the family unit as a whole will be the most rewarding as these will prevent the individual from feeling isolated or that he is becoming a burden, for example ornithology, outings focused on studying wild life and other outdoor interests. Pursuing new interests will not only depend on the individual's physical abilities and interests but also on local amenities and financial resources. For the person who has been a Do-It-Yourself enthusiast, such activities as light carpentry may still be enjoyed if a work area is made suitable for wheelchair use with correct work-bench height and fixed tools.

Gardening can still be encouraged with built-up borders or suitable greenhouse layouts. Some people may benefit from attending Further Education classes, for example in languages, accountancy, art, music, typing and word processing. Involvement in local societies and clubs should always be encouraged, and very often they are keen to involve people with disabilities.

Day Centres run by Social Services may provide a good outlet for some people where new skills can be learnt to maximise ability. The introduction to such centres should be approached with the same tact as the introduction of a wheelchair, as some people could respond badly to seeing people who are more disabled than themselves or they may not be interested in this facility.

A young mother who has multiple sclerosis may benefit from a baby sitting circle or child minding, not only for social contacts but also to allow her time during the day for rest periods.

The divorce and separation rates in families where one member has multiple sclerosis are high, and this needs to be borne in mind by the therapist at all times when advising on leisure pursuits to encourage interaction between the family unit.

Where couples coping with multiple sclerosis are experiencing difficulties with interpersonal relationships, it may be appropriate for the therapist to be involved in counselling to allow feelings, thoughts and issues to be explored. This may need to be undertaken with or alongside other organisations, for example, the Association to Aid Sexual and Personal Relationships of People with Disability (SPOD).

Communication

As social contacts become more difficult for the individual to maintain, he will become more dependent on other means of contact to keep him in touch with family and friends.

Built-up pens and writing boards may help to eliminate difficulties with grip for a time, but if there is an exaggerated intention tremor, the use of an electric typewriter may be the answer. Where speech impairment occurs, the introduction of a speech therapist may be appropriate. With the advent of modern technology some people have learnt to master the use of computers and word processors to overcome any difficulty. The Aidis Trust is a possible resource for obtaining long-term loans of computers and word processors for disabled people.

Telephones designed with disability in mind are available from British Telecom and other telecommunication manufacturers; for example, there are telephones with large buttons which make it easier to dial if tremor is a particular difficulty. There are a multitude of alarm systems on the market and, again, financial help may be available through Social Services or local Housing Departments, or people can be advised on suitable models to purchase.

If the person does not have a telephone, financial help may be provided by Social Services for its installation, especially if he is left alone, living alone or could be at risk without a telephone.

As the condition progresses and the individual is unable to use a telephone, a 'hands off' telephone linked with full environmental controls such as those provided by POSSUM and STEEPER may well be appropriate. These environmental controls are available through the Department of Health and need to be approved by the local assessor within the appropriate Regional Health Authority.

Work

If the individual can continue to work, it will be of great benefit to him, not only physically but also because he will maintain his normal role of wage/salary earner and bread-winner. This is especially important as it helps him keep his self-respect, dignity and one of the key adult roles.

It is often possible for large firms or organisations to transfer an employee internally to an alternative job. This is advantageous to the employer and the individual as he will be familiar with the type of work, surroundings and colleagues, and can also retain any pensionable rights. If a change of employment and employer is necessary, where the existing one is unsuitable, the individual may need the advice and guidance of the disablement resettlement officer about alternative work and possible retraining.

Financial help to enable him to get to work, adaptations at the place of work, for example ramping, access to the toilet and adapted tools may all be needed and are available through the Disablement Advisory Service.

GENERAL HOUSING NEEDS

From the early stages of multiple sclerosis, the occupational therapist must be aware of the problems which may arise from the layout of the home and its locality. Early advice and help with minor alterations will enable the individual to remain mobile and independent at home for as long as possible. For instance, the installation and correct positioning of grab rails in the toilet and bathroom have already been mentioned, but the use of rails in hallways and extra bannister rails on the stairs will help to give him support in more 'open spaces. The positioning of furniture will become important. Stable furniture strategically placed will give support and may eliminate the need for walking aids early on, but at a later stage the furniture may need to be rearranged to allow maximum space for a walking frame and subsequently for wheelchair manoeuvrability. If the person lives in a house, a day's routine will need to be planned so that he does not have to climb stairs more than once a day in order to avoid fatigue. It may be necessary to consider the need for a ground floor toilet, if it is not already in existence.

Long-term planning for eventual wheelchair use will need to be broached at a time when the individual and family are psychologically attuned to accepting that he will need a wheelchair. It is imperative that the physical needs of the individual are taken into account, but not in isolation from the whole family. When considering major adaptations, the therapist will need to discuss what is the normal practice and routine of the household in order to maintain normality as far as possible. For instance, if the major problem is one of gaining access to a first floor bedroom, a single bedroom on the ground floor would immediately split partners which would not only be detrimental to their relationship but enforce feelings of isolation on them both. If they have young children, it would also lead to the person's exclusion from normal bed-time reading and seeing children 'tucked up'. The consideration of a through-floor lift which would give general access to the whole house might be more appropriate.

General access to the home and garden, as well as changes to internal fixtures such as the height of electric sockets, light switches, window openers and appropriate door handles, will all need to be considered.

The therapist will need to advise the family of all possible financial help available to assist with adaptations, whether it be community grants from the DSS, a disabled facilities grant from district councils and/or local social services schemes.

If the person lives in a local council property, recommendations for adaptations under the Joint Circular from the Department of the Environment 10/90 'House Adaptations for People with Disabilities' will need to be made. If, however, the property is not totally suitable, it may be necessary to consider re-housing, bearing in mind that the proximity of friends, good neighbours, schools and work may be of equal if not greater importance.

SUPPORT NETWORKS

The therapist cannot provide all the services which may be required by a person suffering from multiple sclerosis, so it is vital that she is aware of supporting organisations and other professionals who can contribute to the family's overall management and support in order to introduce them at an appropriate stage as the condition progresses. If some services are introduced at too early a stage, the outcome may be one of dependency rather than independence, and the individual may become overwhelmed, frustrated and morose concerning the future. Therefore, the therapist must be adept at introducing assistance and other agencies' and organisations' support at the pscyhologically 'right' time for the individual and his carers.

Statutory agencies and professional helpers other than occupational therapists need to be mentioned — these include the physiotherapist, social worker, district nurse, home care worker and Disablement Resettlement Officer — as does the importance of those networks supplied by the voluntary organisations.

1. Multiple Sclerosis Society

The Society was set up in 1953 for the sole purpose of:

a. promoting and encouraging research into the cause of the condition
b. providing welfare and support for both sufferers and families.

Local branches have been set up nationally to provide practical help within their own community, for example social functions, fund raising for research, respite care and holidays.

2. Carers Association

This is a relatively new association with local branches who give support to the carers, not only of people with multiple sclerosis but of all disabled persons.

3. The Association to Aid Sexual and Personal Relationships of People with Disability

This association provides advice, practical assistance and counselling.

CONCLUSION

The therapist will play a key role in the management of an individual with multiple sclerosis but must also be aware of the need for appropriate input from other professionals and voluntary organisations. The therapist will need to use her practical skills to assess not only the individual's needs but also the requirements of the family in all aspects of daily living. She will need to be a good listener and planner, and resourceful.

USEFUL ADDRESSES

Multiple Sclerosis Society
25 Effie Road
Fulham
London SW6 1EE
Tel: 071 736 6267

(Scotland)
27 Castle Street
Edinburgh EH2 3DN
Tel: 031 225 3600

(N. Ireland)
34 Annadale Avenue
Belfast BT7 3JJ
Tel: 0232 644 914

Carers National Association
29 Chilworth Mews
London W2 3RG
Tel: 081 742 7776

Aidis Trust
18a Fallwood Avenue
Bear Cross
Bournemouth BH11 9NJ
Tel: 0202 571188

The Association to Aid Sexual and Personal Relationships of People with Disability
286 Camden Road
London N7 0BJ
Tel: 071 607 8851

FURTHER READING

Bickerstaff E 1987 Neurology. Hodder & Stoughton, London
Bumphrey E 1987 Occupational therapy in the community. Woodhead–Faulkner, Cambridge
Department of the Environment 1988 Housing adaptions for people with physical disabilities. HMSO, London
Downey P A 1986 Cash's textbook of neurology. Faber & Faber, London

Macleod J, Edwards C, Bouchier I 1988 Davidson's principles and practice of medicine. Churchill Livingstone, Edinburgh
Pedretti L W 1990 Occupational therapy–practical skills for physical dysfunction. C. V. Mosby Co, New York

20

Muscular dystrophy

Jenny Wilsdon

INTRODUCTION

'Muscular dystrophy', a term first coined in the 1890s, refers to certain hereditary diseases which are characterised by progressive degeneration of muscle. It is classified within the group of neuromuscular diseases, that is, among those diseases which involve one or more parts of the 'motor unit'.

A basic motor unit consists of:

- the motor nerve cells (neurones) in the anterior horns of the spinal cord
- their nerve fibres (axons), which run from the spinal cord to the muscles
- the neuromuscular junctions, the points at which nerve impulses are chemically transmitted to muscle fibres
- muscle fibres, highly specialised contractile cells.

Disease or abnormality of function can occur at any of these levels. Myopathies, of which muscular dystrophies are the most significant, develop when failure occurs at the muscle fibres and the muscle fibres gradually die. Some regeneration takes place but cannot combat the amount or rate of destruction; eventually, the muscle fibres are replaced by fibrous tissue and fat.

Not all muscles are uniformly involved. Mus-

Box 20.1 Classification of types of muscular dystrophy by mode of inheritance

---

X-linked inheritance
Duchenne muscular dystrophy
Becker muscular dystrophy
Scapulo-peroneal muscular dystrophy

Autosomal recessive inheritance
Scapulo-humeral muscular dystrophy
Recessive childhood muscular dystrophy
Congenital muscular dystrophy

Autosomal dominant inheritance
Facio-scapulo-humeral muscular dystrophy
Myotonic dystrophy
Ocular muscular dystrophy
Oculo-pharyngeal muscular dystrophy
Distal muscular dystrophy

---

cular dystrophies are classified according to their presenting pattern of affected muscles, as well as by their mode of inheritance (Box 20.1). Many of the muscular dystrophies are rare and unlikely to be seen by occupational therapists other than those in regional centres. This chapter focuses, therefore, on occupational therapy interventions of particular value in the management of the most common of the dystrophies, Duchenne muscular dystrophy (DMD). The treatment aims and techniques relevant to DMD, however, will often apply to other neuromuscular diseases.

The chapter begins by describing the aetiology, clinical features and prevention of DMD. Next, the role of the occupational therapist in assisting the child and his family to cope with the disease is outlined. As there is still no cure for muscular dystrophy, the occupational therapist's role will be to help the individual to retain maximum levels of independent function as his condition deteriorates. Throughout the chapter, this role is described in terms of the 'early', 'middle' and 'later' stages of the disease.

Because DMD is a young persons' disease, its management will involve the entire family unit. Its psychological and emotional impact is therefore examined in relation to the affected child, his parents and siblings. Physical aspects of the home environment are also considered, with particular reference to the types of alterations that may be necessary to accommodate the use of a wheelchair in the home.

Next, practical problems that may arise in relation to personal care are described. This is followed by a discussion of measures that can be taken to enhance the individual's mobility throughout the course of the disease.

The chapter then considers the occupational therapist's contribution in ensuring that the individual's school environment is safe and conducive to optimum participation. Attention is also given to the important role of social and leisure activities. The use of orthoses and indications for surgical intervention in the management of DMD is described, as is the contribution of the physiotherapist and the dietician.

As in any treatment area, the occupational therapist's liaison on behalf of the individual with other members of the treatment team, educators, employers and relatives will help to ensure that a comprehensive and coherent management programme is followed. Her intervention will enhance the person's quality of life in all areas — physical, psychological, intellectual and social — and will extend to all family members. Her involvement, moreover, will not end with the individual's death, but will extend to supporting his family as they make the difficult adjustment to their loss.

DUCHENNE MUSCULAR DYSTROPHY

Duchenne muscular dystrophy (DMD) is a progressive muscular disease characterised by proximal muscle weakness and wasting. It primarily affects boys and becomes apparent between the ages of 2 and 6 years. Progress of the disease is rapid. Walking becomes difficult and by adolescence a wheelchair is usually necessary. The prognosis is poor, death usually occurring during the late teens or early twenties.

Aetiology

DMD is caused by a defective gene which prevents affected children from producing a protein which is essential for healthy muscles. The faulty gene is passed on by X-linked or sex-linked recessive inheritance. The mother carries the defective gene (but is not affected) and passes it on to 50% of her sons and 50% of her daughters. That is, half of her sons will be affected and half of her daughters will be carriers of the defective gene. Occasionally, there is spontaneous mutation (no family history); in this circumstance both boys and girls can be affected. Although the gene can now be identified no cure has yet been found.

Clinical features

Onset is usually around 3–4 years. Signs may be recognised earlier or overlooked, depending on the family history. The muscles which first show signs of weakness are those around the hips, thighs and shoulders. There may be delay in walking or failure of the gait to become steady and coordinated. The child may fall frequently without apparent cause. Navigating steps or stairs is often very difficult. Eventually the gait assumes a characteristic waddle with the feet placed apart and an exaggerated lumbar curve. The child walks on his toes; this allows the line of gravity to fall outside the vertebral column, giving greater stability. Weakness of the shoulder muscles makes lifting the arms above the head difficult. Tiredness is associated with the increased effort required to perform these gross motor tasks.

A characteristic manoeuvre (Gower's) is often seen when the child stands up from lying or sitting on the floor. He will move into a prone position, go into the crawl position (on forearms and knees), extend both arms and legs (into the bear position) and then 'walk' up his legs with his hands until upright.

The affected muscles are often wasted but this may be masked by the accumulation of fat (pseudohypertrophy). This is best seen in the supra- and infraspinati, deltoids, triceps, quadriceps and calf muscles. Atrophy is seen in the glutei, biceps and pectoralis major. Tendon reflexes become progressively diminished and finally cannot be elicited. Sensation is unaffected and pain and cramps are rare.

A number of children with DMD exhibit intellectual impairment, often involving memory and verbal skills. Between the ages of 8 and 12 years, mobility is so restricted that wheelchair dependence is inevitable. Contractures and deformity increase, especially of the spine and trunk. This, in conjunction with the involvement of the respiratory muscles, leads to the increased risk of chest infections. Death is usually from intercurrent respiratory infection or from heart failure due to myocardial involvement.

Prevention

Carrier status

Recent advances in research have made it possible to detect the faulty gene which causes DMD. The geneticist will investigate the family genetic background and take blood samples for the purposes of gene tracking and to test for raised levels of the enzyme creatine kinase (CK). On the basis of these investigations he will determine the prospective mother's carrier status. If her risk is high she has a 50% chance of passing the faulty gene to future sons, who will most probably be affected by DMD.

Prenatal diagnosis

The ability to detect the faulty gene has been enhanced by the development of a technique known as chorionic villus sampling (CVS), whereby a small amount of placental tissue (which contains the same DNA material as the developing fetus) is obtained. This procedure, which has the ability to detect the faulty gene as well as the sex of the fetus, enables prenatal diagnosis of the disease. CVS can be carried out at 8–12 weeks gestation but carries a higher risk of miscarriage than amniocentesis (sampling of the amniotic fluid), which is used in exactly the same way as CVS but which cannot be carried out until 16 weeks of pregnancy. If the tests show that the male fetus has inherited the faulty gene the parents have the opportunity to decide whether to continue with the pregnancy or to consider a termination, though this will be at a later stage if an amniocentesis has been carried out.

ROLE OF THE OCCUPATIONAL THERAPIST

The child with DMD is likely to be referred to an occupational therapist shortly after the diagnosis has been made. It is essential that the therapist liaises with other team members regarding their involvement and, most importantly, that she knows what information has been given to the child and/or his family regarding the diagnosis. From her holistic viewpoint the occupational therapist will identify possible problem areas, whether these be physical, psychological, environmental or social.

The occupational therapist's assessment will be based primarily on an interview with the child and his family combined with the information gathered from the rest of the team. The professionals involved may include:

- local consultants (paediatrician, orthopaedic surgeon)
- regional consultants (paediatrician, orthopaedic surgeon)
- a regional geneticist
- a physiotherapist (local and/or regional)
- teachers
- a family care worker (MD Group)
- an orthotist (local and/or regional)
- a social worker
- a dietitian.

The role of the occupational therapist will be to provide:

- treatment and support for psychological and emotional problems
- advice and information with regard to major adaptations to the home and school
- specialist equipment and techniques to maintain personal independence
- advice and information regarding problems with social and leisure activities and finance.

There are no curative measures or treatments for muscular dystrophy. Management and treatment are, therefore, aimed at maintaining maximum levels of physical, psychological and social function throughout the course of the disease.

Exercise is encouraged to preserve muscle strength and maintain the range of movement at the joints, thereby slowing the development of contractures and deformities. However, the amount of exercise is limited by the necessity not to overtire the person. Surgery is often employed to reduce contractures or deformity, thus enabling the person to achieve a better posture and/or position and so maintain mobility either by assisted walking or wheelchair use. Orthoses and equipment are also provided to achieve these aims.

PSYCHOLOGICAL AND EMOTIONAL PROBLEMS

After diagnosis the family will have to come to terms with the disease and its implications. The acceptance of the diagnosis will depend upon many factors, among which foreknowledge of the previous family history of the disease will be the most important. As DMD is inherited from the mother there will be disturbances in the family dynamics. Relationships between the parents, affected child, siblings and extended family will change, and the occupational therapist must be prepared to be involved with the whole family at various stages during the course of the disease.

The occupational therapist can provide support, advice and encouragement and offer opportunities to express emotions as they arise. She must, however, be aware of her own limitations and make referrals to other professionals as necessary.

Regional and local branches of the Muscular Dystrophy Group (see p. 526) can offer information, support and contact with families in similar circumstances. The occupational therapist should be able to provide her clients with appropriate contact names and addresses.

Early stages

The child

It is unlikely that the child will be aware of the course and eventual outcome of his disease at this stage, unless a relative is or was similarly affected. However, it is important that he is fully involved in all aspects of his treatment so that he feels in control of the situation. He will feel frustration at his inability to perform certain tasks and confusion as to the reasons why. He may be bewildered by changing family dynamics. Play therapy and creative therapies offer outlets for these emotions in a structured, protective environment. The occupational therapist can also reinforce information and treatment given by other professionals.

Parents

Parents will be emotionally shattered by the diagnosis of DMD and its implications, both for the child and the family as a whole. Before the diagnosis is accepted they will go through the bereavement process, mourning the loss of their 'normal', healthy son and of their hopes and aspirations for him and his future. Their relationships with him will change and they may become over-protective. However, they must be encouraged to allow the child to do as much as possible for as long as possible. Once the diagnosis is accepted the future must be anticipated and planned for. This is hard but necessary and the occupational therapist should be honest and factual in order to allow the parents to make well-informed decisions. But, while she should provide information, advice and support, plans and decisions must ultimately be made by the parents themselves.

The relationship between the parents will be strained, particularly if the husband blames his wife for 'giving' the disease to their son. The occupational therapist is often used as an impartial third party in discussions about their relationship; this is a difficult role, however, and may require a more experienced counsellor.

The parents may experience antagonism from the extended family. The paternal side may express anger and detachment: 'It did not come from *our* side of the family.' The maternal side may feel guilt at having passed on the abnormal gene, as well as apprehension that the disease may occur again within the family. All of these emotions will strain family relationships at the very time when support and closeness are needed. Although the prognosis is poor the parents should always be allowed hope and optimism.

Siblings

The early stages of DMD can be very frightening for brothers and sisters, who may not understand the changes that are becoming evident in their brother and in family relationships. They will want to know what is going on, what is wrong with their brother, whether they will catch the disease and what to tell their friends. The Muscular Dystrophy Group produce an excellent booklet for siblings which answers many such questions. Brothers and sisters can offer a great deal of support and should be encouraged to do so.

Middle stages

The young person

The transition from walking to using a wheelchair for mobility will have a great impact on the young person with DMD. The occupational therapist must be positive in her support and encouragement, emphasising the increased independence and new opportunities which a wheelchair can afford. It is important that the person's self-esteem is kept high, possibly by changing objectives and concentrating on what he can do and not on what he can no longer achieve. The change to a wheelchair may also necessitate a change in school, which will bring additional emotional changes and demand the occupational therapist's further support and encouragement. It is important that the home environment is ready for this transition and is 'wheelchair-user friendly'.

During this stage the person will also undergo the transition from child to adolescent (and possibly to adult) and experience the normal physical and emotional changes which this entails. For anyone, this is a time of uncertainty and insecurity, but the person with DMD will also have to cope with the progress of his disease. The occupational therapist must be aware of his development and be ready to offer opportunities to express related anxieties.

Parents

The wheelchair that becomes necessary in the middle stages of DMD presents parents with a constant visual reminder of the eventual outcome of the disease. Again, the occupational therapist must be positive in her approach, emphasising the young person's independence in his wheelchair. She can help the person and his family to set objectives which take into account his change in mobility. There may be a tendency for the parents to look upon their son as a baby, the wheelchair reminding them of the push-chair stage of development. The occupational therapist can make the parents aware of such pitfalls and encourage them to see their son as an emerging adolescent or adult.

Although the young person will require an increasing amount of care and attention, his parents should be encouraged to allow him privacy, both alone and with his friends. It is important for the parents to help in maintaining their son's social circle so that he does not become isolated.

Later stages

By this stage the future will look bleak and it will be difficult for the person and his family to think positively. A reassessment of the overall situation will be required and the occupational therapist can help to set short-term objectives.

Often, two contradictory thoughts are present within the family: first, that time is running out and they have much to do, to talk and to think about; second, that the inevitable is dragging on and that it would be better for the end to come quickly. This creates emotional conflict and may present as anger, guilt, depression or detachment. The occupational therapist must be aware of these emotions and provide opportunities for their expression and discussion in order for the family to feel as comfortable and secure as possible when death occurs.

The person and the family will need support whilst they plan for the final few weeks. The majority of families wish to have the person with them until the end and therefore may require night- or daytime support care. Occasionally, family wishes or circumstances will dictate that the person is within hospital or similar care during these final stages. Whatever the situation, the person and his family will require a great deal of the occupational therapist's time and support.

Aftercare

The person's death does not signal the end of the family's need for help and advice. Support is often provided by a Family Care officer from the Muscular Dystrophy Group; if not, this role should be undertaken by the occupational therapist, who will have been involved with the family throughout the course of the illness and will be well acquainted with their outlook and needs.

Removal of the deceased person's belongings is an important part of coming to terms with his death. The timing of the return of equipment which has been on loan should be considered carefully. Returning equipment too soon or after too great an interval will cause the family unnecessary distress.

Many parents who have received support from the Muscular Dystrophy Group find great comfort in remaining active in the organisation and providing support for others.

HOME ENVIRONMENT

In general, houses are not designed to accommodate wheelchairs. Consequently, turning a home into a place in which a wheelchair user can be independent almost always involves major structural alterations and/or additions.

It is important that the subject of major alterations to the home is broached well before the need for them is apparent. Alterations take time and money and thus require advanced planning. Although this may seem hard and can be distressing for the family, it is essential if the person is to remain independent. The parents will need to know the requirements of a wheelchair user well in advance so that decisions with regard to major alterations or moving house can be made in good time. It is advisable for long-term needs to be addressed in the early stages, as short-term, temporary measures can be costly.

Once a decision to build an extension has been made, approximately two years should be allowed to obtain architects' and builders' plans and planning permission, make financial arrangements, complete building, decorating and equipping, and finally move in.

A ground-floor conversion or extension are the ideal alternatives but alteration to first-floor accommodation with a through-floor lift may be the only practicable solution. Whatever alteration is made must be acceptable to the family after the person has died. An extra ground floor bathroom and toilet are always useful and the bed/sitting room may be used for another child or as an extra livingroom, playroom or study.

The adaptations to the home should provide a bed/livingroom which allows the person privacy. This is very important for an adolescent or young adult who needs his own place in which to be alone or to entertain his friends. There should also be an adjoining bathroom and toilet. Access around the ground floor of the home is also important in enabling the person to remain an integral part of the family. Easy access to and from the house is also vital. Early in the designing of an extension or alteration to ground-floor accommodation the suitability of the ceiling for bearing an overhead tracking hoist system should be considered. This type of system will greatly assist in the care of the person in the later stages.

The family may in fact prefer to move house before major alterations become necessary. The present home may be unsuitable for adaptation. The family may wish to be nearer to a particular school or hospital, or closer to relatives. The family may have been intending to move anyway. In any event, the occupational therapist should be available to advise on the suitability of a new house so that costly mistakes are not made.

Whether the family opts for alterations or for a change of home, the occupational therapist's primary aim will be to ensure that a safe environment (including safe access) is provided. Secondly, she will aim to ensure that the home environment is one in which the person can remain independent for as long as possible. Thirdly, she will try to ensure that the environment offers carers maximum ease of management.

Early stages

The occupational therapist can advise the family on how to make the home easier for the person to move around in freely and safely. A spacious, clutter-free environment will reduce the possibility of falls, and of injury should falls occur. Non-slip floor coverings are more suitable than rugs and deep pile carpets, which may catch the person's feet. Furniture may be used for support as the person moves around, and so should be solid, stable and without castors.

The person should be encouraged to sit on chairs rather than the floor so that he is supported in a good position and can rise and sit down more easily. He may have difficulty in negotiating the stairs; handrails should be fixed to both sides. Alternatively, the person may prefer to revert to sitting (bottom-shuffling), especially to come downstairs. Stairlifts are not advisable as they are expensive for such a short-term solution. A through-floor lift which accommodates a wheelchair may be suitable if the first floor is to be adapted.

Handrails by the toilet and bath will provide additional support. Outside steps should be fitted with interim handrails and replaced by ramps as soon as possible in readiness for wheelchair use.

Middle stages

Space should be sufficient to allow easy manoeuvrability of the wheelchair, with room for transfers to bed, toilet, bath and chair. Light switches and power points should be situated at a height which enables the person to use them with his arms supported by the wheelchair armrests. For safety, alarm cords may be fitted in the bathroom and bedroom, or baby monitors which can be plugged into the mains supply may be used to enable the person to call for assistance.

Work surfaces must be suitable for use from a wheelchair, standing frame or prone stander. Storage cupboards, shelving, wardrobes and drawers should all be accessible from the wheelchair. Room should be available for fitting orthoses and doing exercises. A small, thin, foldable mattress may be helpful.

The bathroom should provide a toilet, basin, bath, shelving and storage facilities. Taps should be of the lever type, as these require less effort to operate and are more easily reached. Further suggestions for equipment can be found on p. 520.

Good heating is essential, as limited mobility reduces the production of body heat and the person will feel the cold more quickly than others do.

Later stages

A ceiling-track hoist is most suitable at this stage as it will provide ease of transfer between bed, toilet, bath and wheelchair. If this is not possible then some type of mobile hoist will be required. A self-operated ceiling hoist is, however, much to be preferred as it provides greater independence during both the middle and later stages. The provision of an environmental control system will enable the person with extremely limited muscle function to be independent within his own environment. The selection of the system will depend upon individual requirements, means of access and availability. Such systems are usually financed through the Department of Health, but the additional provision of such items as page-turners may depend upon charitable sources.

PERSONAL SKILLS

The aims of the treatment and management of DMD with regard to personal skills are:

- to maintain the person's functional independence in personal care for as long as possible (early stages)
- to enable his carers to assist the person with personal care (middle stages)
- to help, advise and support the carers in managing the person's personal care (later stages).

Toileting

In the early stages, strategically placed grab rails can assist with sitting down and standing up.

In the middle and later stages the toilet should be within an adapted environment which allows room for transfer from a wheelchair by assisted transfer or by lifting (using a mobile or ceiling hoist). A toilet seat, chair or moulded insert may be required in the later stages to provide extra support and to accommodate deformities. A urine bottle should be provided for urgent and night usage.

Feeding

As the person's muscle weakness progresses to the trunk and pectoral girdle, the height of the table at which he eats becomes especially important. It should be at just below axilla height so that his elbows can rest on the table, providing support and stability. During the later stages assisted feeding will be necessary.

Dressing

Clothing must be roomy and hard-wearing to allow for various orthoses. Stretchy fabrics and elasticated waistbands will help the person to remain independent. Weakness of the shoulder girdle limits the ability to lift the arms; therefore, front-fastening garments such as shirts and cardigans are more suitable than T-shirts and pullovers.

Bathing

In the early stages the prevention of falls is of paramount importance. The person will be using the family bathroom; therefore, equipment should be discreet and unobtrusive. Grab rails and a non-slip bath mat will help to maintain independence and safety. A small stool can be used to sit upon whilst undressing and when towelling down. A bath board and/or bath seat may be appropriate as weakness increases.

For the middle and later stages of the disease an adapted bathroom is essential. A bath is preferable to a shower, as bathing is safer and more relaxing for the person. However, if a shower is used a shower chair (which may need adaptation) should be provided. Transfer to the bath or shower can be by mobile or ceiling hoist. A special bath insert (inflatable, vacuum or moulded) may be required to support the person in a sitting or reclining position within the bath.

Sleeping

For the early and middle stages the bed should be firm and of a height suitable for transferring to and from a wheelchair. (A transfer board may be necessary.) In the later stages a special bed is often required. It should be remembered that sensation is not affected by DMD and that the person will be unable to change his sleeping posture. This will result in cramps, pressure sores and general discomfort. Some parents set their alarm clocks at regular intervals during the night in order to turn the person. This situation is unacceptable as it disturbs the sleep of both the person and his parents, all of whom need a good night's rest. Various inflatable mattresses are available which regularly change the weight distribution and, thereby, the areas of pressure. Sheepskin pads may protect vulnerable areas of the body. It is well worth considering one of the tilt beds, which not only change the person's sleeping position but offer a tilt facility which can be used for postural drainage. The bed should also offer a variable height facility and be operated by a touch-sensitive switch control so that the person can use it independently.

MOBILITY

The occupational therapist's management programme for the person with DMD should aim to assist him in maintaining independent mobility for as long as possible.

Early stages

The presenting problems related to mobility derive from weakness of the muscles of the pelvis and lower limbs. They include frequent falls, an unsteady gait, lack of stamina when walking, and difficulty in climbing stairs and in rising from the floor. The maintenance of walking ability is greatly facilitated by the use of orthoses (see p. 524) and physiotherapy (see p. 525). Mobility in the home has been discussed on pp. 518–520. If the person finds walking to school tiring, he will be unable to function adequately once he gets there. It may be possible for a parent to take him to school by car, or to arrange for a taxi supplied by the education authority. Alternatively, the person may use a tricycle or a major buggy; here,

however, the psychological effects of returning to a 'push-chair' must be considered. The person's own views on how he wishes to remain mobile must always take precedence.

Middle stages

The decision for the child to move from walking to using a wheelchair as his main method of locomotion is a difficult one for all concerned. It is really a matter of personal preference — first, that of the person with DMD and, secondly, that of his parents. Whenever a decision is taken with regard to wheelchair use the occupational therapist should be ready to offer her full support. Some individuals prefer to continue without a wheelchair, even if this means making difficult and slow progress. Others opt for wheelchair use early in order to increase their independence, especially in social and leisure activities.

Once the decision to become wheelchair dependent has been made the relative merits of self-propelling and electrically powered models must be considered. The main consideration is the upper limb and trunk strength of the person. If the decision is made early he may well be able to cope with a self-propelling wheelchair. The position adopted within the chair is important because of the weakening trunk muscles (see p. 525). The person must be well supported in a symmetrical position; this may entail the use of cushions or other inserts, as a wheelchair which is wide enough to accommodate the pelvis will be too wide to support the trunk. Extensions to the brake handles may be required to increase leverage. Armrests should be of a height to support the forearms without elevating the shoulder girdle (hunching the shoulders).

If upper limb strength is poor, an electrically powered wheelchair will be necessary. As such wheelchairs are expensive, careful assessment and forward planning are needed. The chair must afford room for growth and adaptability for position and control. There is debate as to whether a central or a side control panel is more suitable. A central control panel often inhibits use with tables and other work surfaces, such as desks, kitchen counters, computer stands and sinks. A side control panel may well encourage asymmetrical posturing and, hence, spinal deformity, either because the person leans towards the control or pulls away to gain better leverage.

Later stages

If the adolescent is not already using one, an electric wheelchair will become essential at this stage. Upper limb weakness may be so advanced that a special control unit, such as a micro-switch which is sensitive to small degrees of movement, is required. Position within the wheelchair is still very important: it must provide symmetry, a forward-looking posture and support for the weak trunk. If the person's spine has been internally fixed this will be less of a problem, but a corset or brace may need to be accommodated within the wheelchair. If the person has neither of these supports other methods will need to be employed. An individual moulded insert such as a Derby mould, Burnett body support or Matrix insert may be appropriate. New systems are being developed continually, making careful consideration and assessment essential.

Another problem for the wheelchair-dependent person with DMD is his inability to change position within his chair. He will be prone to developing pressure sores, especially around the sacrum and ischial tuberosities; if spinal deformities are present, bony prominences may also invite pressure sores. A moulded insert will help to prevent sores by providing a continuous weight-bearing area. Alternatively, special cushions or sheepskins can be used. Changes in seating, for example transferring periodically to an armchair, will provide positional variation and help the person to feel part of the family.

SCHOOL

With regard to the person's school experience, the aims of occupational therapy intervention are:

- to ensure a safe environment and advise on adaptations
- to provide support for the person and his teachers

- to advise on special equipment
- together with the teacher, to educate the person's peer group with regard to his needs and problems
- to give advice and support during the transition to other schools.

Early stages

The person's initial difficulties in coping with the geography of the school and participating in certain curricular and playground activities will occur as a result of his unsteady gait, frequent falls and difficulty in rising from the floor. Problems may arise if the school has steps and stairs or if the campus is widely spread. It may be possible to rearrange classes so that movement between rooms is kept to a minimum and rooms which are accessed via stairs are avoided. If steps cannot be avoided then rails should be fitted. Occasionally a school may wish to install either a stairlift or a through-floor lift, in which case the occupational therapist can advise. Often a special friend can be enlisted to help the person. Allowing extra time for travel, possibly by allowing the person to leave each class before everyone else, is another solution. Some of the physical components of the curriculum, for example movement to music, sports and field activities, may be tiring, difficult or unsafe for the person. However, an inventive teacher may be able to adapt certain activities so that he is not excluded. The person will already feel different from his peers so every effort should be made to enable him to join in a wide range of activities.

The psychological stress of coming to terms with the disease may cause behavioural problems and changes in mood or personality. Both the person and the teacher will need support and advice if these occur. However, the occupational therapist must respect confidentiality; the person's actual diagnosis and its consequences can only be disclosed with the individual's and his parents' permission.

As the person is supplied with various orthoses the teacher will need to know what they are, why they are required and how to manage them. At this stage the person should be independent in personal skills; two areas, however, may pose problems. The first is the toilet: if a toilet which has been adapted for people with disabilities is available this can be used; if not, rails should be fitted to enable independence. The second is the dining area: if hot meals are provided the person may need assistance in collecting his food.

The nature and course of the disease make forward planning and preparation for wheelchair use around the school essential. If at all possible, the person should remain with his peer group so that he has their support during the transition from walking to wheelchair use. If, however, transfer to another school is necessary, this should take place before the person makes the transition to wheelchair use so that he can adjust to one change at a time. The ideal solution is to set up a planning team consisting of the person, his parents, school staff, a special needs advisor, representation from the Education Department (preferably from Buildings), the school medical officer and the occupational therapist. The role of the occupational therapist will be to advise on facilities required by the wheelchair user and on the adaptation of the environment to accommodate a wheelchair.

Middle stages

If all has gone according to plan, any necessary adaptations to the school environment will have been made by the time the person becomes dependent upon a wheelchair. 'Teething problems' may occur and the occupational therapist should be available to offer advice and suggest possible solutions. The teaching staff will need to know how to use the wheelchair and how to assist with transfers from the wheelchair to the toilet or to other chairs. Often a teacher's assistant is employed, in accordance with the Education Act 1981, to assist the person with DMD to move around the school. A fire officer will advise on emergency procedures. The policy for accommodating wheelchair users will vary, depending on the education authority; some authorities run special needs units attached to mainstream schools. These offer special needs support in the form of equipment, physiotherapy and hydrotherapy

whilst the person remains within the mainstream system for curricular activities. Other authorities still provide special schools with these facilities. The opportunity to move to a special school is often taken during the transition from primary to senior level. If a change is necessary, support through the transition will be essential. Close liaison among the family, school and health care team aids easier transition.

As muscle weakness progresses to the trunk and upper limbs more problems will arise. The person will need an electric wheelchair if he is not using one already. Weakness of the pectoral girdle will limit upper limb function, especially of the hands, and many activities will become difficult or impossible. The occupational therapist can advise on alternative positions, techniques and equipment. Microcomputers, for example, have greatly increased the independence of people with DMD and helped them to continue their education.

Later stages

The course and speed of the disease will affect the continuance of education and possible employment. Many people affected by DMD will be too weak by mid-adolescence to continue with formal education. With a great deal of support some people may manage to attend special schools, colleges for disabled people and even colleges of further and higher education. Home teachers may be provided for those who are too weak to leave the home; another option is for the person to enrol in an Open University course. A few people are able to maintain employment through the use of microcomputers and home environment systems.

SOCIAL AND LEISURE ACTIVITIES

The person with DMD may experience difficulties in pursuing former sports, social and leisure activities, whether on his own, with his peer group or with his family. He should be actively encouraged to find new interests which require little physical involvement and which can be continued throughout the course of the disease. Starting a collection, playing computer games or studying and breeding small animals, tropical fish or birds may be suitable hobbies. Bird-watching can also be a rewarding pastime; the person can attract birds to a garden feeder, observe them through binoculars, and record their habits. Clubs and societies relating the person's chosen hobby will encourage participation and offer opportunities to meet other people. It is important for the person to find interests in which friends and family can be involved.

In the early stages, participation in selected sports such as swimming and horseback riding is beneficial in maintaining function and providing exercise. Organisations such as the Physically Handicapped and Able Bodied Clubs (PHAB) and therapeutic riding associations may offer local facilities.

The importance of holidays should not be overlooked; libraries and social services departments hold literature about places which cater for the wheelchair-dependent person. Some charitable organisations also offer holiday chalets which have been adapted to accommodate wheelchairs. Social services departments and libraries can also furnish information on access to public buildings, swimming pools and restaurants.

FINANCE

A chronically sick or disabled family member always places additional strain on the family budget. In the case of DMD, financial pressure will build quickly, allowing the family no time to plan or save. In the early stages expenses may relate to frequent visits to the regional treatment centre. During the middle and later stages adaptations to the home and special equipment will be costly. One parent may also need to give up work to care for the person, further restricting resources. Early contact with a social worker from the local hospital, regional centre or the Muscular Dystrophy Group will ensure that advice on allowances and grants is obtained in good time. Fund-raising groups and charities may be called upon to provide expensive equipment such as computers, environmental control systems, electric wheelchairs and special beds. The family will already be under great emotional strain, given the diagnosis and its

implications; therefore, money worries should be alleviated as far as possible.

ORTHOSES AND SURGICAL INTERVENTION

The aims of orthotic and surgical treatment in DMD are:

- to maintain a functional position for as long as possible
- to reduce the development of contractures and deformities to a minimum.
- to support weakened areas.

Early stages

Weakness of the muscles around the pelvic area will cause a forward tilting of the pelvis with accompanying increase of the lumbar curve. This means that the body's centre and line of gravity will be pushed forwards. In order to counteract this displacement and maintain balance in standing and walking the child will flex at the knees and transfer weight through the ball of the foot. As walking on 'tip-toes' is in itself unstable, intervention is necessary to hold the foot plantigrade. Footwear which extends over the ankle joint is essential; Piedro-type boots or 'bumper'-type trainers, for example, are suitable. An ankle-foot orthosis (AFO) which extends from the base of the toes to above the bulk of the calf muscles can be used in conjunction with footwear. Night-time AFOs help to maintain the stretch on the Achilles tendon. As the muscle weakness progresses the child will require knee-ankle-foot orthoses (KAFO) extending from the upper thigh to the foot, followed by hip-knee-ankle-foot orthoses (HKAFO) which combine the former orthoses with a pelvic band. Surgical lengthening of the Achilles tendons is often required at this stage. Finally, a full set bracing system attached to a thoraco-lumbar corset may be necessary if walking is to continue. The extent of the bracing used should be closely monitored and discussed with the person and his parents. The use of orthoses requires great motivation, patience and application; therefore, their provision should not be automatic. It is important to bear in mind that the above-mentioned orthoses are not suitable for all persons with DMD.

Middle stages

When walking becomes too difficult, too tiring or unsafe, even with extensive external support, a wheelchair will be necessary. At this time the trunk muscles are greatly affected; this, combined with limited mobility, produces spinal deformity. The lumbar lordosis becomes fixed with compensatory thoracic kyphosis, often with a scoliosis as the person slumps to one side. As spinal deformities may restrict lung capacity and limit lung function, spinal support will be necessary to reduce the amount of deformity and allow unrestricted breathing. As previously stated, the main cause of death in DMD is recurrent chest infections; therefore, the maintenance of correct spinal position is highly important. There are two main alternatives: external support using a corset, or internal fixation through surgery.

There are many types of surgical corset available but the most commonly used are the lightweight thermoplastic and Neofract types. All corsets are moulded individually to achieve as much correction as possible and are remoulded or replaced as necessary. Body bracing is introduced as soon as scoliosis is detected. The control of the scoliosis is variable; once the curve exceeds 40°–50°, body bracing is usually ineffective in preventing further deformity.

The second alternative is surgical intervention in the form of internal fixation of the vertebral column. The decision to pursue this course is made by the individual, his family and the consultant. It should be remembered that the younger child is more able to cope physically and mentally with major surgery than the older child, and that in earlier stages the curves can be more easily straightened.

The benefits of having a straight spine are not only physical (i.e., concerned with breathing and better sitting and lying posture) but psychological. With a straight spine the individual will be able to look the world 'straight in the eye' again, and his self-confidence will be enhanced by a 'normal' body image.

Later stages

During the final stages of DMD, orthoses and surgery are used to reduce pain and ease management of the person. Special inserts may be required for comfort in sitting and/or lying. These can be made from a variety of materials, for example Hexcelite, vacuum bean bags, Matrix and foam rubber.

OTHER TREATMENT

The physiotherapist plays an important role in the treatment and maintenance of the person with DMD. Contractures frequently occur at the ankles, knees and hips, partly because of increasing muscle weakness and muscle imbalance and partly because children with DMD tend to spend more time in the sitting position than other children of a similar age. The development of contractures is further exacerbated by the child walking on his toes in an effort to keep his balance. Physiotherapy is started before tightness and deformity occur, as a preventative measure.

Initially, a detailed assessment of muscle strength and joint range of movement (both passive and active) is undertaken to provide a precise baseline for treatment planning. The principal aims of the physiotherapist's intervention are:

- to minimise the development of contractures (through frequent passive stretching)
- to prolong muscle strength (through exercise and hydrotherapy)
- to prolong mobility and function (using various orthoses)
- to maintain adequate lung capacity and function (through breathing exercises).

These treatment aims are similar to those of the occupational therapist; therefore, close liaison between therapists is essential.

Another area in which the physiotherapist and occupational therapist must work closely is in the provision of certain equipment. Postural drainage is often necessary in the later stages and the occupational therapist can advise and supply suitable equipment, ranging from foam wedges and tilt frames to a tilting facility on the person's bed. Prone lying boards and standing frames are often used to promote a straight posture and to stretch the spine, hips and knees. These items can be used in conjunction with various activities; for example, the person can use a prone lying board whilst watching television or reading, and a standing frame at a table or work surface of suitable height while writing, doing homework or using a computer.

As weight gain can be a problem, a dietitian is often involved with the person with DMD. The person will have enough difficulty in moving without the burden of excess weight. The dietitian will advise the person, his family and appropriate school staff with regard to diet. The occupational therapist can help by reinforcing this advice and encouraging the person if he experiences difficulty in following the diet.

CONCLUSION

Of the many neuromuscular diseases which manifest as muscular weakness, almost all are progressive in nature. Apart from the muscular dystrophies previously mentioned, these diseases include: polymyositis, dermatomyositis, myasthenia gravis, the spinal muscular atrophies, the glycogen storage diseases, myotonia congenita and the peripheral neuropathies.

Problems associated with the neuromuscular diseases which commence in childhood will be similar to those resulting from Duchenne muscular dystrophy, thus giving rise to similar treatment aims and strategies.

Those neuromuscular diseases which become apparent in adolescence or early adulthood may also give rise to some of the problems typical of DMD and thus to similar management aims. Specific treatment strategies, however, will more closely resemble those suggested for persons with motor neurone disease and multiple sclerosis (see Chs 18 & 19).

USEFUL ADDRESSES

Association for Swimming Therapy
4 Oak Street
Shrewsbury
Salop SY3 7RH
Tel 0743 4393

Muscular Dystrophy Group for Great Britain and Northern Ireland
Nattrass House
35 Macaulay Road
London SW4 0QP
Tel 071 720 8055

Physically Handicapped and Able Bodied (PHAB)
12–14 London Road
Croydon CR0 2TA

Riding for the Disabled Association
Avenue R
NAC
Kenilworth CV8 2LY
Tel 0203 696510

Information available from the MD Group:

- *Adaptations for DMD and allied neuromuscular diseases*
- *Carrier detection and prenatal diagnosis of inherited dystrophies*
- *Children with neuromuscular disease (for professionals)* by Dr Gardner–Medwin MD FRCP
- *Family considerations for surgical correction of spinal deformity in muscular dystrophy*

- *'Hey, I'm here too'*, a guide for brothers and sisters of children with muscular dystrophy
- *The parents' guide to physical management of DMD* by S A Hyde MCSP
- *Weight control in patients with muscular dystrophy*
- *'With a little help'*, a guide to aids and adaptations for people with DMD and allied neuromuscular diseases by Philippa Harpin Dip COT

FURTHER READING

Anderson E M 1980 The disabled schoolchild. Methuen, London

Anderson E M, Clarke L, Spain B 1982 Disability in adolescence. Methuen, London

Department of Education and Science 1978 Special educational needs: report of the committee of enquiry into the education of children and young people (Warnock Report). HMSO, London

Eckersley P, Clegg M, Robinson P 1986 The 1981 Education Act: guidelines for physiotherapists and other paediatric professionals. Chartered Society of Physiotherapy, London

Hegarty S, Pocklington K 1981 Educating pupils with special needs in ordinary schools. NFER-Nelson, Windsor

Levitt S 1984 Paediatric developmental therapy. Blackwell, Oxford

Russell P 1984 The wheelchair child. Souvenir Press, London

Simeonsson R J, McHale S M 1981 Review: research on handicapped children: sibling relationships. Child Care Health & Development 7: 153–171

21

Parkinson's disease

Sybil E. Johnson

INTRODUCTION

Parkinson's disease is a chronic, progressive, neuromuscular condition characterised by symptoms and signs which together may be described as a syndrome of neurological deficits. It is caused by changes in the basal ganglia which manifest as disturbances of motor function distinguished by the slowing and weakening of voluntary movements, including those expressing emotion.

This chapter begins by describing the pathology and aetiology of Parkinson's disease, as well as its principal clinical features, diagnosis, and treatment. The important contribution that chemotherapy has made in alleviating the symptoms of parkinsonism* is described, as well as the much more limited application of surgical intervention. The contribution of the physiotherapist and speech therapist to rehabilitation is then outlined.

There is as yet no cure for the condition, so the occupational therapist's involvement with people with parkinsonism is likely to take place over a period of many years. The chapter describes the aims and approach of this ongoing intervention first in general terms, and then in the context of the 'early' and 'later' stages of the disease. The various facets of the person's needs as they relate

---

* It should be noted that the terms Parkinson's disease and parkinsonism are used interchangeably in this text.

to each stage are described in detail; these include personal care, mobility, home-care and safety, communication, activity and so on.

The needs of family members and carers, especially for respite provision, are given increased attention in the discussion of late-stage intervention, as difficulties in coping are likely to increase as the person's condition deteriorates. However, it is stressed throughout the chapter that Parkinson's disease has profound consequences not only for the person suffering from the condition but also for his family and that the occupational therapist must plan her intervention with a sensitive awareness and understanding of the challenge that Parkinson's disease poses to all concerned.

PATHOLOGY

First described by Dr James Parkinson in 1817 in 'An Essay on the Shaking Palsy', the pathology of Parkinson's disease is still not clearly understood. Onset is rare before 40 and after 65 years of age. The disease affects both sexes equally. Although it can develop at any time, prevalence rises with age; however, its incidence appears to remain stable with increasing life expectancy.

The condition has been shown to be associated with a disturbance of the neurotransmitter systems and accompanying cell degeneration in the dopaminergic pathways in the basal ganglia, primarily the globus pallidus and the substantia nigra (Fig. 21.1). This disturbance, which upsets the balance between the cholinergic and dopaminergic transmission systems, results in three principle characteristics: rigidity, bradykinesia and tremor. Of these three, one may predominate initially, although the others will develop eventually. The disease is insidious in onset. It usually starts unilaterally but tends to become bilateral as it advances. The side on which symptoms first appear remains the worst affected. The individual will often find it difficult to identify the first appearance of his symptoms, but a slow, progressive deterioration over many years will cause a gradual loss of physical abilities. This in turn will lead to a disrupted life-style, eventual loss of employment, a change in appearance, and depression.

AETIOLOGY

The primary cause of Parkinson's disease is dopa deficiency. It is unknown why this deficiency occurs, although theories abound; researchers point to, for example, environmental factors, viral agents, and ageing as possible causes.

The symptoms of parkinsonism reflect the dys-

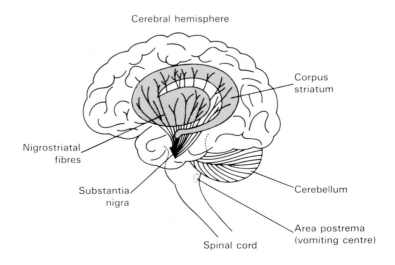

Cerebral hemisphere

Corpus striatum

Nigrostriatal fibres

Substantia nigra

Cerebellum

Area postrema (vomiting centre)

Spinal cord

Fig. 21.1 Left side of the human brain showing schematically the substantia nigra and the corpus striatum (shaded area) lying deep within the cerebral hemisphere. For simplicity, only one side is shown. Nerve fibres extend upward from the substantia nigra and, dividing into many branches, carry dopamine to all regions of the corpus striatum. (Reproduced by kind permission from: P. C. Duvoisin, *Parkinson's Disease — a guide for patient and family*, 'What is Parkinsonism?', p. 5, 1978, Raven Press.)

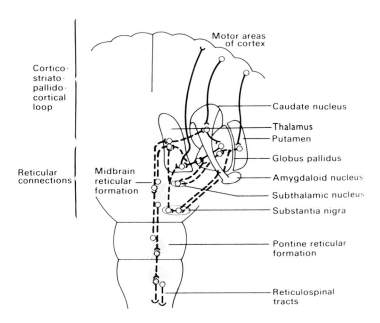

Fig. 21.2   Diagram of the principal connections of the basal ganglia. (Reproduced by kind permission from: R Bannister, *Brain's Clinical Neurology*, Oxford University Press, 1986, p. 336.)

function within the basal ganglia (Fig. 21.2), particularly in the system of nerve cells forming the substantia nigra which produce and store dopamine. The substantia nigra's nerve cells connect with the corpus striatum via long fibres along which dopamine travels. Within the corpus striatum the dopamine acts as a transmitter of chemical messages. When the substantia nigra nerve cells are unable to produce or store dopamine, the striatum suffers a deficiency which, if sufficiently severe, gives rise to parkinsonian symptoms.

Dopamine deficiency may occur in a number of ways. The substantia nigra nerve cells may deteriorate, for example through invasion by a tumour, injury by a CVA, chemical agent damage, drugs, or a virus (encephalitis). If, on the other hand, the striatum nerve cells are unable to receive chemical messages, the effect is the same.

There are two types of Parkinson's disease: idiopathic and secondary. Theories as to causes are described below and summarised in Table 21.1.

Idiopathic Parkinson's disease

This is the most common type in the United Kingdom and studies have investigated a number of theories concerning the suspected causes. There appears to be a family history in approximately 10% of cases, but studies of possible genetic causes have produced conflicting evidence. There is no proof that viral infection precipitates the disease. Vascular and neuronal damage have been investigated but no conclusions have been drawn. At the time of writing, environmental pollutants are being researched. It is thought that these pol-

Table 21.1   Theories of the causes of idiopathic and secondary Parkinson's disease: a summary

Idiopathic	Secondary
Family history	Prescribed drugs (e.g. phenothiazines)
Viral infection	Contaminated drugs (in drug abuse)
Environmental pollutants	Alzheimer's disease
Ageing	Cerebral tumours Severe head injury Continuous cerebral contusion Arteriosclerosis

lutants may induce the disease in people with an inherited sensitivity towards certain toxins.

Secondary Parkinson's disease

This may manifest in several ways, though one is now virtually non-existent, i.e. postencephalitic parkinsonism. An epidemic of encephalitis between 1917 and 1927 resulted in significant numbers of people developing Parkinson's disease in which rigidity was the main feature. The disease as a sequel to encephalitis is now rare and few people who developed the disease following the epidemic survive.

The drug-induced or chemical-induced type may occur as a side effect in those people taking large doses of phenothiazines or, in the latter type, contaminated drugs. Parkinson's disease, or signs resembling the disease, may also develop as part of a generalised condition, for example: Alzheimer's disease; in cases where cerebral tumours affect the basal ganglia; in severe head injuries (post-traumatic parkinsonism); as a result of continuous cerebral contusion i.e. in boxers — the 'punch-drunk' syndrome; or in elderly people who, as a result of several minor CVAs, may experience stiffness which slows movement, a tendency to walk with slow, shuffling steps and difficulty in speaking clearly. These symptoms, plus the slightly stooped posture commonly seen among elderly people, resembles Parkinson's disease and is often referred to as arteriosclerotic parkinsonism.

CLINICAL FEATURES

Parkinson's disease displays three principle characteristics: rigidity, bradykinesia and tremor.

Rigidity

This condition is caused by increased muscle tone throughout the range of movement in the muscle groups of the affected areas. It often affects one hand initially, progressing to one side of the body, then the other, and finally the neck and trunk. Rigidity becomes more pronounced as the condition progresses and the person develops certain characteristics, namely:

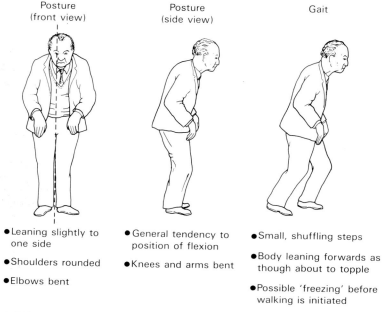

Posture (front view)
- Leaning slightly to one side
- Shoulders rounded
- Elbows bent

Posture (side view)
- General tendency to position of flexion
- Knees and arms bent

Gait
- Small, shuffling steps
- Body leaning forwards as though about to topple
- Possible 'freezing' before walking is initiated

Fig. 21.3 The characteristic stooped posture and hurrying gait of Parkinson's disease.

- a characteristic posture, especially when walking, in which the neck, thoracic spine, hips and knees are flexed (Fig. 21.3). There is a loss of free movement of the limbs, hence the natural arm swing is absent
- impaired spinal rotation
- a tendency towards 'stiff' wrist extension and flexion at the metacarpophalangeal joints and extension of the phalangeal joints.

There are two types of rigidity: 'cog-wheel' and 'lead-pipe'. The 'cog-wheel' effect is felt during passive flexion and extension of the wrist or elbow joint and is characterised by a series of jerky 'giving' movements which are followed by relaxation. The 'lead-pipe' phenomenon produces slow, smooth resistance through the full range of a joint's passive movement.

Rigidity increases with anxiety and concentration. As the condition deteriorates the limitations caused by either type lead to further loss of movement due to contractures and muscular atrophy. If facial muscles are affected the individual develops a mask-like, fixed expression with staring eyes and his emotional responses become extremely slow. Handwriting may become micrographic (very small) and tremulous (Fig. 21.4).

Bradykinesia

This is a slowness and poverty of voluntary movement, in inverse proportion to the degree of

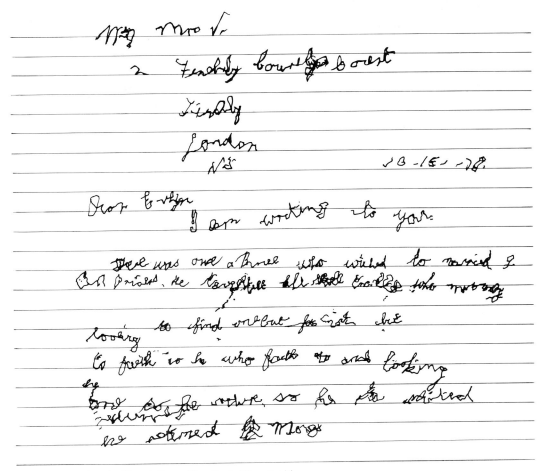

Fig. 21.4 Tremulous handwriting: letter written by a 63-year-old.

rigidity, which results in difficulty initiating and carrying out coordinated movements, for example fastening buttons, writing, walking and turning around. This slowness results from muscle weakness and fatigue and is, perhaps, the most disabling feature of the disease. The individual's general activity level is reduced; he is slow in his actions and has difficulty maintaining his independence. Although activity may begin adequately, movement becomes poor and ineffectual as the person progresses; this is exacerbated by repeated effort leading to fatigue, aching muscles and, in some cases, actual muscular pain. Difficulty in initiating movement will frequently cause a delay between a stimulus, such as a request to sit down, and the subsequent response. The mobility problems caused by bradykinesia include difficulties in and rising from a bed or chair and in getting into or out of the bath. Balance also deteriorates, leading to a tendency to fall easily. The individual's gait may be grossly impaired. He may develop an accelerated gait (festination), walking with short, shuffling steps with a tendency to lurch. He gives the appearance, with his flexed posture, of trying to catch up with his centre of gravity. He will stop slowly, will find it difficult to turn to the left or right and may 'freeze' when he meets a minor obstacle, for example a door threshold.

An interesting phenomenon in Parkinson's disease is that, once movement is initiated, the individual will have less difficulty climbing a flight of stairs than walking on level ground, though descent may be less easy due to his flexed posture and shuffling gait.

It is usual for small muscle movements to be most affected and, as a result, activities such as cutting food and chewing are impaired, with the potential long-term implication of weight loss caused by an inadequate diet. This weight may be regained as the individual becomes less active or is confined to a wheelchair. On the other hand, the person may continue to lose weight as eating becomes increasingly difficult and slow, resulting in reduced quality and quantity of intake.

People with Parkinson's disease often dribble — a feature which they may find most distressing. This is caused by failure to swallow automatically and is exacerbated by poor posture: i.e. the cervical spine is flexed, bringing the chin down so that saliva collects in the front of the mouth.

Speech impairment is not common to all people with Parkinson's disease, but when it is present the voice may be low pitched, slurred and monotonous, with little rhythm or expression but an increased pace. This is often described as 'a fast mumble'.

Bradykinesia combined with rigidity usually results in a very severe reduction in movement, making purposeful activity more difficult. In some very severe cases constant writhing movements will make caring for the individual very difficult.

Tremor

This characteristic is present at rest, though not during sleep, and is inhibited by movement (in contrast to the intention tremor in multiple sclerosis). It usually begins unilaterally in an upper limb and later becomes bilateral. It is rhythmic, commonly affecting the forearm and elbow musculature. The once very characteristic 'pill-rolling' effect between thumb and fingers may be present but has been seen less often since the drug L-dopa (levodopa) was introduced. Initially the tremor may appear periodically, but later its frequency accelerates. Tremor may affect a person's head and jaw and, less commonly, his trunk and lower limbs. It may affect one muscle group after another and will increase with excitement or anxiety, though it can be inhibited temporarily by conscious effort.

Other features

- Despite gross motor dysfunction there is no sensory loss.
- Occasional urinary/bladder dysfunction may be present. This probably results from constipation or as a side effect of chemotherapy.
- Constipation is common and may relate to autonomic dysfunction complicated by immobility and drugs.
- Flushing and excessive perspiration may occur at times, possibly resulting from a

combination of effort and the general effects of the disease.

- The individual will often be depressed and exasperated because his brain functions more rapidly than his muscles. His self-confidence may be substantially undermined.
- The individual's immobility makes his circulatory system less responsive to temperature changes; therefore, he is often cold.
- Parkinson's disease alone does not normally affect intellect but it does slow the mental processes. Studies have shown that approximately a third of elderly people with the disease have some degree of dementia. This may well be caused by other degenerative processes, such arteriosclerosis, as parkinsonism is not necessarily associated with mental disturbance other than depression.
- Dewick and Playfer (1990) state that there is evidence in substantial numbers of people which indicates specific deficits in cognitive function, visuoperceptual mechanisms and memory. Examples of these defects include: difficulty with the interpretation of facial expressions; problems recognising photographs of faces; difficulty with short-term memory processing, including non-verbal and verbal memory.
- The older the person the more likely he is to suffer multiple pathology; for example, in addition to his Parkinson's disease he may also have osteoarthritis, respiratory and/or cardiac impairment and failing senses.

DIAGNOSIS

Parkinson's disease is diagnosed by taking the individual's history and assessing his signs and symptoms. It is important to distinguish parkinsonian tremor from other forms of tremor, for example intention tremor and tremors resulting from hysteria, thyrotoxicosis and poisoning (e.g. by mercury or alcohol). Rigidity must also be carefully examined in order to eliminate other possible conditions or causes, such as lesions in the midbrain, which cause a very different pattern of

rigidity. However, an expressionless face, loss of swing in one or both arms, and often tremor, are so characteristic that diagnosis is relatively straightforward. The poverty and slowness of movement, which will make activities requiring fine movement difficult, will also aid confirmation of diagnosis.

TREATMENT

To date there is no cure for Parkinson's disease. Treatment, primarily chemotherapy and rehabilitation, can alleviate many people's symptoms quite dramatically, enabling them to function relatively well for many years.

CHEMOTHERAPY

The dopaminergic and cholinergic neurotransmission systems assist in the maintenance of normal movement. Parkinsonism is manifest when these two systems are unbalanced. In order to obtain and maintain a balance, drugs (often two or more) may be used in combination.

Drugs act either by replenishing the brain's level of dopamine or by modifying the brain's function in order to compensate for the dopamine deficiency. Dopamine is one of many chemical transmitters in the brain. Acetylcholine, a transmitter for many nerve cell systems, is present in large quantities in the corpus striatum. Although not deficient in Parkinson's disease it has a significant bearing, with dopamine, on maintaining the balance required for normal movement. These two transmitters work reciprocally. Dopamine acts to restrain acetylcholine nerve cells; in parkinsonism these cells are relieved of their restraining influence. This contributes to the disease's symptoms. Drugs which inhibit or block acetylcholine action tend to alleviate the symptoms, whereas drugs which enhance acetylcholine action cause an increase in symptoms. Drugs which block dopamine nerve cell function increase parkinsonian symptoms, whereas drugs which enhance these nerve cells relieve symptoms.

The application of chemotherapy to Parkinson's

Table 21.2 Chemotherapy in Parkinson's disease

Drug	Uses/action	Side effects
deprenyl	Slows progression of PD and delays need for levodopa	
Dopaminergic group levodopa and carbidopa (Sinemet) levodopa and benserazide (Madopar) levodopa (Brocadopa) levodopa (Lardopa) bromocriptine (Parlodel)	Increase levels of dopamine in the brain and reduce rigidity and bradykinesia. Little effect on tremor Stimulates dopamine receptors, useful when maximum levodopa tolerance is reached	Nausea, vomiting, dizziness, faintness, loss of appetite, metallic taste in the mouth, heartburn, confusion, changes in mental state; long-term use may cause dyskinesia (abnormal involuntary movements)
Anticholinergic group amantadine (Symmetrel) benztropine (Cogentin) benzhexol (Artane) orphenadrine (Disipal) procyclidine (Kemadrin)	Block the action of acetylcholine throughout body and brain and control tremor, reduce salivation and decrease rigidity	Dry mouth, nausea, blurred vision, palpitations, constipation, slowness/hesitancy whilst urinating, confusion, memory impairment

disease, summarised in Table 21.2, continues to be developed and evaluated. Current work in the UK suggests that deprenyl may slow the progression of the disease and delay the need for levodopa.

At the stage when levodopa is required, chemotherapy is considered in terms of the reciprocal relationship between dopamine and acetylcholine.

Dopaminergic group

Drugs in this group which contain levodopa may produce almost complete symptom relief in approximately one in five people, particularly in the disease's early stages. The majority show some improvement, i.e. rigidity and bradykinesia may decrease considerably, although tremor is less responsive.

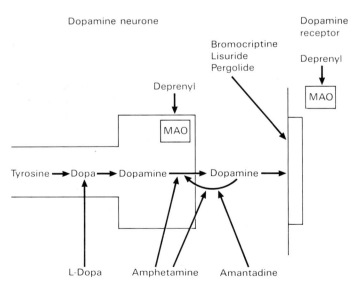

Fig. 21.5 Site of action of dopaminergic drugs. (Reproduced by kind permission from: R Bannister, *Brain's Clinical Neurology*, Oxford University Press, 1986, p. 344.)

The most effective method of improving dopamine nerve cell function is to replenish depleted dopamine levels. Levodopa, which has transformed the natural history of Parkinson's disease (although it has not abolished all of its accompanying problems) converts to dopamine in the brain (Fig. 21.5). It reaches the brain via the circulatory system; therefore, in order to prevent its conversion to dopamine elsewhere in the body it is usually administered in combination with a dopadecarboxylase inhibitor.

Anticholinergic group

These drugs act by blocking the cholinergic transmission at the nerve synapse. They act primarily on tremor and salivation and decrease rigidity. They are useful in the initial treatment of mild parkinsonism and as an adjunct to levodopa preparations.

Cell implantation

Currently the implantation, by injection, of dopamine producing cells is under trial both in the United States and the United Kingdom. Results are, as yet, inconclusive.

The success of chemotherapy in Parkinson's disease is dependent upon the general health of the individual, the severity of his symptoms and the dosage and timing of a drug's administration. Doses have to be monitored and adjusted in order to maximise independence and to minimise side effects. This balance is often difficult to achieve and continuous monitoring and evaluation is required if optimum benefit is to be gained.

SURGERY

Stereotactic thalamotomy is a procedure in which a stereotaxic lesion is made in the globus pallidus or the ventrolateral nucleus of the thalamus in order to reduce tremor and rigidity. It is a comparatively minor operation which used to be common. However, it is rarely used today and recipients are usually younger people whose general health is good and whose disability is primarily one of tremor and rigidity on one side of the body, or those who have very little difficulty with walking or speech. It is still the most effective means of relieving tremor and does not affect subsequent responses to levodopa.

At the time of writing there is vigorous debate and controversy regarding the moral and ethical issues of the implantation of fetal brain tissue into the person with Parkinson's disease. Research to date indicates that it is a potential breakthrough in the long-term alleviation of parkinsonian symptoms. However, moral and ethical concerns may preclude the development of this type of treatment.

REHABILITATION

Despite the depressing picture presented by parkinsonism, rehabilitation can offer much valuable, practical assistance to individuals and their families. The role of occupational therapy is discussed in detail beginning on p. 540.

Physiotherapy

The aim of physiotherapy is to help the person to maintain his independence for as long as possible and to advise carers how to manage as the disease progresses and the person's disabilities become more severe.

Assessment enables the physiotherapist to establish a baseline for her intervention and will include an overall impression of the individual's medical condition and relevant social circumstances and a detailed consideration of his physical state, i.e. posture, balance, gait, functional performance (particularly mobility) and respiration, in relation to his medication regime.

Physiotherapy intervention in the early stages aims to improve functional performance. As the disease progresses treatment will be offered at appropriate intervals in order to deal with specific problems and to assist carers.

Intervention may include the following:

● Specific education in relation to posture and postural awareness in standing, walking, sitting and lying.

- Analysis and correction of impaired movement patterns, including practice in correct voluntary movement utilising auditory and verbal cues if these help. The physiotherapist will emphasise the heel-toe gait to improve the individual's walking pattern.
- Relaxation. This is helpful for some people, particularly if anxiety exacerbates their condition. Physiotherapists and others may prefer to use methods which reinforce postural awareness.
- Exercise. The individual will be advised and encouraged to undertake a programme of exercise at home. This may comprise very specific exercises, continuation of existing physical activity such as walking or a combination of the two.
- Specific respiration exercises which facilitate diaphragmatic breathing with an emphasis on expiration, and proprioceptive neuromuscular facilitation involving the specific manipulation of the muscles of respiration.
- Advice to carers. This forms part of the individual's programme, and may include correct techniques for carers to use in handling and assisting him when he experiences a particular problem, for example in rising from a chair.
- Assessment for walking aids. The physiotherapist will assess for and recommend any walking aids which may be needed although, generally, mobility aids are not as helpful as one might expect. However, a walking stick may help the person who suffers propulsion (spontaneous movement in a forward direction) and a walking frame can help those with poor equilibrium.
- Conductive education. This may be recommended for some people; it involves practising each component of an activity using verbal cues (see p. 546).

Speech therapy

The aim of speech therapy is to maximise the individual's 'available functional speech'; attention is given to pace, initiation difficulties, facial expression, voice intensity, intonation, vocal expression and conversation (Scott et al 1985).

Assessment enables the therapist to identify the nature and degree of any communication difficulty. Check lists and rating scales are used to establish which elements of communication are affected, for example: breathing; swallowing and sucking; musculature of the face and mastication; phonation; emotional behaviour; vocal volume, tone, rate and rhythm. Dysarthria assessments are also utilised, giving a profile of reflex activity function in respiration and in the jaw, lips, larynx and tongue.

Speech therapy utilises both verbal and non-verbal methods in the early and later stages of the disease. The increase in rate and decrease in volume of speech characteristic of parkinsonism is a powerful combination (i.e. the fast mumble) which is difficult to overcome. Therefore, therapy must be adapted realistically to each individual. Specific interventions may include:

- Speech therapists and physiotherapists working together to establish breathing control and patterns which will enhance speech.
- Teaching pacing techniques to enable the individual to monitor the rate of his speech, for example by using a pacing board or by speaking in time (mentally) to a tapping or ticking sound.
- Structuring therapy and the environment to facilitate his continuing awareness and monitoring of his own situation.
- Advice to relatives e.g. to face the person during speech, give him time, make the environment conducive to good communication.
- Group therapy. This may involve intensive courses in which articulation, progressive counting to aid breath control, and social and conversational exercises are undertaken.
- Individual therapy. This is possibly of more value to the younger and/or newly diagnosed person, who may be better motivated to continue exercises away from the treatment environment. Some benefit may be derived from simple exercises, for example dividing up reading passages to control breathing patterns.
- Proprioceptive neuromuscular facilitation involving the specific manipulation of muscles.

This may improve facial expression, voice intensity, respiration and swallowing and is useful at all stages of the disease.

- Prosodic therapy. (Prosody consists of the variations of pitch, timing and volume that give speech emphasis and interest.) This therapy uses exercises which emphasise the affective and prosodic aspects of speech to improve rate, rhythm, intonation, vocal expression and intensity. It is useful at all stages except very late in the disease's course.
- Speech and occupational therapists working together to help the individual with the functional problems (eating, drinking) caused by swallowing difficulties and dribbling (see p. 543).
- Enhancement of non-verbal communication. This may include: more emphasis on gesture and facial expression; communication boards (particularly in the later stages) adapted to suit individual needs; electronic typewriters with assisted keyboards; amplification aids, especially where volume loss is the only disorder; lightwriter (a speech replacement aid with a light touch keyboard and visual display). Speech therapists will utilise exercises for verbal communication along with non-verbal alternatives at all stages of the disease, dependent upon individual needs.

GENERAL HEALTH

The basic rules for general health and fitness are the same for people with parkinsonism as they are for everyone, but they are additionally important for the former group if some of the effects of the disease are to be minimised. The individual should be advised and encouraged to include general health routines in his daily programme. These may include:

- maintaining a sensible, well-balanced diet which includes plenty of fluids and fibre
- eating at regular intervals throughout the day and, if his appetite is poor, taking smaller, more frequent meals
- maintaining the tone and bulk of his musculature, joint mobility, the efficient

function of his cardiovascular and respiratory systems and a good posture. This will require regular exercise, preferably of a type he enjoys, which will encourage him to remain as physically active as possible

- continuing with activity which he finds mentally stimulating, such as the daily crossword or a favourite quiz show
- negotiating medication times to suit his daily routine
- interspersing activity with rest to avoid becoming overtired
- attempting to avoid upper respiratory tract ailments as these will take him longer to recover from, slow him down, and make him extremely tired.

PSYCHOLOGICAL CONSIDERATIONS

By its nature, Parkinson's disease makes the individual vulnerable to depression, anxiety, embarrassment, confusion, loss of motivation, changes in attitude and fear. These feelings, if and when they occur, will also affect his family to a greater or lesser degree.

If he is treated in a positive manner — i.e. if the effects of the disease are explained to him, and if he is encouraged to participate actively in planning his treatment regime and permitted to voice his fears — then his attitude and general emotional state are more likely to remain objective and positive. It is important to identify the person's interests and his key sources of motivation whilst, simultaneously, identifying concerns or problems. In this way a balance can be established which will be realistic, and acceptable, for most people.

Anxiety should be expected and dealt with appropriately. Any anxiety or nervous tension may increase the individual's tremor temporarily and if this is permitted to continue the resulting 'tension equals tremor' pattern will be difficult to overcome. Many people find that relaxation techniques which can be used in a variety of environments can offset the need for further medication.

Depression is a common feature of Parkinson's disease. It should be discussed openly with the individual and his carers and means of counteracting it initiated. It is usually best coped with by maintaining and/or developing interests and activities around and outside the home, as companionship and stimulation often alleviate the depression.

Absent-mindedness and thought block are experienced by most people at some time or another and minor levels of both are found in people with parkinsonism. However, evidence of absent-mindedness or mild confusion do not necessarily mean that the individual's mental function is deteriorating, nor do these 'episodes' lead to serious memory disturbance. Some drugs may cause confusion in older people but, for the majority, making notes or accepting prompts will alleviate the problem.

Fear is usually overcome by encouraging and supporting the individual in his search for information and knowledge about the disease. This enables him to place his fears in perspective, and to make informed choices about course(s) of action which will motivate him, increase his self-esteem, and help him to remain active in his local community.

Embarrassment is another effect of the disease for some people. This, and other problems, must be dealt with on an individual basis in a sensitive and empathetic manner. Establishing the exact cause of the person's embarrassment and utilising a problem-solving, self-help approach with therapy support will often ease the effects.

Learning new skills and recalling what has been learned may be difficult for some. The therapist should use her skill and ingenuity to provide an optimum learning environment, methods which suit the individual, a pace which is realistic and associations which are meaningful. We all learn in different ways and at different speeds; therefore, some experimentation by the individual and the therapist may be needed to ascertain optimum learning conditions.

OCCUPATIONAL THERAPY

Despite advances in chemotherapy and research into fetal implants, the progressive nature of Parkinson's disease will probably require that a person and his family maintain contact with the occupational therapist over a period of many years. Clearly, it is impractical and unnecessary for the individual to receive continuous therapy throughout the course of the disease. Often, following a period of initial assessment, goal-setting and appropriate intervention, the individual will receive short periods of intensive therapy at regular intervals. This pattern should enable him to continue to maximise his functional ability in relation to his life-style and interests and to learn, over a period of time, how to adjust himself to any limitations and to manage life with the disease.

It should be noted that the disease will produce a wide variation in the degree of disability. Some people may have minor symptoms for many years and never become severely impaired, whilst others may become severely disabled and require full nursing care. The treatment required will vary and the therapist must maintain a realistic outlook in relation to the condition's progression and its effect on the individual and organise the intervention programme accordingly. She must also remember that some types of parkinsonism respond more readily to medical intervention than others and that this will affect the outcome of rehabilitation. People with idiopathic parkinsonism, for example, respond well to chemotherapy and are therefore more likely to benefit from rehabilitation. In contrast, those whose condition is attributable to arteriosclerosis gain little from active therapy. Their carers, however, will need much help and advice.

AIM

The occupational therapist's intervention is concerned primarily with maximising residual abilities and compensating for the limitations imposed by the clinical features of Parkinson's disease. More detailed aims are delineated under Intervention, below.

ASSESSMENT

Chapter 7 describes in detail the reasons for assessment, the types of assessment utilised by occupational therapists, and their importance as a baseline from which the therapist and the individual will work.

Initial and subsequent assessment will include all or most of the areas listed below. The therapist, the individual and, where appropriate, his carers will work through these elements at an agreed pace and time, identifying exactly which functions are unimpaired and which need intervention. The assessment may also indicate the type of advice and assistance required and enable the therapist to plan interventions for the short and long term. For example, in the short term she may give advice about transfer techniques and in the longer term initiate modifications to the bathroom and toilet.

Elements of assessment:

- passive range of movement, presence of contractures and the degree of rigidity present
- active range of movement (i.e. full or limited in all joints), coordination, strength, grasp/grip and reach
- characteristics of active movement, i.e. the absence or presence of bradykinesia, rigidity and/or tremor and whether one of these features is worse than the others
- posture, sitting and standing balance, tolerance and the effects of rigidity and bradykinesia on these functions
- general mobility and its characteristics, for example normal gait versus festination
- the presence of pain or any other discomfort caused by repeated effort because of slowness and poverty of voluntary movement
- emotional state — is this affected and, if so, how, for example by depression or anxiety
- intellectual capacity — this requires monitoring throughout the course of the disease
- any degree of deficiency in cognitive function
- the routine effects of medication on function.

Given the progressive nature of Parkinson's disease, a thorough initial assessment and reassessment at subsequent intervals are vital in order to establish a realistic baseline from which to work at each stage. Additionally, occupational therapists may be required to contribute to assessment of a person's ability at other times, for example during the introduction or later modification of

Table 21.3 A summary of pre- and post-chemotherapy functional assessments

Activity	Comment
ADL Walking Stairs (up and down) Dressing Bath (in and out) Chair Turning in bed Eating Drinking	'Independent, with assistance, unable' (or similar) scoring system used and recorded for future comparisons
Dexterity tests e.g. bead-threading, solitaire	Timed and recorded for future comparisons
Handwriting	Timed: copying out a specific poem or passage from a book or writing name and address. Filed for future reference
Drawing	Tracing through a pre-determined maze

chemotherapy regimes. Examples of this type of assessment, which may be used in particular centres rather than in all hospitals, are summarised in Table 21.3.

INTERVENTION

Intervention is based on a multidisciplinary approach, with each profession making a specific contribution to a programme of treatment. Occupational therapy is directed towards assisting the individual in:

- achieving and maintaining as positive an attitude as possible towards his abilities
- maintaining his abilities for as long as is feasible
- modifying his life-style as the disease progresses
- accepting, if possible, the gradual decrease in his functional ability and reliance upon others for selected help
- accepting that routines are increasingly established around medication regimes or vice versa
- balancing activity and rest in order to avoid/alleviate fatigue.

Specific aims will relate to each individual and depend upon his current abilities and needs. Hence, occupational therapy may include:

- education of the person and his carers regarding the need for routine, balanced activity and rest periods, a healthy diet, a problem-solving approach to self-help and exercise and activity which will help to maintain his motivation and mobility
- maintenance of independence in daily living skills in order to alleviate limitations caused by rigidity and/or tremor
- the provision of alternative methods, techniques, regimes and/or equipment to aid self-care and home management
- development of the individual's tolerance to activity and improvement of stamina
- assistance to plan and implement a programme for use at home, i.e. a routine of self-care, domestic activity, work, leisure and creativity which will offer a balanced life-style
- help to increase/modify the person's interests so that his social, physical and psychological needs are met and maintained.

Approach

The occupational therapist and the person with Parkinson's disease jointly identify and analyse what the latter can do, his functional problems and the resolution of these. The therapist and the individual will frequently be working with the symptoms of the disease rather than applying specific neurological theories to treatment; their concern will be to find ways in which the person can live with, or in spite of, his progressive disorder. Therefore, the approach is primarily rehabilitative, utilising problem-solving theory and techniques.

Intervention stages

Identifying specific rehabilitation stages for people with Parkinson's disease is not a straightforward task, given the varying course and effects of the disease. Therefore, in order to provide some indication of the extent of the occupational therapist's involvement the terms 'early stage' and 'later stages' are used.

'Early' is used to describe the stage during which the person is able to benefit from specific rehabilitation.

'Later' is used to describe the period during which there is less emphasis on rehabilitation and more on adaptation, for example in introducing the use of equipment, modifying the environment, and giving assistance to carers.

EARLY STAGE

The general aim of therapy at this stage is to enable the individual to maintain as much of his function and daily life-style as possible, with adjustments when and where appropriate. More specifically:

- The person will need to maintain gross and fine coordination, strength, and concentration, as these are required for self-care.
- Good posture should be encouraged, as should maintenance (or increase) of mobility.
- Activities which encourage specific physical and psychological function and help to maintain self-care, self-esteem, social contacts and productivity will be important.
- The person may need advice and assistance in order to maintain his family, leisure and/or work roles and routines.
- He should be encouraged to continue with his interests such as sports and hobbies, as these will offer him a 'balance' as well as exercise, a creative outlet, and so on.
- He and his family may need advice/information about the condition, its effect on life-style and how best to 'pace' activity.

Personal care

Clothing and footwear, undressing and dressing

- *Clothing.* An individual's choice/preferences in relation to what he wears are important to his self-esteem, dignity, comfort and practical concerns. If his preferences enable him to continue to undress and dress independently, advice will not be required at this stage. If, however, the items of clothing preferred hinder independence he may be reminded that:

— styles which are easier to take off and put on are to be preferred
— fabrics which are warm/cool, lightweight, stretchy, and made of mixed or natural fibres enhance comfort
— wearing several layers of clothing will help him to maintain coordination, range of movement, transfers (standing/sitting) and fine movements; on the other hand, wearing many layers may overtire him
— fastenings should be easily accessible and kept to a minimum, or easily modified in a manner which is acceptable to the individual, for example, by using slightly larger buttons if the button holes/loops will permit this, inserting zips, using velcro 'dabs'.

● *Footwear.* Personal preference must be taken into account. Advice offered at this stage may relate to comfort, support and ease of removal/putting on. Slip-on shoes are ideal, providing they are supportive, and some people may prefer elastic shoe-laces in their lace-up shoes. Both require the use of a shoe-horn.

● *Undressing and dressing* need adequate time and a routine. The individual may find that advice regarding routine preparation of clothing, positions for dressing (e.g. sitting), and special techniques (such as removing/putting on shirts with most of the buttons fastened) may be all that is required at this stage.

Grooming

Activities such as combing or brushing hair, shaving or applying make-up, and caring for finger- and toe-nails should be maintained for as long as possible, as they encourage movement, coordination, dexterity, self-esteem and dignity, and enable the individual to retain control over his appearance. Advice regarding hair-styles, types of razors or make-up applicators and techniques for

nail care may be required, but the individual is often able to resolve any comparatively minor difficulties himself.

Eating and drinking

All three of the main characteristics of parkinsonism may affect an individual's ability to eat, drink and swallow normally. Rigidity tends to 'stiffen' the wrist joint and impair phalangeal joint extension and metacarpophalangeal joint flexion. Bradykinesia affects the movements performed by small muscles and, if it is severe, is likely to impair chewing and cutting actions. Tremor which affects the upper limbs, trunk, head and jaw has implications for eating, drinking and swallowing.

The pace at which a person eats and drinks will slow with time. If he can maintain his routine and pattern of meals, snacks and drinks he should be encouraged to do so. Adaptations, if required, may include:

● taking smaller hot meals more frequently
● modifying the texture of the food eaten so that it is easier to chew
● applying techniques taught by the speech therapist to alleviate early swallowing difficulties resulting from muscle rigidity.

Washing, bathing/showering, care of teeth

People with Parkinson's disease have an oilier skin than usual, particularly on their face, and therefore need to wash and bath more frequently. The following points should be borne in mind:

● Washing at the basin is manageable providing the person assumes a safe position, follows a routine and keeps the items he requires close at hand.

● Care of the teeth depends on whether the person has his own teeth or wears dentures. Toothpaste dispensers, an enlarged toothbrush handle or an electric toothbrush may make the task easier. Denture wearers usually have a preferred method of cleaning their teeth and this should be maintained.

● If the individual is able to get in and out

of the bath safely there is no reason why he should not continue to do so, although he may need a non-slip mat and a strategically positioned grab rail to assist him.

— if he is not safe then he should consider alternatives which retain his independence, such as strip-washes, showering over the bath using a bath board, a walk-in shower cubicle or level access
— he should always test the water temperature prior to washing

● Individuals have preferred methods of washing their hair. Advice on modifications such as a position change may be warranted.

Toileting

Whilst he is still ambulant, the person with parkinsonism will retain much of his independence in toileting, although transfer on/off the toilet may sometimes cause difficulty. (Transfers are dealt with under Mobility, below; the principles of sitting down/standing described there will apply to toilet use.) The therapist should be aware of the following points:

● Many of the parkinsonian drugs cause constipation; therefore, the person is well advised to maintain a fluid intake of up to 3 litres daily.
● Clothing should be easily managed.
● If stiffness and rigidity hinder sitting/standing and technique alone does not resolve the problem the person may need to use a raised toilet seat and/or grab rails alongside or a frame around the toilet.
● The toilet paper holder should be within reasonable reach. If tearing off the required amount of paper is laborious, single sheets or a dispenser may help.
● The toilet-flushing mechanism should be manageable, but if the cistern has a pull-handle this may require slight lengthening to bring it within easy reach.

CASE EXAMPLE 21.1

Mrs B is 82. She lives alone in a ground-floor, warden-controlled flat. Her sister lives in the same block and deals with domestic home care needs of Mrs B and herself.

Mrs B's parkinsonism was diagnosed six years ago. She was recently admitted to hospital as an emergency, following a fall in her bathroom. She presented with increasing lethargy, weakness, unsteadiness, confusion and vomiting and was diagnosed as having a large frontoparietal subdural haematoma. This was drained.

Occupational therapy

Initial assessment

● communication intact
● mobility: unsteady with walking frame, felt unsafe
● transfers: difficulties with all, tendency to fall
● bathing: has shower attachment over bath
● dressing: independent once prompted
● personal hygiene: 'mental block'?
● kitchen: sister performs tasks

Aims

● mobility and transfers: practice to increase confidence and establish safe methods
● home visit: establish home care support to continue (sister) and that mobility and transfers (bed, chair, toilet, bath/shower) can be managed safely
● dressing practice: increase confidence and maintain functional skills

Treatment (daily for 8 days)

● mobility: quite ataxic with lack of confidence. Practice established in conjunction with physiotherapy
● transfers: counting to remember stages, did not comprehend 'safe methods'. Sister and other carers taught methods
● dressing: physically able but out of practice. Seated position recommended. Practice to instil confidence
● sister: advice and education re Mrs B's abilities

Long term

Sister moved into flat with Mrs B. This was facilitated during the home visit (see report). Support from Home Care and Community Nursing service.

OCCUPATIONAL THERAPY DEPT.	REG. NO. _____
HOME ASSESSMENT REPORT	SURNAME __B_____
DATE ____8.6.90._____	FORENAME(S)_____
	ADDRESS_____

TYPE OF ACCOMMODATION	WARD ____N2____ CONSULTANT___RDB_____
Ground floor flat	Label to be used if available

FAMILY & COMMUNITY SUPPORT PRIOR TO ADMISSION	G.P. NAME & ADDRESS
H/H	
Lunchclub - Monday. Sister shops, cooks.	AIDS ALREADY IN USE

ACCESS:

STAIRS:

CORRIDORS/HALLS:

SWITCHES:

SEATING: High seat chair.

HEATING: Central heating.

BED: Low soft single divan, unsuitable for transfers (15ins).

BATHING: Bath 17ins high. Floor to ceiling pole at bottom end of bath.
Bath seat, shower over bath.

TOILET:

KITCHEN: Off living room. Sister responsible for cooking meals.

CLEANING/LAUNDRY: Sister.

EMERGENCY (Telephone, Alarm Cards, Intercom):   Warden. Telephone.

SUMMARY & RECOMMENDATIONS FROM PERSONNEL INVOLVED: COMMENTS	SIGNATURE DESIGNATION

Problems and recommendations.

1. The bed is too low and soft for easy transfers. This has now been changed for the sister's bed which is much more suitable (17ins).

2. Bath: Access to the bath is hampered by the floor to ceiling pole. It is recommended that this be moved to the opposite end of the bath and be used in conjunction with a bath board. The community O.T. will be contacted about this.

3. Transfers: Mrs B. is not yet safe in transfers and needs further rehabilitation to reinforce safe methods.

4. Support: Support will be available on discharge from Home Care Services and District Nurse.

Conclusion

Mrs B.'s sister has decided to live with her on a permanent basis and is making arrangements for this. With this arrangement and the above recommendations Mrs B. will cope at home but she needs further rehabilitation to practise mobility and transfers prior to discharge.

Senior Occupational Therapist

314

Mobility

Mobility and good posture are integral parts of successful function and the achievement of daily tasks. Occupational therapists contribute to each person's overall mobility in relation to transfers, positioning, balance, coordination, posture, exercise, and the modification or replacement of chairs and beds.

● *Walking*. The occupational therapist should reinforce the techniques taught by the physiotherapist, i.e. a relaxed, upright posture, arm swinging, concentrating on a heel-toe gait and auditory cues, i.e. counting or saying 'heel-toe, heel-toe' to himself.

'Freezing' episodes can occur abruptly, often without warning. At such times the person is suddenly unable to continue for several minutes. Many people devise their own methods to help them regain mobility. For example, if he freezes during walking it may help him to step over an imaginary object such as a line on the floor (Fig. 21.6), or over the carer's foot. The 'dog lead' technique may also help: the 'collar' end of the lead is placed around the shoe or around the instep inside the shoe and the lead is passed up the leg and through a small hole in the trouser pocket; the individual holds the end of the lead in his pocket and pulls it to initiate movement in that leg. Sometimes a verbal

command such as 'walk' will be an adequate stimulus. If nothing helps, the individual and his carer must simply wait patiently for the episode to pass. However, advice can be offered regarding the removal of potential hazards such as loose mats and obstructive furniture, which may or may not initiate 'freezing', but will make the environment safer.

● *Conductive education* may be beneficial for those with mild or moderate parkinsonism. This approach totally absorbs the individual in an activity and can make him feel and look physically good while he performs it, thus helping him to be happier and more relaxed. The emphasis is on producing a positive emotional state through group activity; on initiating, executing and completing movements smoothly; and on developing the movement sequence which leads to a function such as walking, whilst working to a rhythmic beat and verbal cues. People who use this exercise mode, or parts of it, find that: the concentration and will-power involved stimulate achievement; their coordination and strength improve; and their fine and gross movement, posture and general mobility benefit.

● *Balance and coordination* are improved by encouraging good posture and positioning in all activities. The person should be advised to forward plan mobilisation and transfers so that voluntary movement and the maintenance of equilibrium are achieved smoothly and safely.

● *Stairs/steps* are usually manageable, as stepping *up* is easier for the individual than walking on level surfaces. If stairs do present a problem, however, the person will need to experiment with safe methods of ascent and descent. Counting may help, as may a conscious effort to step 'up and in' or 'out and down'. Backward descent may be safer for some people and an additional banister rail is often recommended.

Transfers

● *Chair transfers*. The seat height of a chair should facilitate optimum function, and the

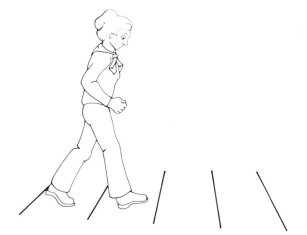

Fig. 21.6 Stepping over imaginary spaced lines may overcome 'freezing' and increase the length of each pace.

overall design should be conducive to its specific use, e.g. relaxing, eating, working at a desk. A chair should have:

— a firm seat which supports the thighs but avoids pressure on the popliteal fossae
— a supportive back; if it is an armchair the back should support the user's head, encouraging him to tip his head back rather than forward
— armrests which support the forearms and facilitate pushing up.

If transfer in and out of the chair is difficult a number of solutions may be tried, e.g.:

— placing a wedge-shaped cushion on the seat (narrow edge to the front) to help the person 'push' his body weight forward if 'bottom walking' to the edge of the seat is difficult
— raising the rear legs of the chair a few centimetres, giving the seat a slight forward tilt
— if the person 'freezes', rocking, counting or a technique change may assist; focusing

on an item at or just above eye level may aid concentration.

The person may also be advised regarding his sitting/standing technique (Fig. 21.7):

— sitting down: with his back to the chair the person feels for the seat edge with the back of his legs; he places his hand(s) on the arms or seat of the chair and lowers himself
— standing up: the 'nose over toes' method involves bringing the bottom to the seat edge and the head forward, placing the feet slightly apart and behind the knees and pushing up on the chair arms or seat.

● *Bed transfers.* Beds should be of an optimum height if possible and have a firm mattress or base. Bedclothes should be lightweight and easy to manage.

At this stage, teaching the individual how to turn over in bed will probably meet most of his bed transfer needs. Figure 21.8 shows the person turning his head in the direction he wishes to move, followed by his knees and his

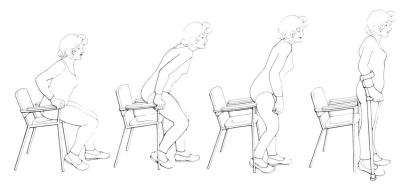

Sit well forward on the chair with both feet on the floor and the weight taken through the stronger (rear) foot—if this is applicable. Hold the arms of the chair firmly. Keep the head up.

Push up with the hands and feet, with the head well forward.

Transfer weight evenly onto both feet, and adjust balance.

Collect aids.

Fig. 21.7 Transfer from sitting to standing.

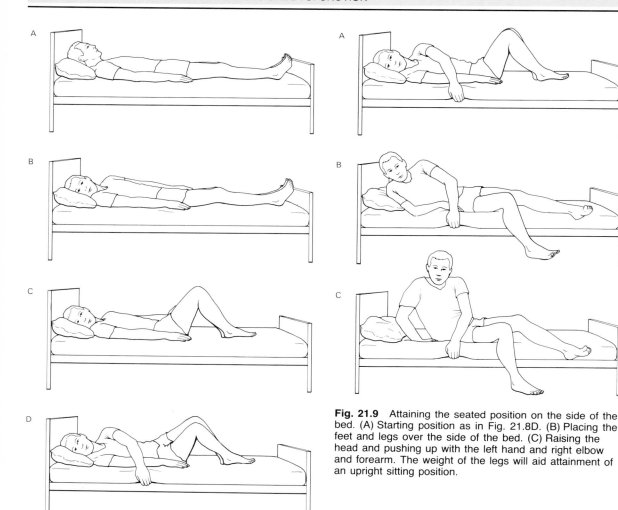

Fig. 21.8 Turning over in bed. (A) Starting position, supine in bed, arms by sides, legs uncrossed. (B) Turning the head towards the direction of the required total movement. (C) Raising the knees and placing the feet flat on the bed. (D) Moving the left arm over the body, towards the direction of the turn.

Fig. 21.9 Attaining the seated position on the side of the bed. (A) Starting position as in Fig. 21.8D. (B) Placing the feet and legs over the side of the bed. (C) Raising the head and pushing up with the left hand and right elbow and forearm. The weight of the legs will aid attainment of an upright sitting position.

'far' arm. In order to get out of bed from the 'turn over' position he puts his feet over the edge of the bed and pushes up on his 'upper' arm and hand, taking his weight on to his 'lower' forearm as shown in Figure 21.9. In getting into bed the procedure is reversed. The person places his bottom as near to the pillow as possible and 'walks' his bottom on to and as far back and towards the centre of the bed as he can manoeuvre. He then lies down, bringing his legs up onto the mattress. In all transfers, the individual should be taught to move his head first as this will influence the position of his trunk and the rest of his body will follow.

Transport

If the person drives he must report his condition to the Driver and Vehicle Licensing Centre. He will have to undergo a medical assessment of his fitness to drive and will be given a license for fixed periods. His condition will be reviewed regularly. It may be wiser for his carer to drive as the condition progresses.

Home-care and safety

Managing and caring for the home, in safety, requires a planned and flexible routine which will maximise the effects of the individual's chemotherapy and conserve his energy for those activities he *wants* to do as well as those he *has* to do to care for himself. He should be advised to remain active and independent at home, maintaining the routines to which he is accustomed when and wherever possible. He must learn to balance his activity so that self-care, home-care, leisure and/or work retain the right proportions.

The routines of shopping and cooking, cleaning and laundry, do-it-yourself and gardening, for example, will need planning in advance and tasks may be reallocated among family members. General advice will probably suffice at this stage and will relate to an individual's abilities and needs. Advice offered may include the following points:

- Ensure that hallways, stairs and work areas are well lit
- Eliminate dangerous floor coverings or provide visual reminders of potential hazards to mobility
- Maintain a warm home for comfort and general health
- Sit rather than stand to avoid overtiring
- Utilise labour-saving appliances for food preparation, laundry, cleaning
- If tremor hinders activity, particularly food preparation, stabilising food or food preparation tools with non-slip mats or clamps may help.

Communication

The Speech Therapy section offers a summary of specific interventions. The occupational therapist can augment formal speech therapy in several ways, and assist the individual to avoid the isolation which may be caused by communication and language deficits in the following areas:

- Verbal
  - Give the person time to express himself
  - Encourage him to utilise the breathing techniques advised by the speech and physiotherapists
  - Advise him to pace himself
- Written
  - The person's writing will have a tendency to decrease in size and to become shaky. Specific exercises (Fig. 21.10) may help some people, but others may find them inhibiting
  - Individuals may be assisted by a variety of means, e.g. rhythmical writing exercise patterns (Fig. 21.11), fibre-tip pens, wide-lined paper, clip-boards to stabilise and angle the paper
- Telephone
  - If the person experiences difficulty at this stage, push-button dialing or the 'Hands Free' facility allowing on-line dialling, supplied by British Telecom, can help.

Remedial activity

Specific activities may be used to encourage coordination, and types of movement and good posture with which the individual has difficulty, for example trunk rotation, limb swing and fine movements. The therapist should encourage the person to maintain his self-care and other routines, such as getting dressed, picking up his clothes to put away and washing and drying dishes, as these activities are conducive to the maintenance of trunk rotation, general upper and lower limb mobility, and coordination.

More specific activity to improve trunk rotation and limb swing can be introduced and undertaken at home with a board game such as solitaire. As illustrated in Figure 21.12, the person sits in a dining-type chair with the board at chest height. As he removes the solitaire pieces he passes them across his body into a receptacle on the opposite side, thus moving his left arm across to his right and vice versa, simultaneously rotating his trunk.

Activity which encourages strength and coordination should be encouraged to help the individual maintain his abilities. These should relate to his interests at home, for example do-it-yourself, gardening, and pet care.

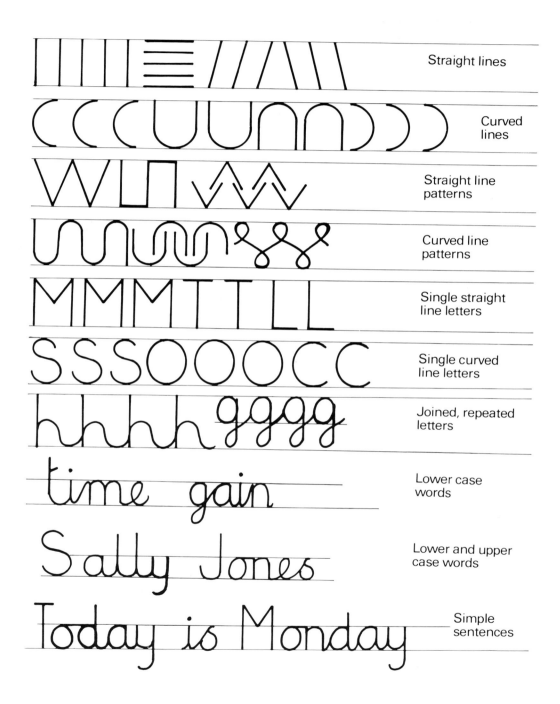

Fig. 21.10 Writing patterns, progressing to letters and words.

Name:

Date:

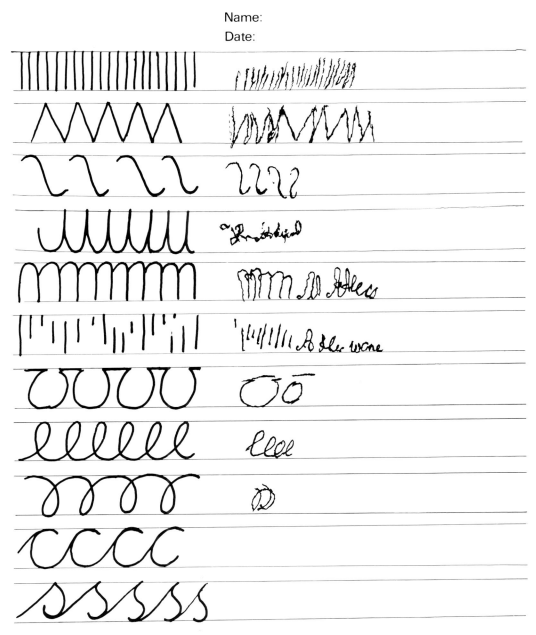

Fig. 21.11 Rhythmical writing patterns.

For the individual who has difficulty with fine movements, the therapist can scale down large activities; for example, a large chess-board used in an occupational therapy department might be replaced with a smaller version such as those used at home. Additionally, daily living activities, such as preparing vegetables, dressing, applying make-up, dusting ornaments and caring for house-plants, are all excellent ways to practise and maintain fine, coordinated movements.

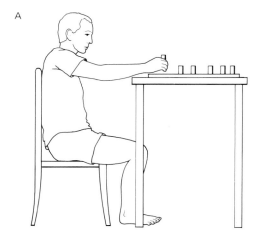

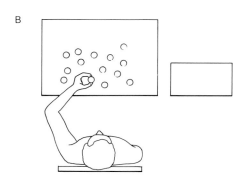

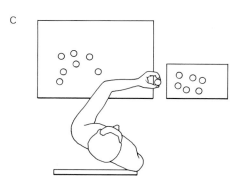

Fig. 21.12 Remedial activity to maintain and improve trunk rotation and upper-limb swing. (A) Starting position: the player sits in an upright chair without arms with the game board at chest height. (B) In mid-position he makes his game move, his upper limb working near the midline. (C) He rotates his trunk and moves his upper limb across the midline to the opposite side to place the game piece in the receptacle.

Certain activities, for example hand-press printing, may be contraindicated as they encourage poor posture, spinal flexion or static muscle work. The therapist must analyse and select remedial activity carefully in order to enhance rather than constrict movement and coordination (see Ch. 6).

Work

If the person is of working age he should continue to work as long as possible, as the discipline of a daily schedule and the physical and mental activity it requires are beneficial. Maintenance of the work role will depend upon the person's particular job and the tasks it involves, and any long-term modifications/changes need to be considered on an individual basis.

Leisure

People with Parkinson's disease should be encouraged to maintain their existing leisure interests and hobbies. During the early stage these interests can offer specific remedial input as well as a creative outlet and should, ideally, provide a balance of physically active pursuits and mentally stimulating activity. If modifications are necessary, they should be made in a way that allows the activity to retain its attraction and rewards.

Education

During the early stage of intervention the education and advice offered by the occupational therapist will be an integral part of her treatment programme. At this stage the individual's drugs will be working well, affording much symptomatic relief; therefore, education and advice should be kept to modest proportions so as not to raise anxiety levels. Advice is usually given 'in passing'; suggestions such as: 'Why not use a chair with a higher seat?', 'Doing it this way may be less tiring', or 'This type of seat will help your posture at work' should be offered as the occasion arises and interwoven with practical rehabilitation.

Personal relationships

Relationships between partners may be adversely affected not only by the disease but by anxiety and fear. Partners should be encouraged to maintain their habits and patterns of hugs, cuddles, kisses and holding hands as well as their normal sexual activity. If they are anxious, they may wish to discuss their concerns with a third party; counselling may be offered not only to allay fears but to advise on means of expressing feelings and love, including possible alternative positions for intercourse. The occupational therapist may be able to offer this advice, but if it is considered more appropriate to involve an independent counsellor, the Association to Aid Sexual and Personal Relationships of People with Disability will be able to advise and help.

LATER STAGES

The general aim of intervention throughout the later stages of Parkinson's disease both is to assist the individual and his carers to modify and adapt their life-style to meet their needs. The therapeutic programme will include:

- education and advice concerning a wide range of needs and activities, with an increasing emphasis on carers' needs
- continuation of relevant early stage activity in order to maintain function
- making arrangements in relation to mobility both within and outside the home
- support, advice and specific counselling when and where role and routine changes may be indicated
- the selection and issue of equipment to assist the person and carers with daily living
- minor and/or major adaptations to the family home, or advice regarding suitable housing if a move is being considered (see Ch. 9)
- enlistment of the services of other agencies and organisations to support and help the family.

Personal care

Clothing and footwear, undressing and dressing

- *Clothing*. The suggestions in the 'early stage' section also apply to the later stages, but carers' needs will need consideration as their relative requires more assistance. The therapist should bear in mind that:

  — fewer layers are easier to manage
  — garments should be lightweight, and warm or cool depending on the season and needs
  — combination items may be helpful, such as bra slips and slipper socks
  — fabrics should be easy to wash to cope with dribbling, any food spillage, hygiene or continence problems
  — the individual's appearance will still be important to him and if he has to modify his choice of style, for example from the more formal to more casual, his comfort and dignity must be maintained.

- *Footwear*. Choice will depend on the person's mobility level. Generally, footwear should be comfortable and supportive. It is useful to remember that:

  — if the person has a tendency to shuffle, a shoe with a leather or hard-composition sole is more functional
  — if retropulsion (spontaneous movement in a backward direction) is a problem, small heels or an inserted heel lift may help
  — low or flat heels may alleviate some of the difficulties caused by propulsion (p. 538).

- *Undressing and dressing*. As the disease progresses carers will become more involved in this activity. As mentioned above, the type of clothing, and the number and combination of garments should be chosen to assist carers as well as to meet the individual's requirements. Additional advice may include:

  — dressing the person in a warm, well-lit room to facilitate comfort
  — using a firm chair, with arms and back

support and a seat height that enables the individual to place his feet flat on the floor
— storing clothing close at hand
— when undressing, preparing items to be worn again the following day by turning them right side out
— encouraging the person to assist, while ensuring he does become overtired.

Grooming

Helping the individual to maintain a satisfactory appearance requires more effort at this stage. Increasingly, relatives will need to assist with nail care, shaving/make-up and hair brushing/styling. Advice, particularly concerning toe-nail care, may be sought. If relatives find it increasingly difficult to manage nail clippers because of the density of their relative's toe nails (and if soaking his feet in warm water first does not help) they should be referred to the local chiropodist, who will be able to advise and assist further. Many health service chiropodists employ foot-care assistants who are able to provide care within the home.

Eating and drinking

The effects of rigidity, bradykinesia and tremor are described on p. 532. Chewing difficulties, dribbling and an increasingly slow pace often result in reduced food and liquid intake, which is detrimental to the individual's general health. Individual needs will dictate individual solutions, but the following modifications to position, routine, crockery, cutlery, technique and food consistency may be used as a guide.

- The person should be assisted to attain and maintain the optimum sitting position so that he can continue to feed himself. This includes maintaining the head and neck in the 'natural curve' position of the spine, thereby discouraging excessive flexion, which inhibits swallowing.
- It may be helpful to reduce the distance between the person's hands and mouth by raising the plate or table.
- Some people will find that using the elbows

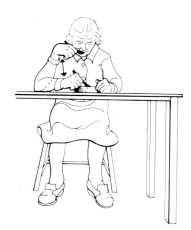

Fig. 21.13 Positioning to allow control of the upper limbs and to use one elbow as a pivot.

as pivots facilitates hand and forearm movement (Fig. 21.13).
- The routine of three meals a day may have to be changed to 5 or 6 smaller, more regular, lighter meals, thus ensuring that the person maintains his intake. Small meals will remain hot and tire the person less.
- For some people smaller, more frequent meals are not an acceptable solution as they disrupt family routine and social contact. Serving a meal on two plates, keeping one warm whilst the person eats the other may be acceptable.
- If he does not wish to use any of the above methods, the person may accept alternatives such as adapted cutlery or may concede that he has to be fed.
- Cutlery with enlarged and/or heavier grips may decrease tremor; sharp knives require less pressure and effort than dull ones.
- Some people may find that weighted bracelets help to control movement and tremor.
- Plate warmers keep food hot whilst it is being eaten.
- Deeper plates and bowls, plate guards and non-slip mats help to optimise poverty of movement.
- Two-handled and insulated mugs (which *must*

be age appropriate) help to overcome the problems experienced with small, one-handed cups and mugs and help to keep drinks hot or cold.

- Alternatively, providing drinking straws or half-filling a cup or mug may help.
- If food spillage or dribbling poses a problem, a large table napkin or apron will protect clothing.
- As swallowing difficulty increases, further advice from the speech therapist should be sought, particularly as lateral tongue movement becomes impaired.
- Advice about chewing, which may be difficult due to impaired lateral tongue movement, may also be obtained from the speech therapist, and the dietitian will advise regarding maintaining essential nutrients and a balanced diet whilst the individual has to resort to softer foods which need less or no chewing.
- Some people may, unknowingly, aspirate liquid during eating and drinking and this can lead to chest infection. The speech therapist will advise on methods of preventing aspiration whilst the physiotherapist will be able to assess lung function and help the individual to cough in order to rid his lungs of any liquid. The occupational therapist may also help if this occurs during treatment.

Washing, bathing and showering, care of teeth

Independence in these activities should be maintained for as long as possible, thus encouraging movement, coordination, dignity and a sense of well-being.

- Washing and other activities at the hand basin may need to be completed from a seated position, with required items close at hand.
- Drug therapy can cause a dry mouth and mouthwashes between as well as after meals can be refreshing, although they do not replace standard dental care.

- Bathing will become increasingly difficult and risky for the individual and his carers. Whilst a bath board, seat, non-slip mat and rails may help for a time, safety should outweigh all other considerations.
- A shower into which a shower chair can be wheeled is a very satisfactory solution for many people, providing the bathroom is warm and the individual puts on a warmed towelling robe or is wrapped in a warm bath towel afterwards.
- The person should be encouraged to wash independently, as far as this is possible, with a carer within calling distance for safety reasons.
- In the very late stages of the disease bed baths will replace showering; assistance from a bath attendant/community nursing service is usually feasible.
- Hair washing and styling will become quite difficult, and carers or a mobile hairdresser will need to help with these tasks.

Toileting

- Constipation will be exacerbated by immobility and may cause some incontinence. Advice should be sought from the local continence service and a programme of regular toileting may help, as slowness and immobility may lead to 'urgency' and accidents.
- Difficulties within the toilet often include

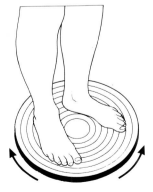

Fig. 21.14 A rotation table can ease turning whilst the person is standing.

turning round to sit down. In this case, particularly if space is confined, a rotation table (Fig. 21.14) can ease the movement for both the individual and his carer.

• Most people with parkinsonism remain continent; however, in the case of the few who do not, the cause should be investigated. If the cause is environmental — linked to poor mobility or to non-medical factors — the occupational therapist can offer practical advice and assistance, such as a routine for day and/or night toileting, commodes, portable urinals and clothing modification.

Mobility

As his disease progresses the person will become less mobile and less inclined to move about his environment; this will result in his withdrawal from many activities. His environment should therefore be utilised as a stimulus to initiate and maintain mobility for as long as possible. Some people's walking is helped by vinyl or carpet patterns, or by the layout of paving in the garden or the pavement. Therapists should reinforce the relevance of maintaining existing movement and mobility to whatever degree possible in order to control any increase in rigidity.

Administering drugs at times that suit the person's daily routine will help him to be mobile when he needs to move about his home. Additionally, adaptations will need to be considered, for example a stairlift or downstairs toilet facilities.

As the later stage advances the person may eventually be confined to a wheelchair and/or to bed. His carers will need much more advice and support as his abilities decrease and the therapist will change the emphasis of her input from the individual to the carers who are managing his daily needs. Psychologically, it is vital that the family are helped to maintain their chosen routines or advised how to modify them in a way which is acceptable to them all.

• *Walking.* Safety is of paramount importance and the occupational therapist should work with the physiotherapist and the family to maintain the required degree of

---

CASE EXAMPLE 21.2

Mr Y is 40. He lives with his wife. Son away from home. He has a short Parkinson's disease history. His first admission to hospital was 18 months ago, on which occasion he was assessed and treated by the occupational therapist. The emphasis of this programme was daily living function.

On his second hospital admission he presents as totally dependent on his wife. He exists from tablet to tablet, during which time he has approximately 10 minutes when he has some function and can help his wife to assist him.

He cannot stand, walk or sit still. His gross, uncontrollable movement patterns make it exceedingly difficult for his wife to manage, for example while feeding him.

Occupational therapy

The immediate concerns are for Mrs Y. A regime of respite care has been initiated. A lightweight wheelchair with head rest has been provided for Mr Y.

Observation of Mr Y's chemotherapy regime in order to optimise the few minutes' function he acquires.

Psychological support for Mrs Y: opportunity to discuss Mr Y's care and care of herself, including her back.

---

walking, standing and balance needed for transfers in particular.

• *Wheelchairs.* The person with Parkinson's disease should require a wheelchair permanently only in the very late stages of the condition, even if one has been utilised for outdoor mobility for some time. Carers should be taught how to use and care for the wheelchair and how to transfer the person from chair to car seat, from bed to chair, and so on. The environment should be modified where necessary, particularly for ease of access to and from the house.

Transfers

Carers will need to be taught back care and the techniques required for their particular circumstances. When and where the individual can still assist he should be encouraged to do so, for example by turning his head, moving his arms, and issuing instructions.

• *Chair transfers.* Whilst the individual can still stand from sitting he should be encouraged to do so. His carer may need to offer minimal assistance, for example by applying gentle palmar pressure on the back of his head.

The person may find a spring-loaded lever-activated (ejector) seat helpful as this will push him up and forward. However, those with poor equilibrium find these seats difficult because they cannot push up *and* step forwards simultaneously; a 'forward flexion' posture may also hinder safe use of these seats.

• *Bed transfers.* Increasingly the bed height will need to assist carers as well as the individual.

When turning over and getting out of bed a focal point on each side, such as a luminous clock-face or a bedside lamp, can help the person to concentrate. If relatives need to help him they should be taught to facilitate his movements with palmar pressure on the head/neck and pelvis as shown in Figure 21.15.

A grab rail attached to the wall beside the bed can be a useful aid to turning whilst others may find an adjustable rail on the side of the bed more helpful (Fig. 21.16).

It will become increasingly difficult for the person to raise his legs onto the bed and in order to relieve carers of constant lifting a leg lifter may be installed (Fig. 21.17).

Once he is confined to bed an electrically operated turning bed will provide a valuable adjunct to the person's care.

• *Hoists.* The need for a hoist will depend upon whether or not the individual remains at home with his relatives in the very late stages of his disease. The idea of using a hoist must be introduced tactfully. Its use must be carefully taught, as hoists require a high degree of skill to operate. Both the individual and his carers must *want* to use the hoist; this will motivate them to learn how to utilise it effectively, as its success within their home will depend on their acceptance of the equipment and the advice and support they are offered whilst learning how to use it.

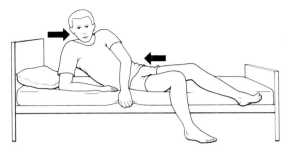

Fig. 21.15 Palmar pressure on the head/neck and pelvis will facilitate sitting up on the side of the bed.

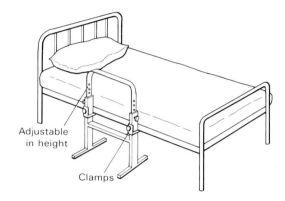

Fig. 21.16 An adjustable bed-rail may assist turning in bed.

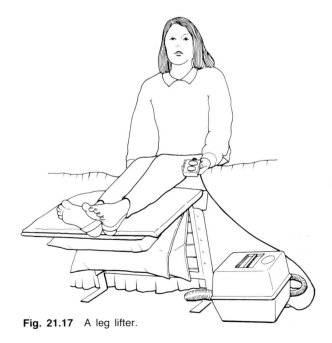

Fig. 21.17 A leg lifter.

Home-care and safety

It will become increasingly difficult for the individual to maintain all his home-care and maintenance functions but he can be involved in the decision-making within his family by being consulted about redecoration, weekly menus, and so on.

As his mobility decreases the likelihood of falls will increase; therefore, safety will assume even greater importance, and advice should be offered about lighting, floor coverings, grab rails and additional stair rails in parts of the house where he may be at risk.

In addition to the home-care suggestions made under 'Early stage', above, the individual might be advised to:

- slide rather than lift kitchen appliances
- fill the kettle from a small jug
- use a trolley *if* appropriate. This particular advice needs to be considered in terms of (a) the individual's posture, i.e. will the trolley push him into an upright position or will it encourage spinal flexion because he pushes too far ahead and therefore overbalances? and (b) the environment, for example, floor surfaces, space to manoeuvre and storage.

As the person's condition deteriorates an alarm call system may become a vital lifeline. Information concerning alarm systems is included under 'Communication', below.

As the person's needs for care increase, his family may benefit from assistance provided by community services such as home care and meals-on-wheels. These should be introduced only if the family wish to receive them and should be seen as supporting their caring role rather than taking it over.

Communication

During the later stages subtle language difficulties and some cognitive problems may emerge, and the occupational therapist must work very closely with the speech therapist if the individual is to benefit from augmentation of formal speech therapy. The following areas of communication should be addressed:

- Verbal
  - Reinforce speech therapy during occupational therapy, allowing the person time to respond to questions and to initiate conversation
  - Word charts/picture charts may help him to meet regular daily needs, for example asking for a drink
  - Posture and position should enhance respiratory capacity, thereby overcoming, to a degree, dribbling and swallowing problems which affect the efficiency of speech
- Written
  - The problems of micrographia will probably be extreme and each individual will need assistance to meet his personal needs and wishes, e.g. if he needs to sign his name he will need a stabilised writing surface and a manageable pen, but if he enjoys writing letters or a diary he will need more sophisticated means of assistance such as an electronic typewriter or word processor
- Telephone
  - The telephone can be a lifeline for some people and British Telecom offer a range of facilities, for example memory for storing numbers, the 'hands free' facility. Other companies will offer alternatives, for example an autodialling alarm facility
- Alarms
  - The variety and range of personal alarms now available is far too extensive to list here. Suffice it to say that the person with advanced Parkinson's disease should have access to an alarm system. This may be one he can wear, or one which is an integral part of an environmental control system.

Remedial activity

At this stage remedial activity will be more closely allied to daily life skills and activities and to the wishes, needs and life-style of the individual than to the encouragement of movement and coordination per se. Therefore, the person will still be encouraged to maintain his abilities, although improvement may not be anticipated. However, any of the daily tasks he undertakes can be utilised to maintain particular movements, strength and coordination, and it is important that these are activities which are of particular interest and importance to him.

Work

The working-age person's desire and ability to continue to work during the later stages of parkinsonism is dependent upon the complexities and demands of his job. Modifications may be made to his working environment or his employer may offer him an alternative within the company. Those whose occupation is heavily manual, or requires speed or great mobility may have to change jobs or cease work. The Disablement Resettlement Officer (DRO), the therapist and the individual will need to carefully evaluate needs, abilities and prospects on an individual basis.

Retiring early, on health grounds, may be a traumatic experience, and the person will need help to consider viable alternatives for paid and unpaid employment, such as working from home or assisting the local community centre in some way. If his partner still works, this may well have a drastic psychological effect on him and opportunities to discuss his feelings may be required. Home-care and self-care routines may also require modification.

Leisure

The person should be encouraged to retain his interests and leisure activities as far as possible, even if modification to scale, working position or environment, for example, is required. If this is not feasible, he may need assistance to select alternative creative and leisure outlets which stimulate, interest and reward him. He should still retain a balance between physical and mental pursuits which offer him variety and family involvement if and when appropriate. The family should endeavour to maintain their holiday pattern even if, at some stage, the type and location has to change.

Some individuals and their families participate in local Parkinson's Disease Society activities and gain much satisfaction from this outlet.

Education

During the later stages education and advice for both the individual and his carers will assume a higher profile. Advice may be offered to carers with regard to:

- encouraging their relative to maintain good posture, movement, and mobility patterns
- relaxation techniques
- when and how to help their relative
- back care and general health
- allowances and benefits
- other services such as community nursing, sitting circles, Age Concern and local church groups.

The therapist should offer opportunities to discuss the disease and its later stages. Carers should be encouraged to:

- maintain routines as far as possible, modifying and adjusting them according to need
- allow more time for activities/tasks
- allow the individual to pace himself, particularly in relation to his drug regime, his abilities and his needs
- maintain a positive attitude
- maintain a balanced life-style which meets all the family's needs and interests.

Respite care

Respite care of a short- or long-term nature may be required in the much later stages of the disease. Both the individual and his carers may find this difficult and upsetting for physical and psychological reasons, but carers do need a break periodically so that they can 'recharge their batteries'.

Respite care should be introduced delicately and gradually. A day a week at a local day centre or hospice may be quite adequate to start with, enabling the family to accustom themselves to this new kind of separation. If the carers need a longer break then residential respite care can usually be arranged, again in a local hospice or respite ward of the local hospital. Facilities and provisions will vary from area to area and the team working with the family will be able to discuss needs, concerns and the respite help available with them.

Carers may wish to stay at home while their relative is in respite care and visit him daily. This offers relief from the physical element of care and is psychologically supportive to those who feel that they are abandoning their relative if they go away on holiday for a few days. On the other hand, families may agree that the carers should take a holiday whilst respite care is provided. The manner in which respite is used will vary according to the needs and wishes of the individual and his family, who should be given every opportunity to select the option which suits them best.

CONCLUSION

Playfer (1990) states that involvement with those who have Parkinson's disease is 'both a rewarding and an exasperating experience'. Parkinson's disease is currently one of the few neurological disorders which respond so positively to chemotherapy. In recent years it has been one of the most researched conditions and results herald a far more optimistic future for individuals with the disease.

Occupational therapists, as members of teams working with those who have parkinsonism, deal with the physical, social and psychological consequences of the condition. Their knowledge, skills, techniques and expertise in function and activity enable them to offer families the opportunity to live successfully with parkinsonism. Adjustments to life-style may be necessary, but the occupational therapist's approach ensures that these are handled in an appropriately sensitive, objective and positive manner in which ability, above all else, retains its importance.

ACKNOWLEDGEMENT

My thanks to Sue Hirst, Senior Occupational Therapist, Royal Hallamshire Hospital, Sheffield, whose help made this chapter enjoyable to write.

USEFUL ADDRESSES

Parkinson's Disease Society
36 Portland Place
London W1N 3DG

SPOD (Association to Aid Sexual and Personal Relationships of People with Disability)
286 Camden Road
London N7 8BJ

REFERENCES

Bannister R 1986 Brain's clinical neurology. Oxford University Press, Oxford
Dewick H, Playfer J R 1990 Cognitive impairment in Parkinson's disease. Care of the Elderly 2(7): 260–262
Duvoisin P C 1978 Parkinson's disease — a guide for patient and family. Raven Press, New York

Geriatric Medicine 1987 Living with Parkinson's disease: a patient's perceptions. Geriatric Medicine (April): 41
Playfer J R 1990 Parkinson's disease — the future prospects. Care of the Elderly 2(7): 263–265
Scott S, Caird F I Williams B O 1985 Communication in Parkinson's disease. Croom Helm, London
Williams A 1990 Cell implantation in Parkinson's disease. British Medical Journal 301(August): 301–302

FURTHER READING

Barker S 1981 The Alexander Technique. Bantam Books, London

Caring 1988 Parkinson's disease explained. Caring (August): 6–7, 26.

Cotton E, Kinsman R 1983 Conductive education for adult hemiplegia. Churchill Livingstone, Edinburgh

Disabled Living Foundation Information Service 1990 Advice notes for people who have Parkinson's disease. ISD 90/1 Disabled Living Foundation, London

Downie P A (ed) 1986 Cash's textbook of neurology for physiotherapists. Faber & Faber, London

Franklyn S, Perry A, Beattie A 1989 Living with Parkinson's disease. Parkinson's Disease Society, London

Hildick Smith M (ed) 1985 Neurological problems in the elderly. Baillière Tindall, London

Hopkins H L, Smith H D 1988 Willard and Spackman's occupational therapy. J B Lippincott, Philadelphia

Pearce J M S 1989 Living with Parkinson's disease. Family Doctor Publications

Sachs O W 1973 Awakenings. Gerald Duckworth, London

Stern G, Lees A 1982 Parkinson's disease — the facts. Oxford University Press, Oxford

22

Peripheral nerve lesions

Annette C. Leveridge

INTRODUCTION

This chapter describes the treatment of people with nerve lesions caused by injury as this is the group most frequently referred to occupational therapists, although trauma is not the most common cause of lesions in peripheral nerves. These can be caused by many factors including, for example, a tumour pressing on the peripheral nervous system or the plaque in peripheral nerves demonstrated in multiple sclerosis.

Injury to the peripheral nerves can be as a result of:

- Direct trauma: lacerations, gunshot wounds, penetrating injuries or burns
- Indirect trauma: fracture fragments may stretch or tear a nerve
- Chronic or acute entrapment: a median nerve can be trapped in the carpal tunnel as a result of a fracture, or inflammatory disease of the joints such as rheumatoid arthritis.

The chapter begins with the classification of peripheral nerves and the anatomy of a nerve. The clinical signs and treatment for nerve injury, the classification and prognosis of peripheral nerve injuries, and specific nerve injuries are then described in some detail. A major section of the chapter is devoted to the role of the occupational therapist during the three stages of treatment — early stage, recovery, and late or chronic stage — and in the specific treatment of lower and upper extremity nerve lesions. In this section, tests used for assessing sympathetic, motor and sensory functions and the management of nerve injuries and retraining necessary for recovery of the above functions are discussed. The applications of different types of orthoses, and activities used for strengthening and sensory reeducation are also covered in this section.

The chapter concludes with a section on the likely social and psychological effects of peripheral nerve injuries on the person and his family, and stresses that a positive and informative approach by the occupational therapist will greatly enhance the rehabilitation process.

CLASSIFICATION OF PERIPHERAL NERVES

Peripheral nerve distribution to the upper extremity

The brachial plexus, formed from the anterior primary rami of the segmental spinal nerves C4 and T1 and 2, supplies the peripheral nerve distribution to the upper extremity. Occasionally the plexus arises one level more proximally or distally. At the level of the clavicle the three trunks formed

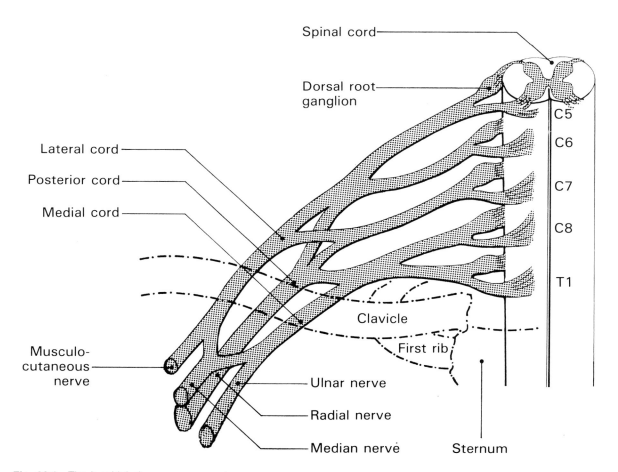

Fig. 22.1 The brachial plexus.

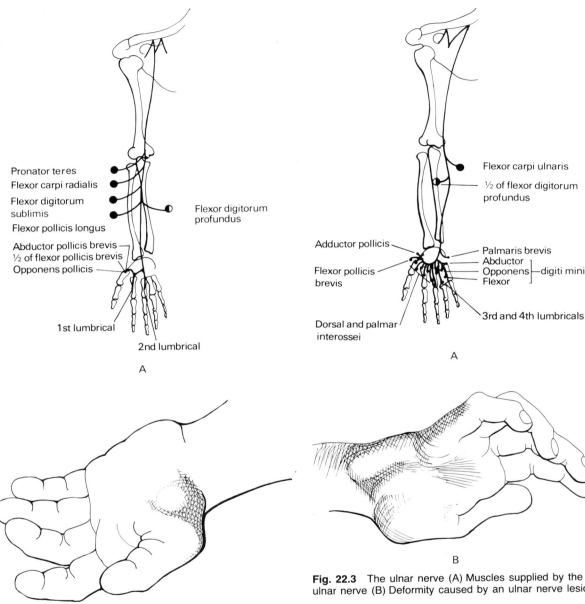

Pronator teres
Flexor carpi radialis
Flexor digitorum
sublimis
Flexor pollicis longus

Flexor digitorum
profundus

Abductor pollicis brevis
½ of flexor pollicis brevis
Opponens pollicis

1st lumbrical

2nd lumbrical

A

Flexor carpi ulnaris
½ of flexor digitorum
profundus

Adductor pollicis

Palmaris brevis
Abductor
Opponens ⎤—digiti minimi
Flexor

Flexor pollicis
brevis

3rd and 4th lumbricals

Dorsal and palmar
interossei

A

B

Fig. 22.2 The median nerve (A) Muscles supplied by the median nerve (B) Deformity caused by a median nerve lesion.

B

Fig. 22.3 The ulnar nerve (A) Muscles supplied by the ulnar nerve (B) Deformity caused by an ulnar nerve lesion.

by union of C5 and 6 roots, C7, C8 and T1 form anterior and posterior divisions which unite to form the lateral, medial and posterior cords (Fig. 22.1) (Lamb 1987).

The median nerve has two branches — the lateral root arises from the lateral cord and the medial root from the medial cord. Figure 22.2 shows the muscles supplied by the median nerve.

The ulnar nerve arises from the medial cord of the brachial plexus. Figure 22.3 shows the muscles supplied by the ulnar nerve.

The radial nerve is a continuation of the

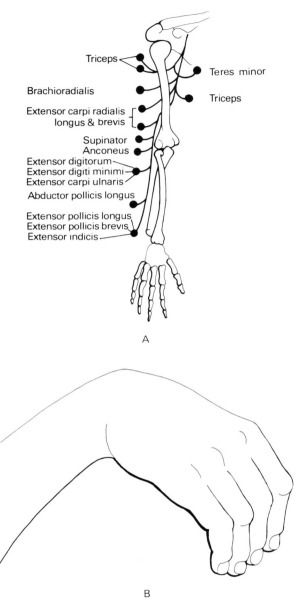

Triceps

Teres minor

Triceps

Brachioradialis

Extensor carpi radialis longus & brevis

Supinator
Anconeus
Extensor digitorum
Extensor digiti minimi
Extensor carpi ulnaris
Abductor pollicis longus

Extensor pollicis longus
Extensor pollicis brevis
Extensor indicis

A

B

Fig. 22.4 The radial nerve (A) Muscles supplied by the radial nerve (B) Deformity caused by a radial nerve lesion.

leave the brachial plexus in one nerve and join another in the arm or forearm. This may cause innervation of muscles that would normally be paralysed at certain levels of nerve injury.

Peripheral nerve distribution to the lower extremity

The nerves supplying the musculoskeletal structures of the lower limb are derived from the anterior rami of the second to fifth lumbar and the first to third sacral spinal nerves forming the lumbar and sacral plexuses.

The principal nerves of the lumbar plexus are the femoral nerve (L2–L4), the obturator nerve (L2–L4) and the lateral femoral cutaneous nerve

posterior cord of the brachial plexus. Figure 22.4 shows the muscles innervated by the radial nerve as it passes through the arm and hand.

At times there is anomalous innervation of the muscles of the hand. It is known that fibres may

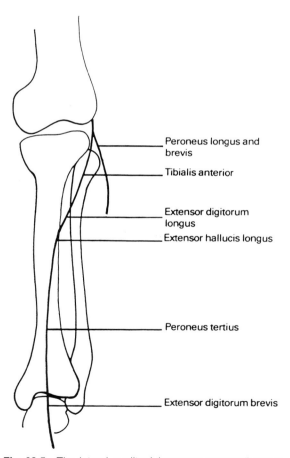

Peroneus longus and brevis

Tibialis anterior

Extensor digitorum longus

Extensor hallucis longus

Peroneus tertius

Extensor digitorum brevis

Fig. 22.5 The lateral popliteal (common peroneal) nerve.

(L2, L3). The principal nerve of the sacral plexus is the sciatic nerve (L4, L5, S1, S2, S3) which is the largest peripheral nerve of the body with a diameter of approximately 2 cm at its widest point. Superiorly and posteriorly to the knee it divides into its terminal branches, the tibial and common peroneal nerves.

The tibial nerve (L4, L5, S1, S2, S3) passes down to supply the posterior leg and the medial and lateral plantar nerves to the sole of the foot. The common peroneal nerve (L4, L5, S1, S2, S3) divides into deep and superficial branches (Fig. 22.5). The deep peroneal nerve supplies the muscles of the anterior-lateral leg region and the superficial peroneal nerve supplies the peroneal muscles.

Anatomy of a nerve

Peripheral nerves carry axons from the cell bodies in the central nervous system to the receptor organs in the motor and sensory endplates. The axon process is the fundamental unit of a peripheral nerve (Fig. 22.6). Sensory axons conduct impulses from peripheral receptors towards nerve cell bodies in the dorsal ganglia, and motor axons conduct impulses from the anterior horn cells to motor end-plates distally. Conduction in axons may occur in both directions but transmission between neurones across synapses is normally in one direction only (Smith 1990). Each axon is an extension of the individual cell within the central nervous system.

A peripheral nerve (Fig. 22.7) consists of bundles of individual fibres, each made up from many fine neurofibrils. Some fibres have a fatty myelin coat; others are thinly myelinated or unmyelinated. All fibres are surrounded by a cytoplasmic sheath, the sheath of Schwann, which is a vital covering in the process of degeneration and regeneration (Boscheinen Morris 1985). Each individual fibre is enclosed by a protective sheath or tube of connective tissue called endoneurium. This protects the individual fibres from stretching.

Nerve fibres form in bundles of varying size called funiculi or fasciculi and each funiculus (fasciculus) is ensheathed by perineurium which provides a protective cushion against external compression. Each funiculus usually contains a mixture of motor, sensory and sympathetic fibres. They are loosely packed in connective tissue called epineurium which forms the outer layer of the nerve. It acts as a protection against stretching of the fibres.

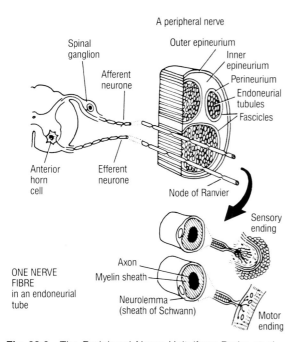

Fig. 22.6 The Peripheral Nerve Unit (from Burke et al 1990).

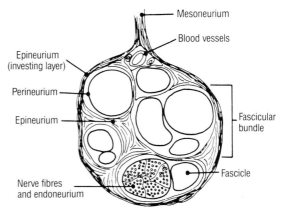

Fig. 22.7 Cross sectional anatomy of a peripheral nerve (from Lamb 1987).

PATHOLOGY OF PERIPHERAL NERVES

Degeneration and regeneration of a nerve

After injury, degeneration occurs to the level of the proximal node of Ranvier. The distal portion of the axon and myelin sheath degenerate and the subsequent debris is removed by macrophages.

Following surgical nerve repair, the proximal and distal ends are united by Schwann cell proliferation, which extends down the endoneural tube along which the axon buds migrate (Boscheinen Morris 1985).

Axons are capable of regenerating at the rate of 1 mm per day, and it is therefore possible to calculate roughly how long the functional recovery of a nerve will take. Clean divisions have the best prognosis, and the more peripheral the lesion, the better the outlook.

CLINICAL SIGNS OF NERVE DAMAGE

Motor, sensory and vasomotor changes may occur after nerve injury.

Motor changes

Paralysis leading to wasting occurs in axonotmesis or neurotmesis. This is evident at 4–6 weeks, develops rapidly at 2 months and reaches its maximum at 3 months. Imbalance of muscle leads to deformity and consequently contracture.

Sensory changes

All modalities of sensation, apart from proprioception (joint position sense), are lost. These are:

- pain
- touch
- temperature
- stereognosis
- two point discrimination.

Vasomotor changes

Circulatory changes occur. Initially the skin is warm due to vasoconstriction paralysis, but after 3 weeks, due to reduced circulation, the skin becomes cold. Trophic changes cause the skin to become dry, shiny and scaly. Skin atrophy and nail changes occur (Boscheinen Morris 1985).

TREATMENT FOR NERVE INJURY

Diagnosis

Diagnosis is assisted by a systematic examination, recording the:

- power of all muscle groups
- distribution of sensory loss
- presence and/or absence of reflexes.

Objective tests such as electromyography or conduction studies help to clarify the diagnosis and assess the prognosis, and are valuable in following the progress of denervation and recovery.

Nerve suture

The aim of a nerve repair is to join as accurately as possible the connective tissue tubes in order that the axons can regenerate down the tubes. Accurate matching of motor to motor and sensory to sensory nerve fibres produces the best results.

Primary repair is indicated where there are clean wounds and cleanly divided nerves and is carried out using very fine sutures passed through the nerve sheath, using microscopic vision.

Delayed repair is preferable for untidy wounds, because the tissues are healed and pliable at 3 to 6 weeks, making it easier to discern the amount of scar tissue to be excised.

The repaired nerve sheath takes 3 to 4 weeks to become strong enough to withstand stress, and during this time the repair is protected by an orthosis.

CLASSIFICATION AND PROGNOSIS OF NERVE INJURIES

Trauma to the peripheral nerves results in the following types of nerve injury:

- *Neuropraxia* is usually due to blunt trauma or compression. Axons remain in continuity and usually recover quickly.
- *Axonotmesis* is damage to individual axons within an intact sheath. This may be caused by direct trauma or by stretching. In the latter case the prognosis is usually worse. Axons regenerate from the proximal end, provided the cell body remains alive, and recovery should be good if the fibres are able to grow down their original neurolemma sheaths.
- *Neurotmesis*. The nerve is completely divided or irreparably damaged over part of its length. Recovery follows the same pattern as for axonotmesis but the reconnection of fibres and end-organs is likely to be much less satisfactory.

Regeneration rarely occurs unless the ends are opposed. The prognosis is better in children.

Tinel's sign is useful for assessing and following recovery. Gentle tapping along the course of the nerve will result in the sensation of pins and needles at the point where the end of the growing axons lie. This growth cone will gradually move distally as recovery proceeds. Nerves may be injured at root, plexus or trunk level. Severe injuries to major plexuses may result in avulsion of the roots from the spinal cord.

SPECIFIC NERVE INJURIES

Brachial plexus

Brachial plexus lesions generally have a poor prognosis, particularly if the injury is proximal to the dorsal root ganglion. Attempts at reconstruction of the plexus are rarely successful.

An avulsion injury caused by violent lateral flexion of the neck and depression of the shoulder may cause a brachial plexus lesion. This injury sometimes occurs as a result of a fall from a motorbike or horse.

Compression of the brachial plexus may take the form of 'Saturday night palsy' which can be caused by going to sleep with the arm over the back of a chair. Other compression injuries of the plexus may result from post-radiation fibrosis or trauma.

Some recovery may occur over the first 1 or 2 years following a severe plexus injury. When this has reached its maximum, reconstructive procedures on the arm may be considered or amputation of the flail limb may be discussed (see Ch. 25).

Radial nerve

A high lesion will result in loss of elbow extension and supination. Where the radial nerve passes through the spiral groove of the humerus it is extremely vulnerable to damage if the bone is fractured. The radial nerve and posterior interosseus branch are commonly damaged as a result of fractures of the radius and dislocations of the elbow.

Damage to the posterior interosseus branch produces weakness or paralysis of finger and thumb extension. Sensory loss is minimal, i.e. it only extends over the dorsum of the thumb web.

Damage to the radial nerve produces loss of wrist, finger and thumb extension, resulting in the characteristic 'drop wrist' (Fig. 22.8).

Direct trauma, such as lacerations caused by glass or knives over the dorsum of the wrist, will cause damage to the extensor mechanism of the hand.

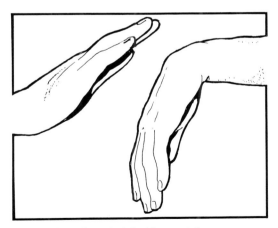

Fig. 22.8 The characteristic 'drop wrist'.

Median nerve

This is most commonly damaged at the wrist and only occasionally in the forearm or at the elbow.

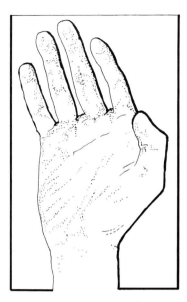

Fig. 22.9 The 'monkey hand' with its flat appearance at the thenar eminence and lack of opposition.

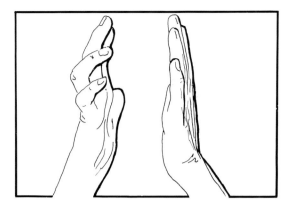

Fig. 22.10 Clawing of the ring and little fingers with flattening in the palm due to loss of interosseous function.

After a median nerve injury, the hand is likened to a monkey hand due to its flat appearance at the thenar eminence and the lack of opposition (Fig. 22.9).

In a wrist-level injury, as well as loss of thumb opposition there is a hyperextension deformity of the index and middle fingers at the metacarpal phalangeal (MCP) joints due to overaction of the finger extensors. This is caused by imbalance across the joints as a result of paralysis of the first two lumbricals.

In a high (elbow or neck) lesion there will be loss of interphalangeal (IP) thumb and finger flexion to the index and middle fingers, loss of forearm pronation and weakness of radial deviation. Sensory loss produces anaesthesia over the thumb, index, middle or middle and ring fingers.

Ulnar nerve

The ulnar nerve supplies the small muscles of the hand with the exception of some thenar muscles. The palmar interossei adduct the fingers, and the dorsal interossei abduct the fingers. In a low ulnar nerve palsy, wasting of the first dorsal interosseus and remaining interossei will be seen. A palmar

view will display clawing of the ring and little fingers with flattening in the palm due to loss of interosseous function (Fig. 22.10). As there may be paralysis of the adductor of the thumb, key pinch can only be maintained by use of flexor pollicis longus. This is known as Froment's sign.

The loss is mainly motor. Damage may occur at any level but is most common at the wrist or elbow. The intrinsic muscles in the hand, when working normally, put the fingers into a position of flexion at the MCP joints and extension at the IP joints.

When these muscles are paralysed by an ulnar nerve lesion, the fingers take up the opposite position (clawing) due to the unopposed pull of the long flexor. Sensation is absent over the little, part of the ring and possibly the middle fingers. This is very inhibiting in activities requiring stability of the ulnar border of the hand such as writing.

Femoral nerve

The femoral nerve is often damaged as a result of penetrating injuries to the anterior thigh, for example with a butcher's knife. This can result in sensory impairment to the upper part of the leg which is supplied by the cutaneous branches, and can also produce a paralysis of the quadriceps, impairing standing and walking. Stairs are a particular problem, as there is difficulty in extending the knee against resistance.

Sciatic nerve

The sciatic nerve may be damaged as a result of fractures of the pelvis and femur, and gunshot wounds of buttock and thigh. The most common injury of the sciatic nerve is compression of one or more of its roots by a lumbar intervertebral disc protrusion, causing pain down the length of the leg to the foot and foot drop. Complete interruption of the sciatic nerve results in total anaesthesia and paralysis of all the muscles below the knee.

Common peroneal nerve

This is frequently traumatised by casts or tight-fitting boots as it rounds the fibular neck just deep to the skin. This results in foot drop — due to the loss of the motor nerve supply to the muscles producing dorsiflexion and eversion of the ankle — and the cutaneous supply producing anaesthesia over the dorsum. Skin-care and vigilance concerning correctly fitting footwear and splints are of paramount importance due to the vasomotor and trophic changes that occur as a consequence of sympathetic and sensory loss.

ROLE OF THE OCCUPATIONAL THERAPIST

It should be the goal of the occupational therapist to maximise motor, sensory and sympathetic function and to help the person to compensate for residual defects, in order that he may retain his vocational role, continue his leisure pursuits and maintain his independence in self-care.

The occupational therapist will use her skills in assessment and evaluation of the injury, and will consider the psychological, social and economic factors that will affect recovery.

Liaison between the occupational therapist, physiotherapist, psychologist, social worker and rehabilitation officer is important, in order that a suitable programme of rehabilitation can be planned.

GENERAL PRINCIPLES OF TREATMENT

Treatment should be planned in three stages — the early stage, recovery and late or chronic stage — and short-term goals will depend on the current phase of recovery.

Early stage

The early stage is characterised by absence of motor, sensory and sympathetic function, and emphasis will be on the prevention of problems secondary to denervation. This stage covers the period immediately after injury and surgery until reinnervation has begun.

Sympathetic function

The therapist should note any signs of decreased sympathetic function such as dryness, temperature or colour changes, early soft tissue atrophy and nail changes. The person should be instructed in skin care and advised to watch out for inflammation or tissue damage. He should also be told how to cope with cold intolerance, by wearing thermal gloves and socks, until adequate sympathetic recovery occurs.

Motor function

The passive range of movement should be assessed and maintained in the absence of muscle power. Active ranges need to be recorded and there should be consistent measuring by the same therapist. Treatment aims to prevent the following problems that can result from muscle imbalance:

- Overstretching of paralysed muscles by unopposed contracture of antagonistic muscles
- Shortening and eventual contracture of soft tissues
- Decreased function of intact muscle due to loss of the synergistic function of paralysed muscles.

Orthoses play an important part in the early management of nerve injuries. An orthosis can be designed to substitute for a paralysed muscle, to improve function and to help prevent overstretching and contractures by restoring the muscle balance (Lamb 1987). Figure 22.16 (p. 575) shows a 'cock-up' orthosis to aid *wrist extension* in radial nerve palsy.

Most people with a single nerve lesion are able to perform self-care activities independently. Multiple, high or bilateral lesions may need provision of adaptive equipment. A functional assessment may be required and suitable advice and equipment given if the person proves to have functional difficulties.

Sensory function

Sensory loss results in a lack of protective sensation so that the person has to compensate visually. There should be an awareness of the dangers of heat, cold and sharp objects. Contact with cooker rings, heaters or lighted cigarettes often results in deep burns on the tips of fingers or the ulnar side of the hand. Insulated mugs, adequately padded oven gloves and long-handled pans should be used as a preventative measure.

Pressure and friction can cause tissue damage when tools or leisure equipment are used, and examination of the skin should be made for signs of inflammation, oedema, blisters or tissue breakdown.

Recovery stage

The recovery stage is characterised by progressive reinnervation — the emphasis being on the restoration of functions within the limits of regeneration — for example from the start of reinnervation to its maximisation (Lamb 1987).

Clinical evaluation of the extent of motor, sensory and sympathetic return is necessary at this stage.

The preventative measures used in the early stage should be continued as long as reinnervation is incomplete. The protective measures utilised will enable the therapist to commence the programme to restore function.

Sympathetic function

There will still be decreased tissue nutrition and slow healing. Until sweating has returned, lanoline or similar oily products should be massaged into the skin to counteract the dryness and cracking of skin which ensues.

A simple method to test the presence or absence of sweating is to rub a plastic pen or biro over the area. If sweating is not present, the pen will slip. Comparison with the same area on the other side will demonstrate the difference, as normal skin will offer resistance to the surface of the pen.

During the recovery stage people may be resuming their former activities. Any blisters, lacerations or wounds occurring as a result of a return to normal occupations using tools and equipment should be treated with care to prevent infection and further injury. The person should continue monitoring the areas.

Motor function

The therapist should be aware of the pattern of recovery of the nerve and recognise trick movements and supplementary action by normal muscles.

Retraining activities to increase strength, coordination and endurance can begin. Until good balance of the muscles is restored, substitution orthoses provided in the early stage will need to be worn when the person is not exercising in order to rest and support the recovering muscles.

Sensory function

Without adequate sensation the person will be unable to use his hand efficiently. Sensory stimuli are initiated as a result of excitation of sensory nerve endings of which there are two kinds:

- *exteroceptive* — occurring in skin, ears, eyes and other internal organs
- *proprioceptive* — occurring in joint capsules, muscle spindles and tendons.

Without sensory feedback from all receptors, a highly skilled and smooth performance of movement cannot be attained.

The stage of sensory nerve regeneration can be assessed by using the *Tinel test* to indicate the progression of regenerating sensory axons. The therapist may thus learn the correct time to start testing for sensory function.

The pattern of return of sensation as regeneration progresses is: protective sensation (deep pressure and pin-prick) followed by moving touch, static touch and discriminative touch.

Touch. Tactile testing is used in order that the therapist may discover whether the skin is anaesthetic, hyperanaesthetic, hypoanaesthetic or normal. This can be performed by using the light touch of the tester's finger or by using a cotton-wool ball. The person being tested is asked to identify whether the touch feels like pins and needles, is normal, or is different in any other way.

Protective sensation can be tested by using a pin-prick, or subjecting the area being assessed to the stimulus of a tube of hot water and a tube of cold water. The person indicates whether the tests are felt and whether or not the sensation is normal compared to the other limb.

After it has been shown that light touch and protective sensation are present, discriminative sensation can be tested by:

- static two-point discrimination
- moving two-point discrimination.

Two-point discrimination is the ability to recognise whether the skin is being touched by one or two points simultaneously. It is developed to a fine degree in the skin at the fingertips.

Further information will help the therapist to decide whether there is a need for sensory reeducation and when it should start. This can be obtained by performing the following tests:

- localisation
- timed pick-up tests.

Localisation is the ability to recognise the exact position of a stimulus on the skin.

During the sensory recovery period the affected skin may undergo a period of hypersensitivity. This can be very distressing and may in turn hinder recovery.

Desensitisation is a programme of graded stimulation to an area to increase its tolerance for tactile input. Stimulation includes rubbing or brushing the area with an assortment of textures which are just past the level of comfort when ap-

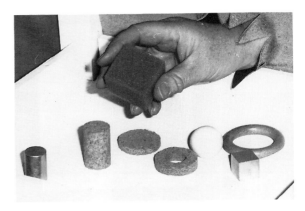

Fig. 22.11 Sensory reeducation.

plied to the area. It can also include tapping or vibration. The tactile input should be followed by active use of the involved area.

Sensory reeducation. The concept of improving sensory function by assessment and reeducation was pioneered by Maureen Salter and Dr Wynn Parry at the Joint Services Medical Rehabilitation Unit at RAF Chessington. As a result of their work it was realised what gross disability can arise from sensory impairment. Many people who have full motor recovery claim that they are unable to work because they have impaired sensation.

The aim of reeducation (Fig. 22.11) is to enable people to make the best use of their recovery by establishing a new bank of codes with which to interpret the altered sensory signals.

Chronic stage

Eventually there is a levelling off of the recovery of motor, sensory and sympathetic function and most people will have returned to their normal life-styles by this time. Those with high or multiple lesions with only a small amount of recovery will need help from the therapist to compensate for residual deficits.

The aim will be to maximise the power of normal muscles, especially those substituting for paralysed ones, and maximise the strength of muscles with return of power.

It may be necessary for the surgeon to carry out

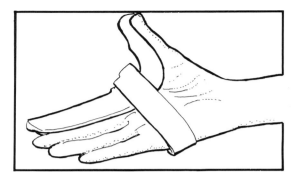

Fig. 22.12 Thumb web spacer.

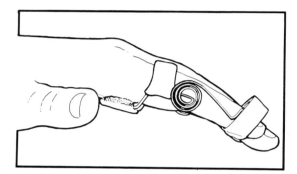

Fig. 22.13 A Capener orthosis.

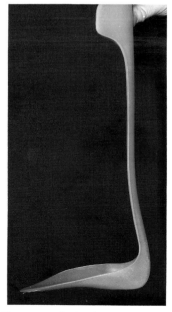

Fig. 22.14 Temporary foot raise.

tendon transfer surgery; therefore the skin and soft tissue will need to be kept soft and the maximum passive range of movement maintained. Deformities should be corrected by orthoses. Examples include thumb web spacers for tight webs (Fig. 22.12); Capener orthoses for proximal interphalangeal joint (PIP) contractures (Fig. 22.13); wrist dorsiflexion orthoses for drop wrists (Fig. 22.16); and ankle dorsiflexion orthoses for foot drop (Fig. 22.14).

During active use of the hand, work orthoses may be needed and a work programme devised to suit the individual. Assessment may indicate the need for modification of the home or work environment; therefore liaison with community services and the person's employer is important, particularly if retraining is required.

The goal of occupational therapy must be to restore the person to vocational, personal and leisure activities to a level which will satisfy his needs.

SPECIFIC TREATMENT FOR UPPER EXTREMITY NERVE LESIONS

Occupational therapy intervention for upper extremity nerve lesions should encompass the following:

- Provision of orthoses and adaptations appropriate to the person's needs at various stages of treatment
- Therapeutic media, for example games, computers with appropriate switches, wood-work and printing, aimed at muscle retraining and strengthening
- Education.

Brachial plexus

If the brachial plexus is ruptured, surgery will be required first, whereas an avulsion or lesion in continuity will only need rehabilitation.

Recovery, if expected, can take up to 2 or 3 years after the lesion occurs. It is important that the person is encouraged to return to his home and work environment as soon as possible. The therapist should see him at regular intervals to assess his progress, orthosis and his functional levels at home and work.

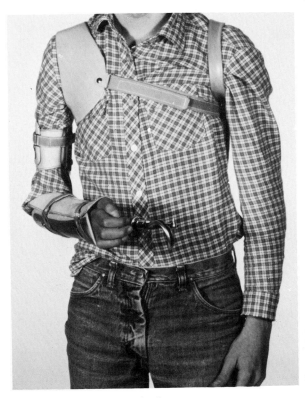

Fig. 22.15 A flail arm orthosis.

Positioning the upper limb in an orthosis supports the shoulder and reduces the risk of subluxation. A wrist extension orthosis or support will stabilise the wrist and hold it in a good position. A flail arm orthosis may be provided for those whose expected recovery will be over a long period or who have total lesions (Fig. 22.15). The severe burning pain characteristic of the brachial plexus lesion can be controlled to some extent by transcutaneous nerve stimulation and anticonvulsant drugs, but distraction is also a very effective method of relief.

People should therefore be encouraged to return to their hobbies and work and, if necessary, retrain for alternative employment. Orthosis-supported activities aimed at maintaining a range of movement throughout the upper limb and preventing subluxation of the shoulder may include:

- large draughts
- stool seating

- sanding
- collating
- cooking
- computer keyboard work.

Radial nerve

The person will be unable to simultaneously extend the wrist and fingers and to radially abduct the extended thumb.

An orthosis is required:

- To assist grasp and enhance grasp strength by providing a stable wrist in extension
- To prevent overstretch of the wrist extensors by unopposed wrist flexion. A simple 'cock-up' orthosis positioning the wrist in extension should be worn during all working hours (Fig. 22.16)

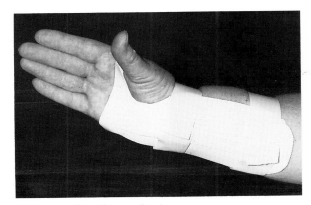

Fig. 22.16 A cock-up orthosis.

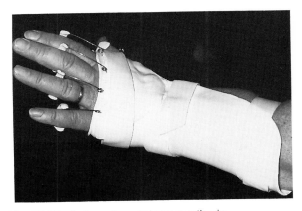

Fig. 22.17 A dynamic radial nerve orthosis.

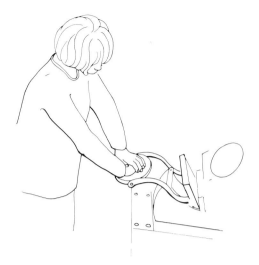

Fig. 22.18   Printing using the wrist-extension board.

- To correct a wrist deformity in flexion, serial 'splinting' or a dynamic wrist extension orthosis should be worn.

A dynamic orthosis will substitute metacarpophalangeal joint extension by elastic or spring traction (Fig. 22.17).

Activities that require muscles to work in groups and therefore facilitate the development of coordination as well as strength should be selected. Those that require a stable wrist during grip, with simultaneous wrist and finger extension, are useful for radial nerve retraining and include:

- pottery — rolling out coils for coil pots
- pastry — rolling it out
- woodwork — sanding and polishing for wrist extension
- printing — an extension board on the printing press for wrist extension (Fig. 22.18)
- games — shoveboard for elbow and wrist extension, wall draughts for elbow and wrist extension
- computer — keyboard games with Myolink and other switches should be introduced (Fig. 22.22).

For later stages, games such as Jacks (five stones) and finger flicking table football are suitable.

When elbow extension and motor control are developing, darts can be used for wrist and finger extension.

Median nerve

The median nerve supply to the hand provides it with a delicate and skilled function due to its excellent motor and sensory supply. Activities such as tying up shoe-laces and writing, and other fine movements, are affected by injury to the median nerve. Orthoses are required to counteract the flat 'monkey palm' deformities that occur due to loss of opposition of the thumb and overaction of the extensor digitorum communis (Fig. 22.19). A thumb rotation strap can be made to dynamically bring the thumb into palmar abduction and opposition to facilitate grip (Fig. 22.20).

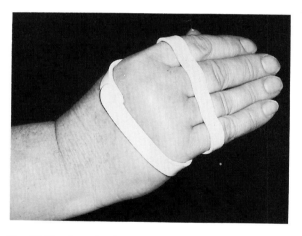

Fig. 22.19   An orthosis is required to counteract flat 'monkey palm' deformities.

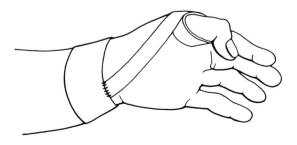

Fig. 22.20   Thumb rotation strap.

After 12 weeks a Capener orthosis can be used to actively extend the IP joints of the index and middle fingers should flexion contractures occur (Fig. 22.21), and thumb web contractures can be counteracted by static web serial orthosis (Fig. 22.22).

People with a median nerve lesion demonstrate clumsiness when attempting to pick up large or small objects due to loss of sensation. Sensory stimulation and sensory retraining are most important. Power grip is affected because the stabilising

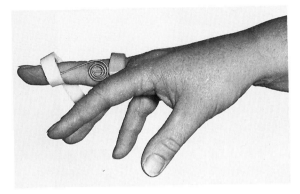

Fig. 22.21 A Capener orthosis for active extension of the interphalangeal joints.

action of the thumb is lost. Loss of palmar abduction of the thumb results in an inability to open the hand to grasp large objects such as a beer glass (Boscheinen Morris 1985).

In the early stages of treatment, activities involving the whole arm should be used. As recovery takes place, attention should be paid to tripod grip.

Activities which can be used include:

- For fine pinch, light pick-ups of small objects graded in size and weight:
  — macramé work
  — pinchpot ceramics
  — light dowel and pin solitaire
  — composing printing.
- For gross pinch:
  — coil and pinch pottery
  — pastry and bread making
  — computer and keyboard games (Fig. 22.22).

Strengthening activities in the later stages of treatment include weight lifting, gardening and woodwork with hand tools.

Residual problems that occur with this lesion may be a permanent lack of thenar muscle re-

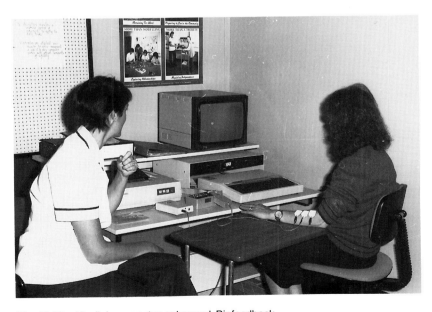

Fig. 22.22 Myolink computer-enhanced Biofeedback.

innervation. An opponens transfer can restore function to the thumb but only if there is sufficient sensation present to ensure that the operative procedure is worthwhile, and rerouting of a tendon will require muscle retraining in most cases. Alternatively the lively thumb opposition orthosis can be used.

Ulnar nerve

A lesion of the ulnar nerve results in a claw hand. This can be controlled by an orthosis which will support the MCP joints in flexion and prevent hyperextension, thus allowing the long extensors to act on the IP joints in the absence of the intrinsic muscles (Fig 22.23).

Loss of stability and power together with loss of coordination are the results of ulnar nerve lesions. These may affect such activities as typing, keyboard playing and sports activities requiring grip of a racquet handle.

Whole arm activities should be used in the early stages, and as recovery occurs, activities involving cylindrical and gross grip, thumb lateral pinch and opposition, and interphalangeal joint extension

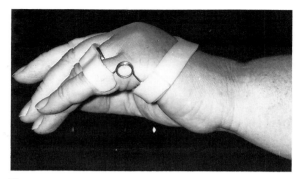

Fig. 22.23 Correction of the claw hand using orthotic support for the MCP joints in flexion.

should be used. Power activities can be used, i.e. syringe blow football for grip strength and woodwork using tools to develop strength and stability of grip. Wall and table board draughts, printing using adapted handles and polishing to assist coordination, are other useful activities. Keyboard work is utilised for finger dexterity and adduction and abduction of fingers, as are slab and coil methods of pottery. Writing practice may be required, due to sensory involvement of the ulnar border of the hand.

CASE EXAMPLE 22.1: MR R. M., AGED 35

Occupation

Cab driver (married), right handed.

Diagnosis

Laceration left wrist: (November '89)
50% division median nerve
99% division ulnar nerve
10% division flexor digitorum sublimis index
  finger
10% division flexor digitorum sublimis middle
  finger
30% division flexor digitorum sublimus ring
  finger
100% division flexor carpi ulnaris
100% division pollicis longus
100% division ulnar artery.

All repaired on day of injury in theatre of Plastic Surgery Unit.

- Kleinert traction to all four fingers with POP backslab.
- Pulleys fitted to produce good line of pull.
- Kleinert traction retained for 6 weeks.

- Referred to physiotherapy from day one for active extension of fingers, elastic traction producing protected flexion, with protective orthosis, monitored by OT department.
- After 6 weeks — active mobilisation under supervision.
- After 7 weeks — flexion of MCPs, but IP flexion minimal. Signs of post traumatic sympathetic dystrophy — needing intensive exercise programme 9 weeks after operation. Improved R of M of fingers with minimal clawing of ring and little fingers.
- Complaining of sensory impairment on ulnar side of hand.
- Hypersensitivity in palm. Some poor quality sensation at tips of little and ring fingers.
- Median side of hand — feeling normal apart from palm.
- Tinel sign up to distal palmar crease on ulnar side.

Twelve weeks after operation
- Remains with no opposition of left thumb.
- Seen by Consultant who concluded that Mr R. M. would require an opponens tendon transfer to bring thumb round into opposition,

although muscle power was thought to be improving in thenar eminence. EMG results after testing (L) hand median nerve produced no movement from the thenar eminence with stimulation of the median nerve, but a very small signal was recorded.

- An Electrical Sensory Threshold test produced a mixed picture of sensation.

To occupational therapy for assessment, workshop activities and orthoses as required.

Assessment

Problems (L) hand (see Table 22.1)
1. Difficulty in opposing thumb to ring and little fingers
2. Non-functional pinch grip
3. Difficulty abducting and adducting fingers
4. Reduced grasp and grip strength
5. Reduced sensation to palm, ring and little finger
6. Hypersensitivity of palm
7. Difficulty flexing MCPs of ring and little finger
8. Difficulty extending PIP of ring and little finger.

Functional difficulties

Work:
Driving — handbrake, gearstick, radio controls,

handling money — all necessary to job as cab driver.
Leisure:
Golf — producing a good grip.

Goal

To have increased functional ability and sensation in hand, which would enable Mr R. M. to return to work, manage activities of daily living and pursue leisure interests.

Aims

- Maintain/improve range of movement
- Maintain/improve muscle strength
- Increase grip strength
- Prevent deformity by using a dynamic opponens orthosis by day and a night-resting thumb post orthosis for opposition
- Increase ability to oppose thumb
- Increase sensibility, especially to ring and little finger
- Improve range of extension of PIP of ring and little finger
- Decrease hypersensitivity of palm
- Increase understanding of condition and precautions needed
- Increase motivation for recovery.

Table 22.1 Activity plan using horticulture

Activity	Tool/positioning	Grading	For problem		Precaution
1. Mixing soil compounds, potting compost, sand, perlite, small gravel, pebbles, marbles	Seated at table Eyes closed/open for identification of compounds/materials	Smoother (e.g. sand) to harder textures (e.g. pebbles) Sieving increases stimulation	(5) (8)	(3) (6)	Skin care *Allergy Hygiene
2. Sowing seeds	* Seated at table — Using pinch grips — Using palmar crease	Large → small sizes. Using tweezers then fingers Using pinch grip easy → difficult fingers	(2) (1)	(7) (5)	
3. Taking cuttings	* Seated at table Using secateurs/scissors Cutting down onto board with knife	Thin → thicker plant material Therapist assisted → independent, large → small handles on knife	(7) (8)	(4) (5)	Care with sharp tools Supervision at all times
4. Watering-can/mister	* Seated or standing	Amount of water Length of time Easy → difficult MCPs	(4) (1) (5)	(3) (6)	Correct positioning of thumb
5. Pricking out	* Seated	Large → small leaved plants Opposing index → ring finger	(2)	(3)	Avoid lateral pinch grip
6. Potting up plants	* Seated	Large → small pots Increase	(3) (5) (7)	(4) (6) (2)	As for soil compounds

NB: Concentration on thumb opposition and finger abduction/adduction where possible
* Using dynamic opponens orthosis

Treatment selected

Orthoses to deformities, and horticulture to improve dexterity and sensation (Table 22.1).
1. Capener orthosis to ring finger fully extended PIP joint within one week
2. Opponens splint worn for activities over 4 weeks.

After one week of activities — hypersensitivity of palm diminishing, but still little sensation on ulnar border of the hand.

After two weeks, sensation returning (tingling to ring and little finger).

Opposition of thumb still absent, so placed on waiting list for opponens plasty.

Ten months after injury

- Excellent progress
- Almost normal sensation in median territory
- Recovering ulnar nerve sensation, with slight weakness of intrinsic muscles
- All FDS and FDP function 100% recovery
- FCU function 100%
- Now good opposition pinch, therefore does not require opponens plasty operation
- He is now working again as self-employed cab driver.

The treatment plan for this man demonstrates the benefit of purposeful activity in improving hand function and sensory return after tendon and nerve injury.

The activity plan using horticulture was devised by a London School of Occupational Therapy third year student, Susan Lynch.

Combined median and ulnar lesions

These lesions produce a very severe disability. When both nerves are divided at wrist level, with accompanying tendon and vessel damage, scarring and fibrosis adhesions between the tendons and nerves may form.

This results in a totally flat claw hand. *Dynamic* orthoses (Fig. 22.24), enabling the person to extend his fingers and improve function, should be instituted. Sensation will be absent on the whole of the volar surface, and over the dorsal surfaces of the tips of all fingers and the volar surface of the thumb (Fig. 22.25). Sensory reeducation is of extreme importance.

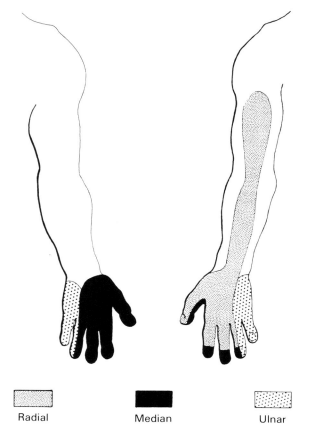

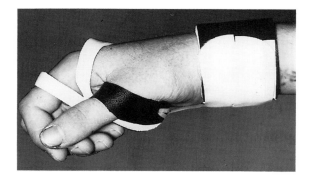

Fig. 22.24 Dynamic orthosis for a combined median and ulnar lesion.

Fig. 22.25 Sensory distribution in the upper limb covered by the median, ulnar and radial nerves.

Sensory reeducation

Stereognosis is the most appropriate means of reeducating sensation. This should commence when sensation of the palm has returned more or less to normal but the finger tips are still hyperanaesthetic.

Sensory reeducation is appropriate after division of the median nerve in particular, because the thumb, index and middle fingers are most commonly used for dexterity in pinch and prehension grips. The ring and little fingers supplied by the ulnar nerve are used mostly for power grip and so do not require the same high degree of sensitivity. The reeducation programme should include specific sensory activities and activities involving functional use of the hand, for example horticulture, potting and planting, and 'Fimo' modelling, clay. 'Fimo' is a coloured modelling material which hardens in minutes in a kitchen oven. To manipulate, rolling and pinching movements are used, and small figures, jewellery and plaques can be formed.

Stereognosis

Stereognosis is recognition of objects through touch stimuli alone. A great deal of concentration is required and therefore the tests should be carried out in a quiet room, with minimum distraction. The person should be blindfolded or should keep his eyes shut during the test (Salter 1987). This is preferable to using a screen or curtain that separates hand and person. He should not see the chart or test items beforehand, in order to eliminate guessing or learning.

External stimuli can be eliminated by covering a table with a layer of foam rubber. A finger stall or cut-out glove can be used to eliminate normal sensation in ulnar-fed digits.

Method

1. The person is given one of several different shaped blocks (Fig. 22.11) and asked to describe it and identify as many properties as possible — for example, is it flat, smooth, cold, square? The object should be simple to identify at first. The person is then asked to open his eyes and describe the object again, adding any properties he missed. He can also repeat the test with his unaffected hand and then try again

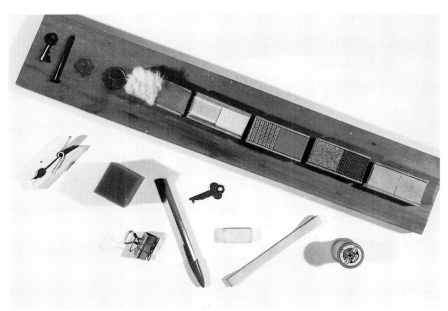

Fig. 22.26 Textures and shapes used for stereognosis.

with the affected one. The time taken for correct recognition is noted.

2. The second stage involves timed recognition of textures, starting with easily identifiable contrasts such as velvet and coarse sandpaper (Fig. 22.26). As recognition improves, textures with only subtle differences can be introduced, and suitable materials include velvet, cotton wool, sandpaper, metal, cork, wool, a scouring pad and fur.

3. The final stage is the recognition of everyday objects such as a nailbrush, electric plug, matchbox or tennis ball. Once these have been mastered, fine objects such as a coin, safety pin, paper clip, button or peg can be used. This can be made more difficult by planting them in containers of rice, lentils, sand or beans (Fig. 22.27), and, additionally, speed tests can be introduced.

Trials undertaken by Maureen Salter showed normal recognition of shapes to be well under 5 seconds, and often 2 seconds. People with median nerve lesions may take over 5 seconds or not identify the object at all.

Documentation of results is important in order that regular assessment and comparison of im-

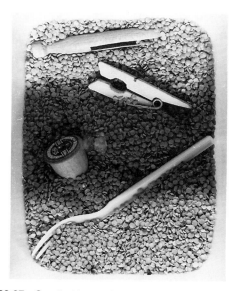

Fig. 22.27 Small objects planted in lentils can aid sensory reeducation.

provement of sensory awareness is recorded and made (Fig. 22.28). Sensory reeducation testing should take place regularly over a short span of time. A session should not last more than three quarters of an hour, otherwise interest and concentration diminish considerably.

Selection of participants for a stereognosis programme

- The age and intelligence of the person affects his ability to recognise objects and textures
- Motivation is vital
- People of different cultures and occupations will recognise familiar items at different speeds
- Expectations have to be realistic
- Functional use of the hand must be encouraged.

Localisation training

Localisation training will usually be necessary after a complete or partial division of a nerve (Salter 1987). Localisation may be altered because not all axons regenerate to their correct end-organs following surgery and so the person will receive false information from his fingertips. Training will correct this as long as he makes continual functional use of his hand.

The person is asked to close his eyes and the therapist touches an area of the volar surface of his hand, using moving finger touch, and asks him to identify the point of contact with the index finger of the other hand. A correct response can be recorded on a hand chart (Fig. 22.29) with a tick, and an incorrect response is recorded by filling in the number denoting the area which was actually touched. If the answer is incorrect the person is asked to look at the testing point to relearn the location. The test should be repeated with the person's eyes open, and then with them closed. This should enable him to recognise the spot where he is being touched. Localisation training should be repeated over and over again during the subsequent weeks.

OCCUPATIONAL THERAPY SENSORY ASSESSMENT

Name: .... Age: .... Record No. ....
Address: ....
Occupation: .... Consultant: ....
Diagnosis: .... Occupational Therapist: ....

Main functional difficulties *Dominant hand*
Work
Daily activities
Hobbies
Stereognosis

Date						
Shapes (Test one section only)	Interpretation	Time	Interpretation	Time	Interpretation	Time
1. Square						
Oblong						
Triangle						
Diamond						
2. Circle						
Oval						
Semi-circle						
Moon						
Average time						
Texture (Test 6 items)						
Sandpaper						
Formica						
Wood						
Rubber						
Carpet						
Leather						
Velvet						
Fur						
Cotton wool						
Sheepskin						
Plastic						
Metal						
Average time						

Fig. 22.28 (cont'd overleaf)

Date						
Coins (Test 3 items)	Interpretation	Time	Interpretation	Time	Interpretation	Time
1p						
2p						
5p						
10p						
20p						
50p						
£1						
Average time						
Objects — large 1. (Test 3 items)						
Sink plug						
Cotton reel						
Plug						
Bottle						
Saucer						
Soap						
Egg cup						
Tea strainer						
2. (Test 3 items)						
Pencil						
Fork						
Metal comb						
Ball point pen						
Screwdriver						
Teaspoon						
Toothbrush						
Paintbrush						
Peg						
Average time						

Fig. 22.28 Chart used to record stereognosis.

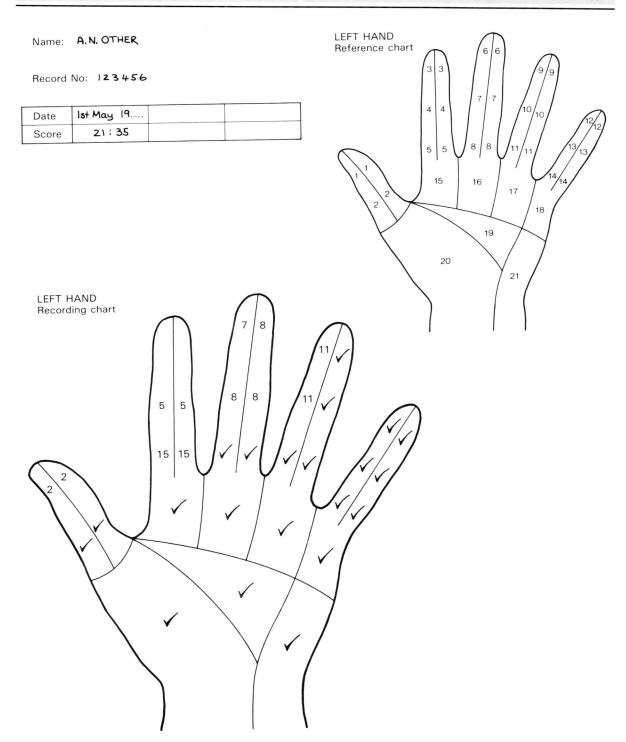

Name: A.N. OTHER

Record No: 123456

Date	1st May 19.....		
Score	21 : 35		

LEFT HAND
Reference chart

LEFT HAND
Recording chart

Fig. 22.29 A localisation chart to indicate areas of absent or affected sensation within the hand.

SPECIFIC TREATMENT FOR LOWER EXTREMITY NERVE LESIONS

After lesions of the sciatic nerve and of the common peroneal nerve (lateral popliteal) it is important to prevent foot drop and contracture of the calf muscles.

A temporary foot-raise should be fitted (Fig. 22.14), and if no recovery occurs it may have to be worn permanently. Sensory loss (Fig. 22.30) demands precautionary measures and foot care. The therapist should ensure that the person understands the necessity for foot hygiene: he should wash his feet daily, carefully drying the skin, and wear clean socks or tights daily. Skin should be checked for rubbing or bruising and the cause removed before further damage occurs.

A static anti-foot-drop orthosis may be required for night use.

Activities for the lower limb should involve use of the whole leg in the early stages of treatment to maintain range of movement and muscle balance. As recovery of the common peroneal nerve occurs, activities are needed to provide active dorsiflexion and eversion of the foot. Games such as foot

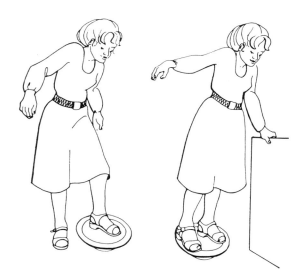

Fig. 22.31 The wobble board used to strengthen the ankles.

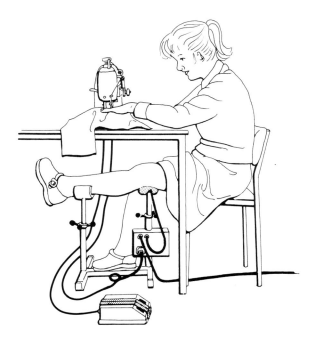

Fig. 22.32 The quadriceps switch.

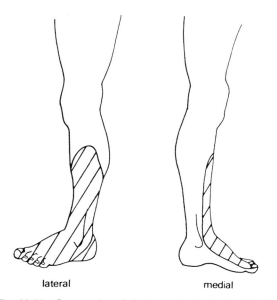

lateral   medial

Fig. 22.30 Sensory loss following a lesion to the lateral popliteal nerve.

draughts and activities providing ankle rotation, dorsiflexion and plantarflexion, for example gardening, workshop tasks and squatting to work, can be utilised. A wobble board (Fig. 22.31) is a useful piece of rehabilitation equipment, and a foot maze marble game can be incorporated to give the board's usage more purpose and interest to the user. General mobility should be encouraged at all times.

Damage of the femoral nerve requires retraining of the quadriceps muscle group. The rehabilitation cycle can be utilised for this, as can the Akron quadriceps switch (Fig. 22.32) harnessed to a tape recorder, computer or other electrical appliances.

After complete division of the nerves of the lower limb, recovery is often slow and sometimes incomplete. It may be necessary to continue treatment for 2 or 3 years. After a pressure neuropathy of the common peroneal nerve, a satisfactory recovery usually occurs in 6 to 12 months.

EDUCATION OF THE PERSON AND HIS FAMILY

Peripheral nerve injuries have psychological implications for the individual which may present in many ways, and reaction may not be proportionate to the extent of the physical injury. Disturbance of body image and loss of self-esteem are of major importance to some, whilst potential loss of function and the social factors implicated will be more important to others.

Factors that may affect the person are:

- disruption of family life due to admission to hospital of the person, whether it be father, mother or child
- temporary or permanent loss of employment
- temporary loss of personal independence
- disruption of leisure pursuits and social contact
- reaction to pain, which may be affected by the person's cultural and religious background.

Motivation can be influenced by:

- the actual degree of the injury and its effect on the person's work and leisure activities
- support provided by family and friends

- psychological state of the person before injury, for example nerve injury after attempted suicide or reactive depression
- level of intelligence, for example the person may not be able to understand or appreciate the importance of relearning skills and their purpose
- language difficulties and cultural background
- attitude of the person to the surgeon and rehabilitation staff.

A positive working relationship between the individual and family and occupational therapist should be established. Fear and anxiety about the future may be alleviated by the provision of as much information as possible about the condition and the treatment involved. Relatives should be encouraged to participate in the rehabilitation process, and instruction about exercise regimes, orthoses and sensory training should be provided for the individual and relatives.

Photographs demonstrating the function that others have achieved with similar injuries may be helpful. A positive approach by the therapist is of paramount importance.

CONCLUSION

Working with people who have peripheral nerve lesions is challenging to the therapist because:

- the causes of lesions are numerous
- surgical intervention is increasingly inventive and skilled, particularly in the field of microscopic surgery
- conservative measures develop as people's needs dictate.

Occupational therapists' assessment, intervention and evaluation contribute practical, realistic and imaginative input into programmes, whether the individual is expected to make a maximum motor and sensory recovery or whether he has to be assisted to compensate and adapt to permanent deficits.

REFERENCES

Boscheinen Morris J 1985 The hand: fundamentals of therapy. Butterworth, London
Burke F D, McGrouther D A, Smith P J 1990 Principles of hand surgery. Churchill Livingstone, Edinburgh
Lamb D 1987 The paralysed hand. Churchill Livingstone, Edinburgh

Salter M 1987 Hand injuries: a therapeutic approach. Churchill Livingstone, Edinburgh

FURTHER READING

Barr N R, Swan D 1988 The hand: principles and techniques of splintmaking. Butterworth, London
Bannister R 1986 Brain's clinical neurology. Oxford University Press, Oxford

Mills D, Fraser C 1989 Therapeutic activities for the upper limb. Winslow Press, Bicester, Oxon
Zeigler E M 1984 Current concepts in orthotics. Unicomp, Chicago

23

Spinal cord lesions

Jane Henshaw

INTRODUCTION

In 2500 BC an Egyptian physician described tetraplegia as 'a mortal condition — an ailment not to be treated'. This view of spinal lesions was held for thousands of years, extending into the early part of this century. During the 1914–1918 war 90% of all people with spinal lesions died within one year of injury and as recently as the 1960s the mortality rate for tetraplegia was 35%.

In recent years, great strides have been made in the medical and paramedical care of people with spinal cord lesions, whose life expectancy is now virtually normal. One very important factor in the treatment of this group of people has been the establishment of centres throughout the country where the individual and his family can be given the specialist care and assistance they need (Fig. 23.1). This chapter examines the important contribution that the occupational therapist can make in the treatment of individuals who have suffered spinal cord lesions.

The first sections of the chapter describe the characteristics of spinal cord lesions, including their causes and classification as well as the complications to which they commonly give rise. The chapter then presents an overview of the kinds of treatment now available to individuals with spinal cord lesions, outlining the aims of surgical inter-

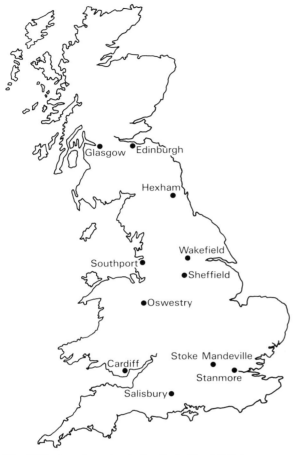

Fig. 23.1 Location of spinal units in Great Britain.

vention, nursing care and physiotherapy as well as the significant role played by the social worker and the psychologist.

The chapter then turns in greater detail to the interventions of the occupational therapist during the 'acute' and 'rehabilitation' stages of care. First, her role in providing psychological support to the individual and his family during the acute or bed-rest stage is described; this includes helping the individual to make productive use of his time while in hospital, providing therapy to maintain hand function, helping the individual to plan for his return to the community, and assessing his specific requirements in the choice of a wheel-chair.

Next, the chapter describes the rehabilitation

stage of treatment, during which the therapist will help the individual to regain maximum inde-pendence in self-care tasks, communication skills, domestic activities, and so on. Various transfer techniques suitable for the paraplegic or tetra-plegic person are explained. Procedures for pre-paring the individual for resettlement at home and in the community are described, and practical con-siderations relating to work and education, leisure activities, driving and sexual function are briefly discussed.

It is evident that a spinal cord lesion can have a profound impact upon virtually all aspects of an individual's life, and that the occupational therapist's involvement in his rehabilitation will be both challenging and extensive. It is important, however, for the therapist to be aware of other sources of support for paraplegic or tetraplegic in-dividuals, and addresses of relevant organisations are provided at the end of the chapter.

CHARACTERISTICS OF SPINAL CORD LESIONS

Causes

The causes of spinal lesion are many and varied, ranging from the bizarre to the mundane. In general, however, they may be described as either traumatic or non-traumatic.

Traumatic causes involve a direct force or impact on the spinal column causing disruption of the vertebral bodies, tearing of the ligaments and damage to the cord or, in a sudden hyperextension injury, 'pinching' of the cord in the narrowed spinal canal. Common causes of injury are: road traffic accidents; accidents at work, such as falling from heights or crush injuries; sporting accidents, for example in rugby, gymnastics, horseback riding and diving; and accidents in the home, in-cluding falling from roofs and falling downstairs — the latter is particularly common in elderly people who have spondylitic changes in the spine. At present, the annual incidence of spinal cord in-juries in the United Kingdom is approximately 10–15 per million of the population.

Non-traumatic causes of spinal cord damage are: infections, such as transverse myelitis, abscess and polyneuritis; tumours which, if malignant, are usually secondary, originating from a primary focus elsewhere in the body; thrombosis in one of the spinal arteries; haemorrhage; demyelinating conditions such as multiple sclerosis; congenital deformities such as spina bifida; scoliosis; or psychological disturbance, as in hysterical paralysis.

Whatever the cause, the presenting signs and symptoms are the same and the effect on the individual concerned is equally devastating. On the whole, people find it easier to accept a disability which can be blamed on a clearly identifiable trauma than one which has resulted from a relatively obscure and difficult to understand non-traumatic cause.

Functional anatomy

The spinal cord is part of the central nervous system, which conducts messages to and from the brain. Any damage to the cord will result in the loss or disruption of messages travelling between the brain and the periphery. The spinal cord has been likened to a telephone cable joining two callers: if there is any damage to the cable the call will be either of poor quality or totally cut off.

Terminology

Damage to the cord above the level of L1 produces the symptoms of an upper motor neurone lesion. Damage below L1 results in symptoms characteristic of a lower motor neurone lesion (Fig. 23.2).

Tetraplegia/quadriplegia refers to a lesion in the cervical cord resulting in loss of motor power and sensory input in the lower limbs, trunk and upper limbs with disturbance of bowel, bladder and sexual function. The degree of upper limb involvement will depend on the level of the lesion.

Paraplegia refers to a lesion in the thoracic, lumbar or sacral levels resulting in loss of power and sensory function in the lower limbs and trunk. The level of the injury will determine the degree of involvement and whether bowel, bladder and sexual function are disturbed.

Complete and incomplete lesions. A complete lesion results in total loss of motor power and sen-

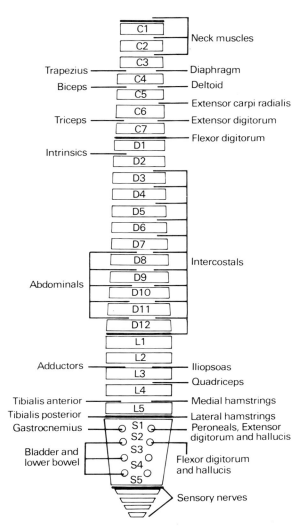

Fig. 23.2 Skeletal muscles and their major spinal segments.

sation below the level of the injury. An incomplete lesion will preserve some motor power and/or sensation.

Classification of lesions

The simplest method of classifying spinal lesions is to define them according to the last functioning nerve root above the injury. For example, in a complete C6 lesion all function above and including the 6th cervical nerve root is retained but functions below that level are lost. An individual with such a lesion would have the ability to move his shoulders, flex his elbows and extend his wrists. He would not, however, be able to extend his elbows, reach above his head, flex his wrists or move his fingers.

In an incomplete C6 lesion, all function innervated by the 6th cervical nerve root and above would be retained, as well as some motor and/or sensory function below that level.

It is impossible for anyone who has not suffered a spinal cord lesion to fully appreciate the devastating physical and psychological effects it has on an individual and his family. The general physical effects have already been mentioned; the psychological effects, although equally profound, are much more difficult to describe and deal with (see Ch. 3).

Signs and symptoms

The most common clinical features of spinal lesions are:

- loss of voluntary muscle power
- loss of sensation to all modalities below the level of the lesion
- loss of sphincter control in relation to bowel and bladder function
- loss of vasomotor and temperature control
- disruption of sexual function.

Complications

Spinal shock

This condition is temporary, starting immediately after transection of the spinal cord. It can best be described as isolation of the spinal cord with total disruption of transmission between the brain and the cord. The duration of spinal shock varies; some reflex activity may appear within 3 days, but may take as long as 8 weeks to reappear. As reflex activity returns, spasticity and increased muscle tone become evident. The full extent of the lesion and any potential recovery cannot be fully assessed until the spinal shock has subsided and bruising of the cord abated. It is usual for signs of recovery to appear fairly early if there are to be any, but there may be a delay of several weeks. Apparent late recovery may follow from the delayed repair of damaged nerve roots.

Autonomic dysreflexia

This is commonly seen in individuals with cervical lesions above the sympathetic outflow but it may be present in any lesion above T6. It may occur at any time after the spinal shock phase and is usually a response to a noxious stimulus, such as a blocked catheter resulting in a full bladder. In such a case the over-distension of the bladder results in a reflex sympathetic over-activity below the level of the lesion, causing vasoconstriction and systemic hypertension.

The individual complains of a pounding headache, profuse sweating, and flushing or blotchiness of the skin above the level of the lesion. This condition should be dealt with as a medical emergency. The cause should be identified and treated and the blood pressure reduced. This may be facilitated by using vasodilators such as nifedipine tablets crushed and swallowed.

Post-traumatic syringomyelia

This is an ascending myelopathy caused by a secondary cyst forming in the cord. This condition is relatively rare, occurring in about 2% of all people with spinal cord injury. Symptoms, which may present from 2 months post-injury onwards, include: pain in the arm, usually unilateral and often described as a dull ache; sensory loss, especially to pain and temperature; and, sometimes, loss of power unilaterally. The diagnosis can be confirmed by computed tomography (CT scan) or by nuclear magnetic resonance imaging (NMR scan). Treatment involves surgical drainage of the cystic cavity; although this relieves pain, there may not be any relief of sensory or motor symptoms.

Para-articular heterotopic ossification

After spinal cord lesion new bone is sometimes laid down in the soft tissue around paralysed joints, especially the hip and the knee. The cause of this is not known. It usually presents with redness and swelling near a joint and can impair movement. If surgical excision of the bone is indicated it should be delayed for about 18 months to avoid further new bone formation.

Contractures

These can result from immobilisation, spasticity or muscle tone imbalance. They may respond to conservative measures such as gentle stretching and orthoses but if this is unsuccessful surgical intervention such as tenotomy or tendon lengthening may be required.

Psychological factors

The psychological effects of a spinal cord lesion can be profound and prolonged. Whilst on bed-rest the individual will experience a wide variety of moods, including fear, anger, frustration, depression and euphoria. Sensory deprivation can result in a high level of anxiety and cause the person to become withdrawn. It is important that the individual and his family are helped and supported and given the opportunity to discuss their hopes and fears. Long-term psychological support may be necessary, as complete psychological adjustment may not be achieved for many years.

Pressure sores

Sores form as a result of ischaemia caused by unrelieved pressure. They affect the skin, subcutaneous fat and muscle as well as deeper structures. They are a major cause of readmission to hospital, yet are totally preventable by simple care routines such as suitable cushioning, correct posture and daily skin inspections.

The general health and well-being of the individual will affect his skin tolerance. A bladder infection will make the individual more susceptible to skin breakdown.

TREATMENT APPROACH

A spinal cord lesion has a profound effect on all aspects of life for both the individual and his family. It is important that a holistic approach is taken to aid his recovery from the psychological as well as the physical trauma and to restore his confidence and self-esteem so that he can live the life that he and his family wish. The most successful way to achieve rehabilitation is to work within a multidisciplinary framework, using the resources of a doctor, nurse, physiotherapist, occupational therapist, social worker and psychologist, as well as of the individual, his family and friends.

MEDICAL AND SURGICAL CARE

The nature and extent of the individual's injuries will determine the exact course of management.

Conservative care

Depending on the level of the lesion the correct alignment of the spine is maintained by cervical traction or lumbar pillows. The individual is then nursed on bed-rest for 6–16 weeks.

Internal fixation

This may be used in unstable and incomplete injuries. In the cervical area a bone graft and/or wires may be used to maintain good positioning of the fracture site. In the thoracic and lumbar regions metal rods and wires are used. In both instances the bed-rest period is significantly reduced.

Surgical intervention in the tetraplegic hand

In the longer term some tetraplegic people may benefit from modern surgical techniques to transfer tendons and restore elbow extension or provide a functional grip. Although the surgery is physically possible, the selection of suitable candidates is critical. They must be highly motivated, as treatment will be difficult and time consuming.

In parts of the USA surgery is being carried out in conjunction with electrical stimulation.

NURSING

The individual should be admitted to a spinal unit as soon as possible, where he will be nursed on bed-rest from one to 15 or 16 weeks. Some people are nursed on electrically-operated turning beds, others on King's Fund beds with pressure-relieving mattresses supplemented by manual, regular turning.

Injuries to the cervical spine should initially be managed using skeletal traction. This will:

- reduce the fracture/dislocation
- relieve the pressure on the cord
- splint the spine.

Traction should remain in situ for 6–8 weeks; at the end of this period the individual will be X-rayed again. If there is sufficient bony union the traction will be removed and a cervical collar used to provide support. Generally speaking, the individual will wear a soft collar whilst lying flat and sitting up to 45° and a firm collar whilst sitting up at 45° and over. The type of collar prescribed depends on the position to be maintained and on whether any other structures, such as the supporting ligaments, have been damaged. People with thoracic and lumbar lesions are nursed flat or with a pillow under the lumbar spine to preserve normal lordosis.

Initially, after injury, all systems are in shock. There may be a temporary loss of peristalsis in the intestines, which could lead to abdominal distension and vomiting. This is known as *paralytic ileus*. Until peristalsis returns and bowel sounds are heard the individual should not be given anything to eat or drink.

Skin care

Initially, turning takes place two-hourly and the individual's skin is inspected for any red marks. Subject to other injuries the turns will be supine, right lateral and left lateral. Positioning of the limbs during the bed-rest period is vitally important, with care being taken to prevent contractures as well as pressure sores (Fig. 23.3). If there is no marking of the skin the length of time between

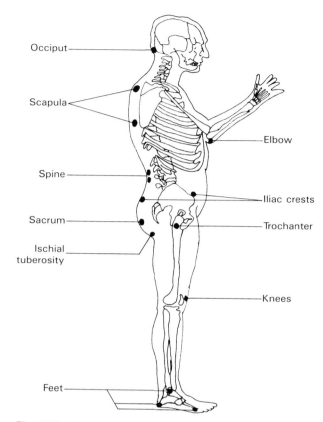

Fig. 23.3 Areas particularly likely to form pressure sores.

turns is gradually increased. The ultimate aim is to enable the individual to sleep through the night without being disturbed.

Bladder management

The basic principle of care is that urine must be removed from the bladder efficiently and with minimum disruption to body organs or processes; an emptying routine that fits the individual's life-style must be established.

It is the advancement in the bladder management of people with spinal cord lesions that has brought about the tremendous reduction in the mortality rate.

Early care

In the newly injured person continuous catheter

drainage is implemented for the first 24 hours. After this period the method of management will depend on the level of the lesion and the age and sex of the individual. A method commonly used is the passing of catheters at regular intervals (intermittent catheterisation). This is usually carried out 6-hourly as an aseptic technique. Fluids are restricted until there is some return of bladder activity.

Videourodynamic investigations will show muscle and sphincter activity as well as pressure and volume during the filling and voiding stages of micturition. These investigations help staff to plan appropriate bladder training programmes.

Bladder training

Wherever possible, individuals are taught to manage their own catheterisation and general bladder care. In a lesion above L1, reflex activity returns as spinal shock subsides. The spinal micturitional reflex is intact, and an 'automatic bladder' which empties regularly and spontaneously can be developed. In lesions below L1, where the spinal micturitional reflex is disrupted, bladder function is obtained by increasing internal pressure, i.e. by filling the bladder. This stimulates the stretch reflexes in the muscles of the bladder and allows urine to flow past the sphincter by overflow incontinence.

Bowel management

While the person is still on bed-rest his bowel is usually managed by manual evacuation and the use of suppositories if necessary. This is usually carried out every other day, and the bowel will learn to respond to this stimulus. When the individual starts getting up from bed his bowels are managed over the toilet if at all possible; this is not only a more natural and dignified position but also makes use of gravity. Initially, nursing staff will give assistance but whenever possible the individual is taught to manage his own routine either by straining or by the continued use of suppositories. The management of the tetraplegic person's bowel is very much dependent on the care services available at home. In order to facilitate bowel management the person's diet should be high in fibre; he should be informed that changes in diet or routine could lead to faecal accidents.

PHYSIOTHERAPY

Physiotherapy commences within hours of the person's admission. During the acute phase the main aims of treatment are:

- To maintain joint range of movement.
Each joint should be put through a full range of passive movement daily or, in the case of the upper limb, twice a day. This prevents contractures by maintaining muscle length. It is extremely important that the full range of movement is maintained in all joints; this will facilitate maximum independence.
- To maintain good respiratory function.
Those who lie flat in bed for any length of time are at risk of developing a chest infection. All people, regardless of their level of lesion should be given prophylactic chest care, including deep breathing, percussion and coughing.
- To improve remaining muscle strength.
Exercises to strengthen remaining innervated muscles may be carried out while the individual is still in bed, providing that the fracture site is not disturbed.

Once the person is out of bed for an hour or more a day his physical rehabilitation can begin. This will include the following:

- Learning basic wheelchair skills. The person is taught how to propel the chair, how to put the brakes on, position the castors, move the footplates and remove the armrests.
- Retraining balance. As he has lost sensation, proprioception and motor power below the lesion, the person will be unable to balance; however, given time and practice he can learn to compensate.
- Strengthening innervated muscles. Any form of exercise, including pulley work, weight-lifting, circuit training and sports can be used to strengthen muscles.
- Learning transfers. This is undertaken with the assistance of the occupational therapist as

well as the physiotherapist and is described fully on pp. 604–610.

- Learning advanced wheelchair skills. These include backwheel balancing, which enables the individual to manoeuvre over rough ground and to move up and down kerbs, and 'jumping' the chair sideways, which enables him to manoeuvre in tight spaces.
- Standing. This is usually facilitated by a standing frame, although initially the individual who is prone to hypotension may use a tilt table that moves him into the vertical position more gradually.
- Walking. People with lesions below the level of T12 may wish to walk using full-length calipers and elbow crutches. This is a slow, exhausting process and few use it as their only means of mobility.

Functional electrical stimulation

Over the years, doctors and engineers have tried to develop systems to stimulate the denervated muscles of paraplegic and tetraplegic people. With the advancement of computer technology, systems have been developed that enable individuals to stand without calipers. Other systems are being devised to give tetraplegic individuals a functional grip. All of these systems are still in their infancy and a long way from achieving their ultimate goals. Alongside functional stimulation there have been improvements in the design of walking braces. In the United States a Reciprocating Gait Orthosis (RGO) has been developed, whilst in the United Kingdom, at Oswestry, the Hip Guidance Orthosis (HGO) has been devised. Both systems offer a more normal walking pattern than conventional calipers and, consequently, conserve energy. The RGO has been designed to be worn under clothing and must be privately funded. The HGO must be worn over clothing and is available through the National Health Service (NHS).

THE ROLE OF THE SOCIAL WORKER

When the individual is first admitted to hospital, the social worker will make contact with him and his relatives in order to offer assistance with travelling expenses and with dealing with the many forms regarding sickness or industrial benefits, Social Security and disability pensions. She will also be able to offer support, a 'listening ear' and counselling. As a team member who is not directly involved in physical care and treatment, she may provide objective explanations and opportunities to discuss treatment and the future.

Contact with the person's local Social Services department should be made as soon as possible and a good working relationship established. This close liaison allows home resettlement to be smoother and easier for all concerned. When a return home is not possible, either because of the individual's age or the age and frailty of the carers, the social worker will make the necessary enquiries for alternative long-term care.

The social worker may be asked to give advice or assistance on a variety of topics, including applying for Mobility Allowance and the Orange Badge Scheme (see Ch. 9). She may offer advice regarding any legal claim, including how to initiate litigation.

Compensation claims

Claims for compensation often follow a spinal cord injury. An individual with a case pending should be encouraged to contact a solicitor as soon as he can so that as little time as possible is lost in this lengthy procedure. Solicitors ask team members, including occupational therapists, to prepare reports for the courts in support of claims for compensation. It is very important that these reports are comprehensive and thorough. The amount of a financial settlement may depend to a certain extent on the team's reports.

THE ROLE OF THE PSYCHOLOGIST

Many units now have access to the services of a clinical psychologist, who is able to offer practical help and advice to staff and carers who are trying to support individuals at a very traumatic time in their lives. Psychologists can also help by suggesting practical ways in which individuals can cope with their anxiety, anger, frustration and feelings of hopelessness.

THE ROLE OF THE OCCUPATIONAL THERAPIST

Successful rehabilitation of people with spinal cord lesions depends on a good multidisciplinary structure of care provision. Occupational therapists play a vital role within the treatment team, using their skills to assess the individual and his environment, plan a treatment programme, and facilitate the development of skills for independent living. Their intervention can be divided into 'acute' and 'rehabilitation' stages.

ACUTE STAGE (BED-REST)

The length of this period will vary, depending on the level of the lesion and on its conservative or surgical management. On average, the person is likely to be in bed for 6–10 weeks. The aims of occupational therapy at this stage are:

- to establish a good working relationship with the individual, his family and friends
- to give psychological support to the individual and his family
- to care for the individual's tetraplegic hands
- to limit sensory deprivation and to provide the opportunity for the person to make constructive use of his time
- to make early contact with community colleagues and begin planning for resettlement at home.

These aims are described in greater detail below.

A good working relationship

It is vital that during the early stage of treatment the occupational therapist establishes a good rapport with the individual and his family and friends. This will facilitate successful rehabilitation. The therapist should learn as much as she can about the individual's life-style and the things that are important to him so that she can plan a treatment programme that is responsive to his needs and desires.

Psychological support

The therapist can do much to reassure those concerned by helping them to understand some of the difficulties which often arise and which may appear threatening at the time. For example, the home environment frequently seems daunting to a newly injured individual and his family, who may begin to panic about how they will cope at home and whether a wheelchair can be accommodated. Talking to the individual and his family about their home and what adaptations can be made may allay some of their immediate worries.

The recognition of depression, fear, boredom and aggression and their causes is of paramount importance. Any reassurance must include the relatives and friends, as should practical activity to help the individual to work through and understand the reasons for his feelings and behaviour.

Care of the 'tetraplegic hand'

Care of the individual's hands is of prime importance and in those units where orthoses are used routinely this should be undertaken as soon as possible after admission. There have been many debates over the years about the merits of splinting and although the policy differs from unit to unit the aims of care are the same:

- to maintain the functional position of the hand, i.e. to
  — support the palmar transverse arch
  — stabilise and support the thumb in abduction and opposition
  — maintain adequate web space
- to maintain good cosmetic appearance of the hand and prevent contractures
- to maintain good range of movement in all joints of the hand and wrist
- to maintain good wrist extension.

Tenodesis or *automatic grip*. This is one of the 'trick' movements which can be taught to a person with C6 tetraplegia and a functioning extensor carpi radialis longus muscle. This grip greatly increases independence, for as the wrist is extended the immobile fingers curl towards the palm (Fig. 23.4) and come into contact with the upward travelling thumb, either at the fingertips

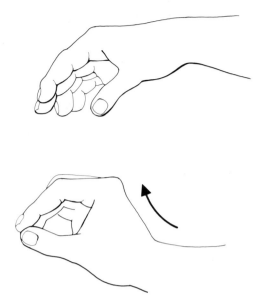

Fig. 23.4 Tenodesis grip. This action at the wrist enables the hand to provide a simple gripping function.

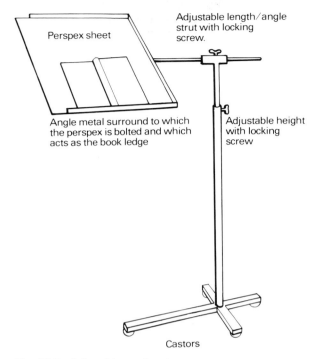

Fig. 23.5 Adjustable reading frame.

or at the side of the index finger. Whilst wrist extension is maintained so, too, is this contact, which can be used as a gripping agent. Practice at picking up objects of varying shapes, weights and textures should be included in the treatment programme and the individual should be made fully aware of the utility of this grip.

Constructive use of time

The occupational therapist can offer assistance, advice and support which may help to make enforced bed-rest more bearable. She should encourage the individual to think and work through his problems. While she should discuss these with him and help him to work out solutions, the person must feel that he is still in control of his own situation, as this will help him to achieve a positive outlook and increase his self-confidence and esteem.

The following equipment may help the individual to make constructive use of time:

● Bed mirrors. One or two mirrors strategically attached to the bed and the over-bed frame will enable the person to see the ward, watch television and see those in adjacent beds.

● Prismatic spectacles. These are usually available from local opticians. The prism enables the wearer to see around the ward whilst looking towards the ceiling.

● Books on tape. Most libraries have an extremely good selection of books recorded on cassette tapes.

● Reading frames. A simple Perspex frame on a height-adjustable stand will enable the person to read a daily paper. This type of frame still needs someone to turn the pages from time to time but is a relatively cheap solution to a difficult problem (Fig. 23.5).

● Electric page turners. These are not ideal whilst the individual is lying totally flat but do work well once he begins to sit up. Several types are available. Some turn pages forwards, others backwards and forwards; some will manage newspapers, others magazines and books.

● 'Overhead computers' enable the individual to work on the computer whilst lying supine.

They can be used to play games such as chess, space invaders and snooker and as word processors enabling people to write and print letters with some degree of privacy.

As increasing numbers of people become computer literate, young people are now able to carry on their education lying in bed, whilst others may enjoy a new medium which may help to boost their self-esteem and confidence and introduce the possibility of future retraining.

Planning for resettlement

During the early stage of treatment it is important that the individual and the occupational therapist consider plans for the future. Whether the aim is to return home, live independently or move into residential care, many months of planning and negotiation will be required. An early start, therefore, is essential. The spinal unit occupational therapist and social worker should make contact with the person's local Social Services occupational therapist and social worker.

Home visit

The home visit should be carried out as soon as a prognosis is clear. A joint visit involving spinal unit and community staff and relatives is recommended at this stage. In some instances, when the lesion is incomplete, it may be advisable to wait until later, when the prognosis is clearer. The home visit may be very distressing psychologically for the family, as it may well reinforce the enormity of what has happened and suddenly face them with reality. It is very useful to take a wheelchair on these visits but care should be taken that introducing the chair does not cause undue distress to the family. Although this visit is carried out whilst the individual is still on bed-rest it is imperative that he is closely involved and consulted, and that any decisions are made with his full participation.

It is always an advantage to have two members of the spinal unit staff on these visits as they can support one another, answer the family's innumerable questions and give help and support if and when the carers are distressed. The home should be assessed with a view to the following:

- Short-term measures: These will enable the individual to go home for weekend leave. Turning circles and doorway widths should be adequate. It should be decided if it is feasible to put a bed into the living/reception room in the short term. The bed height and the suitability of the mattress should be assessed.
- Interim measures. These will enable the individual to live at home before any major alterations are carried out. For example, is there access to a toilet and bath? If not, what temporary measures could be used to overcome the problem?
- Long-term measures. These will enable the individual to live independently or be cared for at home. Alterations frequently include permanent ramping, installation of a stairlift or a through-floor lift, major changes within the bathroom or a ground floor extension.

Once the home visit has been completed, the local authority staff should be invited to visit the unit to meet the individual and discuss the options available for him and his family. He may feel that returning to the parental home is not a good idea and may wish to explore independent living before making any final decisions. The unit and community teams must be willing to discuss all options so that the individual is in a position to make an informed choice about his future.

Wheelchairs and cushions

A knowledge of the manual and electric wheelchairs supplied by the NHS will enable the occupational therapist to prescribe a suitable wheelchair for the individual. His age, size, height, weight, level of lesion and expected use of the chair will all influence the choice (see Ch. 9).

In recent years there have been great strides forward in the design and manufacture of lightweight, high-performance wheelchairs. The range of chairs now available is extensive and the individual should be carefully assessed for the most suitable design to meet his needs. The choice of chairs and optional extras is so great that an individual should be advised to wait until the end of his rehabilitation before purchasing his own chair. By then, he will be better advised and more objective about his long-term requirements.

Cushions

The avoidance of pressure sores is of paramount importance and all individuals should be carefully assessed for the most suitable cushion. Many people are able to sit on a 4″ pincore latex foam cushion with a natural fibre cover and relieve pressure on their ischii by pushing themselves up on the arms of the chair. For others, especially those with higher lesions who are unable to relieve the pressure, other cushioning needs to be investigated. Air cushions such as the Roho and gel and foam cushions such as the Jay Medical are both very good pressure-relieving surfaces.

Pushing gloves

People with tetraplegia need some form of pushing glove when using a manual wheelchair: to prevent pressure sores from developing on their desensitised hands, to provide the necessary friction to push the chair and to protect their hands from the dirt that inevitably collects on the wheels. (Fig. 23.6).

Getting out of bed

Once the person's spine is sufficiently stable he will be gradually mobilised into a wheelchair. This process may take from a day or two to one or two weeks, depending on the level of the lesion and the individual's progress and confidence. Having lain flat for a considerable length of time he will need time to adjust to the change of position and overcome hypotension. He may need to wear anti-embolism stockings and a broad elasticated waistband (abdominal binder) to help prevent the blood from pooling in the lower part of his body. If he continues with symptoms of dizziness and nausea which are not relieved by deep breathing he should be given ergotamine tartrate (Ephedrine) approximately one hour before getting up. He can then sit up gradually on a profiling bed

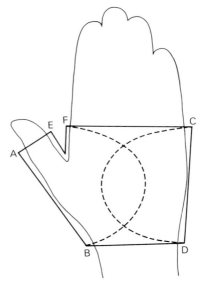

Fig. 23.6 How to make a pushing glove.
(1) Using tracing paper or greaseproof paper draw hand shape with flat palm and thumb in extension. Mark MCP heads of fingers, IP joint of the thumb and wrist joint.
(2) Allow sufficient space around the hand and thumb and draw the pattern shape as shown.
(3) Fold along line AB. Trace the shape of the thumb from A–E–F. From F draw a semicircle to the wrist at B to form an overlap of the glove on the back of the hand.
(4) Fold along line CD. From C draw a semicircle to wrist at D to form the overlap at the back of the hand.
(5) Open out the paper and cut out pattern. Try the pattern on the person's hand to ensure that the thumb width is sufficient and that the overlap at the back of the hand is adequate. Modify if necessary.
(6) Using the pattern, cut out two gloves in firm leather — cut on the bias to prevent the glove stretching when in use.
(7) Cut out palmer pieces to reinforce the palm of the glove and to give traction for pushing the chair — use leather, suede, rubber or pimple rubber.
(8) Sewing. For leather use a strong thread and a leather needle. (a) Sew reinforcement onto the palm. (b) Sew on the Velcro so that 'loop' piece overlaps 'hook' piece. (c) Sew around the thumb web space ¼″ from the edge. Try to match colours of the thread and the Velcro to blend with the leather.

and, once he is in a sitting position, be transferred into a wheelchair. The length of time he is out of bed should be increased gradually from about ten minutes to all day. This may take two or three days for a low-level paraplegic or many weeks for a high-level tetraplegic.

During this period the occupational therapist, physiotherapist and nurse should work closely with the individual, helping to reassure him and build up his confidence. Initially, he will spend the time on the ward, but when he is up for about one hour at a time he will start attending the therapy department for additional elements of his treatment, for example, discovering the versatility of a 'trick' movement, learning how to use a writing aid, or enhancing balance and upper limb strength through heavy workshop activity.

THE REHABILITATION STAGE

The aim of all rehabilitation is to enable the individual to be as physically and psychologically independent as his condition will allow.

The occupational therapist's skills as a problem-solver and her ability to assess and treat an individual in a holistic manner make her a vital part of any rehabilitation team.

People with paraplegia should ultimately be totally independent, depending on factors such as age, sex, motivation and previous level of fitness. However, those with higher lesions will have greater difficulty and their final degree of independence will depend on their level of lesion (Table 23.1).

The description of intervention which follows has particular relevance to the treatment of individuals with high-level lesions.

The following aims may be used as a framework for treatment at the rehabilitation stage:

- to encourage a positive, realistic attitude to the individual's changed circumstances
- to assist the individual to achieve his optimum independence in activities of daily living (ADL)
- to provide daily living aids, adaptations or orthoses needed for independence
- to help strengthen innervated muscles and to encourage the use of 'trick' movements where appropriate.
- to help improve balance and general posture in the wheelchair
- to teach wheelchair skills to the individual and his family
- to assist with resettlement at home and advise on adaptations and equipment

Table 23.1 Functional expectations for a person with complete tetraplegia*

Level of injury	Functional ability
C4	Totally dependent Can use electric wheelchair with chin control Can type/use computer using a mouthstick Needs environmental control system (such as Possum) to turn on lights, open doors etc. — operated by shoulder shrug or mouthpiece
C5	Can feed with a feeding strap/universal cuff and wrist support Can wash face, comb hair, clean teeth — using feeding strap/universal cuff Can give help to dress top half Can push manual wheelchair short distances on the flat providing he uses pushing gloves and capstan rims on the wheels Electric wheelchair needed for functional mobility Unable to transfer
C6	Still needs strap to feed Still needs strap for self-care Can dress top half unaided Can assist dressing the lower half Can propel wheelchair up gentle slopes Can transfer independently into car and onto bed but rarely achieved Can drive with hand controls
C7	Can be totally independent Can transfer, feed and dress independently Can drive with hand controls
C8/T1	Totally independent from wheelchair

* It must be stressed that these expectations are general and depend on the patient's age, sex, physical proportions, physical condition prior to injury, motivation and degree of spasticity.

- to provide information and advice for relatives, carers and friends
- to support and advise with regard to work and/or education
- to offer help and advice with regard to driving, wheelchairs and transport
- to encourage the continuation or development of hobbies, interests and leisure activities.

Personal care

After extended bed-rest and dependence on others

CASE EXAMPLE 23.1

John was a 28-year-old serviceman. At the time of his injury he was on military exercise in Europe and had a water-sport accident. He was taken to the local hospital and then transferred to a spinal unit. A week later he was flown back to the United Kingdom and admitted to a spinal unit.

On examination he was found to have a fracture dislocation of C6/7 resulting in an incomplete tetraplegia below C6, complete below T4. He was a married man, living in his own three-bedroom semi-detached house.

Two-weeks after admission to the unit he developed a pulmonary embolus and needed resuscitating.

He was nursed conservatively with his head in skull traction for 10 weeks. The traction was removed and two days later he began to sit up slowly, using a profiling bed. Ten days after the traction was removed he got out of bed for the first time. At this stage he was in a reclining wheelchair, his neck supported in a firm 'Philadelphia' collar. Within 10 days he was sitting in a standard wheelchair and was attending the physiotherapy and occupational therapy departments, working on balance and neck strengthening and personal ADL such as eating and teeth cleaning.

One month after John got up from bed-rest the collar was removed. Over the next six months he worked at his strength and balance so that by the time he was discharged he was able to roll from side to side and sit up from lying. He could get himself in and out of bed and, using a sliding board, could get in and out of the car. He was able to wash, dress, shave and clean his teeth but found the tasks time-consuming and felt that to keep to a realistic daily schedule he would need some help.

He was able to feed himself, give himself a drink and cook a meal. He had his car adapted so that he could drive. A home visit was carried out while John was still on bed-rest; the house proved to be unsuitable so John and his wife sold it and bought a bungalow which was later adapted to meet his needs.

After leaving the unit John took a computer course at a residential college and has since done work for voluntary organisations. He is still fighting a compensation claim through European courts.

He keeps fit by weight-training and swimming and has recently been on an Outward Bound course in the Lake District, where he took part in activities such as canoeing, horseback riding and abseiling.

John thoroughly enjoys cooking and has used his problem-solving skills to devise ways in which he can prepare and cook food.

Recently John and his wife have separated and although he finds it tiring he is managing to live alone, with care staff coming to help in the mornings and, occasionally, in the evenings if he feels too tired to put himself to bed.

for all care, the ability to be independent in personal care activities will be very important. Initially, adaptations may be necessary but these should be re-assessed regularly and withdrawn as the individual becomes more able. The order in which these skills are attempted will vary from person to person.

Eating and drinking

Eating and drinking are both social activities and it is psychologically important that whenever possible the individual learns to manage independently. Eating can usually be facilitated by using adapted cutlery with individually moulded grips or a universal cuff with an ordinary spoon or fork (Fig. 23.7).

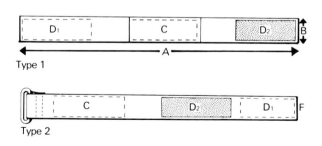

Fig. 23.7 Two types of universal cuff. (1) Straightforward Velcro overlap strap with stitched palmer pocket. (2) Strap end threads through a D-ring to fasten onto Velcro. Measurements: A = width of palm plus fastening overlap. B = width (approx. 2.5 cm). C = pocket; palm width and stitched on three sides. D = Velcro 'hooks' and 'loops'.

The advantage of Type 2 is that one end F can be left threaded, enabling the tetraplegic patient to fasten and release Velcro independently with the teeth.

Initially it may be necessary to use a non-slip mat and a deep-rimmed dish or plate guard but these should be withdrawn as soon as the individual can manage without them, thus keeping specialised equipment to a minimum.

Lack of sensation in the hands and paralysis of the fingers makes drinking from an ordinary cup almost impossible. However, with practice the person may well manage a lightweight insulated mug and, in many instances, a half pint beer mug. It may be necessary for him to use a straw, in which case flexible straws will be useful. Non-return valve straws will prevent an excessive amount of air being swallowed.

Hair

Modern styles which can be maintained simply by washing and towel-drying the hair are generally to be preferred. Grooming the hair is made easier by using a round styling brush, which has a more manageable handle, rather than a comb, and a larger universal cuff will facilitate holding the brush. When necessary, handles of thermoplastic splinting material can be fitted to hair driers and other styling equipment. Individuals should be reminded about the possibility of burning anaesthetic skin with all styling equipment.

Hair washing

Hair is washed most easily in the shower. If it is necessary to wash the hair over a basin, a spray attachment should be used to preclude the possibility of the individual slipping face forward into a basin of water and being unable to lift himself back.

Teeth

The toothbrush can be placed in a universal cuff or adapted with a thermoplastic loop handle (Fig. 23.8). The toothpaste tube can be held between the palms of the hands and the top removed using the teeth. Pump-action toothpaste dispensers and self-pasting brushes can be useful for some people. 'Vanity style' basins with a wide rim

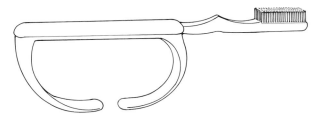

Fig. 23.8 A thermoplastic handle may make it easier to hold a toothbrush.

make it easier for the individual to support himself whilst cleaning his teeth.

Electric toothbrushes may be of some help, although they may be too heavy for some people to manage and the on/off switches are frequently difficult to cope with and difficult to modify.

Dentures can be managed in the usual way by being removed and placed in cleaning fluid.

Shaving

Electric and battery-operated razors can be adapted with a thermoplastic handle or a leather pouch to hold the razor. Wet shaving is possible but a safety razor must always be used. As with teeth cleaning, it may be necessary for the individual to support himself by resting his elbows on the rim of the basin or on some other firm surface.

Make-up

Make-up applicators can easily be adapted to fit a universal cuff. Alternatively, thermoplastic handles can be made.

Washing

The person with a high-level lesion should be able to wash his face and the top half of his body using a flannel mitt.

The basin should be 'vanity style', low enough for the individual to support his elbows and forearms and far enough away from the wall to enable him to push under without hitting his toes or knees on the wall. The taps should ideally be lever style. Flannel mitts are commercially available or can be made by sewing a flannel in half and, if necessary, threading elastic around the opening. Liquid soap or soap-on-a-rope may make washing easier.

Dressing

Once the person with paraplegia has regained his balance he is usually capable of learning to dress himself, initially on the bed, and when he is free of any external bracing, in the wheelchair.

If possible, he should be taught to move around the bed and to dress without the aid of an over-bed pole; otherwise, he will become reliant on the pole and his level of independence will be reduced if one is not available.

Technique (Fig. 23.9)

- The individual sits up in bed. If a urinary drainage bag is worn this is taped to one leg.
- He bends one leg at the knee and lifts it over the other so that the foot is clear of the bed. Socks are put on in this position, ensuring that there are no thick seams to cause pressure on the toes. It should be pointed out to him that socks should be put on before trousers so that there is no risk of him catching his toes in the hems and seams of his trousers.

The action is repeated for the other leg.

- Trousers are put on in the same way as socks and pulled up as far as possible. (Many people chose not to wear underpants; if they are worn, however, care must be taken to ensure that they are not too tight and do not obstruct the leg-bag tubing.)
- The individual then lies down and pulls the garments up, rolling from side to side to pull them over his bottom. This may need to be repeated several times.
- Shoes are put on in the same way as socks.
- The individual can dress his top half whilst sitting on the bed or when he has transferred into the chair.

An individual will soon find methods of his own to make dressing easier. These should be en-couraged, as they will help to build problem-solving skills, self-esteem and self-confidence.

The independence achieved by a person with tetraplegia will depend upon his level of lesion as well as his age, sex and previous physical fitness. He should be verbally independent even if he cannot be independent physically, i.e. he must know how he should be dressed, fed and washed and he should be able teach others how he wishes to be assisted.

Clothing

Advice on clothing should be kept to a minimum so that the individual is still free to express his personality. However, it is advisable that back pockets and studs are removed from jeans and other articles and that practical, natural fibres are worn. Particularly tight clothing should be avoided and care should be taken with elasticated clothing such as socks and bras so that they do not cause pressure marks. Shoes should generally be a size larger than before to accommodate oedema and prevent rubbing.

Transfers

Before the person can learn how to transfer he must learn certain standard procedures, e.g. how to position the chair with the castors forward and the brakes engaged, making the chair more stable. He will learn wheelchair transfers to and from bed, armchair, toilet, bath, car and floor. Most people with paraplegia will be independent in all of these transfers and will also be able to get their chair in and out of the car. Those with higher lesions will be more dependent upon assistance.

Bed transfers

Ideally, the bed and the wheelchair should be the same height.

There are two methods of getting on and off a bed:

1. 'Forwards on' transfer (Fig. 23.10). The wheelchair is placed at right angles to the bed and the person lifts his legs onto the bed one at

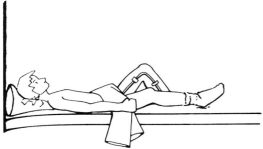

A The bed is lowered to chair height

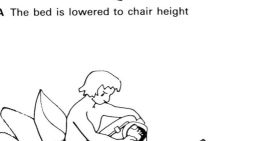

B The heaviest or most difficult leg is dressed first

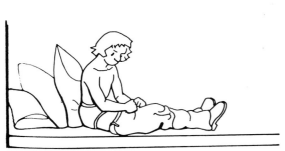

C Garments are pulled up as-high as possible above the knees

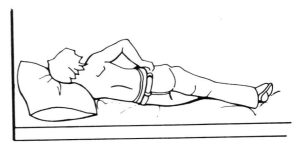

D Rolling from side to side to pull lower garments over the hips

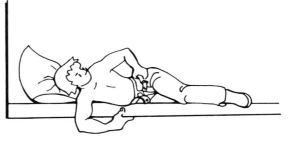

E Holding under the bed side to assist rolling

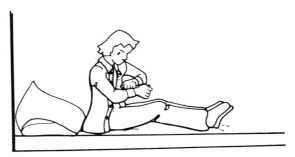

F Top garments may be put on whilst sitting on the bed or in the wheelchair

Fig. 23.9 Independent dressing for the paraplegic individual.

a time. The footplates are swung away and the chair moved closer. The person then moves forwards, in small lifts if necessary. The procedure is reversed for transfer into the chair.

2. 'Legs down' or side transfer (Fig. 23.11). The chair is positioned and the footplates lifted and swung away if necessary. The individual moves forward on the seat to position his feet comfortably on the floor. The near-side armrest is removed and the person lifts his bottom across onto the bed, taking care to avoid the rear wheel. He then lifts his legs onto the bed. The reverse procedure is used to transfer to the chair.

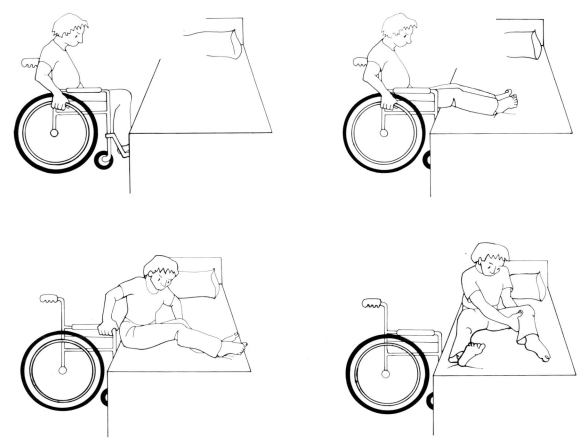

Fig. 23.10 'Forwards on' transfer onto a bed.

Armchair transfers

These are usually achieved by positioning the wheelchair at an angle to the armchair and doing a 'legs down' transfer (see Fig. 23.11).

Toilet transfers

Transferring on and off a toilet is made much easier if the toilet seat is the same height as the wheelchair seat. The toilet seat must always be padded to prevent scrapes or pressure sores. Specially padded seats are preferable to inflatable rubber seats, which tend to perish. The method of transfer will depend on the space available, but where possible the chair should be placed alongside the toilet at a slight angle and a 'legs

down' transfer carried out as shown in Fig. 23.11.

Rails, although useful, should be avoided if possible as the person may tend to become reliant upon them and find transferring difficult or impossible if they are not available.

Shower transfers

Ideally, the shower base should be level with the floor' so that the person can either use a self-propelling shower chair or execute a 'legs down' transfer onto a free-standing shower chair. If the shower base prohibits the use of a wheelchair, then a 'flip down' shower seat on the wall can be used. If a free-standing seat is required it must be noted that it cannot be used with a fibreglass base. In all

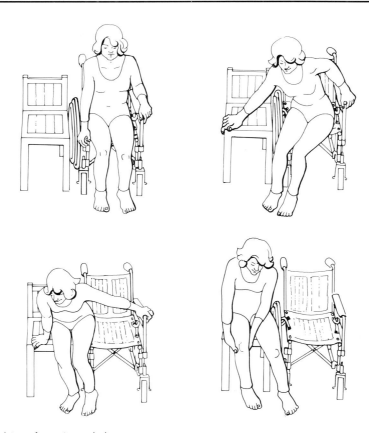

Fig. 23.11 'Legs down' transfer onto a chair.

cases the seat must be padded to prevent pressure sores and the water thermostatically controlled to eliminate any risk of scalding.

Bath transfers

The individual may learn to transfer over the side of the bath or, if it is accessible, over the end of the bath, the same technique being used for both methods (Fig. 23.12).

Difficulty may arise if the person does not have the strength to lift himself back out of the bath. Equipment such as bath boards or seats, and electrically or battery operated bath seats to raise and lower the person may help to overcome this problem.

Safety measures are vital. The water must be run and tested before the person gets into the bath and hot water should never be added once he is in the bath.

Car transfers

The technique used to get in and out of a car will depend on the individual's ability and, to a certain extent, on the make of car being used. It is much easier to transfer into a two-door than a four-door car. Once the car door is open, the wheelchair should be pushed up as close as possible to the door sill. The footplate and the armrest nearest to the car should be removed. The person then moves himself forward on the wheelchair seat and

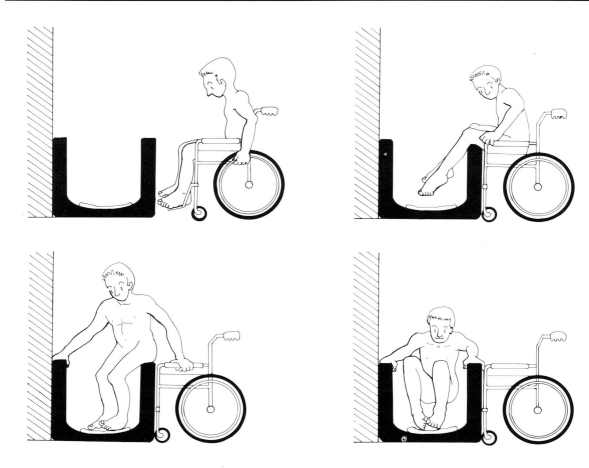

Fig. 23.12 Forward transfer into the bath without aids.

lifts his feet into the well of the car. He then lifts and moves himself across and down onto the car seat, taking care to avoid hitting the steering wheel or dashboard with his legs, making sure he clears the rear wheel of the chair, and ensuring that his head is clear of the door arch. Some people may find a transfer board helpful.

Floor transfers

An individual with paraplegia may fall out of his wheelchair at some time and he needs to be able to get himself back into the chair without help. To do so, he should swing the footplates back and put his cushion on the floor between the front castors. He can then lift himself onto the cushion with his back to the chair. With the armrests removed, he can then lift himself up and back into the chair, swing the footplates back into position and replace the armrests and the cushion.

The easiest way to replace a foam cushion is for the person to sit slightly to one side in the chair, place the cushion next to himself, fold the top of the cushion over, and then lift himself up. The cushion should then spring open and flat under him (Fig. 23.13).

If an individual with tetraplegia falls out of his chair he must rely on carers lifting him back in or on a hoist being used.

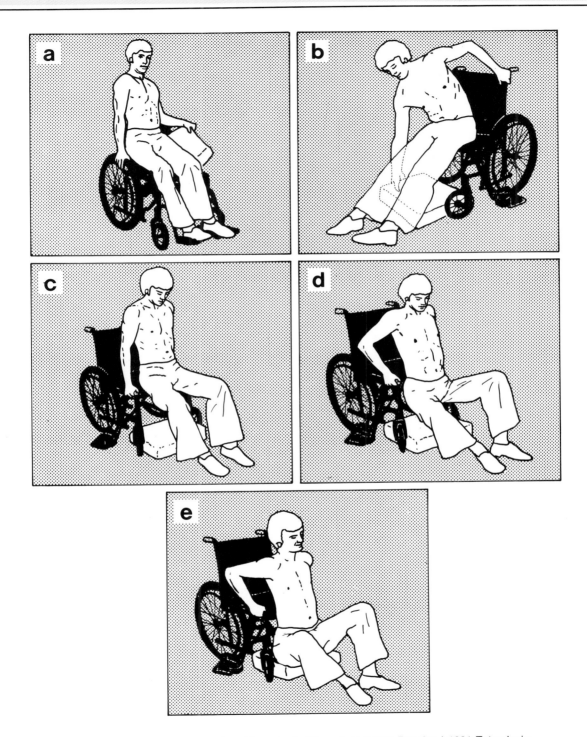

Fig. 23.13 Transferring on and off the floor (cont'd overleaf). (Reproduced from Bromley I 1991 Tetraplegia and paraplegia, 4th edn. Churchill Livingstone, Edinburgh, by courtesy of the author.)

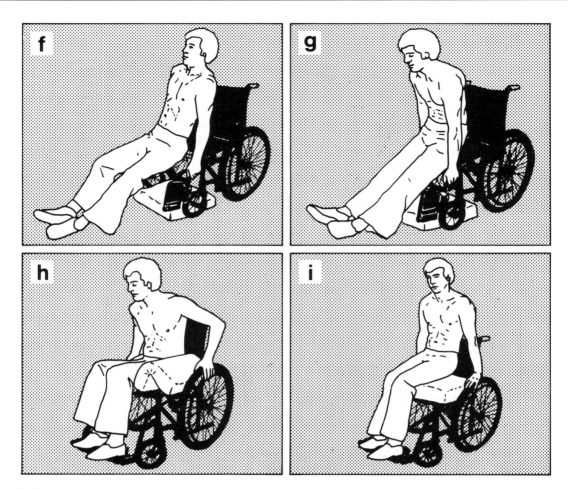

Fig. 23.13 (continued)

Standing transfer

This technique enables one carer to bring the individual to a standing posture and move him from one position to another. It is a method that must be taught carefully and should not be the only method of transfer used (Fig. 23.14). If it is not carried out correctly the individual could be dropped or the carer could hurt himself.

The individual is moved forward in the wheelchair so that his feet are flat on the floor and his knees are at 90°. The carer places her own feet on either side of the individual's feet, preventing them from moving. The carer then blocks the individual's knees with hers and pulls him forward. She puts her chin over the individual's shoulder and, in turn, puts the individual's arms (if possible) and chin over her own shoulder. She then rocks the individual from side to side until her hands are firmly under the ischii. Once in this position the carer is ready to stand up by rocking forward and back. When the carer and the individual are both fully upright the carer 'walks' the individual round until he is in the correct position and then sits him down, the carer pushing the individual's knees back and at the same time pushing her own bottom out. This has the effect

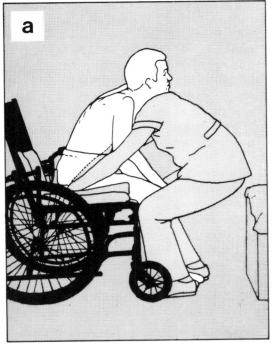

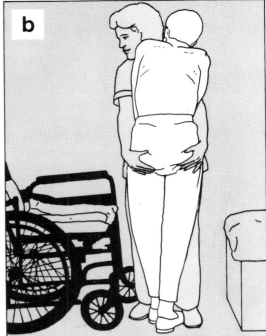

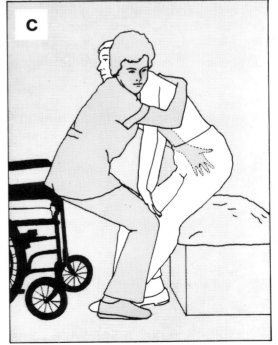

Fig. 23.14 Transferring a tetraplegic person through a standing position. (Reproduced from Bromley I 1991 Tetraplegia and paraplegia, 4th edn. Churchill Livingstone, Edinburgh, by courtesy of the author.)

of pushing the individual's bottom back into the seat.

Hoists

Many tetraplegic people will need to be transferred using a hoist. Great care should be taken with the individual to ensure that the most appropriate hoist and sling are used. All carers should be given training in how to operate the hoist so that they are confident in using it and make the best use of it. A universal or hammock sling should be used so that the individual's trunk is supported and pressure spread evenly across his back. Problems with anaesthetic skin may make it necessary to line the slings with sheepskin. A more detailed description of the use of hoists is given in Chapter 9.

Therapeutic/remedial activity

Attendance in the occupational therapy department is an integral part of the treatment programme. As well as providing a welcome break from the ward, remedial activities entail working to a timetable and encourage social interaction. Occupational therapy presents the individual with the implications of his disability by asking him to participate in normal activity. Activities are selected to use and strengthen innervated muscles to maximum benefit and to initiate a wide and varied programme of work which, whilst being very specific, must also be enjoyable. A relaxed individual who is genuinely interested in the activities offered will participate with more enthusiasm than the individual who is tense or bored and will be able to undertake a more extensive programme of therapy, learning decision-making skills and regaining his initiative.

Heavy workshop activities

Heavier activities such as woodwork and metalwork can provide an additional dimension to a programme designed primarily to improve balance and strengthen muscles. They may provide opportunities for the assessment of work skills and aptitude as well as practice in handling tools and equipment. Men comprise the majority of people with spinal lesions and the traditionally male-orientated working environment of the heavy workshop can enhance self-esteem and confidence by offering the opportunity to 'roll up one's sleeves' and to participate in more male-orientated conversations. Heavy workshop activities, of course, need not exclude women.

Communication

It is important that, regardless of the level of his injury, each person is given the opportunity to learn how to manage pen and paper so that he can communicate in writing as well as orally. Even the most uninterested person should be encouraged to relearn the mechanics of writing, even if only for the purpose of signing legal documents, cheques and greetings cards, or for doing crosswords and puzzles.

A good rapport must be established between the individual and his therapist before writing practice is introduced into the programme, as writing is difficult to perfect and requires interest, patience, practice and perseverance from them both. Gripping and controlling the pen is difficult without finger function. The pen has to be moved across the paper with movement from the shoulder, elbow and wrist instead of by the fingers.

The pen can be held between the fingers and thumb with an adapted holder or with a device that fits into the universal cuff. Alternatively, it can be held between the palms of both hands, or held between the fingers of one hand and steadied by the other. A felt-tip pen should be used initially, as it requires little pressure and can be used at any angle. The paper should be held firmly, either by non-slip matting or a clipboard. It may be more realistic for the individual to master

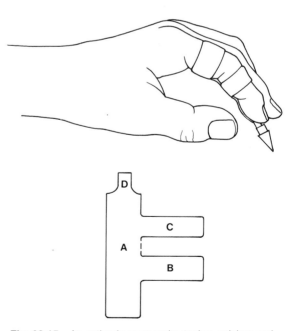

Fig. 23.15 An orthosis may make typing quicker and easier. (1) Cut the pattern out of thermoplastic material and soften in the usual way. (2) Place A along the palmar aspect of the right or left index finger so that D is beyond the fingertip. (3) Fold B and C around the index finger as shown. (4) Place a pencil-top eraser on D.

a word processor for more efficient letter writing, in which case a typing orthosis may be needed (Fig. 23.15).

As computers are becoming more popular and an increasing number of people are computer literate, the demand for sophisticated technology is increasing. The computer technology now available is such that people with severe disabilities are able to communicate, work and run their lives at the push of a button or the blink of an eyelid. Such systems are particularly helpful for people with tetraplegia who want to live independently, or whose family are out during the day (see Ch. 10). Other practical skills related to communication, mobility and independence which should be practised include operating the telephone (pushing buttons, holding the receiver, operating coin boxes and handling phonecards); handling money (coins, notes and wallets or purses); using keys (inserting and turning them and opening doors); and operating environmental control systems.

Domestic ADL

An increasing number of people with spinal cord lesions wish to live independently in their own homes. Wherever appropriate, such individuals should be given the opportunity to spend time in a domestic environment prior to resettlement at home, so that they can learn to handle equipment safely and regain confidence, strength and skill.

Practice related to food preparation should include shopping as well as making beverages, cooking snacks or meals and baking. Wherever possible, it is more appropriate to use modern labour-saving devices as opposed to equipment specifically designed for people with disabilities. Microwave ovens make cooking simpler and quicker and slow cookers enable hot meals to be prepared without lifting dishes in and out of an oven.

Bean-bag trays are useful in an environment where hot plates and cups need to be carried from one area to another.

Washing machines and tumble driers make laundering clothes relatively simple. Control knobs may need adapting to facilitate their operation.

Rotary clothes-lines are simplest, providing they can be reached; alternatively, a system of lowering and raising a washing line has to be used. 'Dolly' pegs can be used by most people with weak grip. A lightweight iron and either a wall-mounted ironing board or a board with space to give knee clearance should be used. People with anaesthetic skin on their hands and arms should take great care whilst ironing. Day-to-day cleaning and tidying should be encouraged; while still in the ward, individuals should, wherever possible, be responsible for making their bed and keeping their 'bed space' tidy.

Resettlement at home

Most spinal units have a training flat or house which enables the individual, with or without his family, to care for himself in a domestic rather than a clinical environment. This sort of facility helps to increase the person's confidence prior to discharge. It is essential that during this stage of rehabilitation he is encouraged to interact with the local community. Trips and visits away from the hospital will help to introduce the individual to the outside world. He will probably have been in the spinal unit for between 6 and 9 months (and in some cases longer) prior to his discharge. He will have become friends with staff and other people in the unit. Generally, he will be keen to go home and look forward to his discharge date. However, he will often need to be prepared for the 'trauma' of loneliness, boredom or frustration, as he will miss the company of the others. He may need help during the first few weeks and months at home, either from local community staff or from the community liaison nurse visiting from the spinal unit.

The individual will be seen at frequent intervals in the spinal unit outpatient clinic, where any problems can be discussed with the consultant or referred on to the appropriate member of staff.

Spinal cord lesions are very emotive and therefore frequently make media headlines, but they are not common and knowledge of their care is not widespread. Therefore it is important that by the time an individual is discharged from a spinal unit he and his family are well-versed in all aspects of his care, as local medical and other care staff may be relatively inexperienced in this area.

Many spinal units have a discharge care manual, a copy of which is given to the individual and his family for reference and to reinforce the teaching given in the unit. The manual explains in relatively simple terms what has happened medically and physiologically and what care should be given. It can be used to teach local staff involved with future care.

In most units relatives are encouraged to spend one or two nights in the unit learning how to care for their relative. They are shown, where appropriate, how to handle him, turn him in bed, dress and undress him, bath him and manage his bowel and bladder. They are encouraged to carry out as much of the care as they (and the individual concerned) feel is appropriate. Whilst most carers gain in confidence and ability through this tuition, some find that the care and commitment required is too great. In such situations the whole family will need to discuss the options available; more care attendant or district nurse help may be in order, or it may be decided that the individual will not return home but will move into independent living or some form of residential care.

This teaching on the wards is frequently followed by a weekend in the training flat or house, where the whole family can work as a unit with the ward staff performing the district nurse role as required.

Work and education

Attitudes to work vary. For some people it is vital, in which case every effort should be made to facilitate a return to some form of paid employment. A period of resettlement at home after discharge is essential and a return to work should be attempted only when the person has readjusted to his domestic situation and can cope with all that work involves. The skills and advice of the Disablement Resettlement Officer (DRO) should be used whenever applicable, for instance in negotiation with previous employers, assessment and retraining, applying for grants and making arrangements for working from home. Young people should, wherever possible, return to their own

school or college to continue their education. However, access and facilities at schools, colleges and universities will vary considerably and should be assessed by the occupational therapist.

Sport and leisure

Sport should be an enjoyable part of the treatment programme for those who are interested. Activities such as basketball, archery and table tennis are frequently played and provide very good upper limb strengthening and balance reeducation. However, some people with spinal cord lesions prefer more sedate activity.

It is possible that the individual will have more leisure time after his accident than he did previously. Every effort should be made to enable him to use his time enjoyably and constructively. There are many sports associations that cater for sportsmen and women with disabilities, either alongside the able-bodied or as a separate group; increasingly, the two groups compete on equal terms.

Driving

Modern technology is such that severely disabled people are now able to drive a suitably adapted car. Most people with paraplegia can drive standard automatic transmission cars that have been fitted with hand controls. There is no need for them to retake their driving test, although they must inform the Driver and Vehicle Licensing Centre (DVLC) and their car insurers of their change in circumstances. It may be advisable for an individual to have one or more driving lessons with a suitably qualified driving instructor who can show him the basic skills involved in using hand controls and who can help him regain his confidence.

The individual with tetraplegia will need more assistance and should be assessed by a driving assessment centre, such as the Banstead Place Mobility Centre or the Mobility Advice and Vehicle Information Service (MAVIS) at Crowthorne. Although he is able to drive, the tetraplegic person will need assistance getting his wheelchair in and out of the vehicle. He does not need to retake the driving test but must inform the DVLC and his insurers.

INCOMPLETE SPINAL CORD LESIONS

The psychological stresses on people with incomplete lesions are great. Their prognosis is ill-defined and although they may make a good recovery they may find it difficult to accept anything less than total recovery. In a unit surrounded by individuals who have complete paraplegic and tetraplegic lesions they are often considered fortunate. Although in many ways this may be true, they still have a disability that prevents them from returning to their previous life-style. These individuals frequently feel frustrated and often feel pressurised to achieve for the other individuals in the unit.

An understanding of the concepts involved in the bilateral approach to neurological conditions (see p. 378) will assist the therapist in her treatment of incomplete lesions.

SEXUAL FUNCTION

Disruption of normal sexual function is often made worse by fear and anxiety. It is important for all staff to be prepared to discuss the issue of sexual relationships sensitively and in a positive and constructive manner. The individual will sometimes broach the subject with someone he feels he can confide in or with whom he has a good working relationship. At other times staff will need to initiate discussion about relationships, explaining the facts and making constructive suggestions about the person's future sex life.

Each person needs to be told what the physical situation is, for example, that a women's fertility is unaffected by her spinal lesion, and although care would need to be taken, she is still capable of bearing children. Male fertility, however, is often decreased because of a reduced sperm count. The individual may also need to be reassured that although his sex life may be altered it is by no means over and he can still have a loving relationship with his partner. Individuals and couples can gain practical advice on aspects such as positioning, and care of the bladder or catheter during intercourse, from organisations such as Association to Aid the Sexual and Personal Relationships of People with a Disability (SPOD) and the Spinal Injuries Association (SIA). Research work is being done, particularly with regard to male fertility and the collection of motile sperm.

CONCLUSION

Therapists working in the field of spinal cord lesions are given the opportunity to use all of their professional skills. During the course of treatment the therapist is likely to work within the hospital setting, out in the community, and in the work environment. She will assess and teach physical skills, help to build self-esteem and self-confidence and encourage coping skills. She will be a facilitator, a counsellor and a friend to the individual and his family.

Advances in modern technology have not only made it possible to treat people with ultra high lesions but have dramatically improved their quality of life. This is an exciting time to be involved in the care of those with spinal cord lesions.

USEFUL ADDRESSES

Association to Aid the Sexual and Personal Relationships of People with a Disability (SPOD)
286 Camden Road
London N7 0BJ

British Paraplegic Sports Association
Ludwig Guttman Sports Centre
Harvey Road
Aylesbury
Bucks HP21 8PP

Disabled Drivers Association
18 Creekside
London SE8 3DZ

Disabled Living Foundation
380–384 Harrow Road
London W9 2HU

Royal Association for Disability
and Rehabilitation (RADAR)
25 Mortimer Street
London W1N 8AB

Spinal Injuries Association
Newpoint House
76 St James's Lane
London N10 3DF

FURTHER READING

Bedbrook G 1981 The care and management of spinal cord injuries. Springer-Verlag, New York

Bedbrook G 1985 Lifetime care of the paraplegic patient. Churchill Livingstone, Edinburgh

Bromley Ida 1981 Tetraplegia and paraplegia: a guide for physiotherapists, 3rd edn. Churchill Livingstone, Edinburgh

Ford J R, Duckworth B 1987 Physical management of the quadriplegic patient, 2nd edn. F A Davis, Philadelphia

Grundy et al 1986 A.B.C. of spinal cord injury. British Medical Journal, London

Malick M, Meyer C 1978 Manual on management of the upper extremity. Marmarville Rehabilitation Centre, Pittsburgh

Morris J 1989 Able lives: women's experiences of paralysis. Women's Press, London

Oliver M et al 1988 Walking into darkness. Experience of spinal cord injury Macmillan, London

Rogers M 1986 Living with paraplegia Faber & Faber, London

Trieschmann, R 1980 Spinal cord injuries: psychological, social and vocational adjustment. Pergamon Press, New York

SECTION 3

Musculoskeletal and vascular problems

24

Introduction to musculoskeletal and vascular problems

Margaret Foster

INTRODUCTION

The human body is a complex mechanism which relies on the smooth interaction of a number of systems in order to function normally. The chapters in this section consider rheumatoid and osteoarthritic disorders, back problems, burns, amputations, fractures and limb injuries. These disorders significantly affect the musculoskeletal and vascular systems of the body. This is not to say that other systems are not involved, but the degree of resulting impairment will generally be less from the involvement of the other systems than from the problems resulting from musculoskeletal and vascular damage.

PRINCIPLES OF OCCUPATIONAL THERAPY

The basic principles for the treatment of the conditions considered in this section do not differ from those that the occupational therapist will use in working with other kinds of disabilities or injuries. However, in a significant number of situations the aims and goals of the interventions described here may be directed towards achieving complete recovery. Following the successful clinical management of the effects of trauma resulting in burns, fractures, limb injuries or amputation, none of the conditions covered in this section is in itself life-threatening.

The occupational therapist is involved in helping people with any of these disorders to achieve maximum potential according to their wishes. This may be in preparation for a total life span in the case of the person with congenital limb absence, or for a considerable number of ensuing years for many others. Where there is residual dysfunction the occupational therapist is involved in assisting the person to make positive adjustments to changed circumstances so that he can meet lifestyle wishes and needs.

THE ANATOMICAL AND PHYSIOLOGICAL BACKGROUND

It may be deduced from the study of the human body that the musculoskeletal system is predominantly concerned with movement and posture, the bones acting as levers and the joints as fulcrums for movement, while muscle contraction and relaxation provides the control for action to occur. Any damage to bones or muscles will therefore result in some disturbance of movement at the affected part. The effect on the person's mobility will differ according to the extent and site of the damage, but the impact on the local affected area will be the same: an alteration in the range of movement.

The vascular system is composed of the cardiovascular (heart and blood vessels) and the lymphatic systems. These are concerned with blood circulation and tissue fluid balance and are important systems in disease or injury:

- in the conveyance of nutrients and oxygen to a damaged site for tissue repair
- in the removal of waste products
- in the coagulation of blood to control fluid loss from a wound
- in the maintenance of homeostasis within the body
- in the production and transport of antibodies to combat infection.

The cardiovascular and lymphatic systems act as

the transporters for the body and interlink with other systems, such as the respiratory system for oxygen and the digestive and urinary systems for waste product removal.

It is virtually impossible to damage one system in isolation. Musculoskeletal injury will have vascular implications and, similarly, a deficit in circulation may starve an area of nutrients, resulting in necrosis of tissues, which will in turn affect mobility.

In understanding health and disease it is important to consider the dependency of the body on the performance of its individual parts. The action of the major organs — the heart and the lungs — is necessary for circulation to occur, and skeletal muscle action is particularly important for venous return.

It is not possible in this text to give a detailed description of these systems, but study of human anatomy and physiology reveals the interplay of the musculoskeletal and vascular systems and their importance in the body's performance in health and disease.

It is important to consider the implications of the anatomical and physiological links between the systems for the occupational therapist's intervention. For treatment to be successful members of the rehabilitation team should understand the effects of the disease or injury on the body, as these will determine the recovery potential and the approaches chosen in the rehabilitation programme. A fracture will not heal without an adequate vascular supply. A disease or injury which reduces mobility will affect circulation, and a defect in circulation may result in secondary complications which reduce mobility. The person with arthritis may have peripheral vascular problems and the individual with peripheral vascular insufficiency may eventually require an amputation because of necrosis of tissue distally.

Occupational therapists frequently use activity as their therapeutic medium. The choice of activity will be dependent on the individual's needs, but any physical activity will obviously affect the motor function of muscles and joints and promote circulatory performance by the vascular system. This principle may form the basis for the choice of specific activities to promote physical improve-

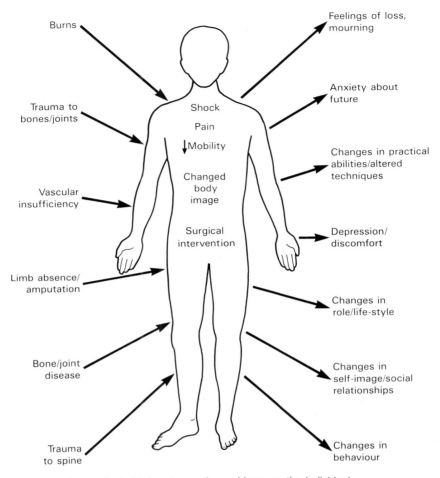

Fig. 24.1 The possible impact of musculoskeletal and vascular problems on the individual.

ment, particularly in relation to the biomechanical approach.

However, occupational therapists are primarily concerned with problem-solving and their role encompasses much more than simply addressing the anatomical and physiological implications of various disorders. While the disorders considered in this section have certain similarities in their physical impact on the body's systems, it is the broader effects of these clinical features on a person's life-style (Fig. 24.1) — the impairments and resulting disabilities — which form the basis for intervention. The following sections will therefore concentrate on other features of these

disorders and their impact on the person, his family and his carers in terms of a changed life-style.

Psychological implications

Back injuries, amputations, fractures, limb injuries and burns may all be the result of an accident or injury. In these instances the impact has been sudden, leaving the individual and those close to him in a state of shock. Physical shock may need intensive specialised nursing if the person is to recover, but the impact of emotional shock may take much longer to overcome.

The stages of recovery from emotional shock

may be similar to the stages of the mourning process described by Kubler-Ross and others, in which the person grieves for what is lost. The person needs to work through the stages of anger and guilt, bitterness, depression, denial and frustration if he is to come to terms with his changed circumstances. He may assign blame for the accident, or feel guilty himself at its occurrence, or be afraid of facing the future. However efficient the process of recovery is, unless the emotional and psychological impact of the bereavement is explored and the necessary adjustments made, the injury or accident is likely to have a long-term effect upon the person's life-style and relationships.

Numerous explanations of the stages of transition from grief to acceptance have been given by psychologists. However, it is now generally recognised that these stages may only reflect the general outline of the process and that the sequencing of the stages may fluctuate. Recovery may level off at a particular stage, causing a return of anger, depression or frustration, and creating a new hurdle to overcome in the rehabilitation process. A sudden memory of something that occurred or existed prior to the accident may trigger a return of mourning, depression or denial. Additionally, the person's response to loss and the process of adjustment is very individual and may be equally dependent on his premorbid personality, family support and security, previous life-style and on the quality of care he receives.

These factors are not unique to the traumatic conditions already identified, but may occur in any situation of loss. However, symptoms are often more dramatic where the loss has been sudden and the person has had no opportunity for gradual adjustment. Those who are affected by a rheumatoid or osteoarthritic disease, or require an amputation for peripheral vascular insufficiency may not experience the sudden initial shock. Nevertheless, many still show the symptoms of the grieving process, mourning the life that is lost or restricted by the disease. There is often a more gradual realisation of the change. In any event, the person must eventually acknowledge the reality of his condition if successful adjustments to residual dysfunction are to be achieved.

The person who has limb deficiency at birth will never have known the experience of life with limbs but in later life may express some anger or bitterness at his loss or limitation. Similarly, it is not unusual for parents to grieve for the 'normal' child they had hoped for at birth, and considerable support may be required to help them with this process.

Age distribution

When comparing or grouping the conditions discussed in this section it is interesting to consider their age distribution. Unlike many conditions seen in occupational therapy, which predominantly affect middle-aged and elderly groups, the disorders in this section have a wide age distribution, the occurrence being highest in young adulthood and early middle age. Only osteoarthritis and amputation as the result of peripheral vascular disease are commonest in those over sixty years. With the exception of congenital limb absence, all the other disorders may occur at any age. Many result from accidental trauma, which occurs most frequently in the young adult.

Age distribution will affect the objectives and goals of therapy. The priorities of many young adults differ from those of the majority of people over sixty years. The potential for physical recovery is usually greater among young people, whose rehabilitation will be directed towards skills which may be actively continued for many ensuing years.

However, on the negative side, the young adult may have less life experience on which to build his rehabilitation than the older person does. This may affect work opportunities or role responsibilities as parent or breadwinner, as well as personal interactions and the social aspects of life-style.

Mobility

Inevitably, damage to the musculoskeletal system will affect movement. This may take the form of short-term loss of movement until recovery occurs, or of long-term movement deficits if there is significant damage or a systemic disorder.

The nature of the problems created by loss of

mobility will vary with the area of the body affected, the extent and cause of the impairment, and the hopes and life-style of the individual. Loss of dexterity and fine finger movement may have similar effects on the life-style and hopes of a computer operator as the amputation of a lower limb may have on an elderly keen gardener. Both will have to consider management of their daytime occupation, either by finding new ways to perform the activity, or by considering alternative activities.

The emphasis on mobility in daily living will vary enormously from one individual to another. A person who is faced with compensating for loss or reduction in movement early in life may learn new techniques more quickly than an older person. However, there may be damage to other areas of the body in the long-term if such techniques redistribute the stresses of mobility onto areas of the body not designed for this purpose. For example, the long-term use of crutches or walking frames may result in osteoarthritic changes in the upper limbs. Many elderly people more readily accept some reduction in mobility as part of the ageing process, but those who have prepared for an active retirement may be just as frustrated as the younger person.

Problems affecting limb movement may cause difficulty with many aspects of personal care, work, and leisure skills, and may inhibit the person's communication through gesture or touch. The loss or limitation of the complex and varied functions of the hands may restrict employment opportunities or affect confidence in making relationships. The hands are highly visible parts of the body, used together in the sight of others to perform everyday tasks. If they are hidden away this may indicate embarrassment at their disfigurement or a reluctance to accept their restricted function.

The lower limbs are the tools of conveyance in the environment, allowing a person to rise from a seated position and move from room to room, level to level and place to place. A lower limb mobility problem imprisons the person in his environment and in so doing restricts social and physical contact. Studies of the physiology of exercise show that a reduction in mobility affects circulation and thereby the person's general health and potential for overcoming injury or disease.

Many members of the rehabilitation team will be involved with improving the person's mobility — most particularly the physiotherapist where physical movement techniques are affected. The occupational therapist may use activity towards furthering these physical improvements, or she may be more concerned with helping people with residual mobility problems to face the challenges of daily living.

Surgery

This may be a sudden intervention as the result of an accident or may be one of a number of techniques in a programme of treatment used to overcome a problem or to improve potential for function. A fracture may require immediate surgery following an accident in order to facilitate bony union. The person who has suffered burns may need repeated skin grafting. The joints damaged by rheumatoid arthritis or osteoarthritis may benefit from synovectomy, arthroplasty or tendon repair. Surgical amputation of a limb may be the culmination of a long period of other treatments aimed to improve distal circulation or healing.

The physical and psychological effects of surgery vary from person to person and the nature of the surgery. Many people take considerable time to overcome the physical effects of anaesthesia. The anxiety of impending surgery may be devastating for some, while others will look forward to the relief from pain and the improvement they hope will result. Advice and education regarding the surgery and the ensuing nursing care can help to relieve some of the person's fears of the unknown, thus engendering a more positive approach to the operation and the immediate postoperative care. If the person can discuss fears and anxieties about the surgery with the team, and question them on the anticipated outcome, he is likely to have a more positive, cooperative attitude, particularly in the early stages of rehabilitation, than those who are fearful and anxious of the success of the surgery and see it as a last hope when all else has failed. A joint replacement for an osteoarthritic hip may make a dramatic positive change to a person's life-style. A laminectomy may relieve pain and the limitations of spinal movement and internal fixation of a fracture will enable the person to achieve early mobilisation and thereby avoid possible complications from prolonged immobility. The surgical amputee who has suffered a long period of pain and limited mobility prior to surgery may see the post-operative stage as a new phase in his treatment which will culminate in an improved quality of life.

Obviously, when surgical intervention is sudden there is little opportunity for education and discussion of fears and anxieties, but studies have shown that where such counselling has been possible the person has been more cooperative in the early post-operative rehabilitation.

Pain

With the possible exception of the child with congenital limb deficiency, all the people with the disorders addressed in this section are likely to experience physical pain. This may be the sudden intense pain from an injury such as a fracture or burn. It may be long-term localised pain from a damaged osteoarthritic joint or from back injury, or chronic generalised pain characteristic of rheumatoid arthritis. People who have had amputations frequently suffer a phantom limb sensation which may at times be physically painful. Damaged exposed nerve endings following burns may retain hypersensitivity and be painful to touch for a considerable time after the accident.

People react differently to physical pain. Some people express the pain openly, avoiding or resisting any activity which is likely to exacerbate their discomfort. Others internalise the pain, stoically continuing activity despite intense agony. It is important for the therapist to recognise the existence and importance of pain and explore avenues of overcoming or avoiding it.

Sudden pain may be a warning. It may indicate:

- over-exertion in activity
- the possibility of infection
- further physical damage which requires investigation.

Chronic pain may destroy both the body and the mind, pressurising the person into changes in life-style, relationships and even personality. The person with chronic pain may:

- lose motivation to perform essential basic personal activities
- be unable to continue domestic, work or social roles
- put pressure on family and carers — practically, emotionally and financially
- avoid close relationships which involve any form of physical contact or other involvement which is likely to cause further pain
- alter behaviour: become withdrawn, tearful, angry, frustrated, depressed or demanding.

By recognising the pain it is hoped that the necessary measures may be taken to control it, or ensure it is of short duration or sufficiently managed to avoid gross inhibition of normal activity. Some clinical members of the treatment team may be responsible for prescribing surgical, chemotherapeutic or other ways of controlling pain, but the occupational therapist should share the responsibility for recognising the pain and encouraging the person to address it positively. In many situations the occupational therapist plays an active role in pain management through her skills in counselling, and by instructing the person in relaxation techniques and compensatory methods to avoid or overcome stressful activities. Such education should include the family or carers to ensure that a positive, understanding approach is maintained in the home environment.

It is also important to recognise psychological pain. This is not unique to people with the conditions discussed in this section, but a considerable number may be affected by it. Psychological pain may be closely linked to the bereavement process previously identified, where it presents as physical pain due to muscle tension, anxiety, fear or frustration. Relaxation and counselling may play vital roles in helping to control such pain.

Some people who have visible disfigurements also suffer emotional pain. This is frequently linked to anxieties regarding acceptance or rejection by others because of changed body image. Such situations require understanding and support to promote assertiveness and help build confidence so that the person can gradually become re-integrated into the community.

THE OCCUPATIONAL THERAPY PROCESS

The occupational therapy process as applied to musculoskeletal and vascular problems is the same as that used in other treatment areas. It consists of assessment, planning, implementation and evaluation. A variety of types of assessment may be used, but the most common are those involving physical measurement, the evaluation of daily living skills and work assessment. Planning and implementation of the intervention will vary according to the disorder, the individual and his particular needs.

As many of the disorders are the result of trauma, much of the early intervention will be clinically based. However, many people may require help on return to the community, either to assist with a short-term mobility problem or, where there is residual dysfunction, on a more long-term basis.

INTERVENTION GOALS

Unlike many areas where the occupational therapist is primarily involved in helping a person to adjust to residual deficit or progressive dysfunction, most of the conditions described in this section have the potential for functional improvement; indeed, with some there may be anticipation of almost complete recovery. Everyone, with the exception of the child with congenital limb absence, will have known normality, so rehabilitation will be a relearning rather than an initial learning process.

There will almost inevitably be some stage in all of these conditions where the person will be required to accept some form of dependency. This may be help with personal care following surgery, or assistance with mobility through the use of crutches or an orthosis. However, to avoid the downward disability spiral, where a short-term impairment becomes a long-term disability, it is important that this dependency does not extend beyond essential need and become an excuse for not making decisions or facing responsibility, or a weapon to gain attention. The treatment team should involve the person and his carers in the intervention programme. Encouraging the individual early on to accept responsibility for decision-making regarding treatment goals may help to prevent a downward dependency spiral. Therapy should aim to achieve the return of the person's maximum physical potential, but should not overlook the emotional implications of the impairment if the body and mind are to work together in unison.

In some instances total recovery will not be possible. Although advances in nursing care and surgical techniques have vastly increased the potential for the individual to return to an active life-style, residual dysfunction will result from such disorders as rheumatoid arthritis and osteoarthritis, and following amputation and severe burns. In these situations management of the deficit is of vital importance. If, despite the impairment, the disability can be minimised to enable the person to achieve his aspirations or goals, a satisfactory adjustment is more likely to occur. It is therefore important to ascertain the person's hopes for the future early in the intervention, to foster realistic objectives and prioritise the goals to achieve them.

A realistic understanding of the value of particular methods avoids later disappointments. The provision of orthoses and pressure garments will reduce the risk of serious disfigurement following burns. However, there will inevitably be scarring and it is important for the person to be aware of this from the start if he is to value these methods positively and not see the outcome as a failure. Modern prostheses, while much improved in design and movement potential over earlier models, will not truly replace the function of the limb and the person will need to accept and adjust to these limitations. A hip replacement can overcome the problems at an individual joint, but cannot positively directly affect the disease process in other parts of the body.

APPROACHES

The occupational therapist may use a number of

approaches when treating people affected by the conditions described in this section. The most commonly used approaches are humanistic, psychosocial, rehabilitative and biomechanical. Frequently there is overlap in the use of these approaches, particular aspects of each being used to attain specific goals at each stage of the programme. Biomechanical principles, for example, are important in the achievement of physical mobility whilst the rehabilitative approach may be more applicable in the early stages following injury or surgery, to compensate for temporary loss of function. This may be gradually phased out in favour of biomechanical principles as recovery progresses. If the improvement is incomplete a return to the rehabilitative approach may be necessary to assist the person to compensate for residual dysfunction.

Humanistic and psychosocial principles are utilised in almost all areas. Occupational therapy is concerned with physical, psychological and social aspects of living and the therapist's philosophy is based in recognition of each person's volition, individuality and potential.

Occasionally, other approaches may be used. These may be specifically directed to psychological processes to facilitate recovery or promote progress. Frequently they are concerned with the acceptance of and positive adjustment to changed circumstances. For example, desensitisation techniques and assertion skills may be of assistance when coping with disfigurement following burns, limb injuries or amputation, and the use of other approaches to promote learning and adjustment may be necessary for the confused elderly amputee, or the person with depression resulting from chronic pain.

CONCLUSION

It is important for all members of the rehabilitation team to view the disorders considered in this section in context. In the past many such disorders have been seen from a predominantly physical perspective — the effects of the damage on the musculoskeletal and vascular systems of the body — and have been treated accordingly. Knowledge of these effects and their treatment is crucial to physical recovery, but equally important is the recognition of the totality of the psychosocial effects of such disorders. The understanding of the mechanics of activity and equipment, the provision of orthoses or prostheses, or the adaptation of techniques and the environment may meet the person's physical requirements, but awareness of his personality, stresses, aspirations, and lifestyle priorities, and of his need for education and emotional support, are equally important for successful rehabilitation.

FURTHER READING

Guyton A C 1987 Human physiology and mechanisms of disease, 4th edn. W B Saunders, Philadelphia
Hopkins H, Smith H 1988 Willard and Spackman's occupational therapy, 7th edn. J B Lippincott, Philadelphia

Kubler-Ross E 1969 On death and dying. Tavistock, London
Versluys H P 1989 Psychosocial accommodation to physical disability. In: Trombly C (ed) Occupational therapy for physical dysfunction, 3rd edn. Williams & Wilkins, Baltimore.

25

Amputation

Jean Colburn and Vivienne Ibbotson

INTRODUCTION

Amputation, the removal of all or part of a limb, may be necessary for a number of reasons and can affect persons of all ages. This chapter discusses the contribution that the occupational therapist can make in assisting an amputee to attain an optimum level of function and independence following limb loss.

The chapter begins by outlining the major reasons for or causes of amputation. (For our purposes, congenital limb absence will be considered as a form of 'amputation'.) General principles of rehabilitation are set out, with specific reference to the role of the occupational therapist in the assessment and treatment of amputees before and after the prescription of an artifical limb. Problems that commonly occur following amputation, such as 'phantom limb sensations', are also described.

Next, the chapter focuses specifically on the rehabilitation of individuals who have lost all or part of a lower limb. Various levels of amputation are described, together with their likely implications for function. Types of prostheses available for lower limb amputees are described and specific problems related to lower limb loss are discussed.

The subsequent sections of the chapter describe the rehabilitation of upper limb amputees. Again, various levels of amputation are described, along with the types of prosthesis appropriate to these. Specific considerations that the therapist should bear in mind during the pre-prosthetic and prosthetic stages of her intervention programme are discussed, and the contribution of other members of the multidisciplinary team is described. Finally, various advantages and disadvantages of using an artificial upper limb are listed.

Throughout, the chapter emphasises that the occupational therapist must be sensitive to the individual needs of each person in planning and implementing her interventions, bearing in mind that the partial or complete loss of a limb has profound psychological implications not only for the individual concerned, but also for those who are close to him.

CAUSES OF AMPUTATION

It is very important for the occupational therapist to know why an amputation has been carried out, as this will influence the goals of treatment and decisions regarding the choice of prosthesis. The most common causes of amputation are outlined below.

Peripheral vascular disease (PVD)

This is by far the most common cause of lower limb amputation, and accounts for about 80% of all cases. The condition primarily affects people in older age groups. Occlusive arterial disease gradually impairs the circulation, causing peripheral ischaemia, and if viable circulation cannot be restored by other means (such as an arterectomy, sympathectomy or femoral bypass) amputation becomes necessary. In such cases cardiorespiratory function may also be impaired, and many people have additional medical problems such as hypertension or diabetes. Because PVD is a systemic disease the overall prognosis is poor. Circulation to the second limb is generally impaired, and many people with PVD are likely to become bilateral amputees in three to five years' time.

Trauma

This is the second most common cause of lower limb amputation and the principle reason for the loss of upper limbs. Most amputations are due to motor vehicle or industrial accidents, but some are secondary to severe trauma such as burns. The amputation may be immediate (limb severed at the time of the accident) or may be necessary at a later date if a badly damaged limb does not heal satisfactorily. In either case there may well be other associated injuries that will affect the outcome of rehabilitation.

Malignancy

Although bone cancer is rare, such cases are always very serious. Radical high-level surgery (such as hemipelvectomy or hip disarticulation of the lower limb, or forequarter amputation of the upper limb) is often necessary as a life-saving measure. Osteosarcomas are the cause of only a small proportion of amputations (5%), but as the disease primarily affects people aged 10–19 years who are usually otherwise fit and active, each person requires skilled care. Attention to social and vocational needs is particularly important.

Congenital limb deficiency

This term is used to describe limb deformities occurring before birth. The actual cause of such malformations is variable, but some contributing factors during pregnancy may be chemicals, drugs, nutritional deficiencies or 'strangulation' of a limb due to the abnormal position of the fetus. Babies may be born with the partial or complete absence of one or more limbs, or with multiple malformations. Such cases occur very seldom but have a tremendous impact on the child's physical, psychological and social development, and on the family unit as a whole.

PRINCIPLES OF REHABILITATION

Amputees require highly specialised, individual

treatment. They have continuing, lifetime needs which can be met only through multidisciplinary collaboration. Teamwork — individuals with special knowledge and expertise working interdependently to attain a common goal — is essential, and the injured person is the most important member of the team. In most amputee clinics the surgeon, prosthetist, physiotherapist, occupational therapist and social worker will deal with day-to-day problems and call on other disciplines for help when needed. Teams may operate within a hospital setting on surgical or rehabilitation wards, or in outpatient units. Regional Disablement Service Centres (DSCs) are responsible for Artificial Limb and Appliance services and the fabrication and fitting of prostheses, and may have facilities for limb training, with physiotherapists and occupational therapists as well as prosthetists on the staff.

The primary aim of treatment is to help each person achieve his maximum level of functional independence, with or without an artificial limb. Psychological support is as important as physical treatment in determining the success of rehabilitation.

All members of the amputee team must be highly skilled, well informed, and able to contribute to a continuing care regime for each individual. The initial period of hospitalisation and prosthetic training is not the beginning and end of care; as conditions change, sockets (or even the type of prostheses) may need to be altered. The 'stump' or residual limb may break down and must be monitored. Community support is often required, and special services will be needed for children, the elderly, and other especially vulnerable people.

THE ROLE OF THE OCCUPATIONAL THERAPIST

Guidelines will be given in the two following sections on Amputations of the Lower Limb and Amputations of the Upper Limb in relation to specific problems of different categories of clients.

The basic principles of assessment and intervention outlined here have general application.

PRINCIPLES OF ASSESSMENT

It is essential that a well-structured and carefully documented assessment is made in all cases so that outcome over time can be properly evaluated. A detailed interview recording factors related to the amputation, personal data, normal roles and responsibilities, skill level, work history and leisure interests is important initially. Work and leisure needs will influence the choice of components for the prosthesis, and also the method of fabrication. Specific assessments (motor, sensory, developmental, cognitive and psychological, as indicated), must be reproducible and standardised as far as possible so that repeated tests will show change over time. Age and level of activity will affect physical status. Some form of standardised functional assessment, such as the Barthel ADL Index, (Mahoney & Barthel 1965) is valuable.

Physical assessment is important and must be well documented, as any loss of range of movement will affect prosthetic use. Goniometry and manual muscle testing should be used to assess both affected and unaffected limbs. Strength is important. For instance, for an above elbow amputee to use a conventional prosthesis he must have good mobility and control of the shoulder girdle on the amputated side, and considerable power in shoulder flexors, protractors and depressors in order to flex the forearm and operate the terminal device effectively. A below knee amputee must have good hip control, full knee extension and powerful quadriceps for normal gait and levels of activity.

Any abnormalities of sensation (either hypersensitivity or diminished sensation) must be recorded and the type, severity and location of pain noted (see p. 632). Other forms of assessment may be needed in certain instances. These will be referred to, where necessary, later in the chapter.

PRINCIPLES OF TREATMENT

Intervention is staged in relation to the status of the stump. Initial healing may be fairly rapid in young amputees, but delayed in people with vascular disease or diabetes. However, the residual limb will initially be oedematous and tender, and a permanent prosthesis cannot be fitted until the stump is reduced to normal size and tissues can tolerate a certain amount of pressure. Consequently, the management of amputees is divided into two clear stages: *pre-prosthetic* and *prosthetic* care.

Pre-prosthetic

The main aims of the therapist's intervention before a prosthesis is fitted are:

* to help the individual to regain independence in self-care
* to teach correct stump care and conditioning
* to help the individual to increase/maintain limb strength and range of movement
* to teach wheelchair management (if indicated)
* to provide or arrange for psychological support and counselling
* to evaluate on an ongoing basis cognition and functional adaptation (in the elderly).

In some instances, pre-operative assessment and treatment may be indicated. In the early post-operative stage it is important to prevent any flexion contractures of the stump, and with lower limb amputees daily prone lying is necessary. The individual should never support the stump on a pillow, or (if a below knee amputee) sit without having the limb fully supported. Special stump boards are needed for wheelchairs. (Instructions for making these are given in the BAOT's *Occupational Therapists' Reference Book* 1990.)

Stump care is of primary importance. Prosthetic fitting is dependent on a good stump shape, and this may be controlled by stump bandaging (Fig. 25.1) using 'shrinker' elasticated stump socks or, occasionally, rigid post-surgical dressings. All techniques require care and expertise. Above all, the person should learn to handle and 'care for' the stump as soon as dressings are removed. The skin must be washed daily and carefully checked with a mirror for any signs of skin

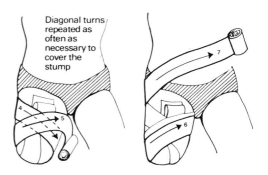

Fig. 25.1   Stump bandaging. Above knee amputation — used infrequently to control oedema because of the difficulty in ensuring the bandaging is applied evenly, exerting equal pressure on all aspects of the stump.

irritation or abrasion. Gentle massage may help to desensitise the limb, and will help the person to adjust to limb loss. Initial reaction to the sight of the amputation may be one of distress, or even disgust but the person's assumption of responsibility for his own self-care will help him to adjust to his changed body image and accept his loss. It is also important for a family member or princple carer to be involved in the early stages of treatment. Reactions of carers are critical and can affect the person's motivation for rehabilitation. Group treatment, and the opportunity for family members to attend support groups with amputees, can be advantageous at this stage.

Prosthetic

The therapist's main aims following the introduction of a prosthesis are to help the individual to:

* increase standing tolerance and improve weight transference and gait control (lower limb)
* increase wearing tolerance and unit control (upper limb; e.g. terminal devices, elbow locks, etc.)
* attain independence in all Activities of Daily Living (ADL) and in the care and use of the prosthesis

- gain proficiency in advanced functional activities, and in work and leisure skills.

Her role at this stage also includes:

- providing or arranging for psychological support and counselling as necessary
- arranging for the provision of support services where indicated.

It is imperative to monitor the person carefully through all stages of prosthetic training. The stump is still vulnerable and can easily break down if the prosthesis does not fit properly and causes skin friction or local pressure areas. This can only be checked by the individual wearing the prosthesis for short periods of time at first (30 minutes to an hour) and then examining the stump critically for signs of pressure, redness or local discomfort. The time tolerated can be increased daily, as can the demands of the activities that the person undertakes. Group activities with other amputees can be helpful, as they allow for expression of feelings, and encourage people to learn problem-solving techniques from one another. The occupational therapy department can be used to simulate a wide range of normal daily activities, such as homemaking, workshop or clerical skills. Learning through play is the technique adopted for children.

Self-management

Above all, individuals must learn how to look after themselves and protect the stump. Specially tailored seamless stump socks must always be worn with a prosthesis, and underwear (of natural fibres) is necessary to protect the skin if any form of suspension or harness is worn. Good prosthetic use requires effort and a good deal of persistence. Continual practice is necessary to achieve semi-automatic movement responses and this is best accomplished on a full-day regime in occupational therapy.

The final stages of treatment should focus on work-related skills and social activities. Some adaptation may be needed in a number of areas. High-level lower limb amputees will certainly need a wheelchair for outdoor mobility, and transport-ation and use of public facilities generally should be checked.

APPROACHES TO TREATMENT

The occupational therapist will utilise aspects from a variety of treatment approaches in both her pre- and post-prosthetic intervention programmes.

Biomechanical principles may be used to build up joint range of movement and muscle strength in the proximal parts of the affected limb in order to prepare for prosthetic training. Activities to build up range of movement and strength in the other limbs may assist the person to maintain or regain mobility and bilaterality.

The rehabilitative approach will be utilised to compensate for functional loss and some aspects of a cognitive approach may be used to educate and inform the individual and the family regarding treatment processes, mobility techniques and the importance of particular practices in limb care.

In all areas, the occupational therapist will adopt a humanistic approach, recognising the needs and wishes of the individual and respecting personal drives and circumstances.

PROBLEMS RELATED TO AMPUTATION

Four particular problems related to amputations need some consideration. These are: phantom limb sensation, phantom limb pain, psychological trauma and peripheral neuropathy.

PHANTOM LIMB SENSATION (PLS)

This occurs in virtually all cases of amputation. Amputees have the sensation that the missing limb is still present and 'normal'. It often seems to move and may feel hot, cold, or sweaty, especially in highly innervated areas such as the hands and feet. In most cases this phantom limb sensation is present immediately after surgery and lasts for a variable amount of time (weeks, months, even years). Understandably, it is very disconcerting to the individual. It is important that this phenomenon is clearly explained before surgery, otherwise the individual may be reluctant to discuss the problem and will believe he is reacting in an abnormal way.

PHANTOM LIMB PAIN (PLP)

This is a more serious problem. It usually affects only a small number of amputees, but has considerable functional implications. Sufferers experience pain — often described as 'stabbing', 'burning', 'squeezing' or 'crushing' — which is variable in frequency, intensity and duration. Onset may not occur for weeks or even years after the amputation. It has been found that PLP can be precipitated by tiredness, minor injuries to the stump and tissue breakdown, and that it is exacerbated by emotional stress or cold weather. The condition is difficult to treat and may become chronic if it persists for more than six months. It is vital to find the pain 'triggers' for each person as well as ways of alleviating discomfort (such as heat, rest, distraction), so that individuals can learn self-management techniques. Psychological counselling can help to reduce stress and anxiety related to PLP.

PSYCHOLOGICAL TRAUMA

All individuals will have an emotional reaction to amputation, and this will vary in relation to age, sex, culture and personality. When individuals have good patterns of coping with stress or loss they may adjust more easily, but it has been found that reactions to amputation are similar to those for bereavement. Amputees are likely to have a sense of numbness and restless pining and to be preoccupied with thoughts of loss as they mourn the amputation and the diminution of their self- and body-image. Raphael 1984 found that adjustment is more difficult for individuals who have rigid, compulsively self-reliant personalities, or who have experienced prolonged illness or some other recent significant loss such as retirement or unemployment.

Even where amputation does not significantly affect function, it can have an enormous impact on self-esteem. Individuals may project their own disgust with their changed appearance onto others, becoming overly concerned about loss of sexual attractiveness or inadequate personal relationships, and may react by becoming depressed or more demanding. It is important to recognise that, just as with other forms of bereavement, it takes time to adjust. Counselling is important, and group techniques in occupational therapy can be very beneficial. Ongoing support groups for amputees and family members may be of value.

PERIPHERAL NEUROPATHY

This condition is often present in people who have diabetes and PVD, but may also occur in trauma. Sensory, motor and autonomic nerves may be impaired, leading to: decreased awareness of pain, heat and other critical protective sensations; motor weakness causing foot deformity or maldistribution of pressure over the soles of the feet; and dry, cracked skin. In each instance there is an added risk related to skin breakdown of the stump and of the unaffected limb.

In addition, it is important to realise that sweating will be increased in relation to loss of body mass and that another cause of skin breakdown is maceration, i.e. softening caused by moisture. It is therefore essential for stump socks or undergarments to be changed daily (or several times a day in hot weather), to make sure the skin is always dry. Stump socks must always be clean, as any build-up of body salts can cause skin friction.

AMPUTATIONS OF THE LOWER LIMB

LEVELS OF AMPUTATION

The actual level of amputation is very important in relation to prosthetic function. It is essential to preserve as much limb length as possible, as this will provide better leverage for acceleration in gait and will reduce the energy cost of ambulation. At a normal walking pace the increased cost of energy

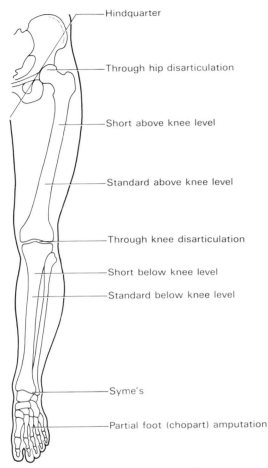

— Hindquarter

— Through hip disarticulation

— Short above knee level

— Standard above knee level

— Through knee disarticulation

— Short below knee level

— Standard below knee level

— Syme's

— Partial foot (chopart) amputation

Fig. 25.2 Levels of lower limb amputation.

for a below knee (BK) amputee is 15%–20%; for an above knee (AK) amputee 50%–70% and for a bilateral amputee as much as 300%.

Terms used for lower limb amputees are descriptive of the level of amputation (Fig. 25.2). The significance of loss, in mechanical terms, is cumulative. The following components of ambulation are affected:

- forefoot leverage for 'push-off'
- ability to accommodate to uneven ground (in/eversion)
- kinesthesia and proprioception of knee joint
- power and mechanical leverage (this will change in relation to the length of the

residual limb)
- centre of gravity (this will change in relation to the loss of body mass, affecting balance and righting reactions).

Normal walking is an 'automatic' learned response, based on sensory regulatory mechanisms. All amputees lose some sensory awareness as well as power, and have to relearn walking patterns and balance reactions. The loss of the knee joint is functionally very significant.

PROSTHESES

Considerable advances have been made in the design and fabrication of artificial limbs in recent years, but standard fittings are still often heavy and cumbersome. Only three of the most common types of prostheses are illustrated here: the Below Knee (BK), Above Knee (AK) and Through Hip Prosthesis (THP) (Figs. 25.3–25.5).

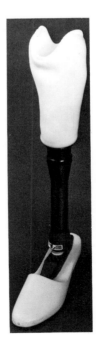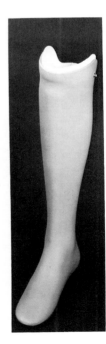

Fig. 25.3 Definitive below knee prostheses. Endolite Patella Tendon Bearing limb — without and with cosmesis. (Photograph by courtesy of Chas A. Blatchford & Sons Ltd.)

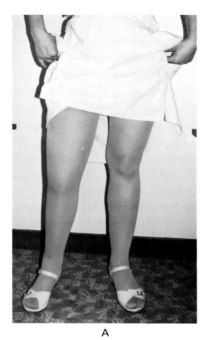

A

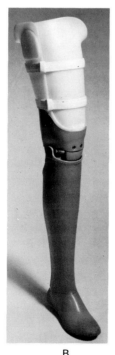

B

Fig. 25.4 (A) Endolite above knee limb. (B) Above knee prosthesis. A PRIMAP limb. (Photographs by courtesy of Chas A. Blatchford & Sons Ltd.)

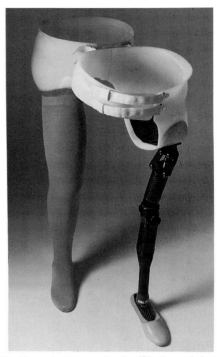

Fig. 25.5 Through hip prosthesis. (Photograph by courtesy of Chas. A. Blatchford & Sons Ltd.)

It is important to note that, with the exception of Syme's and through knee prostheses, no weight can be taken on the end of the stump. Designs of sockets are primarily determined by the distribution of body weight. BK amputees have patella tendon bearing (PTB) sockets in which weight is taken through the patella tendon and the medial and lateral flares of the tibia (Fig. 25.3), while AK amputees are supplied either with a quadrilateral socket, taking weight mainly through the ischial tuberosity, or with a narrow 'medial-lateral' socket in which weight is distributed over the medial and lateral aspects of the femur. Quadrilateral sockets may cause skin irritation of the ischium and pubis, and discomfort in sitting. In the case of hip disarticulation the patient is fitted with a rigid socket suspended from the iliac crest on the opposite side of the pelvis to the site of the amputation, and weight-bearing is through the ischial tuberosity and the bulk of gluteus maximus on the amputated side. The hip joint is set forward to ease sitting and give more stability in standing — the centre of gravity, passing behind the joint, assists hip extension (Fig. 25.5).

Specialised components for prosthetic feet and knee joints can allow lower limb amputees to take part in athletic events. A new energy-storing prosthetic foot (ESPF), for instance, is specially designed to respond to a downward force in heel strike with a mechanical 'rebound' to simulate the push-off phase of running and fast walking.

The amputee team will discuss with the prosthetist the design and components best suited to each person's needs. It is therefore important for the occupational therapist to be well informed about available prosthetic options so that these can be matched with the individual's functional requirements.

All lower limb prostheses consist of: an inner socket (made by the prosthetist from a plaster cast of the person's stump and designed to control weight-bearing areas); an outside shell to provide normal leg length; a replacement knee joint if necessary; and a prosthetic foot. A soft cosmetic cover is provided. Most elderly people need some form of auxiliary suspension such as a waist band or shoulder strap to keep the limb in correct alignment. Younger people with a good, muscular stump may be fitted with a total contact suction socket which is held in place by suction only. This gives more freedom of movement but puts more stress on the tissues of the residual limb.

SPECIAL CONSIDERATIONS FOR LOWER LIMB AMPUTEES

Peripheral vascular disease (PVD)

People admitted for amputation caused by PVD will have had a gradually deteriorating condition for some years and may well have had previous vascular surgery in attempts to save the limb. Symptoms of advanced ischaemia will have been present for several weeks with severe, burning pain and sleepless nights, so the person will generally be exhausted and in poor physical condition when he comes into hospital. Therefore, a period of pre-operative assessment and treatment is necessary.

Pre-operative stage

Aims for the therapeutic team at this stage are:

- *detailed assessment*: physical, psychological, cognitive, overall functional status and living situation
- *physical treatment*: correction of hip, knee flexion contractures, increase of strength and range of movement of upper and lower limbs and trunk and improvement of overall exercise tolerance
- *self-care*: learning of basic transfer techniques and wheelchair management
- *education, support* regarding reasons for amputation, type of prosthesis and training programme. It is important for the individual to develop trust in the team and to have realistic expectations of treatment outcome.

Elderly amputees may have cardiorespiratory problems, arthritis or other medical conditions as well as poor sight or hearing. In addition, they may be slightly confused and forgetful. This will affect their capacity to learn. Pinzur et al (1988) believe that psychological testing for PVD amputees over the age of 60 is essential. They identify a number of cognitive factors needed for successful prosthetic use: attention, concentration, memory, organisational skills, and perceptual skills. In a study using a number of cognitive and psychological tests (such as the Test of Mental Function for the Elderly, Auditory/Verbal Learning Task, Key's Complex Figure and the Minnesota Multiphasic Personality Inventory Test), they were able to predict correctly who could be successfully fitted and trained with a prosthesis. It is very important for amputee teams to keep detailed records and to follow the outcome of rehabilitation in all cases, in order to develop their own criteria of suitability for prosthetic training.

There are two options for elderly PVD amputees: prosthetic training and wheelchair living. If the person is likely to become proficient in the use of a prosthesis the preferred level of amputation is BK. (Saving the knee has been found to increase the potential for ambulation in elderly persons by 50%.) If the person does not have the mental or physical capacity for independent ambulation, an AK amputation may be performed. Careful assessment at the pre-operative stage is therefore very important.

Pre-prosthetic stage

The specific focus for PVD amputees is independence in self-care and home management. Considerable time must be spent on practising ADL such as transfers, dressing and hygiene. Functional independence can only be regained by a *relearning* process; this takes time and repetition. Overall tolerance will be low, and there may initially be post-operative confusion. It is important to note any changes related to the preliminary assessment, and to evaluate emotional reactions to the amputation. Depression or withdrawal is not uncommon.

In order to be effective, self-care routines *must* be habit forming and therefore applied in a consistent, ordered manner. Safety is of paramount importance, and the person will have to learn to adjust to poor balance and position sense and to impaired sensation. If phantom limb sensations are present it is easy to forget that the limb has been amputated. Individuals with PVD may fall at night when they get out of bed to go to the toilet if they do not have a night-light and a bedside commode. Training in all home routines should be instituted in hospital.

Above all, individuals with PVD must be taught specific care techniques for their stump and remaining limb. Some general principles are:

- *dressing*: keep limbs warm with woollen socks; wear lace-up shoes with toe room for support and natural fibres next to the skin. Avoid tight elastics, stretch socks, slip-on shoes or sandals and always wear socks with shoes even when stockings are not worn.
- *hygiene*: wash residual limb daily using mild soap and patting dry with soft towel. Check skin with a mirror. Check skin folds carefully, and inspect foot for abrasions, cuts, scratches. Take care with toenails. (Regular visits to a chiropodist are advisable.) Check water temperature carefully, and if wearing a

prosthesis bathe at night (bathing in the morning may cause 'puffing' and make the prosthesis tight). Do not walk about barefoot.
- *toileting*: if there is a tendency toward incontinence, urgency or frequency, build in routines of regular toileting, control of fluids, and regimes for bowel care re bathing and dressing.
- *transfers*: generally, use standing pivot transfers. Must have firm seat and mattress to avoid 'dragging' and appropriate toilet and bath aids. Stools will be needed for basin and bath, as well as grab rails.

A large number of PVD amputees are diabetic. Malone et al 1989 found in a controlled study of 203 patients that education in foot care reduced the risk of a second limb amputation by about one third.

Prosthetic stage

A temporary prosthesis may be used to evaluate potential for a permanent prosthesis, using crutches or a Zimmer frame. In any event, a PVD amputee will need to train for the additional physical exertion of walking. As oxygen consumption goes up, heart rate and blood pressure will increase to accommodate the effort of ambulation. Early weight-bearing is important with the elderly to prevent loss of normal movement patterns, muscle atrophy and joint contractures.

The entire focus in occupational therapy should be on functional activities and safe home management techniques. Tasks in the kitchen unit give an opportunity for controlled weight-bearing, problem-solving, and the use of aids such as trolleys or perching stools. It is important to evaluate the person's capacity for safely 'planning and doing', and a visit to a local shop (using a wheelchair for outdoor mobility) may be advantageous. Critical decisions must be made prior to discharge on the person's capacity for independent living, the support services needed, and the regime to be followed at home. In some cases, if an individual has insufficient support at home, alternative accommodation will have to be found.

Trauma (BK, AK)

Pre-prosthetic stage

The particular focus for young people who have suffered amputation as a result of trauma is on physical restoration. Treatment in physiotherapy and occupational therapy is aimed at gaining maximum strength and range of movement in the residual limb and affected leg, and increasing general physical tolerance.

Treatment can be rapidly progressive (unless there are complications from associated injuries), and weight-bearing can start within a few days with an early post-surgical prosthetic fitting (EPSF). Individuals may be provided with various types of prostheses, such as a plastic air splint to control post-operative oedema and promote healing, or a pneumatic pylon (PPAM-Aid). This can be used 5–7 days post-operatively before sutures are removed for partial weight-bearing with crutches. Young amputees will have an intensive treatment programme.

BK Amputees need to strengthen quadriceps and regain full extension of the knee. Resisted activities for the unaffected leg with the stump supported in a sling (such as the treadle lathe, Fig. 25.6) will give static quadriceps exercise with reciprocal innervation, and will strengthen the un-

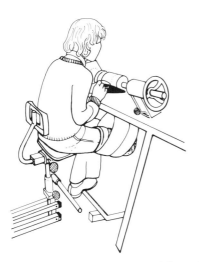

Fig. 25.6 Using the lathe to encourage static work of the quadriceps in the slung limb.

affected limb and trunk muscles at the same time. The quadriceps switch may also be of value, as initially many people will not wear a temporary limb all day.

Prosthetic stage

Intensive treatment, carefully monitoring stump tolerance, should lead to rapid progress at this stage. Workshop activities provide excellent opportunities to increase standing tolerance and improve weight transference. Recreational activities that encourage spontaneous movement responses (such as table tennis, darts and bowls) will help to increase self-confidence. Work-related skills and problem-solving tasks (such as managing rough ground and inclines, lifting and carrying) should be included in the late stages of treatment and advice given on leisure pursuits. Special limbs can be provided for swimming, skuba diving and other sports activities.

Trauma, malignancy (Hip disarticulation or hemipelvectomy)

Pre-prosthetic stage

The main difference between high level and low level amputations of the lower limb is that there is little, if any, post-operative oedema in the former. The pre-prosthetic stage is therefore quite short, possibly only three or four weeks, ending as soon as healing is sound.

People should be mobile as soon as possible, and can stand on the sound leg within two or three days. In most cases of malignancy, amputees are young and fit, and it is important to prevent muscle weakness, loss of balance and loss of self-confidence. They can generally get about well with crutches, and will hop on one leg for short distances.

Initial emphasis is again on self-care. It is most important to protect the skin and to adapt clothing. A tailored body stocking is the preferred garment to wear under a prosthesis, but an alternative is a cotton vest. Clothing with a prosthesis should be easy to put on and take off (as a track suit), and it is important to wear flat, lace-up shoes.

Prosthetic stage

Most young amputees will choose to wear a prosthesis rather than accommodate themselves to wheelchair living, but ambulation is necessarily limited so a wheelchair may be needed for outdoor mobility.

The design of a high level prosthesis presents a number of problems. The rigid socket round the pelvis causes some abdominal pressure, so many people have some problems with distension after eating and drinking, or (in women) with premenstrual tension and fluid retention. Initially there are difficulties with digestion and elimination, but individuals can be taught bladder and bowel routines, and can control diet in terms of the size and frequency of meals. Sweating can present difficulties, too, as the prosthesis must be close fitting.

Tolerance to wearing the prosthesis can only be built up slowly. Gait training is carried out in physiotherapy, while occupational therapists help the person to achieve independence in self-care and basic home management techniques.

Psychological aspects are extremely important, and must be taken into account throughout treatment. Every effort must be made to help each person achieve *his* goals and live life as fully as possible despite his disability. Constructive use of leisure time is vital for all lower limb amputees as a focus for exercise as well as pleasure. Many high level amputees participate in sports such as skiing with adapted equipment, so all former interests need not necessarily be discontinued after surgery.

No information on children with lower limb deficiencies or amputation or bilateral amputees is included in this section. Both groups require very specialised intervention, and more detailed information can be obtained in texts listed under 'Further Reading'.

AMPUTATIONS OF THE UPPER LIMB

The number of people affected by upper limb amputation, whether congenital or acquired, is relatively small. The ratio of lower limb to upper limb amputees seen for the first time at the Sheffield DSC in 1989 was 19:1. This figure reflects the statistics available at other DSCs throughout the country. Therefore, because of the small total number of upper limb amputees, it takes longer for the occupational therapist to gain experience and confidence in treating the varied needs of this group of people.

LEVELS OF AMPUTATION (Fig. 25.7)

Forequarter

This involves the removal of the whole arm, part of the scapula and most of the clavicle, usually because of a malignancy. Fortunately this kind of amputation is rarely necessary and is usually carried out only as a life-saving measure. Because of the residual shape of the torso, the artificial arm has to be attached to a shoulder cap which has been built up to assume the natural shoulder contour.

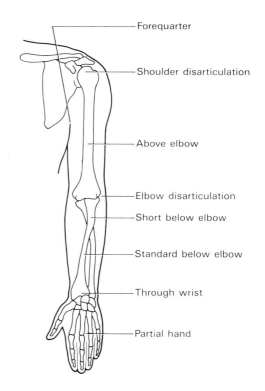

Fig. 25.7 Levels of upper limb amputation.

The individual may find the prosthetic arm restricting, heavy and uncomfortable and resort to the wearing of a shoulder cap only. The cap will, at least, allow clothing to sit more correctly on the shoulders.

Shoulder disarticulation

Again, this type of amputation does not occur frequently but can be caused either by disease or trauma, particularly road traffic accidents. Although it is possible to fit a limb, there will be limited residual movement with which to obtain good function. Many such amputees find it preferable to use their prosthetic limb passively.

Above elbow

Depending on the residual length of the arm, considerable function is achievable following this level of amputation. A highly motivated individual can make good use of the prosthesis and terminal devices.

Below elbow

Generally, this is one of the least complicated levels of amputation to which an artificial limb can be fitted. However, the remaining length of forearm can be critical. If it is extremely short there may be difficulty in securing the socket; if extremely long there may be difficulty in accommodating the wrist unit without making the whole arm too long. The success rate of rehabilitation within this group should be high.

Elbow disarticulation

This type of amputation is not commonly seen, as it is difficult to successfully fit either a cosmetic or a functional prosthesis at this level.

Through wrist

Following this level of amputation pronation and supination are retained, but because of the necessity to fit the prosthesis a good way up the forearm, valuable sensation is lost. The artificial limb can be extremely functional but rather clumsy unless care is taken with the type of socket prescribed. Unavoidably, the affected limb is usually longer than the unaffected limb after the prosthetic wrist unit is fitted.

Partial hand

Amputations of this kind are usually the result of an injury, for example catching the fingers in moving machinery. They are all dealt with according to individual need, especially as any area from mid-palm to the ends of the digits can be affected. Frequently, no device is provided as the remaining part of the hand provides considerable sensory feedback which is inevitably lost once covered by any form of prosthesis. However, cosmesis on occasion may provide an essential psychological boost and should not be overlooked. A basic opposition plate can provide a degree of function if desired.

TREATMENT
Pre-prosthetic
Congenital

Despite research, no reason has yet been found to account for the fact that babies are still being born with limb deficiencies. It is essential that these children and their families are referred as early as possible to a Limb Centre. A firm relationship with the rehabilitation team, comprised of the doctor, prosthetist, occupational therapist and nurse, built on trust and confidence and promoting a positive attitude, can then begin. In many cases a prosthesis will not be prescribed until the baby is approximately 6 months old. (This varies from Centre to Centre.) However, the parents can be supported, counselled and helped in every way possible to come to terms with what they will inevitably feel to be a failure on their part in not producing a perfect child.

The need for parents to be given the opportunity to discuss hopes and fears for the future, even at such an early stage, should be recognised. Often the best people to help with this situation are parents who are already coping with a limb deficient baby. They will be aware of what the family is experiencing and can supply first-hand knowledge of problems and possible solutions.

Regular contact with the rehabilitation team at the Centre is important, even if a limb is not to be prescribed for some months, as the family should not be left to feel isolated or uninformed. Support for the families of limb deficient children is also available through 'Reach', the Association for children with hand or arm deficiency'.

Acquired

It is not always possible for the occupational therapist to be involved in the individual's care pre-operatively, particularly if the amputation is an emergency procedure following trauma as opposed to elective surgery necessitated by disease. More frequently, amputees are referred to the occupational therapist after discharge from hospital, when healing has occurred and the limb is ready for the first prosthesis.

If a referral is received pre-operatively, it is necessary to assess each individual case most carefully. A realistic approach, together with a positive outlook, should be adopted, and support and counselling should be offered to both the amputee and his family. It should always be remembered that everyone close to the person is affected by the amputation and that they should therefore always be included in the management of the situation.

Surgery will try to produce an area where the skin is in good condition on the remaining part of the limb, with sensation as close to normal as possible. The scar tissue should be located in the best position available, where the prosthesis will not cause undue discomfort or pressure. The bone needs to be stable, secured by muscles, with sufficient soft tissue cover to form a protective pad. To avoid future problems from hypersensitivity, nerve endings are buried as deeply as possible. However, it must be remembered that circumstances do not always allow for all the preferred criteria to be met, particularly when the limb is severely damaged during trauma.

Following surgery, the 'stump' should be firmly bandaged to help control oedema. As the amputee is usually not able to do this for himself, the process is often abandoned on discharge from hospital because of the inconsistency in techniques used by other people. Provision of a length of Tubigrip to form a sock can be a useful alternative. The fit should be such that the sock does not roll down, forming a garter.

Mobility should be retained in the remaining part of the limb, through activity which demands a full range of movement. This will promote good circulation and assist the healing process whilst building up the muscle strength necessary for early acceptance of a prosthesis.

It is not always necessary to provide a temporary prosthesis or gauntlet, as it may be possible to fit a prosthesis as soon as the wound is fully healed. Should there be a prolonged period before a prosthesis is prescribed, however, the therapist should discuss this with the amputee to explain the necessity of providing a gauntlet as a temporary measure. This will enable the early return of bimanual activities and an improved level of independence.

If the dominant hand has been affected the person is usually advised to commence activity to promote a change in dominance in fine dextrous activities as soon as possible. The individual will need to develop skill in controlling his new dominant hand, as well as the artificial limb; therefore, the earlier rehabilitation is initiated, the better the outcome is likely to be.

All aspects of personal ADL should be assessed. This is an important area directly related to the person's independence and one in which he can achieve early success and a boost to morale.

Prosthetic

Congenital

When the baby is approximately 6 months old, many doctors recommend the fitting of the first artificial limb. This will take the form of a light plastic one-piece socket and fixed hand, fitted onto the baby's arm with an elastic cuff to prevent it slipping off easily. The fitting of this arm immediately completes the baby's body image and will encourage him to be two-handed. At this early stage he will be able to hold large toys in both hands and will begin to become accustomed to the

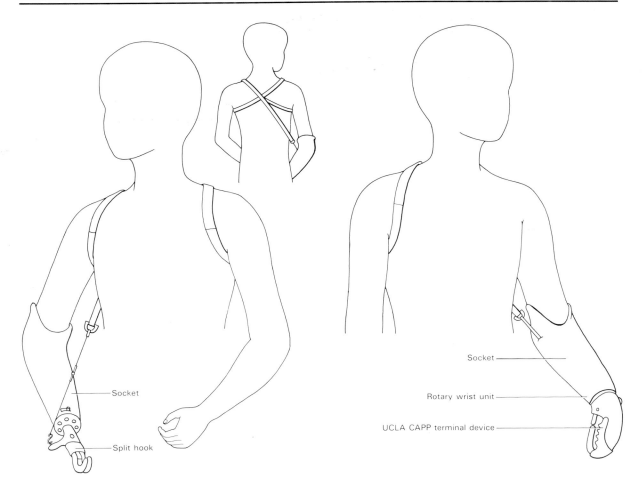

Fig. 25.8 Child's below elbow prosthesis.

idea of having another hand to help when playing. It will help reduce stares from strangers when away from home, as the baby will appear two-handed.

It is considered appropriate for a functional prosthesis to be introduced from approximately 18 months of age onwards. It is important to recognise that a child cannot fully operate a prosthesis until he has reached the appropriate stage of 'developmental readiness', so developmental testing is an important component of prosthetic training. For a below elbow absence there are two basic designs of limb, although research and development are constantly being devoted to the upgrading of these devices. The two designs are:

1. The child's version of an adult body-powered functional limb, comprising a socket, a wrist unit and a terminal device — either a small hand or a small plastic-covered split hook, both of which rotate and lock into any one of several positions on the wrist rotary.

2. The 'Child Amputee Prosthetic Program' (CAPP), which originated in the USA. Although very different in appearance, it offers the same advantages of function as the limb described above. However, it provides a better gross grip.

Both types of limb are attached and activated by a somewhat complicated strap arrangement (Fig. 25.8) which passes across the shoulders and under the opposite armpit. Once a prescription for a limb has been decided upon a cast is taken, as described on p. 642.

Objects can be picked up and dropped by using shoulder movement to open and close the hook. At this stage, several training sessions will be arranged to encourage full use of the limb and to show the family how best to supervise activities at home between sessions.

Regular appointments are recommended to monitor changes in needs, particularly as the child grows and develops.

Acquired

Once the wound has healed and most of the oedema has subsided, a referral will be made to a Limb Centre for general assessment. This will be carried out by members of the rehabilitation team. The most important team members, however, are the amputee himself and members of his family who attend the initial visit.

At this point, the individual may be feeling extremely vulnerable, frightened and worried, although he will probably not admit to this until much later when recalling his initial feelings. It is therefore important to establish a relaxed, informative relationship whilst instilling confidence for future visits to the Centre. Both the prosthetist and therapist provide valuable lines of communication between the amputee and doctor, as in many instances there is still an aura of authority surrounding the medical profession which may inhibit a free flow of feelings.

SEQUENCE OF EVENTS

At the first visit to the Limb Centre, the residual limb, known as the 'stump', will be fully examined. The therapist should be aware that people frequently dislike the term 'stump' and prefer to refer to their 'right' or 'left' arm as before. The term 'little arm' might be used where children are involved.

Provided the stump is not excessively swollen, the type of limb to be prescribed will be discussed and if possible a similar limb demonstrated.

It is important to establish the amputee's aspirations and requirements regarding a prosthesis so that due consideration can be given regarding its prescription and, looking further ahead, to training requirements. At this point the prosthetist will take over the manufacture of the artificial limb.

THE PROSTHETIST

On receiving the doctor's written prescription, the prosthetist will begin by taking a negative plaster cast of the stump. It is extremely important that this is taken correctly, as the end product, and thus the success or failure of the use of the prosthesis, relies on the accuracy of this initial stage.

This cast will form the basis of the inner socket, which fits snugly over the stump. There will then be an outer socket, suitably contoured to match the remaining arm. A below elbow amputee will sometimes have a self-suspending socket, that is, one without an appendage or strap, although this will not usually be recommended for the first limb. More frequently, a system of straps is required to ensure the prosthesis stays firmly in place and offers a means of attaching the operating cord in the case of the functional prosthesis (Figs 25.8–25.11). These differ according to the level of amputation and the type of limb prescribed.

In the majority of cases an appointment is given for an intermediate visit for fitting; at this session any problems can be ironed out and alterations made, prior to completion of the prosthesis.

At delivery the amputee will be shown how to put on and take off the prosthesis and its relevant suspension system. The various parts will be named and described, and the functional aspects of the limb will be demonstrated. It usually takes from 4 to 6 weeks after the first visit to the Centre for the prosthesis to be delivered. From this stage, the occupational therapist will take over the main part of treatment and education.

THE ROLE OF THE OCCUPATIONAL THERAPIST

As always, the occupational therapist's ultimate aim is to rehabilitate the individual to a maximum level of independence. In working towards this end, the therapist will, of necessity, adopt various approaches which frequently overlap. With regard to the physical aspects of the disability, the rehabilitative approach is implemented

A

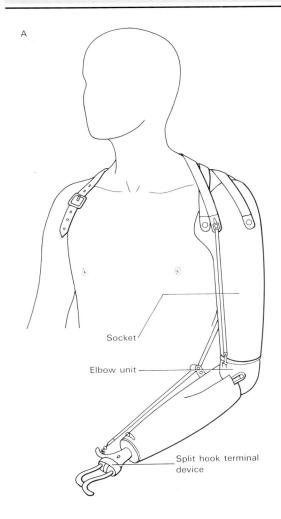

Socket

Elbow unit

Split hook terminal
device

B

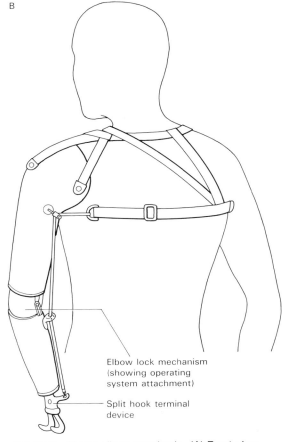

Elbow lock mechanism
(showing operating
system attachment)

Split hook terminal
device

Fig. 25.9 Above elbow prosthesis. (A) Front view.
(B) Back view.

throughout, although the success of this will
depend considerably on how the individual's
psychological and emotional stresses are overcome
through the therapist's use of a humanistic
approach.

Biomechanical principles may also be utilised to
maintain or improve function in the proximal parts
of the amputated limb, and developmental techniques
will be used with children.

It cannot be stated too strongly that every person
is an individual and should be treated as such.
The amputation is only a part of the whole problem
to be faced and it is incumbent upon the
therapist to take a sensitive and realistic overview
of the situation.

Although this discussion has focused on the
provision of functional artificial limbs, occasionally
an amputee will need to achieve independence
either with a purely cosmetic prosthesis or without
a prosthesis at all, and it is equally important to
support, counsel and advise this group of people.
Congenital amputees have particular concerns at
each stage of development — schooling, adolescence
and vocational training — and need
continuity in care and guidance.

Initially, practice in using an artificial limb aims
to reinforce the information given by the prosthetist.
This ensures an understanding of the limb,
its parts and how they work, and the best method
for the individual concerned for putting on and

A

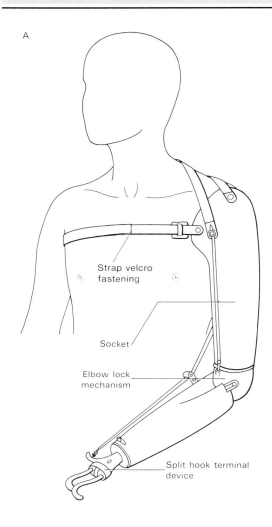

Strap velcro
fastening

Socket

Elbow lock
mechanism

Split hook terminal
device

B

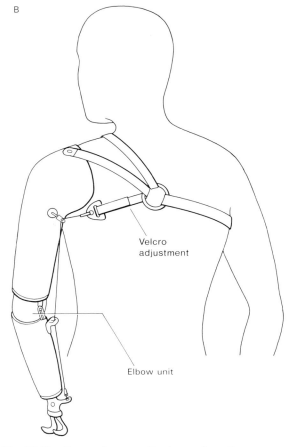

Velcro
adjustment

Elbow unit

Fig. 25.10 Above elbow prosthesis — alternative suspension system. (A) Front view. (B) Back view.

taking off the prosthesis. Care of the limb, particularly hygiene of the socket, is also stressed.

Once understanding of the hardware is achieved the next stage is to learn how to gain control of the limb and its terminal devices, using it effectively, naturally and appropriately. A programme of practice and learning ensues. The time taken will vary with the individual, although general guidelines are as follows:

- Below elbow: approximately 12–16 half-day sessions
- Above elbow: approximately 16–24 half-day sessions.

A double amputee will take considerably longer to achieve competence with prostheses. In all cases, the time required will be greatly affected by motivation, home circumstances, available transport and travelling distance.

TRAINING

The therapist should be able to demonstrate the full potential of the limb and terminal devices through realistic activities. She must bear in mind throughout the programme that tolerance to the limb varies from person to person and will need to be gradually increased over a period of time. It is advisable to utilise the arm mitts provided by the Limb Centre over the stump to improve com-

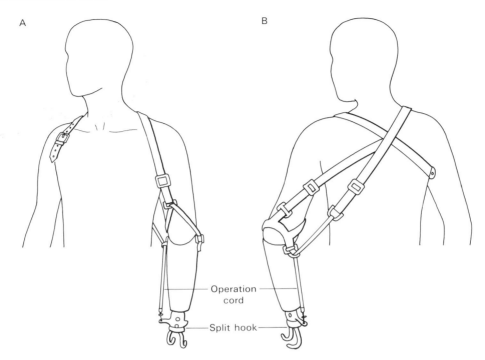

Fig. 25.11 Below elbow prosthesis. (A) Front view. (B) Back view.

fort at the socket. Wearing a T-shirt can also prevent the straps rubbing on the skin during the initial stages.

It is usual to begin learning control of the limb through using a split hook. This is operated by exerting tension on a cord attachment by means of the amputee's own body power.

Whether the affected limb is the dominant or non-dominant arm, control of the prosthesis needs to be learned primarily using one-handed activities with the artificial limb. This can be gained by providing a series of objects of different dimensions to be gripped. Initially the tasks set should be easy to complete, thereby affording immediate success and building confidence.

Progression continues through activities graded from light to heavy, thick to thin, and large to small, working in different planes. Ultimately, the amputee should be capable of holding an egg or slicing a tomato without crushing the shell or skin.

Once achieved, a basic level of control can be put into practice in a project involving a variety of manipulative skills. Woodwork, for example, would require the drawing and measuring of a pattern, cutting out, sawing, planing and sanding wood, and many other tasks using both limbs in a natural, functional manner. The individual's continuation of hobbies and pastimes should be discussed, as this is as important as the maintenance of routine daily activities.

Future prospects should now be considered regarding returning to work, if this has not been previously discussed. It may be necessary to involve the Disablement Resettlement Officer (DRO) for guidance on retraining possibilities. Contact with previous employers may be relevant here.

When good control has been gained and a level of confidence achieved, only perseverance in practising at home will improve speed and efficiency with the prosthesis. Provided motivation is good and there are no problems with the prosthesis and its comfort, the amputee will be well on his way to becoming a regular wearer and user.

TERMINAL DEVICES

This is the term used to describe the detachable implements which can be fitted into the wrist section of the prosthesis. A number of different grasping, manipulating and holding movements are carried out by the complicated and sophisticated mechanism of the human hand. Unfortunately, these movements cannot be reproduced by any one terminal device; therefore, a large number of different devices have been devised to assist in a considerable number of activities ranging from fishing and golf to digging and driving (Fig. 25.12).

When assessing a new limb-wearer the therapist should bear in mind that the fewer devices required, the less frustrating limb-wearing will become. One device may perform several tasks, thereby necessitating fewer changes and reducing the amount of 'luggage' to carry from place to place.

The most useful terminal device by far is the split hook. Usually this is the first one to be provided. Its simplicity of design and multiplicity of uses is unsurpassed by any of the other devices.

Often it is almost the only tool an amputee will use. It is made of aluminium alloy, stainless steel or carbon-fibre and is comprised of two curved, rubber-lined jaws, one fixed and one movable, both tapered at the end to provide a fine grip. Grip strength is determined by the number of rubber bands attached to the hook, each one providing approximately $1\frac{1}{2}$ lbs of force. (This does not apply to the carbon-fibre hook.) The hook, as with other actively controlled devices, is opened by exerting tension on the operating cord and closed by relaxing that tension.

By pre-positioning the hook into any one of the twelve wrist positions, the wearer can use it for holding, carrying, pushing or picking up objects.

Assessment with and provision of tools such as quick-grip pliers, a universal tool holder or spade grip may enable a return to previous employment. Emphasis should be placed on the fact that these are tools, much the same as tools previously used in employment, even though they operate by slightly different means.

As always, assessment for terminal devices must be geared towards provision for individual requirements (Figs 25.13, 25.14).

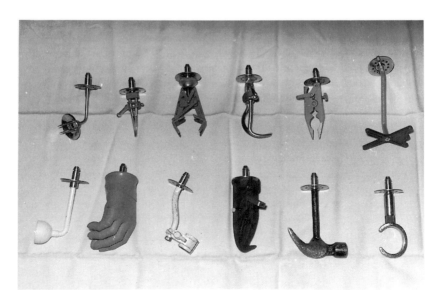

Fig. 25.12 A variety of terminal devices frequently in use. Top row: potato holder, tweezers, universal tool holder, split hook, long-nose pliers, snooker cue rest. Bottom row: driving appliance, mechanical hand, golf appliance, carbon fibre split hook, claw hammer, Williams 'C' hook.

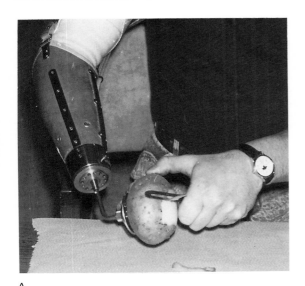

A

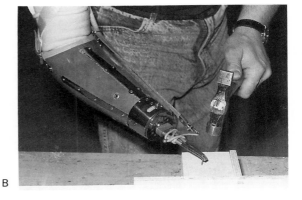

B

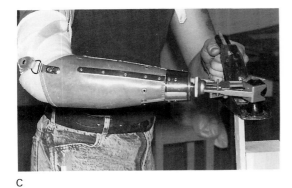

C

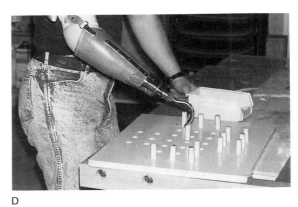

D

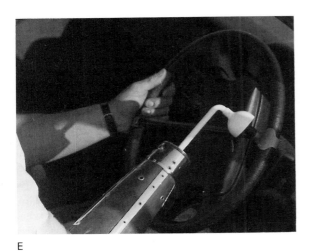

E

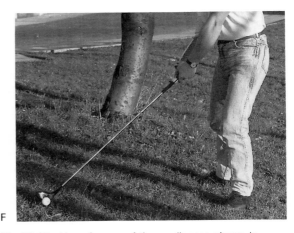

F

Fig. 25.13 Use of some of the appliances shown in Fig. 25.12. (Note: the user is wearing a heavy-duty socket, rather than the more commonly prescribed lightweight socket.) (A) Potato holder. (B) Tweezers. (C) Universal tool holder. (D) Split hook. (E) Driving appliance. (F) Golf appliance. (G) Carbon fibre split hook. (H) Claw hammer.

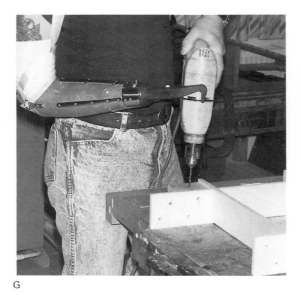

G

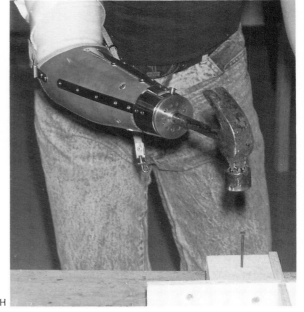

H

Fig. 25.13 (continued)

PSYCHOLOGICAL ASPECTS

Although the psychological impact of amputation has already been discussed in general terms (p. 632), there are certain considerations of specific relevance to upper-limb amputees.

In addition to the obvious practical problems that result from being born with limb absence or from losing part of an arm, many people in these circumstances are burdened by unresolved psychological problems. These are frequently well hidden as the years pass, but are nevertheless tucked away ready to reveal themselves on unforeseen occasions.

The immediate shock and worry occasioned by the birth of a baby with a limb deficiency is taken on board by the parents. As the child grows towards adulthood there will be the inevitable questions to be answered — if answers can indeed be found — as to 'What happened?' or 'Why me?' or 'How do I cope?' However, many of these children grow up to be quite remarkable adults, coping with everyday activities in the only way they know how, achieving independence by sometimes unconventional methods, but nevertheless achieving it.

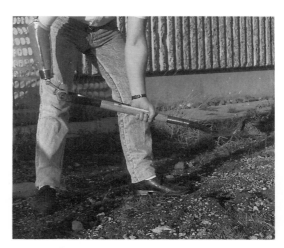

Fig. 25.14 Gardening using the spade grip attachment.

To lose an arm or part of an arm in later life takes on a different meaning because one is losing a part of one's body that has functioned in everyday tasks quite automatically. How to carry on in the same way must seem an insurmountable problem. This may be particularly difficult when there has been, as in most cases, no time to at least try to prepare for this shattering event. Suddenly the body is noticeably incomplete; gestures of anger, frustration, caring and comforting are less easy to implement. From carrying out daily activities independently one is suddenly dependent on someone else for even the smallest task.

Allowance must be made for a period akin to grieving over the death of a close friend or relative. Support and counselling should be available to help work through this period, in which the person must feel that he has no future.

Goals should be realistically set, and a positive outlook encouraged from the beginning. It should never be assumed that anyone other than the amputee knows what it is like to have suddenly lost a part of his body or what effect this is likely to have on life in the future.

As and when necessary, the therapist should, in a sensitive manner, provide as much information as is available, together with practical help with coming to terms with the loss and subsequent use of an artificial limb.

If the situation lends itself to this, introducing the individual to another amputee with a similar background (e.g. with regard to age, sex, level of loss or circumstances leading to the loss) could be of great value. This should not be entered into lightly as it could do more harm than good if the timing is wrong or the choice of amputee is not made with care.

PHANTOM SENSATIONS

The majority of amputees will experience a degree of phantom sensation and pain, as described on p. 632. The duration, severity and form of PLS and PLP vary considerably and there is no acknowledged framework by which these feelings can be explained. Sometimes, if the amputation is due to trauma, the hand can be 'felt' in what seems to be its last position prior to the moment of impact. Other sensations range from 'pins and needles', itching and cramp to simply a feeling that the absent part is still there.

Occasionally, these sensations become so extreme as to be described by the amputee as actual pains, although the pains are more likely to be felt in the stump. Care must be taken to identify the nature and extent of these feelings and, if they

persist, it may be necessary to arrange for further physical or psychological treatment, after consultation with the relevant medical staff specialising in this field of work.

However, in the majority of cases where such sensations do remain, they settle to a manageable level which can be tolerated and accepted. Early exercises in stump desensitisation often help considerably in alleviating this disturbing reminder of the amputation.

FURTHER CONSIDERATIONS

Brachial plexus lesion

This is usually caused by trauma (often a motor-cycle accident) and predominantly affects young men.

In the majority of people, the damage is irreparable because of stretching, tearing or avul-

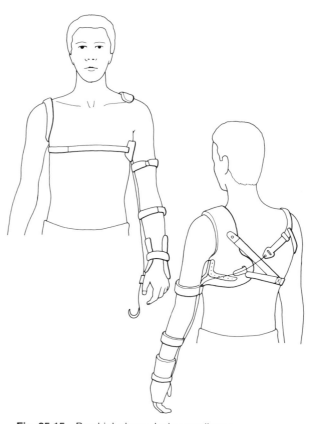

Fig. 25.15 Brachial plexus lesion appliance.

sion of the roots directly from the spinal cord. Upper trunk lesions are more common than lower lesions.

At some stage, where further recovery seems unlikely, a flail arm orthosis may be indicated. This appliance will enable the hand to be brought into a functional position and will supplement elbow flexion. The ability to continue with bimanual activities will thus be maintained and, ideally, employment prospects improved (Fig. 25.15).

Occasionally, where there has been complete avulsion, it may be necessary to consider amputation as an alternative option. This should, wherever possible, be discussed at length with the person affected and the implications of leaving the flail arm intact and of amputating made known. If surgery is decided upon, the management will be the same as for other amputees.

Myoelectric controls

Myoelectric controls for upper limb prostheses have so far been used only to a limited extent in Great Britain, although they have been available to amputees in North America and other European countries for 20 to 30 years. Major trials began in Britain in 1978 when powered hands with myoelectric controls were provided for pre-school children. These proved successful and this type of prosthesis is now available to those adults most likely to benefit from the system.

Myoelectric control systems can be used to operate any device such as a powered hand, wrist rotation unit or elbow unit. Surface electrodes embedded in the socket pick up minute electrical impulses from voluntary muscle contractions in the stump. Each signal is then amplified and processed to act as a control mechanism for a selected function. For instance, with an electric hand one muscle site is needed to open the hand and another to close it. Power for all functions is provided by a battery which is either worn externally (attached to a belt with young amputees) or incorporated into the socket (Figs 25.16 and 25.17). Batteries must be regularly recharged (with continual usage this may be necessary every 24 hours).

An important advantage with this type of prosthesis is that an amputee can often have a self-suspended socket without any additional straps or 'harness' (Fig. 25.17) which aids freedom of movement and comfort in wearing, and the most satisfactory results have been obtained with short below elbow amputations. The main disadvantages with this type of limb are the increase in weight (mainly located in the powered hand), and delayed movement response. Operation of a split hook requires only one brief movement, whereas the myoelectric hand depends on the muscle signal activating the electrode and this signal being amplified and processed before operating the mehanism of the hand. Hand movements, too, are relatively slow to give the amputee control of the grasp/release mechanism. There is no sensory feedback with a powered hand, and it is not (at this point in time) interchangeable with any other terminal device. Trials are being carried out with a two-speed powered split hook, activated in the same way as a myoelectric powered hand, but this device is not yet available to suppliers.

Myoelectric control systems are sophisticated and expensive, and with a growing child there are additional problems related to the need for continual modification of the socket. A careful team assessment of all individuals who might benefit from such a prosthesis is necessary before any decision is made. This must be based on a realistic appraisal of needs and functional potential. Unless the amputee is able to look after the prosthesis properly it can break down and require a great deal of maintenance. It is therefore important not to raise expectations too high.

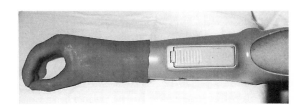

Fig. 25.16 Myoelectric controls for powered hand with battery incorporated into the socket.

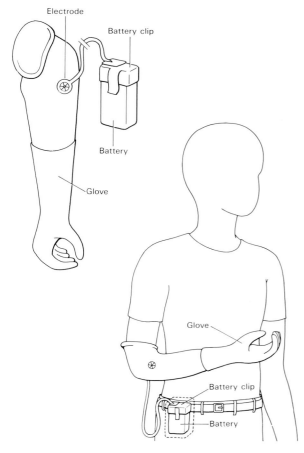

Fig. 25.17 Self-suspended below elbow prosthesis with myoelectric controls for battery powered hand (battery is attached to belt).

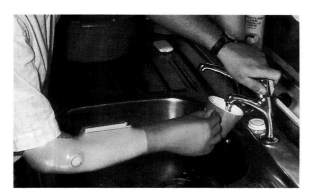

Fig. 25.18 The myoelectric hand used for everyday tasks.

Advantages and disadvantages of upper limb prostheses

Below is a short list of some of the points to consider regarding the wearing of an artificial arm, applicable to both congenital and acquired amputees:

Advantages

- An artificial limb completes the body image and prevents people staring
- Whichever side is affected, it will provide a non-dominant hand
- Bimanual activities can be learned or recommenced
- A return to work may be accelerated by using the limb
- If expertise is gained with an artificial arm, an amputee will still be reasonably independent should anything happen to the remaining arm
- Where a limb has been provided for a congenital absence, the child will grow up with an image of himself as being two-handed. It will also provide experience upon which he can base a later decision as to whether an artificial arm is, or is not, beneficial to his life-style.

Disadvantages

- Depending on the site, important sensory feedback and sometimes movement can be impeded
- The limb and straps may be heavy, hot and uncomfortable, particularly in hot weather
- A skin reaction may arise from the materials used or an existing skin condition may be aggravated. This can usually be resolved but it takes time and perseverance to find the satisfactory solution
- Self-consciousness may be increased, especially in teenage years when many individuals are particularly sensitive concerning appearance and performance
- Frequent visits to a Limb Centre will be necessary, especially during the growth years

of children and the initial stages of rehabilitation of adults. This may cause problems if there is difficulty with travelling arrangements or obtaining time off work.

One of the strongest arguments for wearing and gaining expertise with an artificial arm is the desirability of the amputee reaching a level of independence whereby he would not become totally dependent on others should he, for example, fall and fracture his remaining arm. However, account must always be taken of the amputee's feelings and aspirations before realistic intervention strategies can be put forward by the rehabilitation team.

CONCLUSION

Information in this chapter is applicable to relatively straightforward cases of recent amputation. The main ingredient to successful rehabilitation is motivation. Without this, it is extremely difficult to encourage maximum potential with or without a prosthesis. However, in certain circumstances, motivation may not be enough. If a limb has been amputated because of disease, the type of treatment in progress for that disease may influence the timing of referral to a Limb Centre. In such cases all efforts will be focused on controlling the disease itself, and the amputation itself will fade into the background. The individual will still need support and encouragement, however, in gaining expertise and confidence with the remaining limb. As much information as possible should be provided regarding the future.

At times the ageing process brings with it problems such as rheumatoid arthritis, Parkinson's disease or circulatory disorders. Conditions such as these will have a bearing on the level of independence the amputee can achieve. Difficulties may also arise if the amputee has lost a partner who used to assist with some of the more difficult aspects of daily routine.

It is therefore necessary to assess the potential of the new amputee and to reassess the situation of the long-standing amputee who is facing a change in circumstances. It is essential to approach each amputee with a flexible and realistic attitude, and with an awareness of individual needs.

ACKNOWLEDGEMENT

Grateful thanks to Ron Hutchinson LBIST, SRN, RMN and Mrs Pat Hutchinson for their help and support.

USEFUL ADDRESSES

British Limbless Ex-Servicemen's Association
185/187 High Road
Chadwell Health
Essex RM6 6NA

Disabled Living Foundation
380/384 Harrow Road
London W9 2HU

National Association for Limbless Disabled
31 The Mall, Ealing
London W5 2PX

Reach: Association for children
with hand or arm deficiency
(Contact the local DSC for
current details of secretary)

Royal Association for Disability and Rehabilitation
25 Mortimer Street
London W1N 8AB.

REFERENCES

Mahoney F I, Barthel D W 1965 Functional evaluation: the
Barthel Index. Maryland State Medical Journal 14: 61–65

Malone J M, Snyder M, Anderson G et al 1989 Prevention
of amputation by diabetic education. American Journal
of Surgery 158: 520–524

British Association of Occupational Therapists 1990
Occupational therapists' reference book. Parke Sutton,
Norwich

Pinzur M S, Graham G, Osterman H 1988 Psychologic
testing in amputee rehabilitation. Clinical Orthopaedics
and Related Research 229: 236–240

Raphael B 1984 The anatomy of bereavement: a handbook
for the caring professions. Hutchinson, London

FURTHER READING

Atkin D J, Meier I I, Robert H (eds) 1989 Comprehensive
management of the upper limb amputee. Springer Verlag,
London

Banerjee S N (ed) 1982 Rehabilitation management of
amputees. Williams & Wilkins, Baltimore

Department of Health and Social Security 1986 Review of
Artificial Limb and Appliance Centre services, Vol I, Vol
II—Annexes to. DHSS, London

Engstrom B, Van de Ven C 1985 Physiotherapy for
amputees: the Roehampton approach. Churchill
Livingstone, Edinburgh

Friedman L W 1978 The psychological rehabilitation of the
amputee. Charles C Thomas, Illinois

Kosterik J P 1981 Amputation surgery and rehabilitation:
the Toronto experience. Churchill Livingstone, New York

Krebs D (ed) 1987 Prehension assessment: prosthetic
therapy for the upper-limb child amputee. Slack, New
Jersey

Lamb D W, Law H T 1987 Upper limb deficiencies in
children: prosthetic, orthotic and surgical management.
Little, Brown, Boston

Mensch G, Ellis P M 1986 Physical therapy management of
lower extremity amputations. Aspen, Rockville

Robertson E 1978 Rehabilitation of arm amputees and limb
deficient children. Baillière Tindall, Eastbourne

Setoguchi Y, Rosenfelder R (eds) 1982 The limb deficient
child. Charles C. Thomas, Illinois

Trevan R 1989 Peripheral vascular disease: occupational
therapy in peripheral vascular disease of the lower limb.
British Journal of Occupational Therapy 52(4): 132–134

Vitali M, Robinson K P, Andrews B G, Harris E E 1978
Amputations and prostheses. Baillière Tindall, Eastbourne.

Wynn Parry C B 1981 Rehabilitation of the hand.
Butterworth, London

Young H 1989 Peripheral vascular disease; arterial disease of
the lower limb and venous disorders of the lower limb.
British Journal of Occupational Therapy 52(4): 127–132

26

Back pain

Doreen Rowland

INTRODUCTION

Back pain has a wide spectrum of presentations ranging from a mild ache in the small of the back, causing only a small degree of discomfort, to chronic disabling problems. The back pain office of Health Economics in 1985 reported that there were over 22 million episodes of back pain in the UK each year. Only a small number of people affected enter hospital, the majority being treated in the community by general practitioners. A high proportion of people seen in outpatient clinics also present with back problems. Dixon (1980) reported this to be as high as 25% of the total number seen in 1980. The number of work days lost in the UK due to back pain is thought to be over 30 million each year.

The first sections of this chapter describe the major types and causes of back pain and briefly review the wide range of treatment methods available to back pain sufferers. The role of the occupational therapist in the multidisciplinary back care team is discussed, and the main approaches that she might take in the treatment and management of back pain are outlined. This is followed by a discussion of the process of assessment by which the therapist gains an understanding of the impact of back pain upon all aspects of the individual's daily life.

Next, the chapter considers the nature of the occupational therapist's intervention, with particular attention to the invaluable advice and education she can offer with regard to good posture and correct techniques for carrying out Activities of Daily Living (ADL). Different methods which the therapist might use in promoting awareness of back care are described. Finally, practical considerations in the use of specific activities in the rehabilitation programme are described.

PRESENTATION OF BACK PAIN

It is important to distinguish cases of mild back pain from those which are more severe, taking into account the site of the pain, the type of pain and its intensity. Back pain can present anywhere from the base of the neck to the buttocks. It can be divided into pain which arises directly from the muscles, fascia, dura, dural root sheaths, ligaments, periosteum and apophyseal joint capsules, and that which arises indirectly when the nerves are compressed, irritated or overstretched. It can be referred from another part of the body served by the same nerve root, as in low back pain associated with gynaecological problems. Mechanical back pain may result from overuse of the spine (with resultant muscle fatigue), direct or indirect trauma, spinal tumours, stress or degenerative changes in the spine. Radicular pain or referred pain may result in associated leg pain. In some situations stress or tension may cause psychosomatic back pain when there is no identifiable medical or organic cause.

It is important for the clinician to discover from the back pain sufferer certain detailed information on the pain he is experiencing. This may be determined through an interview and questionnaire and should aim to ascertain where the pain is felt, its type and duration, what eases the pain or makes it worse, and how the pain affects everyday life (Stoddard 1979).

Acute pain

Acute back pain is one of nature's ways of warning that something is wrong with the back. Altering activities or avoiding a specific movement often reduces the pain. However, a prolonged decrease in the range of movement of the spine can lead to muscle weakness and poor posture, which in turn may have functional implications for the back pain sufferer.

Chronic pain

Chronic pain may be defined as that which lasts more than three, or in some instances six, months. This can result in general loss of mobility and a reduction of independence in personal care, work and leisure activities. This may lead to reduced self-esteem, poor motivation and depression. There may be social implications, such as the loss of role as breadwinner or home organiser. There may be financial implications related to being off work for long periods, and rehousing may be necessary if the loss of mobility is permanent.

Chronic pain syndrome is the term usually used to describe pain which lasts longer than six months and has ceased to perform a useful protective function against injury.

Psychological factors

Psychological responses to illness or disability vary from one individual to another. People react in different ways to pain, frequently as the result of the childhood example of parents or others, either to 'be brave and carry on', or to respect the pain and give it attention. Chronic pain can change the personality. Lack of comfort and sleep, together with a loss of activities and roles can cause withdrawal, introversion and depression, and may lead to anger and aggression. Pain perception is more devastating in some people than in others. Engel (1959) attributed this to a possible 'pain personality'.

Pain may also be used to advantage as a way of avoiding other difficulties to be faced at home, at work or socially. Relaxation techniques and counselling may help the person to control the pain and face some of the underlying issues. By addressing the basic problems and reducing the requirement for secondary gain through the back pain, a more positive approach to activity may be achieved. Where the problems are complex or severely inhibit function, referral to a psychologist or psychiatrist or enrolment in a behavioural back pain programme may be necessary.

CAUSES OF BACK PAIN

Back pain can result from injury or occupational hazard or may be the result of a degenerative, hereditary or congenital problem. Abnormal vertebral curvatures, described below, are illustrated in Figure 26.1.

Kyphosis

Kyphosis, or forward curvature of the thoracic spine, may result from muscular pull or prolonged stooped posture such as that adopted by some people with Parkinson's disease. Kyphosis may also occur following bony damage, for example ankylosing spondylitis, osteochondritis or osteomalacia.

Lordosis

An exaggerated lumbar curvature, lordosis may result from forward tilting of the pelvis, which

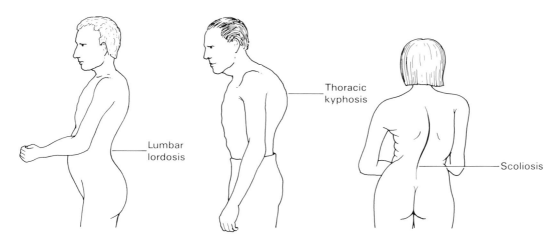

Fig. 26.1 Abnormal vertebral curvatures.

Scoliosis

Scoliosis, or sideways curvature of the spine, is a condition which may present as an irreversible structural curve, with or without twisting of the vertebrae. It may also be a non-structural problem caused by posture or muscle pull which can be reversed on lying or sitting. Its causes vary from destructive lesions to the vertebrae and soft tissue contractures of the chest wall to bone disease. It may also occur as the result of other disease, for example poliomyelitis or muscular dystrophy. Surgery to correct or stabilise the curvature may assist positioning, but is not always successful in relieving back pain.

may occur as a natural habit and cause poor posture or may result from predisposing conditions such as obesity and pregnancy. Lordosis also occurs in some children with Duchenne muscular dystrophy but this rarely causes severe back pain, and may be encouraged in some children to reduce the risk of the development of scoliosis.

Spondylolysis

A degeneration or dissolution of a vertebra, spondylolysis sometimes leads to spondylolisthesis, a forward slip of one or more vertebrae on the one below. Mechanical pain can result from this problem or there may be pain resulting from compression or overstretching of a nerve root. Surgery to stabilise the spine (spinal fusion) or to release a compressed nerve may be necessary either as a long-term solution or an emergency procedure to prevent secondary neurological damage. In some cases conservative treatment may adequately correct displacement.

Stenosis

Stenosis, or narrowing, of the spinal canal can result in nerve root compression by bone, the intervertebral disc or by some other intrusion, such as a tumour or osteophytes. Surgery is required to remove the offending cause of the compression and release the nerve roots. Occasionally this may not be possible and paralysis will result.

Disc disease

When a disc bulges or ruptures the annulus fibrosus or part of the inner gelatinous nucleus pulposus can press on the nerves. The bulge or pieces of ruptured disc debris can be removed by surgical intervention. This usually follows a period of investigation or a course of conservative treatment, consisting of, for example, bed-rest, epidural injection and manipulation or traction to reduce pain and ascertain the extent of the damage to the disc.

Tumours

Tumours cause a relatively small proportion of cases of back pain. They are classified by their position in the spine and may be primary growths or secondary to those occurring in other areas of

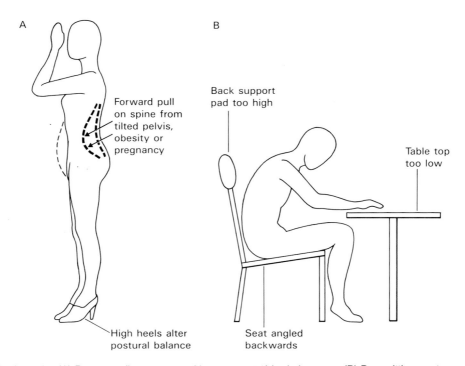

A

Forward pull on spine from tilted pelvis, obesity or pregnancy

High heels alter postural balance

B

Back support pad too high

Table top too low

Seat angled backwards

Fig. 26.2 Back strain. (A) Poor standing posture with accentuated lordotic curve. (B) Poor sitting posture with forward-flexed, C-shaped sitting position.

the body (Hayward 1980). Treatment methods include radiotherapy, steroids or surgical intervention. Following surgery, chemotherapy, further radiotherapy or endocrine therapy may be indicated.

Ankylosing spondylitis

This condition is characterised by ossification of the spinal ligaments and stiffness of the sacroiliac joints. It can cause minimal loss of movement or may progress to complete loss of range of movement in many areas of the spine. Treatment to prevent long-term problems from poor fixed postures relies on the person maintaining a good exercise regime and attention to correct posture to minimise or prevent fixed deformities. Anti-inflammatory drugs may be used. Surgery is rarely recommended. Physiotherapy has a major role in offering advice and implementing suitable exercise regimes.

Muscular back strain

By far the commonest cause of acute back pain, muscular back strain may be the result of a specific stressful action, for example lifting or performing a sudden stretching or jarring movement. It may also be the progressive outcome of prolonged back strain through poor postural habits and accompanying muscle weakness which can occur in obesity, pregnancy or in daily activity in the home, at work or at rest. In most instances conservative measures are the initial choice of treatment (Fig. 26.2).

Other causes

Back pain can also result from bony, muscular or neurological damage resulting from wider disorders, for example osteoarthritis, rheumatoid arthritis, multiple sclerosis or spinal injury. It is frequently difficult to identify the specific cause of back pain because of the diversity of modes of presentation, especially in secondary referred pain. There are numerous diagnostic methods, among which investigation of the person's history and observation of responses to conservative treatment play an important part.

TREATMENT METHODS

Many methods of treatment have developed over the years, some conservative, others invasive. Because of the diversity of the aetiology and presenting symptoms, there is no one universally accepted method of treatment.

Bed-rest

For most people in acute discomfort, bed-rest is initially recommended, especially when there is evidence of nerve root compression and acute muscle spasm. The commencement of careful mobilisation is allowed only when the symptoms subside. An isometric exercise programme is recommended when bed-rest extends beyond a few days.

Relaxation

This is an increasingly successful method of treatment and is discussed on page 672.

Traction

This may be used to relieve acute back pain. A constant stretching force applied while the sufferer is lying down relieves pressure on intervertebral discs. More powerful intermittent stretching may be performed under the close supervision of a physiotherapist.

Manipulation

Treatment is directed to the specific area of spinal involvement. Pressure is applied manually to rotate the spine or effect anterior, posterior or lateral movements of the spine.

Massage

This is often used in conjunction with other techniques such as manipulation, heat and exercise. It aims to relax tense muscles and thereby reduce pain and is used most frequently with people with acutely strained muscles.

Heat

This also aims to promote muscle relaxation and thereby relieve pain. It can be a useful antecedent to other forms of treatment.

Exercise

Exercise has two main aims:

1. gradual stretching to restore movement to the normal range
2. muscle strengthening to improve muscle tone and thereby reduce strain on bones and joints.

Graded exercise programmes are directed by the physiotherapist, taking account of the person's pain problem, stage of treatment and lifestyle. Exercises which induce pain should generally be avoided, but in some cases it may be necessary for the person to work through the pain, especially when he has been experiencing hypersensitive chronic pain.

Spinal surgical supports

The exact function and value of these has not been fully proven. However, it is believed that by limiting range of movement and increasing abdominal support they reduce the spinal load. Continuous use can easily lead to dependency and should be avoided except in special circumstances, for example following a spinal fracture. Short-term use in the acute stage may relieve symptoms and the support may be used intermittently when the person is performing particularly heavy activity.

Orthoses

Occupational therapists may be involved in the fabrication and provision of support orthoses. These are usually for short-term use and made from thermoplastic materials (see Ch. 11).

Chronic pain sufferers, who may require long-term orthotic support, will usually be provided with a commercially manufactured support.

Acupuncture and acupressure

There are many ways of stimulating acupuncture points: by inserting needles, by applying pressure, heat, or electrical current, and by vibration, ultrasound or lasers. *Acupressure* refers to stimulation without the use of needles. All these techniques have proved useful with some people; in most cases it is found that the greater the stimulus, the greater the response.

Transcutaneous Electrical Nerve Stimulation (TENS)

This technique transmits electrical energy across the skin surface to stimulate nerve response. This has the effect of masking the pain and can be a valuable tool in enabling chronic pain sufferers to cope with everyday living.

Chemotherapy

A variety of drugs can be used for pain control. If prescribed with bed-rest many have dramatic positive effects upon acute pain. Muscle relaxants, analgesics and anti-inflammatory agents may all be used with beneficial results. If the pain is localised, anaesthetic injections may be given directly into the pain area. Epidurals and nerve blocks may control severe intractable pain. Additionally, chemotherapy can be used to dissolve damaged discs and treat tumours of the spine.

Yoga and meditation

Some centres use one or both of these techniques, particularly with chronic pain sufferers, to encourage a state of control of mind and body in order to relieve anxiety and tension, promote muscle relaxation and facilitate controlled mobility.

Surgery

Surgical intervention may be corrective, as in the case of spinal fusion to correct scoliosis, or ameliorative to relieve pressure by removal of the offending cause. Surgical intervention techniques include laminectomy, microdiscectomy, fenestration and spinal fusion (Hayward 1980).

Chiropractic

This treatment concentrates on mechanical back problems. It involves manipulating the vertebral joints to improve posture and relieve pain.

Osteopathy

Sudden strong force is applied to the affected area following exercises to stretch or relax the muscles around the joint. This method is used particularly with acute mechanical pain.

Physiotherapy

The physiotherapist is the key worker in the management of back pain. Heat, massage, TENS, manipulation, exercise, advice and education may all be within the physiotherapist's expertise.

Psychological support

People with organic and non-organic back pain will benefit from some psychological support. This may be provided by simple support and advice given with other treatment techniques. More in-depth counselling may be required, particularly for those who suffer long-term pain. Behavioural psychotherapy may help people suffering pain with no structural cause to work through the pain.

THE ROLE OF THE OCCUPATIONAL THERAPIST

Occupational therapy intervention is of value to everyone suffering from acute or chronic back pain, whatever its cause. The wide range of skills that the occupational therapist has to offer should not be underestimated; her work involves more than simply providing equipment to assist people with a decreased range of movement. An occupational therapist's training enables her to offer help and advice addressing the needs of the whole person. Her role may include:

- providing a detailed assessment of the presenting problems at home, at work and during leisure activities
- offering advice, education, training and practice on correct static and dynamic working postures and on correct techniques for performing everyday activities
- advising on equipment to improve independence and posture when appropriate
- helping the person to improve muscle strength, activity tolerance and range of movement through purposeful activity
- offering counselling to help resolve specific psychological or personal problems
- offering individual relaxation training to assist the person to control his pain and ease anxiety and tensions
- reviewing the person's work prospects
- liaising with other professionals to ensure that a comprehensive approach is taken to the individual's problems.

THERAPEUTIC APPROACHES

Because back pain has a wide variety of presentations and causes, the occupational therapist must have a thorough understanding of each person's diagnosis and circumstances before she can provide realistic and appropriate intervention. She will need to be familiar with functional anatomy, ergonomics and the effects of pain, and will need the skills to gain each person's confidence, especially as some back pain sufferers may be sceptical of yet another treatment method in a long line tried over many years. Some people may be aggressive or uncooperative during initial contacts.

The occupational therapist must be sensitive to each person's limitations. In the majority of instances people with acute pain will not be able to participate in active rehabilitation activities to the level anticipated of those attending occupational therapy just prior to return to work. Likewise, the person with a progressive disorder, such as a spinal tumour, will require a totally different approach from the person with resolved acute disc damage.

The therapist should also be aware of the effects of the *setting* of her intervention upon the individual's progress. Ward-based work may be more common and appropriate in the acute stages of the problem or immediately following surgery, but will be less suitable in the later stages. Rehabilitation departments or specialist centres are often specifically designed and equipped to provide heavier and more work-related activities than departments based in general hospitals. Advice, education and work-station design are all vital components of rehabilitation in the community both at home and at the work location.

In all cases the occupational therapist should adopt a humanistic approach in her recognition of the individual needs of each person and in her choice of purposeful activities and sensitive intervention strategies.

The rehabilitative approach

This approach may be employed in the treatment of people with residual limitations in activity tolerance, strength, or range of movement due to back injury or disease, and may be used to compensate for limitations in the early stages of care following acute damage to the back. Taking this approach the therapist may provide equipment to assist in the performance of essential tasks, offer opportunities to practise alternative techniques to avoid back strain, and modify the environment for ergonomic advantage.

The biomechanical approach

This approach may be employed in treating those who have a particular weakness which may be overcome through specific mobilising or strengthening exercises. Such exercises may be used to improve spinal muscle or joint action or to build up abdominal or lower limb muscles to promote good posture or correct lifting techniques.

The educational or cognitive approach

This approach is used in almost all cases to inform the individual (and, where appropriate, his family or carer(s)) about the back problem and ways of managing it, with the aim of engendering informed responsibility for future back care.

ASSESSMENT

It is essential for a detailed initial interview and full assessment to be carried out. Preliminary observations by the occupational therapist on how the person moves, and on his posture, gait and facial expressions can yield useful information on the extent of his back problems. For example, a bias to one leg when standing may indicate pain or discomfort or a postural deformity, and the way in which the person moves can indicate whether posture is tense or guarded.

Accurate assessment of the person with back pain is an essential forerunner to positive intervention, and concise recording of the findings forms the basis for intervention planning and monitoring.

Initial interview

This should include a brief history of the person's back problems, how long he has had them, the possible cause and other previous treatments, and how the problems affect his everyday life now. In addition to providing clinical background, this helps the therapist to gain insight into how the sufferer views his problems and what attitude he has towards them. Details of any current treatments should also be obtained.

The interview also enables the therapist to further explain her role and enlist the person's cooperation.

Pain

It is impossible to measure pain objectively. A statement often heard in pain clinics is 'Pain is whatever the person says it is'. It is, however, necessary to identify the type of pain experienced, how it presents, and what, if anything exacerbates or relieves it. Pain identification charts may assist the person to describe the site and type of pain (Fig. 26.3). The therapist should discuss how the pain affects positions and movements such as

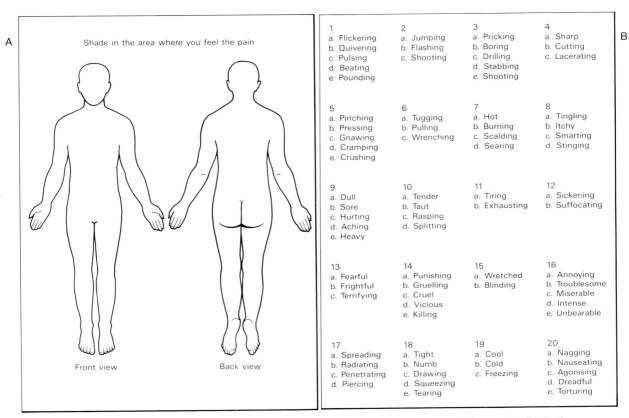

A

Shade in the area where you feel the pain

Front view   Back view

B

1	2	3	4
a. Flickering	a. Jumping	a. Pricking	a. Sharp
b. Quivering	b. Flashing	b. Boring	b. Cutting
c. Pulsing	c. Shooting	c. Drilling	c. Lacerating
d. Beating		d. Stabbing	
e. Pounding		e. Shooting	

5	6	7	8
a. Pinching	a. Tugging	a. Hot	a. Tingling
b. Pressing	b. Pulling	b. Burning	b. Itchy
c. Gnawing	c. Wrenching	c. Scalding	c. Smarting
d. Cramping		d. Searing	d. Stinging
e. Crushing			

9	10	11	12
a. Dull	a. Tender	a. Tiring	a. Sickening
b. Sore	b. Taut	b. Exhausting	b. Suffocating
c. Hurting	c. Rasping		
d. Aching	d. Splitting		
e. Heavy			

13	14	15	16
a. Fearful	a. Punishing	a. Wretched	a. Annoying
b. Frightful	b. Gruelling	b. Blinding	b. Troublesome
c. Terrifying	c. Cruel		c. Miserable
	d. Vicious		d. Intense
	e. Killing		e. Unbearable

17	18	19	20
a. Spreading	a. Tight	a. Cool	a. Nagging
b. Radiating	b. Numb	b. Cold	b. Nauseating
c. Penetrating	c. Drawing	c. Freezing	c. Agonising
d. Piercing	d. Squeezing		d. Dreadful
	e. Tearing		e. Torturing

Fig. 26.3 Tools to help the individual describe the site and type of pain. (A) Diagram to indicate pain distribution. (B) Word list to aid description of pain type.

lying, sitting, standing, walking, bending and lifting.

Movement

Movement assessment should be undertaken with care. In the acute stage following injury or surgery all spinal movements may be contraindicated. The consultant or practitioner's views should be obtained before any physical assessment is begun. Any unnecessary measurement should be avoided, for example by consulting recent measurements obtained by the consultant or physiotherapist. If, however, the therapist needs to make specific measurements the number of changes of position the person is required to perform during the process should be minimised by assessing a number of movements in one position.

Spinal movement

Spinal movement will often be restricted or instigate pain. A number of methods of assessment are available but the simplest and most frequently used will be described here.

Forward flexion can be measured in centimetres from the extended fingertips to the floor when the person bends forward to touch his toes from an upright standing position while keeping his knees straight. It is important to ascertain whether he has ever been able to touch his toes in this way. The therapist should check that the person is not flexing forward from the hips alone by observing whether the lumbar lordotic curve is reversed when bending.

Lateral flexion can be measured to both left and right by asking the person, from a standing position, to slide one hand down the outside of the same leg as far as he can reach without bending foward. The distance from the floor to the extended fingertips is measured. Repetition of the action on the other side of the body provides a measurement for comparison.

Rotation may be estimated by asking the person to turn the shoulders to left and right while seated with his arms across his chest. This is a purely observational assessment, as accurate rotational measurements are difficult to obtain.

Extension may be assessed by asking the person to lie prone and then raise his upper trunk off the couch as far as possible. This may be measured with or without the use of the arms to assist in raising the trunk.

Lower limb movement

It may be necessary to assess this prior to a full programme of remedial activity. Of particular importance is the strength of the muscles of the buttocks and thighs for lifting and mobilising. Any significant weakness or wasting of muscles of the lower limb may indicate nerve involvement and affect posture and gait.

Neck movement

A restriction of neck movement may occur in conjunction with damage to the thoracic vertebrae or may be an indication of more generalised disease affecting the spine. Where there is severe pain in the neck and limited mobility it may be necessary to measure upper limb and hand function to see if there is any possibility of involvement of the brachial plexus.

Tolerance to activity

This is often poor among back pain sufferers, especially in such static positions as sitting, standing and kneeling. Tolerance can easily be assessed by occupying the person with a familiar pleasurable activity in each of the positions and noting the length of time before the pain increases and distracts him from the task.

Work tolerances for manual tasks should be assessed, particularly in the later stages of intervention when the therapist is aiming to facilitate return to domestic tasks, work, or leisure pursuits.

Activities of daily living

This is a major area of involvement for the occupational therapist. She should note the person's social and domestic situation and role, and the demands these make on ADL. A thorough assessment of any activity which causes difficulty should be made to identify the extent and specific nature of the problem.

Work

Note should be made of the person's work history and of the environment and the postural and activity requirements of his present job. Any particular occupational demands such as prolonged sitting, heavy lifting or long-distance driving should be identified. Attention should be paid to sick leave if the person is currently employed, or to whether he has been medically retired. Referral to the social worker for advice on benefits or to the Disablement Resettlement Officer (DRO) may be recommended.

If back pain is the result of an accident it is important to discover whether any compensation claim is pending as this may have a negative effect on some people's attitudes to intervention and recovery. However, compensation may equally be a source of much-needed financial help, especially if the person is permanently disabled.

Assessment for benefits such as invalidity, mobility and constant attendance allowances can lead to conflict in the person with chronic pain. He may be in a situation where he is now only able to perform very limited work, in terms of either duration or remunerative level, and may have to remain disabled, and thus eligible for benefits, in order to retain anything resembling his previous income.

Leisure pursuits

These should be noted in terms of what leisure pursuits the person has, to what level he participates and how enthusiastic he is to return to them.

Psychological factors

The therapist should note the way in which the person presents and by asking pertinent questions identify mood — whether he is anxious, depressed or despairing, or whether he is hopeful for the future. Formal help from the psychologist or psychiatrist may assist people with serious negative responses. Pain may affect socialisation and personal relationships and sensitive counselling may be indicated for some people.

Other treatments

The occupational therapist should identify any other treatments the person is currently receiving, noting their progress as well as details of any past treatments and their outcome. She should also ascertain what he hopes personally to gain from treatment in order to more accurately identify his aspirations and his understanding of the situation.

OCCUPATIONAL THERAPY INTERVENTION

ADVICE AND EDUCATION

Posture

The aim of advice and education is to inform the person about correct posture and habits and to engender awareness of the back when performing activities or at rest — in other words, to promote a 'think back' attitude.

Lying posture (Fig. 26.4)

A firm mattress and bed base will help the person to maintain a good posture in bed. Purchase of a new, expensive 'orthopaedic' bed can be avoided

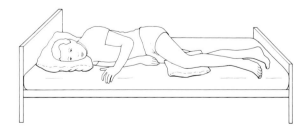

Fig. 26.4 Good lying posture. Side lying in bed with one pillow under the head and a small pillow under the forward knee.

by placing a firm board between the mattress and the bed base. Side lying (the first aid recovery position) is the posture most recommended. The head pillow should be just deep enough to fill the gap between the shoulder and the back of the head. Those with pain in the upper spinal region may use special orthopaedic pillows or soft cervical collars to support the neck.

Standing posture

A good standing position is attained when an imaginary line dropped from the ear will pass through the top of the shoulder, the middle of the hip joint, the back of the patella and the front of the malleoli of the ankle joints. The angle of the pelvis and the lordotic curve are important factors to consider. Some professionals recommend maintenance of the lumbar lordosis at all times. Others recommend flattening of the lordotic curve when

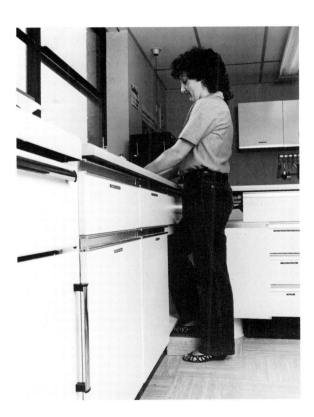

Fig. 26.5 Good standing posture: one foot forward and slightly raised to reduce lumbar lordosis.

standing, believing that by concentrating on maintaining it a person is likely to accentuate it and thereby increase stress on the dorsal lumbar region. Obesity and pregnancy also accentuate lumbar lordosis. All agree that abdominal and buttock tone should be maintained when standing. When prolonged standing cannot be avoided a small footstool or brick may be used to alleviate pain by allowing the person to flex one hip by placing the foot on the support, thereby promoting a more relaxed position. The ideal height of any work surface to be used when standing is 5 cm (2") below the level of the elbow. Low-heeled or flat shoes are also advisable in preference to high heels, which tend to accentuate lumbar lordosis.

Sitting posture

This is important for both working and resting positions. Poor sitting positions and seating are major factors contributing to low back pain and limited sitting tolerance. The ideal seat height and depth allow the person to place both feet flat on the floor when the back is fully supported. The angle of the backrest will depend on the task being undertaken and the purpose of the chair. When relaxing in the chair, reclining the backrest slightly promotes a comfortable relaxed posture. This, however, would be impractical when working at a desk, when a more upright position is required. A reading slope or frame on the desk may also improve the working position by overcoming the need to lean forward over the desk, but it should not incline above 45° (Fig. 26.6). In any chair, if the lumbar spine is correctly supported armrests or a higher backrest support will be unnecessary, except where the back pain extends to the upper spine or neck. Where armrests are provided they should support the forearm with the elbows flexed and the shoulders relaxed. A similar height is recommended for a work table. Working at a table which is too high leads to shoulder elevation and increases fatigue. A table that is too low, on the other hand, encourages the user to lean forward and strain the lumber spine.

A wide variety of seating is available for home or work. The therapist may give advice on a suitable type of chair to purchase or on modifications to an existing chair. Low soft seating which flexes the hips above 90° and promotes a slouched-forward C-shaped spinal curve (such as a beanbag or soft deep lounge chair) should be avoided. A small, firm, wedged cushion placed under the back of the cushion in such a lounge chair may assist temporarily by altering the seat angle to the floor, provided it does not significantly alter the backrest recline angle. Many specially designed chairs are adjustable to meet individual requirements. Alternative seating which alters weight-bearing to include the knees as well as the ischial tuberosities,

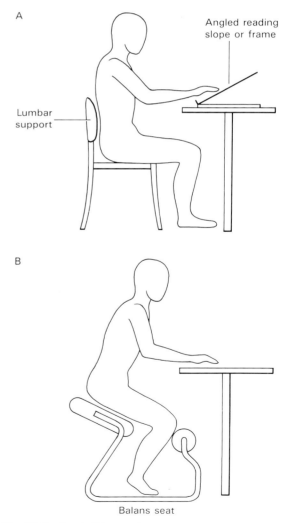

Fig. 26.6 Good sitting postures.

for example the Balans chair (Fig. 26.6), may benefit some people by promoting lumbar lordosis and encouraging good spinal muscle tone.

Long sitting with the legs extended forwards is contraindicated for most people in the acute stages of back pain. The main points to remember are to maintain the natural curves of the spine, to keep the back straight and to avoid side tilting, hunching or sagging. It is not advisable to maintain a static position for long periods of time. Frequent changes of position should be recommended.

Bending, lifting and carrying

These activities should be avoided by back pain sufferers whenever possible and no one should be encouraged to bend forward with the knees straight. Dropping onto one knee, or full kneeling, may enable activities to be performed at a low level. The correct lifting technique (Fig. 26.7) is as follows:

- Visually assess any load before attempting to lift it to ensure that it is manageable in terms of size and weight.
- Stand close to the load, facing the direction of travel, with the feet slightly apart and the toes angled outward.
- Keep the head up and the back straight.
- Bending at the hips and knees, grasp the object to be moved firmly at the base, keeping it close to the body. In this position the hip extensors are mechanically advantaged. The quadriceps group of muscles assist the lift and simultaneously tense the iliotibial band to which the glutei are attached.
- Test the weight by raising the object slightly before making the full lift.
- Lift by straightening the knees.
- Keep the back straight at all times, and do not twist when bending, lifting or putting an object down.
- Carry loads close to the body, using the arms to hold the item at waist height. It is better to distribute weight evenly, for example by carrying two equal loads rather than one heavy load (Fig. 26.7).

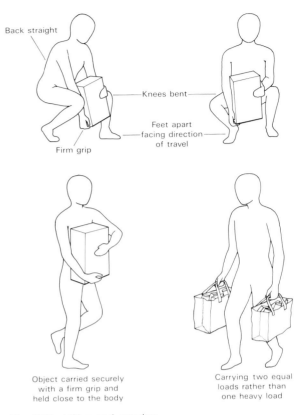

Fig. 26.7 Lifting and carrying.

It may be advisable for some people to wear an abdominal or spinal brace when lifting, to encourage correct posture and reduce the risk of strain to the lumbar region.

When the load appears to be too great, alternative methods for moving it should be pursued, for example pushing, pulling, obtaining help or using a mechanical aid. Before the load is moved it is also vitally important to ensure that the route of moving and the place where the load is to be deposited are clear.

Activities of daily living

Many people experience difficulties in this area. Everyday activities can become major problems because of pain and decreased range of movement. Many people will have developed coping strategies to overcome particular difficulties before they begin to work with an occupational therapist. It is important for the therapist to check these strategies to ensure that activities are not being undertaken in a way that will lead to further long-term problems. On the other hand, some people may have coped with their difficulties for some time and may have developed beneficial coping methods which the therapist might learn for use with others.

It is rare for a person with back pain not to achieve some functional ability in personal and domestic tasks, although full independence may not be possible. Education in ergonomics, practice in alternative techniques, provision of equipment and reorganisation of work schedules may assist the individual to manage his daily activities. However, on a simpler note, reminding him that 'Rome wasn't built in a day' and encouraging him to take two or more days to complete tasks previously achieved in one may assist him in coming to terms with the restrictions resulting from the back problem. The therapist may discuss changing roles and patterns of activity with other members of the family; this may further assist the individual to make the necessary adjustments to reduced activity levels.

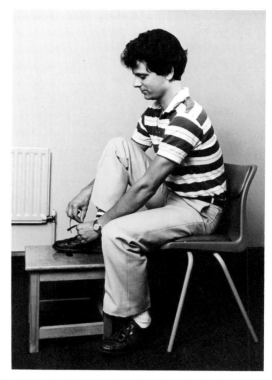

Fig. 26.8 Assistance when dressing: placing foot on a stool and flexing from the hip.

Mobility

The person with back pain should undertake transfers from lying to sitting from a side lying position at the edge of the bed. The feet should be lowered to the ground while the trunk is raised by pushing through the arms onto the mattress and keeping the back straight. To lie down the process is reversed.

Standing may be possible from a seated position on the edge of a chair or bed by leaning forward, taking the weight through the legs and pushing up on the armrests or mattress with the hands. If the legs are weak and there are no arms on the chair, rising can be assisted by placing the hands on the thighs and pushing down through the legs. When reversing the procedure in order to sit, the person should first make sure that he can feel the edge of the bed or chair behind his knees.

Dressing

The lower half of the body presents most difficulties because of limited reach. Reaching the feet can be facilitated by standing or sitting and placing each foot in turn onto a footstool (Fig. 26.8). Alternatively, some people find it easier to reach the feet from a sitting position by flexing the knee to bring the heel of the foot up onto the edge of the chair and extending the spine to reach the back of the lower leg and foot. Equipment to extend reach, for example a long-handled shoehorn, may be beneficial. Some people prefer to dress lying supine on the bed and raising each leg in turn to reach the feet.

Personal hygiene

The greatest and most frequent problem for people with back pain is getting in and out of the bath.

This should always be attempted with care and a non-slip mat is essential. Sitting with knees bent, kneeling or standing are preferred methods; long sitting in the bath is to be avoided. Having filled the bath, it is possible for the person to step in by standing sideways at the side of the bath, reaching across to the wall or the other rim with the nearest hand for support, and lifting the nearest leg over the side of the bath by flexing the hip and the knee. Keeping the back straight, the person can then step in with the other leg. Taking the weight through the arms by holding on to the bath sides, he can lower himself onto one knee and, maintaining support with the arms, bring the legs through into the sitting position. This movement will be assisted by the buoyancy of the water. To get out of the bath the procedure is reversed. A shower obviously presents fewer difficulties, but for those who feel anxious standing in a shower, a shower chair, (or bath board if the shower is over the bath) may be safer.

Shaving, washing, cleaning teeth and washing hair all involve forward flexion over the washbasin which may cause pain. Alternative methods which may be considered include sitting at the washbasin on a stool, or on the side of the bath if it is close enough to the basin.

A useful method for hair washing is to kneel at the side of the bath, leaning over the edge, and use a jug to ladle water, or a hand-held shower attachment. This position should also be adopted when cleaning the bath.

Domestic tasks

Many different problems present themselves in this area as a result of reduction in range of movement, limited reach, poor activity tolerance or restricted ability to lift objects. Problems may be exacerbated by the design of household equipment or furnishings. Assistance may be required with heavy tasks such as floor cleaning, bed making, vacuuming, shopping and looking after small children. The general rule, especially in the acute stages, is to avoid activities which accentuate or cause pain. During recovery correct use of equipment with good posture is essential to avoid further back strain.

When cleaning floors with a mop or hoover, or mowing a lawn, the person should hold the handle of the equipment at hip height; it is important that he walk forward with the equipment, rather than remaining stationary and leaning forward. Twisting movements should also be avoided.

Reorganisation of storage may be beneficial. Large or heavy regularly used items should be easily accessible, not kept at the back of high or low cupboards. Top-loading washing machines are easier to use for most people with back pain. Lowering washing lines and using a prop to raise them prevents overreaching, and placing the laundry basket on a trolley or chair overcomes the need for regular bending. Castors fitted to heavy furniture facilitate easier moving when cleaning.

Sexual problems

Back pain may negatively affect sexual activity. Many people are reluctant or embarrassed to mention sexual problems, despite the limitations the back pain may impose on their relationships. Severe or long-term pain may destroy any pleasure gained in sexual activity and may lead to avoidance of close contact situations or intercourse. This may create feelings of hostility or rejection in the partner as well as frustration in the person experiencing the pain. Fear of further injury to the back during intercourse may further impede relationships.

Open sharing of feelings between partners can facilitate greater understanding. Advice from professionals regarding the medical implications of intercourse can clarify concerns regarding risks. Discussion of positions to adopt to attain comfort together in bed, including alternative postures for sexual intercourse, may help. Some people prefer to read such information privately rather than discuss it, so guideline booklets may be useful. Specialist guidance and counselling about difficulties with sexual relationships may be obtained from the Association to Aid the Sexual and Personal Relationships of Disabled People (SPOD).

Child care

Many new mothers suffer back pain as the result

of the strain imposed on the lower spine during pregnancy from added frontal weight, poor posture and muscle stretch. This frequently results in problems with lifting and bending when caring for the baby and his siblings.

Advice on lifting techniques, lightweight equipment or alternative techniques may overcome some of the difficulty. Kneeling to change nappies on a plastic sheet on the bed or cot rather than on the floor reduces bending. Small children may be encouraged to climb onto an armchair or the bed for assistance with dressing, and the use of simple reins enables the mother to retain contact with the small ambulant child when out shopping if stooping to hold hands or manoeuvring a pushchair causes pain.

Postnatal abdominal and pelvic floor exercises should be encouraged to counteract the onset of a prolapsed womb, which may cause long-term back strain internally.

Driving

This is frequently a very painful activity because of the limitations of car seat design, the demands made when getting in and out of the car, movements required when driving and the need to remain seated. The car seat may require modification. Except in the more expensive range of vehicles, which have lumbar adjustments, many car seats tend to encourage a forward-flexed C-shaped position which adds to stress on the lower spine. Backward tilting thigh support and the absence of lateral support also exacerbate the strain. The transmission of jarring, swaying or swerving driving movements further adds to the discomfort.

The driver who suffers from back pain should be advised to relax and sit well back in the seat, adjusting the angle of the backrest to a position of comfort while retaining good vision. The seat should be positioned so that the steering wheel, gears and controls can be easily reached without stretching forwards. The legs should be comfortably flexed when using the pedals. A lumbar roll or seat insert, such as the Back Friend, may provide added seat support. Drivers should avoid long continuous periods of driving, and should adopt the habit of taking regular breaks, leaving the car and taking a short walk, at least every hour.

When getting into the car the person should commence with the seat well back, step into the car with one foot, lower himself gently into the seat and then lift the second leg into the car. When comfortably seated he should move the seat forward into the driving position (Fig. 26.9). The procedure should be reversed when stepping out of the car.

Driving should be avoided for four to six weeks following spinal surgery, and anyone wearing a cervical collar is usually advised not to drive. If spinal range of movement is severely limited then driving, particularly reversing the car, may become impossible. Weakness of limbs, particularly that affecting the lower limbs may reduce control of pedals and reaction speeds which may affect safety, and advice should be sought from the medical officer before recommencing driving. In certain jobs which involve a significant amount of driving, special seating may be provided and financial assistance may be obtained from the employment agency where the DRO is based.

MODES OF GIVING ADVICE AND PROMOTING EDUCATION

A variety of methods may be used by the therapist to support her advice and promote education on beneficial methods of management of back pain. A considerable amount of information can be conveyed on a one-to-one basis through assessment, discussion, demonstration and the provision of opportunities to practise techniques. Group teaching and learning may be used in some areas. This may involve a short course of sessions which enables a small group of people with back problems to learn and practise together, and to share information concerning particular problems or techniques and equipment which they have found to be successful. Such group work can be psychologically supportive for the individual in that it helps him to recognise that his difficulties are experienced by others. It also offers the practical gains of shared information and learning.

To promote continued learning many therapists recommend particular texts which provide infor-

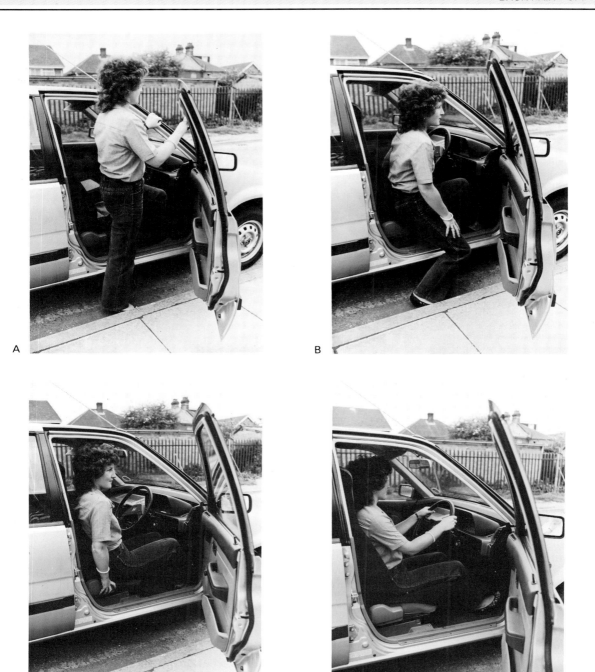

Fig. 26.9 Getting into a car. (A) Facing forwards, step into the car. (B) Flex hips and knees simultaneously and lower body weight onto the edge of the seat. (C) Push up on hands to move to the centre of the seat without twisting. (D) Correct driving position. Position of the arms minimises strain on the back and neck. Reverse the process for getting out.

mation and advice to which the person can refer following specific treatments; one example is D. Devlin's *You and Your Back* (1977). Therapists have also produced guidance leaflets, many with a large number of diagrams to which the person can refer at a glance for further information. Advice may also be provided in video form, which may be used in classes and discussions, or at home for reference and continued education. One such video offering exercise guidance is *Mind Your Back*. Therapists have also been involved in the production of educational videos to provide guidance in the prevention of back injury, particularly in lifting and handling techniques, for carers, industry and other groups.

Relaxation

Relaxation techniques may be taught by various members of the treatment team, including the occupational therapist. Relaxation skills should be taught in a way which allows them to be put into practice in everyday life, so they can become part of the daily routine. Relaxation may be taught in a number of ways, using voice and music, and the person should be taught to relax in a number of different postures. A number of relaxation tapes are available which may be used at home following relaxation training.

Back schools

In many areas of the country back schools are recognised as an efficient means of managing the large numbers of people who suffer back pain. The emphasis is on providing a multidisciplinary approach offering a comprehensive programme of education, advice and practice. Various personnel may be involved and the classes are organised on different patterns of attendance. One such school is run at the Wolfson Medical Rehabilitation Centre in Wimbledon. The Wolfson programme is by a team of occupational therapists, physiotherapists, nurses and psychologists, with input from the DRO and a dietician. The programme extends over a period of four weeks, for a class of twelve people.

The overall aim of the back school is:

- to enable individuals to become responsible for the management of their own backs
- to provide education in anatomy, posture, exercise programmes and lifting techniques
- to advise on seating, ADL, driving, work and leisure
- to improve self-management of pain during any activity, exercise or daily task
- to improve individual tolerances in static and working positions.

A questionnaire completed before attendance at the school enables the team to understand each person's back problems from his own perspective, including how it affects everyday life at home, at work and during leisure activities. Education sessions in a group setting stimulate interaction, as well as offering support, advice and help from peers. Advice, education, exercise and opportunities to try out equipment and daily tasks are provided. In the latter stages of the course activities may be upgraded to meet requirements for return to work or some other activity.

SPECIFIC TREATMENT ACTIVITIES

A wide variety of biomechanical techniques may be used to increase range of movement, strength and tolerance in the spine and limbs. Activities may be used to assess work potential and to prepare the person to return to work or the domestic role. Successful participation in purposeful, pleasurable activity may promote a sense of well-being and thus help to reduce the invasive constraint imposed by pain on activity as a whole.

All treatment activities should be based on the aims and goals identified following assessment, recognising the age and life-style of the person and his existing problems, strength, pain-free range of movement and stamina. Activities chosen may reflect domestic needs, or may be workshop based. Such equipment as the treadle lathe or rehabilitation cycle may be used to strengthen lower limbs. Bench work may be used to promote standing or sitting tolerances and may be adapted to promote particular spinal movements. Heavy activities such as outdoor gardening or sawing and planing wood may promote activity tolerance for those employed in manual work.

All activities should be perceived by the individual to be purposeful and should allow for specific grading to meet his evolving needs and abilities. Working positions should be monitored and the person should become involved in self-monitoring during activity, as an introduction to his personal responsibility to 'think back'.

Activities may be used for work simulation. Work tasks should be analysed and the work environment simulated as far as is practicable. The activity should be broken down into manageable stages, alternating light and heavy, high and low, simple and complex actions wherever possible (see Ch. 6). Emphasis should be placed on decreasing stress and increasing efficiency while maintaining good posture (Fig. 26.10). The person should be encouraged to change positions frequently and to put into practice the lessons learned in the education sessions. Posture, correct positioning and storage of equipment, and suitable seating and working heights should all be addressed. Correct postures and use of the limbs, together with self-monitoring, should facilitate increased activity tolerance and, through alerting attention to back care, reduce the risk of further damage. If modifications may be required to the workplace the support of the DRO should be sought.

For those not in employment, attention to leisure activities may be given through specific activities which relate to previous interests or through introduction to alternative leisure pursuits which do not place undue strain on the spine. Activities which involve a considerable range of spinal movement or any form of impact to the body should generally be avoided. Supported controlled movements, such as those used when swimming the breast stroke, are preferred.

CONCLUSION

The occupational therapist has an important role as a member of the multidisciplinary back care treatment and management team in both the

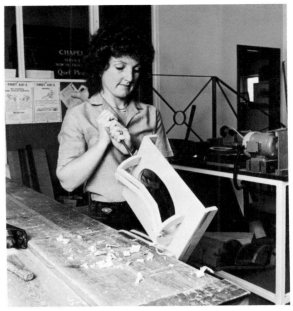

A

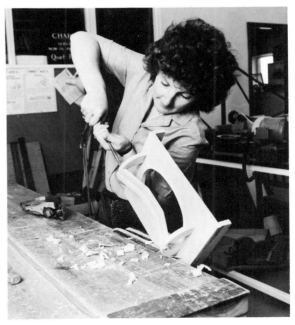

B

Fig. 26.10 Working positions. (A) Correct — spine position is correct, minimising back movement through proper use of arms. (B) Incorrect — strain is placed on the spine and upper limbs are used inefficiently.

hospital and community setting. Her role includes provision of individual activity programmes to promote anatomical function in order to overcome an acute episode and education in back care to reduce the risk of a reoccurrence of the problem. For people who suffer long-term chronic back problems, education, about the nature of the pain, together with advice and assistance in its management, may facilitate continued participation in self-maintenance tasks, role duties and leisure activities.

An additional role for all members of the team is that of prevention. Along with the physiotherapist, the occupational therapist gives advice on lifting techniques and good posture. Both professionals may be involved in the production of educational material for back care and in aspects of equipment and work station design.

The value of health education should not be underestimated. *Prevention is better than cure*, especially when one considers the cost of chronic back pain to the individual and his family, and the cost to the nation in terms of lost productivity and the provision of care.

ACKNOWLEDGEMENT

I would like to thank:

Marie Sammons, Head Occupational Therapist, Elderly Services, Richmond, Twickenham and Roehampton and previous author of this chapter, for allowing me to use her text and the photographs provided by Richard Bolton of the Department of Teaching Media, Southampton General Hospital.

Romayne Price, Senior Occupational Therapist, Atkinson Morley's Hospital, Wolfson Medical Rehabilitation Centre, for her advice and support while writing this chapter.

D. G. Jenkins, Consultant in Rheumatology and Rehabilitation and Medical Director of the Wolfson Medical Rehabilitation Centre for reviewing this chapter.

USEFUL ADDRESSES

Back Pain Association
Grundy House, Somerset Road
Teddington, Middlesex
TW11 0AB

The Royal Society for the Prevention of Accidents
Cannon House, The Priory Queensway
Birmingham B4 6BS

SPOD
Association to Aid the Sexual and Personal Relationships of Disabled People
286 Camden Road
London N7 0BJ

REFERENCES

Devlin D 1977 You and your back: how to cope with back pain and how it can be avoided. Pan Books, London
Dixon A St J 1980 Diagnosing low back pain. In: Jayson M I V (ed) The lumbar spine and back pain. Pitman Medical, Tunbridge Wells, pp 135–155
Engel G 1959 Psychogenic pain and the pain prone patient. American Journal of Medicine 26: 899–918
Hayward R 1980 Essentials of neurosurgery. Blackwell Scientific, Oxford
Liarg M H 1988 Low back pain: diagnosis and management of mechanical back pain. Primary Care 51(4): 827–847
Mind your back: how to relieve, recover from and prevent back pain. Produced by Videology, Ltd. (Obtainable from The Back Shop, 24 New Cavendish St, London WIM 7LH)
Stoddard A 1979 The back: relief from pain. Posture Health Guides, Martin Dunitz, London

FURTHER READING

Adams C J 1976 Outline of orthopaedics, 8th edn. Churchill Livingstone, Edinburgh

Bannister Sir R 1978 Brain's clinical neurology Oxford University Press, London

Bartorelli D 1983 Low back pain: a team approach. Journal of Neurological Nursing 15(1): 41–44

Bickerstaff E R 1978 Neurology, 3rd edn. Hodder and Stoughton, London

Brunswick M 1984 Ergonomics of seat design. Physiotherapy 70(2): 40–43

Byway C, Fletcher B, Hayne C R 1990 Fight back — a self help programme for back pain sufferers. Back Schools of Southern Derbyshire and Nottinghamshire District Physiotherapy Services, Spencer (Banbury)

Caslette R 1981 Low back pain syndrome, 3rd edn. Davis, Philadelphia

Flower A, Naxon E, Mooney V, Jones R 1981 An occupational therapy programme for chronic back pain. American Journal of Occupational Therapy 35(4): 243–248

Frederick B, Brown B E, Nelson–Allen C E, Amble D S, Clark V L 1980 Body mechanics, introduction manual, a guide for therapists. BAFCA Enterprises, PO Box 3192, Lynnwood, Washington 98036, USA

Griffiths B L 1987 Back pain — why bother. Journal of Professional Nursing 3(3): 280–284

Hayne C R 1984a Ergonomics and back pain. Physiotherapy 70(1): 9–13

Hayne C R 1984b Back schools and total back care programmes — a review. Physiotherapy 70(1): 14–17

Health Service Advisory Committee 1984 The lifting of patients in the Health Service. HMSO, London

Humphries M 1989 Back pain. Routledge & Kegan Paul, London

Jayson M I V (ed) 1980 The lumbar spine and back pain, 2nd edn. Pitman Medical, London

Jayson M I V 1981 Back pain: the facts. Chaucer Press, Bungay, Suffolk

Lucois P R 1983 Low back pain, symposium on orthopaedic surgery. Surgical Clinics of North America 63(3): 515–527

Mandal A C 1984 The correct height of school furniture. Physiotherapy 70(2): 48–53

Rothman R H, Simeone F A 1975 The spine. Saunders, Philadelphia, vols 1, 2

Rudinger E (ed) 1978 Avoiding low back trouble. Consumers' Association, London

Sammons M 1987 Back pain. In: Turner A (ed) Practice of occupational therapy, 2nd edn. Churchill Livingstone, Edinburgh

Willer A P, Rowland D 1985 Back to backs — a guide to caring for your back after surgery. (Obtainable from A P Willer, Physiotherapy Clinic, Wilton Grove, Wimbledon, London SW20)

27

Burns

Patricia M. Riley and Rosemary Cooper

INTRODUCTION

The occupational therapist's work with people who have suffered burn injury is both demanding and challenging as it encompasses a wide range of concerns and addresses the needs of all age groups. The person who has a burn injury may need help in all spheres of life — physical, psychological and social — and in various environments, whether at home, at work, or in school.

This chapter aims to illustrate the stages of occupational therapy intervention as it applies to the treatment of burn victims from hospital admission to discharge and aftercare. The first sections of the chapter explain the classification of burns by type, depth, extent and cause. The team approach to burn treatment is then outlined, followed by the general aims of the occupational therapist's intervention. The specific stages of the occupational therapy process — from assessment, through early intervention, to post-grafting care — are described, along with various practical and psychosocial factors to consider in domestic and work rehabilitation. The chapter then turns to the needs of children who have suffered burn injury, with particular attention to the involvement of parents or carers.

Next, various types of orthoses that can be used to aid the healing process are described, together with their applications to various parts of the body. The use of pressure garment regimens in reducing hypertrophic scarring is also outlined.

Finally, the chapter returns to the psychosocial aspects of burn injury and the management of emotional problems that may arise during rehabilitation and reintegration into the community. Throughout, the chapter stresses the importance of the involvement of family and friends in the rehabilitation programme to its final outcome.

BURN INJURY

The skin is the body's largest organ. It is a sensory organ and acts as an environmental barrier, helping to regulate pressure and reduce loss of essential fluids. When a burn occurs the skin and some underlying structures may be damaged, thus potentially producing a life-threatening situation.

CLASSIFICATION OF BURNS

Burns may be categorised by the following criteria:

- the type of burn
- the depth of burn
- the percentage of skin surface involved.

These categories can be further subdivided according to their cause, as follows.

Type of burn

- Thermal
  — flame
  — steam
  — hot liquid
  — hot metal
- Chemical
  — acid
  — alkali
- Electrical
- Radiation
- Friction.

  N.B. Exposure to extreme cold (e.g. liquid

nitrogen) may produce the same effect as exposure to extreme heat. Frostbite is a type of burn.

Depth of burn

- Superficial. Involves the epidermis, resulting in erythema, pain and blistering. Healing usually occurs spontaneously, normally within 7 to 10 days.
- Partial thickness. May be referred to as dermal or deep dermal, depending on the thickness of dermis involved. Granulation tissue may form, although grafting is often necessary, especially with deep dermal burns. Scarring will occur.
- Full thickness. Extends to subcutaneous tissue and may include tendon, muscle and bone damage. Spontaneous healing is not possible and skin grafts are always necessary. Scarring will occur. Reconstructive surgery may also be required over a period of years, depending on the site and severity of the

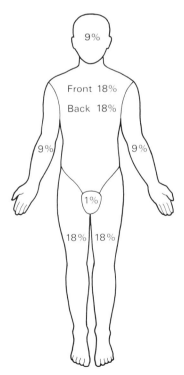

Fig. 27.1 Wallace's Rule of Nines.

burn, particularly in the case of growing children.

Percentage of skin surface injured

Wallace's Rule of Nines is usually used to give a quick estimate of the area of the body surface affected by burn injury. This divides the body into areas of 9% or multiples of 9% (Fig. 27.1).

People who have incurred burns involving over 15% of the body surface are usually transferred immediately from Accident and Emergency to a specialised burns unit. The Lund and Browder chart for estimating the severity of the burn wound is then used to give a more accurate percentage of the body surface involved (Fig. 27.2).

Individuals who have suffered burn injuries of less than 15% are commonly treated on plastic

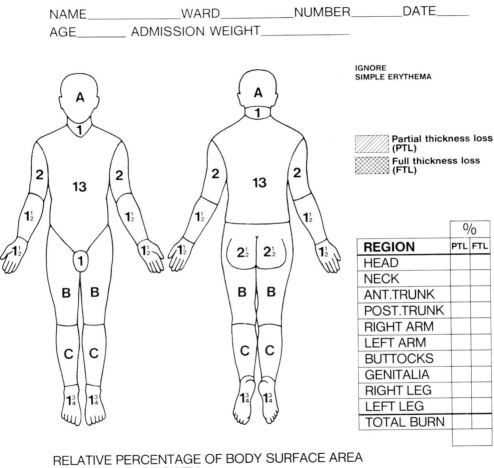

NAME_____WARD_____NUMBER_____DATE_____
AGE_____ ADMISSION WEIGHT_____

IGNORE SIMPLE ERYTHEMA

Partial thickness loss (PTL)
Full thickness loss (FTL)

REGION	PTL	FTL
HEAD		
NECK		
ANT.TRUNK		
POST.TRUNK		
RIGHT ARM		
LEFT ARM		
BUTTOCKS		
GENITALIA		
RIGHT LEG		
LEFT LEG		
TOTAL BURN		

RELATIVE PERCENTAGE OF BODY SURFACE AREA AFFECTED BY GROWTH

AREA	AGE 0	1	5	10	15	ADULT
A=½ OF HEAD	9½	8½	6½	5½	4½	3½
B=½ OF ONE THIGH	2¾	3¼	4	4½	4½	4¾
C=½ OF ONE LEG	2½	2½	2¾	3	3¼	3½

Fig. 27.2 Lund and Browder chart for estimating severity of the burn wound (by courtesy of Smith and Nephew)

CASE EXAMPLE 27.1

Mr A, a 37-year-old right-handed man, sustained a 35% partial thickness flame burn. He is a motor mechanic and his injury was the result of a petrol explosion at work. He is married with a one-year-old child.

Stage	Problems observed	Treatment plan	Occupational therapy intervention
Early	Burns extending across the joints of the hands and knees Fear, anxiety, pain and shock	Provide orthoses to prevent contractures. Provide reassurance	Hand orthoses Knee extension orthoses Introduce self to Mr A and his relatives. Explain procedures
Grafting	Grafts extending across joints Depressed about dependence on staff Anxious about medical procedures Passive behaviour	Provide orthoses to protect newly grafted areas ADL assessment Promote independence Provide reassurance	Hand orthoses Knee extension orthoses Teach relaxation Supportive counselling Advice and information booklets Provision of equipment: • large-handled cutlery • book rest • insulated beaker • non-slip mat Introduction to an outpatient in similar circumstances Provide opportunities in daily tasks to encourage decision-making
Post-grafting	Anxiety re: • physical function • finance • return to work • concern for relatives Lack of confidence Fear of meeting people	Explore psychological problems	Supportive counselling Liaise with: • social worker • psychologist Socialisation programme Gradual introduction of visits outside the hospital Discussions with Mr A and his wife with regard to a return to the home Discussions re work assessment and activities Introduction to support group Discussions re the need for outpatient care
	Scarring Hyperaesthesia of scars Limited flexion at MCP and IP joints Slight contracture of right thumb web	Plan for scar management	Show 'before and after' pressure garment photographs Provide information booklets Provide opportunity to talk to outpatient wearing pressure garments Provide pressure garments with silicone inserts
		Assess: • hand function • ADL • work Plan activity programme	C-bar serial stretch orthosis with silicone insert Graded programme to improve hand function and reduce sensitivity Programme of work activities including a work visit and visits to petrol stations Introduce a work project to build sense of achievement

CASE EXAMPLE 27.1   (Cont'd)

Stage	Problems observed	Treatment plan	Occupational therapy intervention
Outpatient	Fear of petrol and work situation	Explore Mr A's fears	Establish desensitisation programme
	Irritability towards wife and intolerance of young baby	Identify current problems in family relationships	One-to-one discussion with ● Mr A ● his wife Encourage discussion in support group Liaise with clinical psychologist
	Reluctance to return to work with less than full hand function	Reassess hand function	Upgrade activity programme including simulated work activities Project to further improve sense of achievement Reassurance as to his abilities
	Lack of energy	Education of effects after trauma	Establish home activity programme with achievable goals and monitor.
	Frustration regarding use of pressure garments	Reevaluate fit of garments Reinforce benefits More frequent outpatient appointments	Alter design of pressure garments Show 'before and after' photographs Discussion with another patient and within the support group

surgery wards in general hospitals or as outpatients through Accident and Emergency departments.

Incidence of burns

Most burn injuries result from accidents and the groups most likely to be at risk are the elderly (especially the frail elderly), the physically disabled, young children, those people with mental health problems and people working in potentially hazardous situations.

MEDICAL MANAGEMENT OF BURN INJURIES

The initial medical management of burns involves the treatment of shock following the injury. There is an increase in the permeability of blood vessels and a loss of valuable electrolytes and plasma proteins. Fluids need to be replaced. The volume of fluid necessary is calculated using various for-

mulae based on the extent of the burn and the weight of the person. Where granulation tissue does not form skin grafting is required, and reconstructive surgery may be needed over a period of years, depending on the severity and the site of the burn (Settle 1986).

The team

It is essential that all members of the team work together to ensure cohesion of the intervention programme. The consultant is responsible for medical management but relies upon specialist nurses to implement the fluid balance programme and maintain pain control. Nurses are also responsible for wound care to avoid further wound damage or infection and for the maintenance of positioning to minimise or prevent contractures. They are also frequently required to provide emotional support.

A dietician may give advice on a high protein, high calorie diet to counteract hypermetabolism and to support tissue repair. The physiotherapist aims to encourage and maintain mobility both in the injured and non-injured areas. Exercises to promote good breathing may be beneficial for those who have inhaled hot air, smoke or other gases, or who have been ventilated. In the later stages of rehabilitation the physiotherapist is usually involved in the prevention of hypertrophic scarring and its effects.

The psychologist and social worker are frequently members of the team. Relatives and friends, whose reactions play an important part in the recovery process, should also be educated and supported in order to become positive members of the treatment team.

OCCUPATIONAL THERAPY INTERVENTION

The occupational therapist may be involved with the person from shortly after his admission to a burns unit or ward up to and beyond his discharge. The person may continue to attend the hospital as an outpatient for up to 18 months following the injury, and may require help in the community for some years.

The injured person and, whenever possible, his relatives should be involved with programme planning. The individual's perspective on his own needs and priorities will help to determine treatment goals.

Progression of treatment is dependent on wound recovery and the person's psychological state. Specific goals will vary from person to person, but the general aims of treatment are:

- To reduce oedema and maintain range of movement
- To prevent deformity from contractures by correct positioning and the use of orthoses
- To minimise the effects of scarring by using pressure techniques
- To maintain functional independence
- To increase tolerance to fatigue and improve muscle strength
- To assist with psychological adjustment to the injury and its after-effects

- To educate with regard to skin care, including sensory retraining following nerve involvement, desensitisation of grafted areas through graded activity, and development of a good skin care regimen which includes lubrication and massage
- To resettle the person in the community and at work.

Medical management of the injured person is the priority on admission. The occupational therapist's emphasis at the early stage is to prevent deformity and to maintain range of movement by the provision of orthoses (see p. 685).

ASSESSMENT

Background information on the injured person is also needed at this stage. This may include:

- details of the type of burn
- an estimate of the percentage area of the burn
- knowledge of the depth and location of the injury
- any secondary factors to be considered
- the person's past medical history
- an indication of the person's functional ability prior to the injury
- the circumstances of the accident
- details of the person's family and social roles
- an indication of the person's previous psychological status.

As healing progresses, assessments should be used to provide a more detailed baseline for treatment planning. These may include measurements of joint range of motion, oedema, sensation and muscle strength as well as functional assessments.

EARLY INTERVENTION

Custom-made orthoses may be required in order to prevent deformity (see p. 685).

It is important that the person be given every opportunity to maintain his independence. The occupational therapist may need to provide adapted or specialised equipment, e.g. large-handled cutlery, lightweight beakers, an enlarged TV switch, an alphabet communication board, etc.

Any treatment that involves providing equipment or making orthoses must be carried out with regard for the control of infection, in accordance with the policy of the burns unit and/or the hospital.

It is important for the occupational therapist to explain her work to the person's relatives so that they understand the principles of treatment and can become actively involved. Developing rapport with the relatives at this stage is beneficial in:

- providing support and encouragement to the relatives
- helping the relatives provide support and encouragement to the person with the burn injury
- providing accurate information about long-term care, which will help reduce anxieties about the future. Written information is particularly helpful here.

POST-GRAFTING STAGE

It is usually at this stage that a more thorough assessment can be made. Range of movement and sensation can be tested. Self-care activities can be assessed and appropriate equipment provided.

Graded purposeful activity, progressing from gentle unresisted to resisted work, can be used to improve range of movement and muscle strength using a biomechanical approach.

Desensitisation of grafted areas using activities graded from 'soft' to 'hard' may be used. Care must be taken regarding vigorous activity and shearing forces on newly healed skin, which is delicate and may break down easily.

Participation by the person in planning treatment and setting his priorities, together with his involvement in activities which require a gradual increase in the amount of decision-making and use of initiative, will help to increase self-esteem. A gradual programme of socialisation may be needed, particularly for those whose scars are visible. The burns unit or ward will have become a safe environment for the person where staff and relatives are used to his appearance. The first visit to the occupational therapy department may need to take place at a quiet time, as the person will have to come to terms with the reactions of others gradually.

Domestic rehabilitation

The following concerns surrounding the person's return to home life may need to be explored:

- Practical considerations:
  - Safety in the home, e.g. use of fire and cooker guards, coiled safety flexes, testing of temperature of domestic hot water, storage of household fluids such as bleach and caustic soda. Leaflets on safety are available from gas and electricity boards, social services, health education departments, etc.
  - Use of specialised equipment, e.g. bath aids, electric can-openers, long-handled utensils, wheelchairs
  - Financial concerns
- Psychosocial considerations:
  - Fears associated with using appliances such as kettles, chip pans, garden mowers, barbeques; use of car — especially filling petrol tank
  - Anxiety regarding ability to resume previous roles within the family and/or community
  - Avoidance of situations which may cause anxiety, e.g. going to the pub, sexual relationships, going swimming, lighting the gas fire
  - Over-dependency on others or inability to accept help
  - Social isolation.

The person may need to make a preliminary home visit in order to prepare for discharge. Day visits and weekend leave can assist this process.

Work rehabilitation

The persons' ability to resume his previous employment will need to be assessed. Areas which may need to be considered include:

- muscle power and range of movement, e.g. ability to stand or sit for long periods or to use heavy tools or equipment

- the work environment, e.g. dust or dirt levels, exposure to chemicals
- stamina
- tolerance to noise
- anxiety, especially if the accident happened at work. Early visits to work may help to allay this
- concentration
- hand function
- access to and within the workplace.

It may be necessary to involve the Disablement Resettlement Officer (DRO), particularly if alterations to the workplace or specialised equipment are required. The DRO will also be helpful in cases where the nature of the work needs to be modified or if the person requires formal work assessment, or retraining. Information regarding disablement resettlement services is available in all Job Centres.

THE BURNED CHILD

In the case of an injured child the occupational therapist will work with the child's parents/carers as well as with the child. In order to promote understanding of treatment techniques and activities and to reduce anxiety, clear explanations must always be given to both the child and the parents/carers about the importance of the procedures and what will be involved. Role play may be introduced to assist the child to accept interventions. For example, orthoses and pressure garments can be tried out on a doll or soft toy, or a parent, first.

The child in hospital

Some regression is expected in the child during hospitalisation, but if prolonged this may necessitate the intervention of a psychologist. Regression is usually indicative of a need for love and attention in the face of anxiety, fear and pain in strange surroundings. Regression can be extremely distressing for parents who are attempting to cope with their own feelings of guilt regarding the injury. Support for the parents to provide love and care without over-indulgence is necessary to enable the child to return to his previous developmental level. Discussion with other parents, either in a support group or individually, can be very helpful.

The value of play

Play is an important part of recovery for the child, and the occupational therapist can provide suitable toys which serve a therapeutic purpose. In selecting toys to use in her programme, the therapist might look for:

- toys which require and thus help to maintain upper limb range of movement and bilaterality
- toys which require different grips, thus helping to maintain hand function
- toys and floor games requiring lower limb mobility, thus helping to maintain lower limb strength and range of movement.

Parents can be actively involved in incorporating toys into the child's rehabilitation programme.

Children also use play to act out frightening experiences, for example by role-playing reactions to a fire or the incident relating to their injury. The occupational therapist, parent, and any other member of the treatment team can help the child with this process. Role play can give the child the opportunity to practise the coping strategies he will need in dealing with questions about his scars, for example, or in returning to school.

After discharge

Parents will need support and encouragement as they implement the pressure garment regimen. They often find support in talking to others in similar circumstances. If the child has been treated on a regional burns unit it may be too far for the parents to return to the unit to meet other parents, especially as travelling may involve bringing a small child and siblings. It can, therefore, be very beneficial for parents to keep in touch with other parents by telephone or through letters. The occupational therapist can often facilitate these contacts through outpatient clinic appointments and arrange face-to-face groups for those able to travel.

Liaison with the local health visitor or social

worker in the community may be necessary to assist with the pursuance of prescribed treatment practices after discharge. The child will need to return to the hospital at regular intervals for replacement of the pressure garments.

ORTHOSES FOR BURNS

Orthoses are used to:

- maintain range of movement
- prevent contracture and deformity
- maintain functional position
- immobilise grafted areas.

Orthoses should be applied whenever a burn extends across a joint, taking into account the depth of the burn and the exercise regimen and working practice of the unit or ward.

It is important to mould the orthosis individually on each person, as close to the skin surface as possible, and usually on the flexor aspect of the body. Areas regularly requiring orthoses include:

- joints of the forearm, wrist and hand
- the neck
- the axilla
- the elbow
- the knee
- the ankles
- joints of the feet
- planes of the face, especially around the eyes and mouth.

Static orthoses are applied unless otherwise indicated.

Joints of the forearm, wrist and hand

The hand is frequently injured because it is one of the most exposed parts of the body and is used to protect the face or extinguish a fire. Burns on the dorsum of the hand can result in a 'claw hand' deformity. This consists of hyperextension of the metacarpophalangeal (MCP) joints, flexion of the interphalangeal (IP) joints of the fingers, adduction and extension of the thumb, and radial deviation at the wrist. It also results in flattening

of the palmar longitudinal and transverse arches, producing a non-functional hand.

The extensor mechanism of the hand is poorly protected, particularly across the proximal interphalangeal (PIP) joints. Any flexion, either passive or active, may be contraindicated if there is a partial thickness burn to this area. In the early days boutonnière deformity may occur due to the rupture of the central slip of the extensor tendon at the PIP joint.

Palmar burns are less common, as the palm is more protected and the skin is thicker. Burns to the palm result in tightening of the palmar fascia and flexion and adduction of the fingers and thumb.

To counteract a pull towards claw hand deformity the orthosis should provide the following position:

- Wrist — 30° extension
- MCP joints — 70° flexion
- IP joints — full extension
- Thumb — opposed and extended
- Web space and palmar arches — maintained.

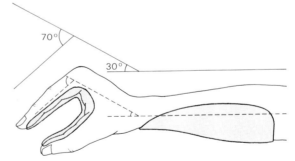

Fig. 27.3 Optimum position for the wrist and hand to prevent contracture.

Dynamic orthoses may be applied if there is tendon damage (Fig. 27.3).

The neck

The neck should be supported in the natural extended position, maintaining the joint space under the chin and along the jawline (Fig. 27.4).

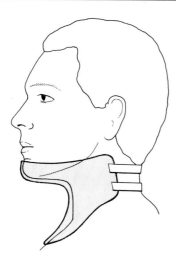

Fig. 27.4 Neck support position.

The axilla

The axilla should be supported with the arm abducted at 90° to the body, and with a 10° forward flexion at the shoulder (Fig. 27.5).

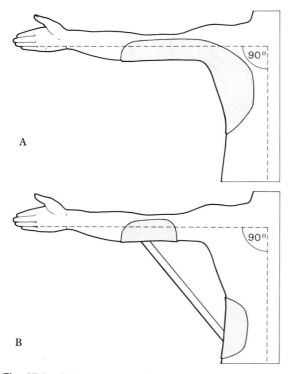

A

B

Fig. 27.5 Axilla support position. (A) Enclosed support. (B) Open support.

The elbow

The elbow should be maintained in extension with the forearm in the neutral position between pronation and supination. Orthoses usually take the form of a gutter orthosis or a three-point extension support (Fig. 27.6).

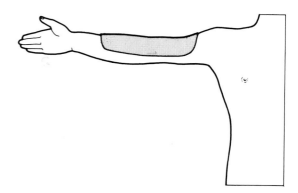

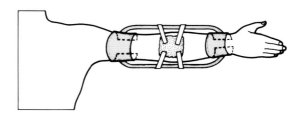

Fig. 27.6 Elbow orthoses. (A) Gutter support. (B) Three point extension support.

The knee

Where possible the knee should be supported in full extension, ensuring the orthosis has a contour fit into the popliteal fossa at the back of the knee (Fig. 27.7).

The ankles and joints of the feet

The foot should be positioned in a neutral position, i.e. at a 90° angle to the tibia, allowing the sole of the foot to be placed flat on the floor when mobilising. There should be no pressure on the dorsum of the heel or the medial and lateral malleoli of the ankle. Metatarsophalangeal and interphalangeal joints should be held in extension and the arches of the foot maintained (Fig. 27.8).

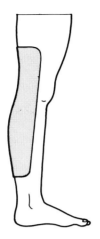

Fig. 27.7 Knee extension gutter support.

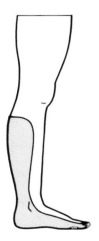

Fig. 27.8 Ankle/foot support in neutral position.

Planes of the face

The face is a complex structure which is highly mobile. Burns scarring may result in contracted tissue, particularly around the mouth and the eyes, which limits mobility and produces deformity.

Pressure face masks may be used in conjunction with silicone inserts (Gollop 1988). These may be applied to the full face or on small areas, for example around the nose (Fig. 27.9) (Malick & Carr 1980). Semi-rigid transparent face masks may also be used to help flatten scar tissue. These are usually made in conjunction with a maxillofacial

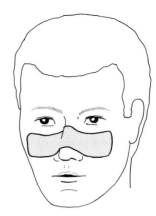

Fig. 27.9 Nose pressure conformer.

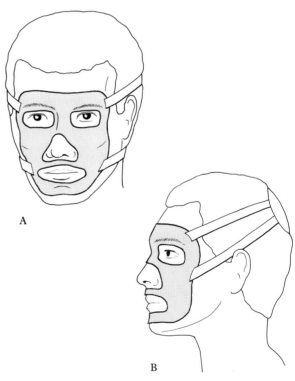

Fig. 27.10 Full face mask. (A) Front view. (B) Side view.

prosthetic technician (Fig. 27.10) (Powell et al 1985).

Partial or full thickness circumferential burns of the mouth may contract, causing microstomia un-

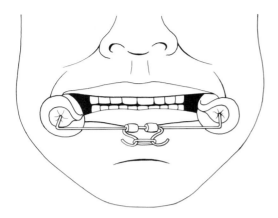

Fig. 27.11 Microstomia splint.

less opposing force is applied. Full stretch of the mouth needs to be maintained by use of a microstomia splint (Fig. 27.11) (Heirle et al 1988).

Orthotic materials

The materials chosen should be easily washable, conforming, easily adjustable and suitable for bandaging on to the affected part in the early stages.

There is a wide range of low-temperature thermoplastic materials available on the market. Sometimes it may be necessary to increase pressure over a raised scar using one of a range of silicone materials available — Silastic foams and pastes, silicone elastomers, or silicone gel sheeting (Gollop 1988). All of these can be individually moulded to the area and taped in place, positioned in the orthosis or placed under the pressure garment.

All orthoses should be regularly reevaluated, adjusted and, if necessary, redesigned as the person progresses. Immobilising orthoses may be necessary once grafting has taken place.

In the early stages most orthoses are bandaged on, but once oedema has been reduced straps may be applied. It is important to remember that simple alternatives to traditional orthoses may be used. For example, the person may find that a foam roll for the neck is very useful in maintaining neck extension when lying supine, particularly in the early stages. A piece of thick foam bandaged around a small child's arm may serve the same purpose as a thermoplastic elbow gutter.

If contractures do occur, serial stretch orthoses may be required, often in conjunction with the pressure garments.

The success of any orthotic regimen depends on:

- appropriate prescription
- the expertise of the occupational therapist when making and fitting the orthosis
- appropriate choice of style, design and materials
- compliance of the person, his relatives and the entire treatment team.

TREATMENT OF HYPERTROPHIC SCARRING

Immediately after healing a burn wound may appear quite flat. However, over the ensuing months hypertrophic scarring may develop. The scars become cherry red, hard, lumpy and raised, and if left untreated may cause contractures and deformity.

Pressure garment regimen

The application of controlled consistent pressure using pressure garments keeps the scar flat, smooth and pliable. Garments are usually required when the wound has taken longer than 2–3 weeks to heal spontaneously. For the best results the following points must be adhered to:

- The garment must be applied as soon as healing has occurred.
- The garment must be worn 24 hours per day, being removed only for massage, creaming and bathing.
- The person must attend regular outpatient clinics to enable progress to be monitored. Adults are usually seen every 6–8 weeks, but children are seen more frequently.
- The garments should be hand-washed daily, following the manufacturer's instructions, to maintain the elasticity of garments.
- The garments should be worn for 12–18 months, until scar maturation, i.e. when the scar is soft, flat and pale, pink or white.

Each pressure garment is custom made, and accurate measuring is essential to ensure a good fit. The most commonly used material is Lycra. The garments are either commercially available or made in the hospital. Two or three sets of garments are usually provided and generally need to be replaced approximately every three months. Heavy use or, in the case of a child, a growth spurt may necessitate more frequent replacement. Gloves may need to be replaced every six weeks depending on the person's life-style.

In order to ensure the compliance of the burned individual and his relatives or carers it is essential to explain clearly the pressure garment regimen to all concerned. 'Before and after' photographs may be used to promote a realistic understanding of the outcome. Information booklets may also assist, some of which are provided by the manufacturers.

The fitting and removal of the garments initially requires practice. Added support and encouragement are needed in the early days, particularly with parents of small children. Once the benefits can be seen or felt, the person and his family are usually self-motivated and assume an active role in the pressure garment regimen.

At the end of pressure garment treatment camouflage make-up creams can be shown to the person so that he may choose if he wishes to conceal a scar; similarly, parents may wish to know what is available for their child in the future. These creams are available on prescription. It is important to be realistic about their value so that the person does not build up false expectations.

PSYCHOSOCIAL ASPECTS OF BURN INJURY

The injured person may have one or more of the following initial emotional responses to his injury.

Fear

Often accidents have occurred in places or situations which were previously considered safe. The person may be afraid to face the situation of the accident again after recovery. The actual treatment of the injury involves painful procedures which may cause fear. The person can see and feel the damage to his body and may be apprehensive about others' reactions to him. He may fear that the success of the healing will be limited. In hospital, children are frightened at the strangeness of the environment and the procedures which may be necessary; despite love and reassurance they may feel abandoned by their parents, who allow such treatment to happen.

Isolation

The person may be nursed in isolation, and this can appear to be a punishing situation, especially for children. The person is unable to see how others are reacting to pain, disfigurement and treatment techniques, and is often unsure how to react himself. He may emotionally try to isolate himself from the situation, and not see or accept the reality of his predicament.

Frustration

The person is inactive and dependent. The recovery is slow and it is difficult for him to envisage the whole of the treatment programme. Hand injuries can initially be especially frustrating and traumatic as they are clearly visible to the person concerned and they emphasise his dependence on others.

Guilt

The accident may have been the injured person's fault and others may have been hurt. The person often worries that he has caused problems for others to cope with. The parents of a child who has been burned often have deep feelings of guilt and need to be well supported throughout the whole of the rehabilitation period. Often parents tend to compensate the child for the injury by becoming over-protective and over-indulgent or by not imposing any discipline or structure on him. This tends to result in the child becoming more dependent on the parent and often causes unwillingness to participate in the treatment programme. Establishing a trusting relationship helps parents come to terms with the situation to allow the child some independence. In certain cases individual counselling or psychotherapy for the parents may be beneficial.

Loss/grief

Parents commonly grieve for the loss of their 'perfect' child because the child is permanently scarred. This has a particular tendency to occur when the child is very young at the time of the accident.

Adults may grieve at the loss of their previous physical image and at the implications this may have for their social life.

Signs of emotional problems

The person may show a number of reactions to this emotional crisis. These may include:

- attention-seeking behaviour
- regression of normal abilities
- loss of appetite
- anger with self and the treatment team
- unpredictable or aggressive behaviour
- passive behaviour
- depression.

Management of emotional problems

All members of the treatment team need to be aware of the person's emotional crisis and will be involved in helping him come to terms with reality following his bereavement. The occupational therapist plays a valuable part in this process and must support both the injured person and the family during the lengthy treatment programme. Developing rapport with the person and gaining his trust by using an empathetic and non-judgemental approach is initially the most important aspect to consider. It is essential to encourage the individual to live in the present in a positive way. Counselling may be necessary in order for the person to come to terms with his altered body image and all the implications this has for him in his personal, social and sexual life.

Truthful and realistic explanations must be given to the person regarding the treatment procedures to be carried out, and the family needs to be involved at all stages. Relaxation, role play, socialisation and desensitisation techniques may all be of value during the rehabilitation programme. Good assertion skills need to be developed as the person has to adapt to other people's reactions — their questions, their stares, their avoidance. The person may gain some benefit from membership of support groups and nationally linked networks organised for those who are disfigured and disabled.

CONCLUSION

A burn is a sudden, painful, distressing event which can change a person's life for ever. Occupational therapy intervention aims to minimise the impact of the injury on the person's physical, social and functional status, and assist the person to make practical and psychological adjustments.

The length of the intervention period frequently extends up to and over two years. The final physical outcome is dependent on the person's cooperation and perseverance in the treatment regime. The final psychosocial outcome depends on:

- the person's own personality and coping strategy
- the response of his family, friends and community
- the quality of help and support provided by the treatment team.

REFERENCES

Gollop R 1988 The use of silicone gel sheets in the control of hypertrophic scar tissue. British Journal of Occupational Therapy 51(7): 248–249.

Heirle J A, Henly J A, Keely G P, Cramm A E, Hartford C E 1988 The microstoma prevention appliance: 14 years of clinical experience. Journal of Burn Care Rehabilitation 9(1)

Malick M H, Carr J A 1980 Flexible elastomer moulds in burn scar control. American Journal of Occupational Therapy 34(9): 603–608

Powell B W E M, Haylock C, Clarke J A 1985 A semi-rigid transparent face mask in the treatment of post burn hypertrophic scars. British Journal of Plastic Surgery 38: 561–566

Settle J A D 1986 1986 Burns — the first five days. Smith & Nephew, Welwyn Garden City

FURTHER READING

Allsworth J 1985 Skin camouflage — a guide to remedial techniques. Stanley Thornes Publishing, Cheltenham

Bernstein N R 1976 Emotional care of the facially burned and disfigured. Little, Brown, Boston

Bernstein N R 1989 Coping strategies for burn survivors. Praeger, New York

Cason J S 1981 Treatment of burns. Chapman & Hall, London

DiGregorio V R (ed) 1984 Rehabilitation of the burn patient. Churchill Livingstone, New York

Fisher S V, Helm P A 1984 Comprehensive rehabilitation of burns. Williams & Wilkins, Baltimore

Hill C 1985 Psychosocial adjustment of adult burns patients — is it more difficult for people with visible scars? British Journal of Occupational Therapy 48(9): 281–283

Hooper W 1989 Life after a burn: how to cope at home. Available from Jobst Division of Zimmer Surgical Specialities, Swindon, Wilts

Kemble J V H, Lamb B E 1987 Practical burns management. Hodder and Stoughton, London

Malick M H, Carr J A 1982 Manual of the management of the burn patient. Harmarville Rehabilitation Centre, Pittsburgh (available in UK from Smith & Nephew, Welwyn Garden City)

Mason S, Forsham A 1986 Burns aftercare — a booklet for parents — your child at home after injury. Burns 12: 364–370

Mason S, Turner H, Foley A 1986 Burns aftercare — a booklet for patients at home after injury. Smith & Nephew, Welwyn Garden City

Pedretti L W, Zoltan B 1990 Occupational therapy: practice skills for physical dysfunction, 3rd edn. C V Mosby, St Louis

Porter J 1982 The therapist and the burns patient. Therapy Weekly, April 8th: 4

Quinn K J, Evans J H, Courtney J M, Gaylor J D S 1985 Non pressure treatment of scars. Burns 102–108

Rivlin E, Forshaw A, Polanyj G, Woodruff B 1986 A multidisciplinary group approach to counselling the parents of burned children. Burns 12(7): 479–483

28

Limb injuries

Kate Abbott, Ruth Sampson and Glenys R. H. Crooks

INTRODUCTION

Injuries to the limbs are extremely common, affecting people from all social classes and age groups. Young adults tend to suffer the more severe limb injuries, which may occur at work, during sport or on the roads. For the most part they suffer short-term debility and are looking for a recovery to near-normal function. Problems are not related to a degenerative disease process and treatment can be active and vigorous.

This chapter examines the role of the occupational therapist in helping people with limb injuries to regain maximum function and independence. The first half of the chapter is devoted to the treatment of injuries to the joints of the upper and lower limb, and begins with a discussion of general aims of treatment, i.e. pain control, oedema reduction, the maintainance of bilaterality, sensory reeducation and the development of activity tolerance. Upper limb injuries are then discussed in detail, focusing on the shoulder, elbow and forearm, wrist and hand in turn. The rehabilitative goals pertinent to each structure are outlined along with special equipment, remedial games, therapeutic activities and orthoses that the therapist might use in her programme. Next, the therapist's intervention in lower limb injuries is considered, with particular attention to the recovery of mobility. As with upper limb injuries, treatment aims and techniques are discussed with reference to particular sites — i.e. the hip, knee and ankle — and the use of equipment, games, activities and orthoses is discussed in relation to each.

The next section of the chapter turns to the management of fractures, tendon injuries, ligament injuries and crush injuries in relation to specific sites on the upper and lower limb. The customary treatment (whether surgical or conservative) for each injury is described, along with the responsibilities that the occupational therapist will assume in ensuring that the prescribed management regime is maintained and integrated with the individual's daily life. Treatment aims relevant to each injury are defined, and contraindications for particular positions and movements are pointed out with reference to the use of orthoses and exercise.

The final sections of the chapter discuss the therapist's intervention in cases of reflex sympathetic dystrophy (RSD), tenosynovitis and repetitive strain injury (RSI). Although the pathological basis of RSD and RSI is still being debated, the occupational therapist's role in helping the individual to cope with these conditions is none the less a significant one.

As always, the importance of a multidisciplinary team approach in ensuring quality care for the injured person is emphasised. However, it is ultimately the individual who, with professional support and guidance, must accept responsibility for himself in making a successful recovery. Although the occupational therapist's approach to the treatment of limb injuries will principally be a biomechanical one, she must recognise the psychological impact of the injury upon the individual and his family. As in all areas of care, psychological and social considerations must affect the planning and implementation of her therapeutic programme.

PRINCIPLES AND METHODS OF TREATMENT

Most limb injuries are of an acute nature although a minority are caused by chronic problems such as joint instability. It is nevertheless important to emphasise the whole person in the treatment of such injuries. Careful assessment of the person's domestic, social and work situation should form the basis for the direction, goals and priorities of treatment. As well as applying humanistic principles, the occupational therapist will employ a predominantly biomechanical approach to overcome the physical impairments resulting from limb injury. In planning a treatment programme a great deal can be gained by measuring the person's range of motion and performing a functional assessm... the limb. Checks should be made for 'trick'... ...nts, and any difficulties ... be fully invest... tion o...

UPP

Injur...
funct...
and ...
actio...
mani...
comr...

As ...
limb...
the a...
are ...
is se...
imm...
ible...
max...
mer...
imp...
fect...

T...
app...

Pa

Th...
jur...
pai...
use...
a v...

Distraction is also an important weapon in the fight against pain, especially where it is intractable. Purposeful, constructive and creative activities may be of particular value in maintaining the person's interest as he progresses through different stages of treatment.

The therapist may also use transcutaneous electrical nerve stimulation (TENS) where pain so dominates the picture that the person is reluctant to participate and negligible improvement is made. In more major injuries the therapist should help the person come to terms with the reality of pain. Often there will be some residual pain as well as cold intolerance. Awareness of this fact needs to be held in balance with the hope of a pain-free limb.

Oedema reduction

Oedema reduction should be a first priority. Elevation of the affected part during rehabilitation and the use of pressure gloves, sleeves or finger stalls are expedient. Treatment should be regular and persistent, and care should be take not to introduce too much activity too soon, as this might cause further swelling. Periods of activity and exercise can be alternated with periods of rest, possibly with the injured part splinted in the optimum position. An OB Help Arm to support the limb against gravity and the use of elevated activities will also help reduce oedema.

Maintaining bilaterality

Where a person has injured an upper limb it is important to counteract any tendency to become one-handed. The inclination to favour the affected part should be offset by encouraging functional use, with or without the help of equipment, as early as possible. The person's natural protective tendencies need to be overcome in order to maintain a bilateral body image and facilitate function in the injured part.

Sensory reeducation and desensitisation

Damage to the peripheral nerves is often seen in combination with limb injuries, especially those caused by crushing. A complete peripheral nerve lesion is perhaps less common in these situations than axonotmesis or damage to digital nerves, though the functional deficit is much the same in the short term.

A fuller account of sensory reeducation and desensitisation can be found in Chapter 22.

Tolerance to activity

Activity tolerance must be developed by gradually increasing the duration and frequency of an activity. This applies both to tolerance to certain movements and to skin tolerance. If skin has been extensively scarred, grafted or has simply lost its normal toughness during the time the individual has been off work, time will be required to harden the tissues. Progress should be closely monitored so that there is no risk of skin breakdown. Increasingly tough materials can be used for progressively longer periods of time in therapy.

The shoulder joint

The wide range of movement at the shoulder enables the hand to be placed in a variety of positions. A strong shoulder also stabilises the distal joints, allowing fine work to be done efficiently. Disturbance of this system results in impaired function for the whole arm. Most activities are performed with the shoulder in some degree of flexion and abduction, the maintenance of which is the goal of the early stages of treatment unless the nature of the injury contraindicates this. Bilateral activities will encourage controlled use of the injured shoulder; care must be taken that the individual takes advantage of such activities and does not let the injured part become a 'passenger'. Bilateral movements also prevent compensatory trunk rotation.

An OB Help Arm or a system of suspended slings and springs will eliminate the effects of gravity, reducing pain and thereby enabling the person to work for longer periods in the desired position with less muscular effort. Activities should be lightweight and positioned so that the person stretches, but does not stress, the joint. A table that enables height adjustment according to the person's needs should be used. Remedial games such as draughts, the span game, solitaire and sliding puzzles, and activities such as baking, pottery, light woodwork (sanding and varnishing) and using a guillotine will promote shoulder mobility.

As shoulder strength and range of motion improve, treatment can be upgraded by reducing support, increasing the length of treatment sessions, adding resistance, increasing the complexity of the activity and changing the working position. Middle-range abduction and flexion should be established, and greater emphasis on shoulder extension and rotation should be considered. The height of activities can be increased or the person's position in relation to the activity changed so that a particular movement is isolated (Figs 28.1, 28.2, 28.3).

Use of an adjustable long handle on a wire twister produces a good middle range of all shoulder movements. Body positioning, however, is crucial, as the person will naturally twist, seeking to make the exercise easier by using trunk and elbow movement to compensate for the stiff and painful shoulder.

A tall span game can be introduced to promote the outer range of abduction and flexion, with the advantage that it encourages limited rotation (Fig. 28.4).

A wall board with adjustable height and angle is a useful piece of equipment on which to mount

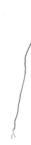

Fig. 28.2
to shoulder

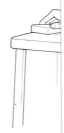

Fig. 28.3 E
top by chang

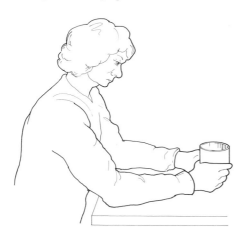

Fig. 28.1 Early stage shoulder flexion: activity just above waist level.

activities.
light sawi
gradually
creases. S
(Fig. 28.5)

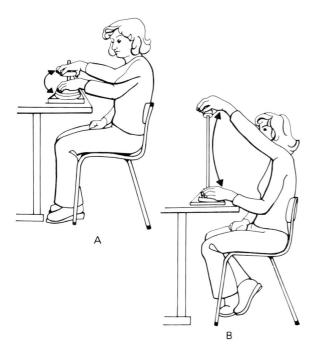

Fig. 28.4 Shoulder flexion (A) Using a standard span game (B) Flexion is increased when the dowel rods are lengthened. (Note: the height of the board can still be altered according to the range of movement required).

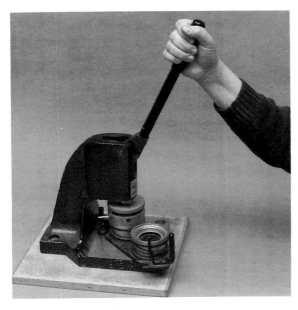

Fig. 28.5 Badge making.

bar all provide shoulder exercise, as do many domestic cleaning tasks.

Towards the late stages of treatment the aims are to strengthen the muscles around the joint and increase their tolerance to repeated activity. Treatment media used in earlier stages can be upgraded as the person works to achieve a stable and strong joint. Work assessment followed by specific treatment to simulate work-related activities should be given priority.

The elbow and forearm joints

These joints can be considered together because of the proximity of the head of radius to the elbow joint. Assessment will reveal that a person rarely presents with a problem elbow without some degree of supination/pronation deficit. Functionally, it is important to achieve enough flexion to be able to take the hand to the face and enough rotation to enable placing of objects (the forearm in pronation) and carrying and receiving of objects (the forearm in supination).

The injured elbow must be treated with respect, as the danger of myositis ossificans (the ossification of muscle) is always present. This is so especially where the joint is 'forced' into extension. Treatment should be gentle and active, without passive stressing of the joint. Progress may well be slow and if any myositis ossificans occurs range of motion may be a permanently reduced. The risk of myositis ossificans should be explained to the person to dissuade him from trying to passively straighten the elbow or to carry heavy weights.

Initially, the aims of treatment are to reduce oedema and increase joint movement in the middle range of flexion/extension and pronation/supination. Extension may be promoted through activities which encourage the person to push out into controlled extension, as in sanding, pottery, clay or pastry rolling, elevated games, and games positioned such that the person must stretch the forearm away from the body.

Although both pronation and supination are needed for normal function, supination is often the slower to return, and thus may require more attention early in treatment. The activities mentioned above as well as remedial games, badge making and light woodwork may be used to promote specific pronation or supination as required. The FEPS apparatus (designed to treat flexion, extension, pronation and supination) can also be used in conjunction with other activities and equipment (Fig. 28.6).

As improvement occurs, stool seating and use of the wire twister with a long handle or FEPS attachments may be introduced, offering more resistance and an increased range of motion. Printing can be initiated carefully, ensuring no sudden stress is placed on the joint and that the person does not 'cheat', using the body weight to operate the press and thus forcing passive extension at the elbow. Table tennis, darts, coits and table football, or Labyrinth and 'Star Wars' type games (both with FEPS attachments) can also be employed. A tendency to use the shoulder to compensate for restricted elbow movement can be counteracted by having the person place a piece of card between the arm and chest. This will encourage him to maintain the shoulder in adduction in order to prevent the card from moving (Fig. 28.7).

Home-based activities such as ironing, polishing and dusting or light gardening activities such as

Fig. 28.7
inhibits s
forearm.

weeding
elbow a

Tow
woodw
printing
bar to
creased
used w
sion. T
and res

Whe
thus m
the elb
it is pa
toleran

Ofte
a plate
point a
range
slowly
tinued

The

Like t
sidered
joint a
injury

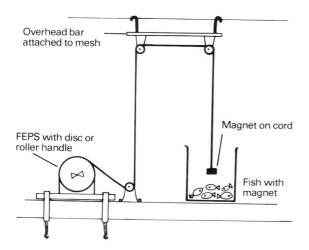

Fig. 28.6 FEPS apparatus in use with the magnetic fishing game. The apparatus can be used for several different activities. Resistance varies for each activity and can also be added to the apparatus itself by means of a screw adjustor.

tension, pronation and supination. The wrist also permits radial and ulnar deviation, allowing positioning of the hand in different planes and at different angles. Since the tendons and neurovascular supply to the hand cross the wrist, the secondary effect of wrist injury is pain and reduced movement in the hand. The position of the wrist affects the working length of the finger flexors and extensors. Wrist motion acts as a fine adjustment of function in these tendons and governs tenodesis or 'automatic grip' (see Fig. 23.4). Thirty degrees of wrist extension is necessary for optimal function in the digital flexors. The normal wrist will always extend during firm grasp.

The aims of treatment for injuries affecting the wrist are to obtain maximum flexion, extension, pronation, supination, grip strength and full mobility of the hand. Ulnar and radial deviation are not treated specifically, except in the case of individuals who use these movements very specifically as part of their job.

Joints distal to the wrist often show marked oedema; this is treated in conjunction with the wrist. Where swelling and pain in the wrist and hand are severe the first aim may be simply to achieve some sort of gross functional grip, thus paving the way to detailed exercises for achieving specific movements.

Use of the FEPS apparatus and remedial games such as the marble game (Fig. 28.8) will promote both flexion and extension. The sliding puzzle game (Fig. 28.9) can be used to achieve passive extension. Pronation and supination can be encouraged using the span game, solitaire with tongs, and FEPS activities. Creative activities such as light woodwork, pottery, baking and gardening will help achieve all wrist movements and encourage functional use of the hand, improving both mobility and grip strength.

As improvement occurs, treatment can be upgraded to include activities to increase the range of movement and provide increased resistance. Printing (with or without an extension board), use of the wire twister, stool seating, woodwork (sawing, planing, drilling and screwdriving), cookery and remedial games (table tennis, puff football, and Labyrinth or 'Star Wars' with FEPS attachments) can be used.

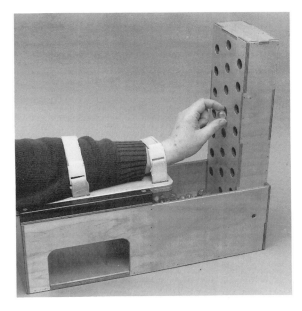

Fig. 28.8 Marble game.

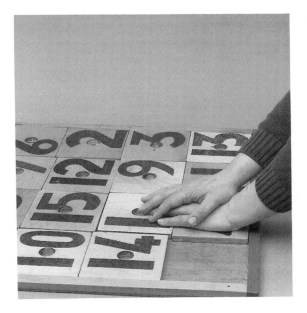

Fig. 28.9 Sliding puzzle.

The person is often discharged at this point, continuing to exercise at home. While this may be acceptable in the majority of cases, some people will need further rehabilitation to attain work or sport fitness. Activities used at this stage can be more generalised, concentrating not on isolated movements but on tolerance and strength. For example, heavy gardening, concreting, and woodwork projects involving sawing and planing may be used for those requiring particularly strong function in their employment or leisure.

The hand

The hand is a complex, delicately balanced structure allowing both great strength and very fine manipulation. It is a highly integrated structure, so that injury to one part always affects others. For this reason detailed and accurate assessment of the hand as a whole is necessary (see Ch. 7). Each affected joint should be measured and overall functional ability assessed, so that a baseline for treatment and progress can be established.

Reduction of oedema around the small joints of the hand is of primary concern. Swelling in the hand causes a characteristic posturing with the thumb adducted in the plane of the hand, metacarpophalangeal (MCP) joints extended and interphalangeal (IP) joints flexed. This position must be corrected if mobility is to be restored to the hand.

The hand must be treated as a functional unit during the rehabilitation process. The injured parts should work with the whole in everyday use, the particular movements which need to be regained should be specifically isolated and practiced.

Flexion

The aim of treatment is to achieve both gross grip and individual digit flexion. The two are inextricably linked — as IP joint flexion improves, so does grip — and the two must be developed in tandem so that the maximum potential improvement is made. Many treatment activities will enhance both flexion and grip, but the therapist should ensure that specific rehabilitation of individual digital flexion is not overlooked.

Remedial games may be used to isolate specific movements. MCP and IP joint flexion of fingers and thumb may be encouraged through the use of tongs or an isolation splint with remedial games or

fine pin
or splir
to be m
The go
that is
digital fi
start wi
nails or
(Fig. 28
encourag
are pick
of the ha

A FEI
will also
helpful
mello, m
and pincl

Grip a
from gro
games, la
smaller p
the flexio
weighted
woodwork
cluded in
activities
making als

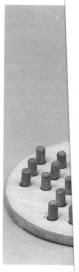

Fig. 28.10 Fle
flexion.

Handles on tools and aids can be modified to obtain the specific grip size required or to promote a particular joint movement. With imagination the therapist can find many and varied activities to maintain the person's interest and motivation in accordance with his individual needs.

Therapeutic putty may be used very effectively in warm-up exercises to promote grip strength and isolate specific joint motion. Suppliers produce a booklet illustrating its application.

Orthoses have a vital role to play in restoring flexion but can never replace specific treatment by the physiotherapist and occupational therapist. Although their styles and applications are too numerous to describe comprehensively here, some basic uses are illustrated in Figures 28.11–14.

Extension

Although the general tendency is for therapists to focus on flexion in the early stages of treatment, maximum extension is also vital for function. Extension is required to release objects, in manipulative work and for everyday hand dexterity. Given the anatomy of the extensor muscles, it is more difficult to isolate specific digit extension than specific digit flexion. Therapeutic putty exercises are useful here as warm-up activities (Fig. 28.15).

Remedial games played with extension tongs, bagatelle, pottery, baking, scissor work, making elastic band pictures and games where pieces are

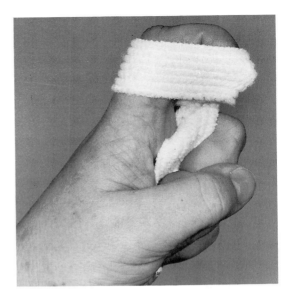

Fig. 28.12   Elastic bandage orthosis to promote IP flexion.

lifted against Velcro resistance can all promote active extension.

Passive extension can be achieved by using an extension board or printing press with the injured hand held beneath the other; a similar strategy can be used with sanding, polishing and sliding puzzles.

Orthoses, including serial night extension orthoses to stretch joint contractures or adhesions, may be used. Dynamic orthoses may be required to achieve improved specific joint extension.

Adduction and abduction

Many of the activities suggested above for use in promoting pronation and supination will also encourage adduction and abduction. FEPS discs will help the person spread the injured hand, as will elastic band games and pictures and remedial games which require pieces to be picked up between the fingers. The 'intrinsic frame' may also be used. This is a wooden frame with interwoven elastic bands which allows the person to exercise his intrinsic muscles. (The intrinsic frame may also be useful in improving flexion, extension and opposition.)

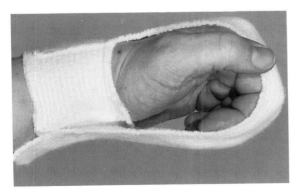

Fig. 28.11   Flexion orthosis. Elastic bandage with Velcro fastenings provides semi-dynamic pull to encourage MCP and PIP flexion.

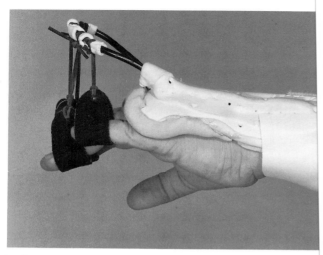

Fig. 28.13 Outrigger orthosis to provide resistance to active finger flexion

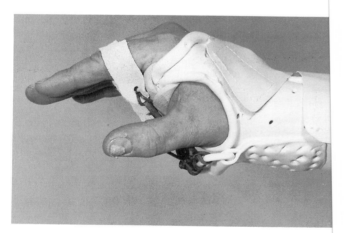

Fig. 28.14 Dynamic MCP flexion orthosis.

Opposition

While this movement is encouraged in the treatment already outlined, specific attention should be paid to its return to ensure that good thumb-to-fingertip pinch is realised. Serial C-bar orthoses may be required to stretch a contracted first web space. Any activity which facilitates pad-to-pad pinch can be used to gain opposition.

Manipulative skills

As range of motion improves the person will need

to be giv
pecially if
The perso
simulated

LOWER

The main
is its effect
ability to l
be given t
and distal

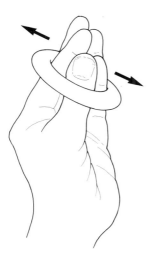

Fig. 28.15 Warm-up extension exercises using therapeutic putty.

easily lead to back pain and deformity, and to many other secondary problems.

Where multiple injuries have occurred, normal progress may be impeded by the involvement of an upper limb. This can make the use of walking aids a major problem, and may even necessitate confinement to a wheelchair in the early stages of rehabilitation.

When treating a person with lower limb injuries it is important to consider stability at the joints before increasing the range of movement. Stable joints are essential for weight-bearing and subsequent safe mobility.

Occupational therapists are involved in treating a wide range of problems, including fractures, soft tissue injuries and neurological conditions. Following thorough assessment, treatment will centre on improving stability and increasing the range of movement at the hip, knee and ankle joints, with attention to all the relevant muscle groups.

The hip joint

The hip joint facilitates an erect posture, the swing-through phase in walking, and sitting. The power and volume of the muscles around this joint reflect these functions. If this joint is unstable the resulting uneven gait will affect the person's balance and posture.

The therapist's role in treating hip injuries in the elderly is primarily concerned with independence in daily living. Helping the person to regain the ability to transfer from sitting to standing safely and confidently should be the foundation of treatment, as these individuals rarely require outpatient therapy once this has been achieved.

However, younger people may benefit from additional workshop activities. Initially, such activities are likely to be non-weightbearing. The main aims of treatment are to:

- maintain and increase the muscle bulk in the thigh
- maintain and improve the range of movement at the hip joint, with particular attention to flexion and abduction. These movements may be most affected due to surgical lateral incisions and disruption of musculature following trauma.

Whilst the joint is painful, stiff and non-weightbearing, effective early quadriceps muscle strengthening can be achieved by using the following:

- Reciprocal activities. The wood turning lathe, for example, can be used with the affected leg in a sling, and the unaffected leg treadling, causing reciprocal quadriceps contraction in the slung leg (Fig. 28.16).
- Remedial games with the person seated and moving lightweight draughts or noughts and crosses by elevating the affected leg. This type of activity also encourages abduction.
- A quadriceps switch (Fig. 28.17) with the person seated, the hip in flexion and knee in extension. The switch is activated by quadriceps contracture.

As the person progresses to weight-bearing, these exercises can be upgraded and new ones introduced. The electronic cycle, for example, can be used bilaterally to increase the range of movement at the hip and knee, thus promoting an even gait and increasing muscle bulk and strength (Fig. 28.18). The foot-powered lathe can be used with a Camden stool to enable a progression from reciprocal exercise to the use of both legs.

It is important to consider the individual's work

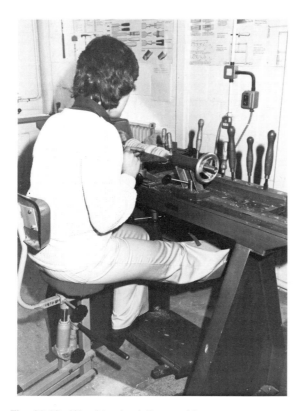

Fig. 28.16 Wood-turning lathe used to encourage reciprocal action of the quadriceps in the slung leg.

Fig. 28.17

The kne

The knee
lower limb
virtue of
mobility.
ment prob
knee, the
treatment

- to elimi
- to elimi
- to increa

The treatm
also help to

It is imp
between th
of extensio
straighten tl
ability to rai
knee straigh
tension can
knee in flexi
the joint ca

situation in the middle and late stages of rehabilitation and to plan his treatment accordingly. A maintenance fitter, for example, may need to crouch and to climb ladders in his job. Consequently, in the occupational therapy department these activities should be assessed and simulated using work benches of varied heights and by having the person work in confined spaces, e.g. under the bench. Job analysis and visits to the workplace can assist the therapist greatly with planning this part of the programme.

In the later stages of recovery, when the individual is fully mobile, some attention may also be given to leisure interests. Sports activities emphasising hip and knee mobilisation can be used as treatment media, the competitive element in team games encouraging maximum effort and participation.

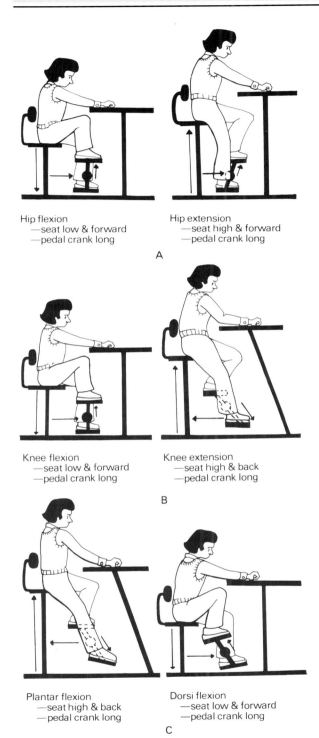

Hip flexion
—seat low & forward
—pedal crank long

Hip extension
—seat high & forward
—pedal crank long

A

Knee flexion
—seat low & forward
—pedal crank long

Knee extension
—seat high & back
—pedal crank long

B

Plantar flexion
—seat high & back
—pedal crank long

Dorsi flexion
—seat low & forward
—pedal crank long

C

Fig. 28.18 Use of the electronic cycle to increase (A) hip movement (B) knee movement (C) ankle movement.

usually the result of quadriceps muscle wastage and weakness.

The treatment approach for both extension problems is the same, and may include the use of a quadriceps switch, reciprocal work with cycle or lathe, and remedial floor games, such as noughts and crosses (see Fig. 10.11B). However, full weight-bearing should not be encouraged on the affected leg before extension lag is eliminated. In the later stages of recovery, activities performed while standing, such as printing, benchwork and cookery, can be included in the programme.

Activities to increase flexion include the use of the electronic cycle, potter's wheel and treadle fretsaw. In the later stages work- and leisure-related activities are also used. Previous equipment is upgraded by adjusting seat heights and working positions, and by using different materials, for example, thicker wood, which adds resistance to the saw blade can be used with the electronic cycle.

The ankle

All age groups sustain ankle injuries requiring rehabilitation, ranging from sprains and strains to complicated fractures. The occupational therapist is often involved very early in the treatment programme in more than one capacity.

Accurate assessment of range of movement may be aided by the use of an ankle measuring box. However, before assessment and treatment planning it is important for the therapist to recognise that the individual's expectations regarding the injury may be unrealistic. Ankle rehabilitation is often a lengthy process with no guarantee of complete recovery. Residual problems of prolonged swelling, loss of movement, pain and long-term weakness may be experienced.

Orthoses

The individual may require orthoses for several reasons, which are described below.

● Lightweight supports may be needed to improve stability in strains and sprains. For example, a stirrup-type orthosis allows plantar- and dorsiflexion whilst preventing inversion and eversion.

- Back slabs may be required to maintain a good position, offer protection, and reduce swelling following internal fixation or in an extensive soft tissue injury. Initially they are worn continually, except for gentle exercise, but in the later stage they fulfil the role of night support. In situations where dorsiflexion is impaired, back slabs can be successfully used serially. They are unsuitable for weight-bearing. Traditionally, removable back slabs were made of plaster of Paris, but lightweight, remouldable materials such as Fractomed have proven to be more comfortable, harder wearing and, in the long term, more cost effective.

- Below knee cast braces have been successfully used in the treatment of ligament and tendon disruptions. A range of ankle hinges are available to aid in the correct manufacture of this type of orthosis.

- Below knee zipped casts (e.g. Neofract casts) give protection during mobilisation and, later on, in weight-bearing, whilst allowing continuation of physiotherapy techniques such as hydrotherapy. These give more support than a back slab for fractures where surgical intervention is not appropriate. The foot can be easily immobilised in the required position.

- Various sports-type supports are readily available and often serve a useful purpose in providing support and pressure after removal of below knee plasters and in giving the person confidence as he returns to work and leisure activities. They may also be used successfully to support the ankle following a minor injury which does not require full immobilisation.

- Moulded insoles can be used effectively to alleviate a wide range of problems when the individual becomes weight-bearing. Their shock-absorbing properties help to relieve some discomfort. The incorporation of arch supports and lateral borders encourages full use of proprioception to help stability and promotes an even gait. Heel pads serve a similar purpose for Achilles tendon injury and fractured os calcis.

In the

In the
bearing
must be
individu
review,
to be as
recovery

Reme
directed
reeducat
ment. Ex
of rice o
moved th
whilst re
Other eq
clude the
either slu
treadle se
dorsiflexic
Space Inv
dorsiflexic

Group a
the treatm
valuable t
experience
tions and i

Foot pa
bines exer
introduced

As the i
the prograr
tional equip
particular e
of the tread
range of mc
should be
hobbies and
exercises us
progressing
are of bene
uneven surf
ground.

In the fina
be upgraded.
rotator, may
son. In addit

to work assessment and simulation. Gardening or building, particularly on rough ground, is valuable, whilst crouching and low benchwork can also be helpful for those who have to work in difficult positions or in confined spaces.

SPECIFIC INJURIES

BASIC PRINCIPLES OF FRACTURE MANAGEMENT

Diagnosis is usually through history of the injury, clinical examination and X-ray. Symptoms such as deformity, swelling, bruising, tenderness, localised pain, impaired function and crepitus may indicate a fracture. Fractures heal through callus formation but reduction and support may be necessary to facilitate healing. This may take the form of casting or orthoses to support the fracture site in a good anatomical position and protect other structures such as nerves or blood vessels which may be at risk if bone movement occurs. Fractures may also be immobilised by internal or external fixation.

Rehabilitation falls into two categories:

- maintenance of movement of all uninvolved joints to preserve their function throughout fracture healing
- mobilisation of joints proximal and distal to the fracture after union has occurred, together with restoration of maximum function of the whole limb.

The occupational therapist may be involved in applying orthotic techniques for immobilisation or rehabilitation. Practical activities are important in enhancing the healing process and preventing or reducing the risk of permanent disability. Since many fractures interfere with everyday function, attention must be given to independence in daily living activities throughout the rehabilitation programme, most particularly in the early stages. However, it is equally important that as treatment progresses and more active movement is encouraged, any superfluous compensatory equipment is gradually withdrawn.

Upper limb

Clavicle, scapula and upper part of the humerus

The precise nature of the occupational therapist's intervention will depend upon the mode of support or immobilisation for the fracture and the age and needs of the person. These fractures are usually treated by means of a sling to support the weight of the arm, but some may be reduced by means of a figure-of-eight bandage or an abduction orthosis. All will affect the use of the arm in daily living activities and the individual will need to learn techniques for maintaining independence while he has the use of only one hand. Following the removal of the support, gentle active exercise to promote shoulder movement should be encouraged and the use of any compensatory equipment for daily living activities reevaluated. Therapeutic activities chosen should be relevant to the needs of the individual and gradually upgraded to increase range of movement at the shoulder joint and gradual return of strength to the whole limb. The elderly may need practice with domestic duties to regain confidence in their bilaterality.

Shaft of the humerus

The type of fracture incurred at this site often depends on the nature of the accident. A fall on the outstretched hand frequently results in a spiral fracture, whereas direct force or a fall on the elbow is more likely to cause a transverse fracture. If the person is upright and the arm is supported in a sling the effects of gravity will usually reduce the fracture. A plaster U-slab is often applied to the upper arm to prevent angulation when the person is sitting or lying. After one week the initial oedema will usually have been reduced; the fracture can then be held more effectively in a functional brace. If the occupational therapist is involved at this stage she should encourage the individual to use the arm for light activities involving a pendular movement of the shoulder. Abduction of the arm, however, should be avoided. The support provided by the brace should be checked regularly as the oedema subsides.

After six weeks, it is usual for the brace to be

discarded and for active shoulder mobilising activities to be introduced. Some fractures are internally fixed by plating or intermedullary nailing and active shoulder mobilising may usually commence at three weeks post-fixation. It is not unusual for the radial nerve to be compromised by the fracture. A dynamic orthosis is usually supplied and wrist and hand function are encouraged alongside shoulder mobilisation. In some elderly people, particulary those with pathological fractures, bracing may be used for long-term support.

Forearm

There are a number of different fractures which may occur in the forearm but almost all are treated by reduction and immobilisation in a plaster support. Depending on the type and site of the injury, the plaster may enclose the wrist joint and forearm and, in the case of fractures to the upper part of the radius and/or ulnar the elbow joint may also be immobilised. Internal fixation with plates and screws may also be used, but plaster is usually still applied.

The support may be worn for a period of 4–8 weeks, depending on the injury and the method of fixation. In some cases the plaster may be replaced with a functional brace after two weeks.

The therapist's role is to maintain mobility in the non-immobilised joints of the whole limb, to reduce any oedema in the hand and to retain maximum independence in personal care activities. The therapist should also be alert for any signs of median or ulnar nerve involvement.

Following removal of the immobilisation, treatment aims to restore mobility to the elbow, forearm and wrist joints. Extension of the wrist is particularly important for grip, and restrictions in forearm pronation and supination will affect many everyday activities.

Scaphoid bone

Scaphoid fractures are relatively common and may take 6–8 months to heal. Fractures of the middle one third or waist of the scaphoid are notorious for delayed or non-union. If the fracture is displaced, open reduction with a screw is preferable; other-

wise, th
forearm
the prox
may be
moulded
flexion
support
and may
work sit
to the f
couraged

Metaca

Metacarp
result of
Reductio
through
support,
wiring o
angulatio
alignmen
finger de:

Rehabi
full mobil
individual
through
activities
oppositio

Lower I
Pelvis

Fracture o
through gi
and may t
factor ca
Undisplace
or traction
open redu
nal fixatio
of treatme
face a pro
rehabilitati

Neck of

Fractures o
commonly

of osteoporosis) and are often the result of a fall. In younger people, they can occur as a result of direct trauma. Whatever the person's age, treatment usually involves surgical intervention, varying in nature according to the level of the fracture. In some cases pins and plates are required, while in others a partial or total hip replacement is necessary. Given the advanced age of the majority of people suffering this type of fracture, early mobilisation is important in order to minimise the risk of secondary complications.

Shaft of femur

In order to fracture a normal shaft of femur a considerable force is required. This injury is probably most often sustained in road traffic accidents, and all age groups are at risk. As with fractures of the pelvis, the type of intervention used may be determined by the nature of any concurrent injuries. Treatment is now often surgical and the fracture is held with an intermedullary nail. However, if the fracture is comminuted or if shortening of the femur due to malalignment is likely, the individual may be treated initially with traction and then a cast brace may be fitted in order to commence mobilisation.

Lower end of the femur, the patella and the tibial plateau

Fractures at these sites affect the stability and mobility of the knee joint. They may be treated surgically by internal fixation or patellectomy or by conservative means. The knee joint can be immobilised in a plaster cylinder or may be treated by traction and cast bracing.

Rehabilitation initially aims to maintain or restore full active knee extension and stability. Once this is achieved, activities are introduced to promote knee mobility and build up adequate strength in the whole limb for full weight-bearing and a return to work and life activities.

Shaft of tibia and fibula

Tibial and fibular fractures are commonly caused by road traffic and sporting accidents. They are treated in a variety of ways, depending on their position and severity. For undisplaced or easily reduced simple fractures a full-leg plaster of Paris cast may be used. For displaced, comminuted or compound fractures internal fixation with pins and plates or an intermedullary nail may be necessary.

Alternatively, an external fixator may be applied. This allows easy access to open wounds and skin grafts in order for dressings to be changed. External fixation has the added advantage of allowing adjustment of alignment at the fracture site, thus helping to prevent shortening.

Tibial fractures are notorious for having a long healing period and therefore early mobilisation is encouraged where possible. A Sarmiento-type cast brace may be applied after the external fixator or plaster has been removed. This allows knee and ankle movement while the fracture site remains protected.

Ankle, talus and calcaneum

Fractures at these sites may be treated conservatively in a plaster cylinder or by internal fixation with wires, screws and plates. Rehabilitation aims to promote stability of the ankle joint, to extend the range of active plantar- and dorsiflexion for normal gait and to increase standing tolerance and the ability to walk over uneven surfaces. Particular activities may be necessary to increase tolerance of specific postures or actions for work or leisure pursuits. For example, the plumber or engineer who works in a restricted environment may require particular strengthening of the ankle and forefoot to tolerate prolonged periods working in a squatting position.

TENDON INJURIES

Upper limb

Tendon injuries occur most frequently in the hand or lower forearm. Often only one or two digits will be affected, but occasionally damage is widely spread, with tendon injuries to all digits or at several levels. Most are the result of accidents, but repairs to ruptured tendons (often associated with rheumatoid arthritis) can be considered in this group. A sound basic knowledge of the anatomy of the flexor and extensor system is essential in assessing and treating a person with these injuries.

There are many different methods of mobilising a tendon repair. Early active motion may be appropriate in some cases, whereas only passive movements may initially be indicated in others. Some injuries should be totally immobilised for several weeks. Surgeon and therapist together should discuss the pros and cons of each method and decide on a regime for the individual concerned. All treatment protocols aim to restore full function to the injured tendon by:

- reducing adhesions
- preventing joint stiffness/contracture
- restoring tendon glide.

Treatment should be targeted on the injured flexor or extensor tendon in order to restore the 'pull through'. The use of an isolation orthosis with remedial games such as solitaire (Fig. 28.19), or with remedial activities such as typesetting, will enable the person to use the injured tendon to its full potential. Resistance to activities should be gradually increased as the tendon strengthens, timing being dependent on the chosen treatment regime.

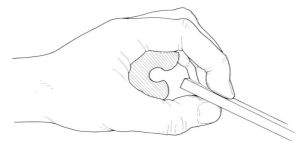

Fig. 28.19 Solitaire using an isolation orthosis to achieve specific IP joint flexion.

Flexor tendon injuries

People who have had flexor tendon repairs are generally seen one to three days post-operatively in order to remove bulky dressings so that the exercise programme can commence. They are usually fitted with a thermoplastic orthosis. The wrist and hand are held in flexion so that the flexor

Fig. 28.20

system is
the sutur
is 30° of
with IP j
of MCP a
their coll
prevents
prolonged
relaxed. (
and MCI
position i

Kleiner
be added
position c
on the el
full active
the band s
ive tensior
is flexion,
joint contr
achieved r

Whatev
therapist v
of exercise
affected jc
the regime
to periodi
achieved.

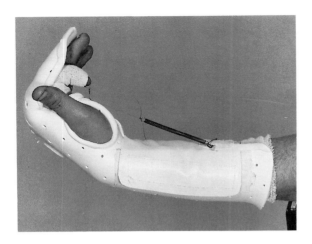

Fig. 28.21 Kleinert traction.

Extensor tendon injuries

Rehabilitation following extensor tendon injuries tends to be less complex than that involving the flexor system. The hand is generally supported in an extended position according to the site of injury and is then mobilised to regain active extension and flexion at the appropriate time. Extension lag (a deficit between passive and active extension) is most commonly caused by the tendon healing in slight attenuation. Night orthoses in full extension and treatment activities designed to encourage full active extension will help to eliminate lag.

A dynamic extension orthosis may be used at any stage in order to allow active flexion against the elastic band traction, while the extensor system is rested and allowed to heal in a satisfactory position. This is called reversed Kleinert traction.

Lower limb

The Achilles tendon is the most frequently injured tendon in the leg. It may be strained or partially or wholly torn. In all cases the ankle should be rested with the foot plantar-flexed and the tendon in its relaxed position. A heel raise pad will achieve this for a minor injury, whereas a long leg cast may be required for a partial rupture. In cases where the tendon is completely ruptured, surgical repair is usually carried out, after which the affected leg is placed in a plaster of Paris cast.

Occupational therapy treatment after removal of the cast involves gently exercising the ankle to increase mobility of the joint (most particularly dorsiflexion) and to increase calf muscle bulk.

Treatment has to be very carefully upgraded in order not to cause further damage to the tendon. Initially, it may be necessary for the individual to have a heel raise on the shoe but this can be reduced as improvement occurs. It may also be necessary to restrict the person to partial weight-bearing for a short time.

Tenolysis

If a person achieves a good passive range following tendon repair, but adhesions limit active movement, the surgeon may consider a tenolysis of the tendon 4 to 6 months post-operatively, once collagen has matured. Intensive rehabilitation is needed to obtain maximum benefit after this procedure.

As it is important for exercises to start as soon as possible following surgery, the person needs to be well motivated to work hard and to master the pain. Initially, the tendon is exercised very gently through the full flexion and extension range with minimal resistance. Treatment concentrates on the tenolysed tendon's movement. TENS may be of value in relieving pain in the crucial early stages.

Improvement in active motion tends to be achieved in the first two or three weeks. Subsequent rehabilitation is aimed at maintaining and improving the quality (power and function) of this range of movement.

Tendon transfers

If a tendon is irreparably damaged, its motor unit has been paralysed or its primary repair has failed, a tendon transfer may be considered. The tendon chosen for the transfer is divided distally, rerouted to produce its new function and sutured to the damaged distal tendon stump. The surgery may be preceded by an initial operation in which a Silastic rod is implanted for several months in the position of the intended transfer, making a mature adhesion-free bed for the new tendon. Orthotic and rehabilitative strategies are similar to those used in the case of repairs, but include an emphasis on reeducation of the transfer to its 'new job'. Constant practice and functional use will help the brain to integrate the tendon's new role into everyday activity.

LIGAMENT INJURIES

Ligament injuries will require more lengthy immobilisation than tendon injuries if joint stability is to be regained. Some mobility may have to be sacrificed for the sake of achieving a stable joint. The ligaments surrounding a joint are an integral part of the joint capsule and injuries to them will be considered in this section.

Upper limb

The collateral ligaments of the MCP joint of the thumb and the PIP joints of the fingers are those most often damaged. Primary treatment may be conservative or surgical, depending on the severity of the problem, and is followed by the use of orthoses to protect the joint from lateral movement for several weeks (Fig. 28.22). An orthosis which allows some movement in acceptable directions will help to reduce potential joint stiffness (Fig. 28.23).

The lengthy immobilisation necessary to achieve a stable and therefore functional digit may result in joint stiffness. Passive stretching of the joint is not usually recommended until later stages of treatment so that the healing ligament is not jeopardised. Likewise, care must be taken at all stages in treatment not to use an activity which will stress an injured ligament by stretching it. Treatment should aim to restore full active range of move-

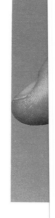

Fig. 28.2
allows 75
stability.

ment to
some re

Injur
quently
which t
the joi
protecti
proxima
that sho
mal PIP
(DIP) jo

It is r
in assoc
ments.
instance
side to l

Froze
has its
shoulder
unaware
painful a
and rhy
further i

Lower

Tears of
the knee
or road

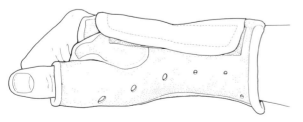

Fig. 28.22 Orthosis to protect MCP joint ligaments of thumb.

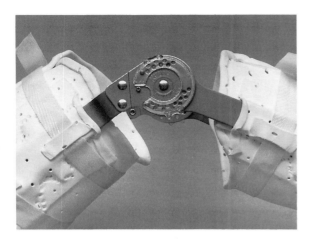

Fig. 28.24 Cast brace with restricted hinges.

severity of the tear, they may be treated conservatively or surgically repaired with or without the use of Dacron, carbon or autogenous fibres. Initially, a plaster of Paris cast is applied with the knee held in 30° flexion. The knee may be treated in a cast brace with restricted hinges defining the amount of motion allowed and protecting the injured ligament (Fig. 28.24). For example, a tear of the anterior cruciate may be treated in a cast brace allowing a 30°–60° range of flexion.

The surgeon will advise when the person can transfer from the cast to a brace adapted to the appropriate range, allowing maximum movement while protecting the healing ligament. This can be modified to allow a progressively wider range of movement as recovery occurs.

Initially, the person may be treated whilst still wearing the brace. Exercises can be devised which use the range of movement available and build up the leg muscles. It is important to monitor exercise very carefully after brace removal in order that the person does not over-stretch the repaired ligament. As stability improves at the knee, more vigorous activities can be introduced to achieve a full range of movement and increase quadriceps muscle bulk.

CRUSH INJURIES

These can be sustained to a single digit or the whole of a limb. Even where there is no fracture, rupture of tendons or injury to neurovascular structures, soft tissue damage will lead to gross oedema and considerable pain. Scar tissue will form, with the consequent danger of adhesions causing profound limitation of movement.

It is sometimes tempting to regard a person with no specific diagnosis beyond a soft tissue crush injury as poorly motivated when he presents with a painful, stiff hand and fails to make a swift response to rehabilitation. In fact, such injuries often take more hard work and commitment on the part of the individual and therapist than those with a specific diagnosis or in which surgical intervention is required. Damage to soft tissues is frequently widespread, involving all systems. The person will need encouragement and support, especially in the early stages when progress is slow and hard-won and pain rules the tolerance to activity.

In major crush injuries fractures, amputations and severe damage to tendon and neurovascular systems may occur. There may be skin and muscle loss. A person involved in such a mutilating accident will be shocked and may well go through a bereavement reaction. While surgeons are able to revascularise and reconstruct a severely damaged digit or limb, the decision to do so must be balanced against the likely functional outcome and the person's own agenda and priorities.

Compartment syndrome may occur following a severe crush injury, particularly in the lower limb. To relieve the pressure in the muscle compartments a fasciotomy is performed. Skin grafting is usually necessary. The therapist is involved from the early stages in applying orthoses, facilitating sensory adaptation, increasing range of movement and muscle bulk and aiding mobilisation. Provision of pressure garments may be particularly valuable in some cases.

The psychological 'backlash' of losing part or all of a limb and any disfiguring scarring is as vital a symptom for treatment as physical dysfunction. Both the individual and his relatives will need care, support and a listening ear if they are to adjust well to a new body image and its implications. It is important to remember that people's reactions and ability to cope vary greatly and while one person may hide a whole hand from view, having lost only a fingertip, another may lose a whole hand or live with terrible scarring and cope amazingly well, both functionally and emotionally.

Early orthoses are aimed at resting the injured part in a good position for recovery. Shoulder and elbow injuries are rested with the forearm supported in a sling, while those to the wrist or hand are immobilised in the 'safe' position with collateral ligaments out to length to reduce the risk of joint contractures.

The ankle is rested in a neutral position to prevent foot drop. The knee is held in 5° of flexion, allowing normal swing-through gait. In many cases oedema will already have caused poor positioning and serial orthoses may be necessary to reach the optimum position for recovery.

If surgery has been performed the timing of mobilisation will be an individual decision made by the surgeon in discussion with the therapist. It will be based in part on the quality of the repair, especially where microvascular surgery has been employed.

In any crush injury the first aim is to reduce oedema and encourage active movement. The two are inextricably linked: as oedema is reduced, active movement is facilitated; as range of motion improves, oedema is pumped out.

Assessment of daily living skills and provision of help as necessary is particularly appropriate for people who have suffered severe crush injuries which will incapacitate them for some time. The benefits of assistive equipment should be carefully weighed against the need to encourage bilaterality and controlled use of the injured part. The therapist should bear in mind that early facilitation of a degree of independence can be a considerable boost to the injured person's confidence.

REFLEX SYMPATHETIC DYSTROPHY (RSD)

This is an umbrella term used to group together a number of conditions, including Sudeck's atrophy and shoulder-hand syndrome. It is characterised by pain disproportionate to the original injury and has three intrinsic stages:

- *Acute phase* (first 3 months). Disabling,

vicious circle of pain and disuse. Orthoses to improve passive and active ranges of movement and maintain a good resting position have an important role, but should not be allowed to substitute for hard work by the person and his therapist.

TENOSYNOVITIS AND REPETITIVE STRAIN INJURIES (RSI)

Tenosynovitis is simply the inflammation of a tendon. This may occur following an injury but is often caused by repeated movements which cumulatively lead to damage to a particular tendon or group of tendons.

For simple cases, rest of the aggravated tendons in an orthosis (positioned with tendons in a neutral or relaxed position) for several weeks followed by gradual return to use of the affected part works well. There is, however, a tendency toward recurrence of the problem.

Tenosynovitis is most often seen in the abductor pollicis longus and extensor pollicis brevis tendons (De Quervain's syndrome), in the flexor or extensor groups at the wrist, at the common extensor origin at the elbow (tennis elbow) or in the Achilles tendon.

In acute cases the limb is supported with the affected tendons in a resting position. A steroid infiltration to the affected area is often of benefit. Mobilisation should be graduated, taking care not to aggravate the recovering tendons and cause a relapse.

The medico-legal debate about the diagnosis of RSI continues to rage. Many believe it to be a fashionable disease with psychological origins, seen mainly among bored or disadvantaged workers.

RSI sufferers do not necessarily present with inflammation or crepitus. Their main symptom is pain and weakness of grip. A period of rest followed by graded rehabilitation is sometimes of benefit. Occasionally, assessment of the person's work environment will reveal poor ergonomic design (e.g. with regard to tools, posture, temperature or working heights) that could be modified to relieve the problem.

Whether or not there is a sound pathological basis for a diagnosis of RSI, those who suffer from it can become substantially disabled. Sensitive treatment and counselling may enable people with this diagnosis to come to terms with their discomfort and expand their functional horizon.

CONCLUSION

When treating limb trauma the occupational therapist predominantly uses a biomechanical approach to overcome physical impairments. However, she should not lose sight of the needs and wishes of the individual and the use of the limb in the fuller context of living. The objective of rehabilitation is to minimise the long-term effects of the injury and to promote maximum functional activity along with adjustment to any residual dysfunction. In the upper limb, mobility and dexterity are particularly important for everyday tasks, while in the lower limb strength and stability are vital for weight-bearing and ambulation.

Any trauma will have psychological implications for the individual and his close relatives and these should be respected and addressed to help the person to attain a realistic and positive approach to therapy. Activities should be appropriate to the needs and wishes of the individual and provide specific anatomical exercise for the injured part and the limb as a whole. As recovery occurs, regular assessment and evaluation of the limb will enable the individual and the therapist to measure change and adjust activities accordingly. In the later stages of treatment, activities should aim to promote return to role duties and leisure pursuits. For many people, physical recovery from a limb injury may be almost total. Where this is not possible, the therapist should help the person to attain his maximum functional potential and to adjust to any residual deficit.

FURTHER READING

Adams J C, Hamblen D L 1990 Outline of orthopaedics, 11th edn. Churchill Livingstone, Edinburgh

Burke F D, McGrouther D A, Smith P J 1990 Principles of hand surgery. Churchill Livingstone, Edinburgh

Caillet R 1976 Neck and arm pain. F A Davis, Philadelphia

Caillet R 1976 Shoulder pain. F A Davis, Philadelphia

Caillet R 1982 Hand pain and impairment. F A Davis, Philadelphia

Caillet R 1985 Knee pain and disability, F A Davis, Philadelphia

Conolly W B, Kilgore E S 1979 Hand injuries and infections. Edward Arnold, London

Dandy D J 1989 Essential orthopaedics and trauma. Churchill Livingstone, Edinburgh

Hunter J M, Schneider L E, Mackin E J, Callahan A D 1984 Rehabilitation of the hand. Mosby, St. Louis

Lamb D W, Hooper G 1984 Hand conditions. Colour aids series. Churchill Livingstone, Edinburgh

Lister G
 Churc
Macnico
 hand.
Macnico
 Surge
 proble
McRae
 Churc
Putz-An
 manu
 Taylo
Salter M
 Churc
Wynn F
 Butte

29

Osteoarthritis

Jane James

INTRODUCTION

Osteoarthritis affects the majority of people by the age of 55. It is the most common form of arthritis, affecting men and women equally, except for primary generalised osteoarthritis, which is ten times more common in women. For some people, osteoarthritis is a severely disabling condition, causing considerable functional impairment; for others, it never reaches a stage where treatment is required.

Osteoarthritis is a degenerative disease which causes the normally smooth articular surface of the joints to become damaged. This is turn restricts the range of movement of the joints and causes pain and stiffness. Osteoarthritis can affect any joint. However, the large weight-bearing joints in the hips, knees and spine are particularly at risk. Primary generalised osteoarthritis most commonly affects the first carpometacarpal and metatarsophalangeal joints.

Osteoarthritis cannot be cured but the restrictions it causes can be minimised or reduced in various ways to enable the person to continue living an independent and fulfilling life and to cope emotionally with any remaining impairment. Surgical intervention is becoming more effective as new techniques evolve; however, people treated surgically require further rehabilitation to ensure maximum potential is reached. The occupational therapist, along with other members of the primary health care team, has a vital part to play in encouraging people to reach their goals for independence. Her role includes advising and counselling people just prior to surgery and she may often be involved in treating, advising and counselling people receiving conservative management. An occupational therapist working at a person's own home can provide useful advice on joint protection, safer or easier methods of carrying out some household tasks and can be a useful source of information. As a member of a team the occupational therapist should always be aware of the other professionals' roles and should work in cooperation with her colleagues for the benefit of the person and his carer(s).

The first section of this chapter describes the clinical features of osteoarthritis — its signs, symptoms, pathology and causes. Next, the two main areas of treatment are outlined, namely, conservative management and surgical intervention. The role of the occupational therapist in each of these areas is then described, beginning with areas in which the therapist can offer advice and assistance to the person in a programme of conservative management: safety at home, indoor and outdoor mobility, equipment and techniques for daily living activities, and protection of the affected joints. Next, the therapist's role in facilitating rehabilitation following surgery is discussed. Finally, a typical therapeutic programme that might be applied to someone who has undergone a hip replacement is outlined, demonstrating in practical terms the vital role that the occupational therapist has to play in the rehabilitative process.

HOW DOES OSTEOARTHRITIS AFFECT A PERSON?

CLINICAL FEATURES

Osteoarthritis usually begins in one joint. Onset is gradual, taking place over months and years, unless the condition is caused by trauma, in which case onset may be fairly rapid.

Phys

- Insta
  ostec
  arthr
  loss (
  also t
  tissue
- Bony
  the os
- Tende
- Increa:
  in the
- Crepitu

Sympto

- Pain wit
  graduall
  with trai
  worst at
  night.
- Stiffness
  stiffness i
  greater da
  movemen
  results in
  morning; t
  gentle mov
  getting-up
- Deformity,
  the knees o
  leg caused |
- Referred pa
  involvement
  sciatic pain
  affected the
  shoulder or ;
  nerves as the
  muscle tensio

Typical diag

Some people wi
their general pra
referred to a hosp
diagnostic investig

- Radiological ex:

of joint space. There may also be sclerosis of the underlying bone, subchondral cysts, osteophytes and irregularity of the joint surfaces.

- The synovial fluid appears clear yellow and non-inflammatory, although some debris may be present.
- Laboratory tests are normal, and blood tests are normal unless the osteoarthritis is due to a biochemical condition such as gout or a rheumatic disease such as rheumatoid arthritis.

Clinical examination includes investigation not only of the apparently affected joint but of the whole person, to establish limitations of movement, pain level and loss of power of the limb as well as the effect of the condition on the individual's work, social, emotional and domestic life.

Pathology of osteoarthritis

As previously mentioned, any joint may be affected by osteoarthritis, although the weight-bearing joints of the lower limbs and spine are most commonly involved. The articular surface becomes rough and the cartilage in the affected area degenerates, particularly at the points of greatest pressure, eventually flaking away to expose the underlying subchondral bone. This then becomes thickened, dense and eburnated (polished), whilst at the margins of the joint buttressing osteophytes are formed. Where the bone is denuded, synovial fluid may enter and form cysts within the bone.

The lubrication mechanism of the joint is affected and it may become dry and creaky, even to the extent of the individual being able to hear the joint moving and creaking (crepitus).

The muscles close to an affected joint may spasm as a protection mechanism to prevent painful movement. They may waste if a protective posture in an unusual position is habitually adopted by the person as, for instance, when the hip is held slightly flexed with some internal rotation and adduction.

CAUSES OF OSTEOARTHRITIS

Osteoarthritis is a degenerative disease which may be primary or secondary in cause.

Primary osteoarthritis occurs in joints for no known reason, although there may be some familial tendency.

Secondary osteoarthritis may develop in response to a number of different factors.

For the person affected, the implications of primary and secondary osteoarthritis are identical and the therapist will not usually need to differentiate between the two types. The main causal factors may be congenital or acquired.

Congenital causes

If dislocation of the hip was undetected at birth or some other bony deformity was present the resulting abnormal stress on the joints could cause osteoarthritis to develop in later life.

Acquired causes

- other conditions leaving a damaged joint surface, for example Perthes' disease of the hip, haemophilia, avascular necrosis
- trauma, such as fractures where there has been subsequent malalignment of the joint, or where the joint itself was involved and damaged. Additionally, it may result from loose fragments of bone or cartilage remaining within the joint
- repeated trauma, particularly related to certain occupational diseases. This may affect the upper limbs, lower limbs, or spine.
- septic or other arthritis where the articular cartilage is destroyed
- obesity over a prolonged period, which causes extra wear and tear on the weight-bearing joints, particularly the hip and knee.

WHAT CAN BE DONE FOR PEOPLE WITH OSTEOARTHRITIS?

Osteoarthritis cannot be cured, but considerable

improvement can usually be gained through treatment. Benefits of treatment include the following:

- Pain may be reduced or eliminated
- Range of movement can be extended
- Mobility can be improved
- Personal independence can be enhanced
- Work prospects can be improved
- Social and leisure activities can be enjoyed again
- Further deterioration may be prevented or slowed and general quality of life can be vastly improved.

Treatment is usually either conservative or surgical in nature. Rehabilitative techniques are important in both types of treatment and, as always, the active involvement of the person and his carer is essential. Results will almost always be improved when the person has had the opportunity to discuss his treatment and has been given clear answers to his questions. Good communication will help the person to feel more confident in both the team as a whole and in the individuals carrying out the treatment. The person will also have an understanding of the importance of his own contribution and will be better motivated and less anxious about the process.

CONSERVATIVE TREATMENT

Included in the conservative treatment of osteoarthritis are:

- rest or a moderation of activity
- drug therapy for relieving pain, including a local injection of steroids where necessary
- remedial therapy by the various team members, including provision of equipment such as walking aids
- diet and exercise regimens to improve general level of health
- joint protection advice and possibly orthoses for support
- manipulation under anaesthetic.

It is useful to remember that these techniques will not influence the damage already caused by the osteoarthritis. However, they may make life for the individual and his carer much more

bearable
is encou
a reduc
result. 1
pain and
ment. T
activities
healthier
and the
of impro
chronic (
pain.

SURGI

Surgical
where os
physical a
is affecte
with con
ceased to
relief.

A num
developec
While the
variable,
larly succ
different
surgeons.

Main su

*Joint ar
joint*

This usua
with artifi
joints for
many diff
over 100 f
may be re
occupation
joints of tl
metacarpa
replaced. J
elbow and
ankle join
replaced.

Replacement techniques do not always involve inserting a complete joint. In the hip the femoral head and the acetabulum may be smoothed and a highly polished cup inserted into the acetabulum to provide a new joint lining which will allow free movement of the femoral head and which will not deteriorate and become rough or restricting. Partial replacement may also be the chosen technique for the patella or for the carpal bones.

Replacement joints may be made of metal, polythene, special ceramic material or a combination of these. Joints may be constructed of a single element or may be made up of different sections which can be selected and fitted by the surgeon according to the individual's requirements.

Joints may be fixed using special cement or screws and plates, or by ensuring a very precise push-fit of the prosthesis which is then packed closely with pieces of bone to fit the joint. The natural process of ossification then assists the formation of new bone to hold the prosthesis in place.

In very occasional cases a new joint may be created by excising the head and neck of the femur and the upper half of the wall of the acetabulum and replacing these with a mass of soft tissue such as the gluteus medius muscle. This then acts as a cushion between the remaining bones and is known as a 'Girdlestone pseudarthrosis'.

Osteotomy or the cutting of bone

This technique is used to correct deformity, relieve pain and improve stability of the joint. An osteotomy may be performed at the hip if there is considerable shortening of the limb (together with pain and a lack of stability of the joint) causing difficulties of mobility. The femur is divided between the greater and lesser trochanter and the shaft is displaced to correct the deformity. The bones are then fixed, usually by screws and plates. Further natural healing processes usually continue the repair, causing the articular cartilage to thicken. Osteotomy of the neck of the scapula may reduce the effect of osteoarthritis in the shoulder.

Arthrodesis or permanent fusion of the joint

This may be the option chosen if complete relief from pain is desired, or if a prosthesis cannot be inserted. The joint is fused in a position which is appropriate for the particular limb involved and which will accommodate the requirements of the person in everyday life. There is no rigid ruling for positioning as mobility of other joints and the general age and fitness of the person will be taken into consideration. Arthrodesis of a single joint which is particularly painful can cause surprisingly little disability and can be easily adapted to.

Complications following surgery may include deep vein thrombosis, infection of the wound and loosening of the new joint or the fixings used to fuse the bone. If the new joint was fixed in cement it may be necessary either to replace it or to remove it and leave a pseudoarthrosis. Dislocation of a joint may occur and must be guarded against; the person must realise the importance of being aware of the possibility and needs to have a clear understanding of the movements which might cause problems; for example, adduction, internal rotation and flexion of the hip beyond 90° are contraindicated in the first few weeks following hip replacement.

WHAT ROLE DOES THE OCCUPATIONAL THERAPIST PLAY?

Following surgery or in conservative management the general aim of rehabilitation should be the person's return to an improved home and daily life, with the highest level of independence and confidence possible within his capability. The occupational therapist is part of the team who will be working with the person and his carer both initially in the hospital and then possibly at home to achieve satisfactory rehabilitation. Sometimes occupational therapists work across these two areas so they can follow the individual through the process, but frequently the hospital therapist needs to liaise with her community colleague to assure continuity in the later stages. It is important for the stages of treatment to flow smoothly, and cooperative working procedures for the occupational therapists employed in different areas are essential if duplication and omissions are to be avoided.

Whether the person is to take part in a conservative programme of treatment or is to undergo surgery, the occupational therapy process of assessment, planning, implementation and evaluation will be exactly the same. The process should be recorded and may often be discussed with the person and his carer. In fact, legislative provision ensures the right of individuals to view their local authority records (Access to Personal Files Act 1987). As a result of this legislation some community occupational therapists provide copies of parts of their records for the person and have found that many people appreciate this improved knowledge. The occupational therapist should consider the individual person and his carer and should plan a balanced programme of intervention which recognises the person's particular circumstances, provides a challenge, and sets goals which are both realistic and relevant to the person.

The aims of intervention should be:

- to improve mobility and strength of the joints
- to reduce pain
- to maximise independence in everyday life (work, domestic, social, emotional)
- to educate the person and his carer and ensure they have a good understanding of the condition in order to further assist in the achievement of the above aims.

GENERAL PRINCIPLES OF CONSERVATIVE INTERVENTION

It has already been noted that osteoarthritis can have very different effects on people. Consequently, the part played by the occupational therapist will vary according to the severity of each individual's impairment. When daily problems are relatively simple she may concentrate on giving advice, possibly recommending simple pieces of equipment (such as a long-handled shoe horn, Fig. 29.1) to assist in daily living activities. The therapist should consider all aspects of the

Fig. 29.1
flexing of

person's
his prop
problems
his cond
many oth
count in
intervent

The oc
treatment
a team, e
It is imp
sistent ad
the therap
on peopl
tations a
proach. S
relationsh
feel free
Elderly p
ask for ad
then are
hardship
they anti
quently n
elderly pe

range following assessment; during this time the person and his perhaps equally elderly carer or spouse is put under extra pressure because of the urgency of the help needed.

It is generally accepted that full involvement of the person and his carer during the assessment, planning, and implementation stages of the treatment programme will make progress much easier for everyone. The following sections describe areas in which the therapist can offer advice and, with the cooperation of the person and his carer, introduce adaptations to the person's environment that will enhance his quality of life.

Safety in the home

Loose rugs, worn carpets and slippery floor surfaces can be changed or eliminated to minimise the hazards they present. Stair rails and banisters should be securely fixed to ensure people can rely safely on them. The rails should provide a comfortable grip (see Fig. 29.2). A 'mop-stick' rail is preferred, fixed with brackets which allow the hand to pass easily along the rail without hitting the wall or the fixings. The height of the rail should either match an existing rail or banister or should be measured to suit the individual. Build-

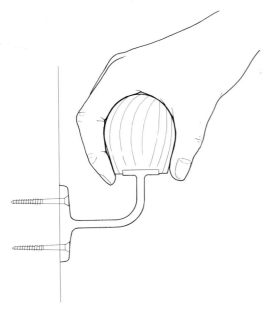

Fig. 29.2 Mop-stick rail.

ing regulations recommend a minimum height of 840 mm but this may be a little high for a smaller person, so the therapist should discuss the matter with the person and his carer and agree on a suitable height. It will always be important for the therapist to adopt a sensitive approach to suggesting changes to a person's own home; a careful and clear explanation of the reasons for the proposed changes will usually result in agreement.

Bathrooms and kitchens can be areas of risk particularly when floors are wet and slippery. However, the dangers can be reduced if care is taken when walking and if loose mats are removed or secured. Non-slip tiles or vinyl with a special non-slip surface may be recommended. Waterproof carpeting may prove a safe and warm alternative.

Safe lifting techniques are important in protecting both the affected joints from further strain and any unaffected joints from damage.

Mobility — indoor and outdoor

The physiotherapist may have recommended a walking aid and given instruction on usage and posture. In her own work with the person, the occupational therapist should ensure that the physiotherapist's recommendations are adhered to. Much of the advice that the person will receive about mobility is linked to practical and safety aspects. The occupational therapist should try to impress upon him the need for care when walking outside, particularly in wet weather. If pain is experienced the person may already be taking great care to protect the affected joint. Different surfaces may become slippery when wet and the gradient may add to the difficulty, particularly when a walking aid is used. The ferrule(s) on a walking aid should be in good condition to ensure the safest support. The occupational therapist should point this out to the disabled person and his carer, emphasising the importance of checking ferrules regularly and replacing them when necessary.

Access to the home should be assessed and if possible a home visit made with the person and his carer present. Steep steps can sometimes be made more easily negotiable by the addition of a half-

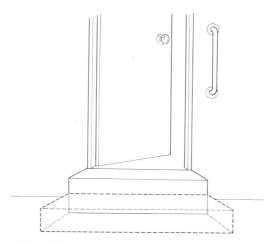

Fig. 29.3 Half-step and grab rail at entrance.

step (Fig. 29.3). This may be constructed of wood, firmly fixed to the existing step and covered with a safe non-slip surface, or may be permanently made out of concrete or using firmly fixed slabs. A grab handled fixed near the door (Fig. 29.3) may also be of assistance.

Problems associated with a longer flight of steps may be more difficult to overcome but properties may have an alternative access not usually used by the person or there may be a way to reroute the usual access. Rails beside the steps can assist but should be constructed of suitable material to withstand weather and should be measured to a convenient height for the person.

Inside the home mobility may be more difficult if the property has internal steps (apart from the stairs). Strategically placed grab rails can be helpful but the occupational therapist should discuss these carefully and should avoid making homes look like hedgehogs sprouting rails at every opportunity. Too much furniture can create problems of space and hinder mobility with a walking aid. Large heavy objects can form good hand-holds for the person walking without equipment. Some doorways may be exceptionally narrow, which can make it difficult to pass through them with a walking frame; bathroom and toilet doors are the most common examples of this problem. The occupational therapist may need to consider an adaptation to widen the doorway or it may be feasible to provide a narrower walking frame.

The
usually
home
vices
departr
or a co
son wi
work t
alterati
authori
occupat
the cri
usually
and su
occupat

Many
provisic
These
mittee
mendat
cupatio
make a
ance of
of disab
This ca
about w
or desir
this pro

Equip

The oc
recomm
strain o
alternati
may be
handled
and elast
and pain
avoid fle
person sh
angles (F
height fo
ing the se
importan
fixed to
using a

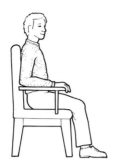

Fig. 29.4 Chairs should be firm and high enough for easy rising.

creasing the length of the legs because this will reduce the chair's back length and, in an armchair, can leave the person with little arm support for getting up out of the chair.

Bathing

This can be difficult whether the osteoarthritis affects the upper or the lower limbs, so equipment such as a correctly fitted bath board, bath seat and non-slip mat can, with proper instruction for use, be considered (Fig. 29.5). The therapist should ensure that any plastic-type bath is strong enough to support such equipment.

If the person has a shower fitted over the bath, the bath board can be used to sit upon as a safer alternative to standing, (see Fig. 29.6); if the

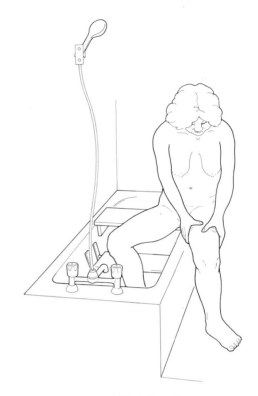

Fig. 29.5 Typical use of bath board.

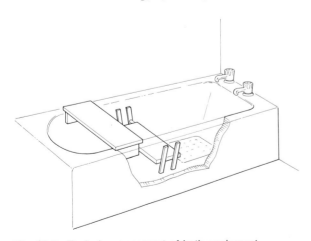

Fig. 29.6 Typical arrangement of bath equipment (cut-away bath panel for illustrative purposes only).

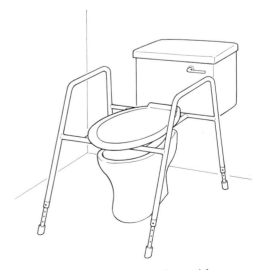

Fig. 29.7 Toilet with combined raise and frame.

shower is a separate cubicle the therapist may suggest a seat. This may be a free-standing chair or stool (providing the shower base is strong enough to withstand the pressure from the legs) or may be a wall-mounted seat.

Using the toilet

This poses difficulty if the toilet is low but various means can be taken to raise the seat height and provide assistance in rising. An example of a combined raised toilet seat with rails is shown in Figure 29.7. This can be free-standing or fixed to the floor. A separate seat raise can be provided and should be fitted to the toilet securely. A grab rail or frame might also be required.

Dressing

The therapist may advise the person to be seated at a comfortable height whilst dressing and to make use of long-handled equipment and easy fastenings.

Other equipment

For the person with osteoarthritis in the lower limbs, standing to carry out kitchen tasks may be painful; provision of a high perching stool (Fig. 29.8) can help ease pain and reduce dependency on carers.

More complex equipment may be relevant for those people with greater impairment, particularly if surgical treatment is not possible or has not succeeded. Hoists can greatly assist transfer of a wheelchair-bound person and help to relieve his carer (see p. 259). Special beds can greatly assist in easing the pain caused through immobility, by enabling the person to change his own position during the night. Such beds can also contribute towards reducing any swelling by elevating the legs, and may assist nursing care by raising the person's height. As beds tend to be fairly expensive items, and since the features offered in different models vary, careful choice should be made before purchase.

Fig. 29.8

Diet a

As men
will put
possibly
normal
weight l
may be
the dieti
to plan r
ming. Us
exercise
or centr
therapist
activities
range of
muscles b

Joint p

The pers
and infor
know wh
pational t
resting or

hands or may provide working orthoses for hands. Spinal supports may also be requested to assist posture.

Work and leisure

The occupational therapist should discuss with the person whether the joints affected have been causing problems for him at work (if he is still employed) and, if so, whether any change may reduce the strain. If machinery can be altered or if a supportive chair would help it may be possible for the Disablement Resettlement Officer (DRO) to help organise this or other adaptations. If the job is not adaptable or if there is very great impairment the DRO can provide advice on assessments for retraining and future prospects.

The therapist should discuss the person's leisure activities with him and may make suggestions regarding equipment to help the person continue a favourite hobby. Alternatively, she may suggest a new interest which accommodates his disability.

The occupational therapist needs to have a basic knowledge of the welfare rights system in order to advise people on claiming benefits. This is a very complex area in which not many therapists are expert, but a general knowledge will prove invaluable, particularly for people who have to leave work or who become more disabled and require care from someone else.

The occupational therapist should also be alert to other information the person might find useful, for example that relating to support groups and local services such as Home Help. Section 9 of the Disabled Persons (Services Consultation and Representation) Act 1986 describes the requirement of the local authority to provide relevant information to disabled people. The local authority therapist should have a system for ensuring she gives people this information.

REHABILITATION FOLLOWING SURGERY

The time spent in hospital following surgery has become shorter so the occupational therapist must ensure that the essential elements of treatment are instituted quickly. The person must start rehabilitation as early as possible in order to gain the most benefit. Styles of treatment vary according to the type of operation and the regime of the surgeon. However, the occupational therapist's four main aims will be exactly the same as those listed on page 722.

The occupational therapist will be working with the rehabilitation team to provide a balanced programme of treatment which gradually increases strength, mobility and independence whilst ensuring that activity is carried out safely.

The occupational therapist should plan her programme of treatment (following assessment of the person's needs) so that the activities complement the treatment being carried out by other team members. The whole programme should form a comprehensive package designed to meet the goals agreed on with the person and his carer.

Treatment should be implemented at a rate which is sensitive to the rate of progress of the person, but which continues to challenge and encourage performance to the maximum. The therapist should be aware of factors that can lead to slow progress. An older person, for example, may progress more slowly after surgery purely for reasons of reduced physical ability associated with ageing or as a result of anaesthesia. Similarly, a younger person might be poorly motivated to work at the rehabilitation because of an emotional problem at home. Another reason for slow progress might be a lack of understanding by the person. He may have taken part in a discussion with the surgeon about the operation but because of anxiety may have remembered little of what was said. Consequently he may be unable to appreciate the reasons for the activities, advice and precautions prescribed by the rehabilitation programme. However, the occupational therapist should have the communication skills to clarify such matters and the sensitivity to adapt her approach to suit the person.

The occupational therapist's role is to work with the person and the carer to identify any areas of difficulty and then to plan a course of action to try to alleviate the problem so that treatment can be most effective.

It is important for the person to receive a clear explanation of the precautions to be observed following surgery. The occupational therapist, even if she is not actually responsible for giving this explanation, must be very familiar with the particular precautions for different kinds of surgery. The other rehabilitation team members and the surgeon should be approached to clarify any areas of uncertainty concerning a particular operative procedure.

General precautions

Precautions should be taken to:

- prevent dislocation of the new joint
- prevent infection (both of the wound and generally) for the first few weeks
- avoid forcing the range of movement of the joint
- avoid aggressive exercise initially
- maintain good posture.

There may be other specific precautions for particular types of prosthesis so it is always necessary for the occupational therapist to familiarise herself with local procedures. Some units prepare written advice leaflets about what should be avoided but a growing number of therapists also prefer to give verbal explanations, including the reason why the advice is important. It is recognised that if the person has a better understanding he will be more inclined to follow the therapist's advice. A reminder list might be provided for use by the person and the carer.

A typical programme

The following outlines the stages of treatment through which the occupational therapist might guide an individual undergoing hip replacement.

1. *Discussion*. The therapist should explain the treatment process to the person prior to surgery and discuss his home circumstances, taking note of any areas of concern.

2. *Surgery*.

3. *Some bed rest*. This may be only two days but is occasionally longer, depending on the type of new joint involved.

4. *Return to weight-bearing*, using a walking aid such as elbow crutches, a frame or a walking stick. The therapist should teach

correct
advice i
compler

5. *Aa*
hip shou
rotation

6. *De*
will pro
so advic
ways to
risk will
allowed
suitable
dress wh
at a suit
knees an
floor. Up
problem.
movemer
avoided.
garments
Good use
extends r
stocking
(Fig. 29.
flexion w
the hip.
interested
be encou
involveme

The pe
discussed
concern,
the home
noted pric
contact w
therapist
possible n
occupation
advice on
as comfor
which will

Bathing
included i
interventic
getting int
29.5. Initi
rather thar
the hip (se

be helpful here. If the person has a shower cubicle, a seat will preclude the difficulty of prolonged standing. Use of a toilet which is too low can be facilitated with a combined frame (Fig. 29.7) or with separate seat raise and frame components. Such equipment must be securely fixed, and the person and his carer should be briefed about how it can be removed for cleaning and replaced safely.

Chairs should be at the correct height, as discussed on page 725; arm rests will assist in rising and are especially helpful for an older person.

It is essential for most people to regain domestic skills and confidence before returning home. The occupational therapist should provide the opportunity for practice with adaptive equipment. A high perching stool (see Fig. 29.8) will ease the strain of standing for long periods. Long-handled equipment can be of use in the kitchen to reduce bending or stretching. Trolleys can be helpful in moving items (Fig. 29.9) but before recommending their use at home the therapist would be wise to check thresholds, as these can restrict the use of trolleys.

7. *Improvement of mobility*. The physiotherapist and nursing staff will be involved in promoting mobility. The occupational therapist should emphasise the need for good posture and a correct walking gait. If time permits, activity to improve strength and movement at the affected joint will be beneficial. This might take the form of practice in domestic tasks or table activities which promote walking and standing tolerance without strenuous lower limb exertion.

8. *Return home*. The arrangements for returning home will vary according to the person's circumstances, particularly age and the support networks in existence. An elderly person living alone will probably require more consideration than a younger person with a partner. It is always important for the therapist to feel confident that the person has achieved a safe level of independence before discharge. The older person may require involvement of various community support services, e.g. district nurse, home care, meals-on-wheels.

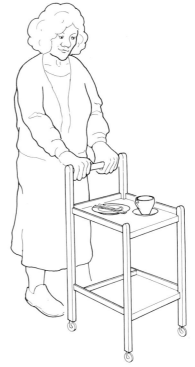

Fig. 29.9 Trolley for carrying items.

It is generally accepted that a joint home visit prior to discharge, with the relevant professionals, is the best way to ensure a safe return home. Staircases commonly cause problems and it may be necessary to temporarily move a bed downstairs and provide a commode for the first few weeks following discharge home. The home visit should be arranged so any essential work or pieces of equipment can be provided before the person arrives home. This needs liaison among the professionals concerned and may mean rearranging discharge dates to allow completion.

9. *Follow-up*. Any necessary follow-up should be clearly explained before discharge and arrangements made to return equipment which may only be needed over the initial period; bathing equipment for a younger person, for example, may be needed only for the first six weeks. An older person might attend an outpatient department or day centre for some weeks so that his progress can be monitored and his satisfactory rehabilitation ensured.

Surgery and rehabilitation should result in the person being able to return to everyday life and carry out work, social, domestic, emotional and leisure activities in a more active way.

CONCLUSION

Even though osteoarthritis cannot be cured the effects of any impairment may be minimised by sensitive and realistic treatment. Advice and education about the condition will assist the process of rehabilitation and enable the person to continue to function to his maximum potential. The occupational therapist must consider that an

older p
other a
lung ca
ditional
impairn
function
most in
individ
not det
cupatio
conside
implica
establis
life. T
tailorec
most
everyd

ACKNOWLEDGEMENT

My thanks to all of my colleagues at the Leicestershire Social Services Department and Leicestershire Health Authority for their invaluable consultation.

FURTHER READING

Adams J Crawford 1986 Outline of orthopaedics, 10th edn. Churchill Livingstone, Edinburgh
Department of the Environment 1978 House adaptations for people with physical disabilities: a guidance manual for practitioners. HMSO, London
MacDonald E M 1976 Occupational therapy in rehabilitation. Baillière Tindall, London

30

Rheumatoid arthritis

Elke Small

INTRODUCTION

Rheumatoid arthritis is one of a large number of diseases of the connective tissues. It affects the joints but may have other, systemic implications.

A significant number of people diagnosed as having rheumatoid arthritis may experience few long-term problems, suffering only one or two exacerbations which spontaneously subside. However, for many people the disease follows a pattern of exacerbations and remissions over a number of years. Such people will require intermittent therapeutic intervention in response to changing impairments and needs.

This chapter begins by describing the characteristics of rheumatoid arthritis and the impact that the disease is likely to have upon an individual's psychological, physical and social well-being. The range of treatments available for rheumatoid arthritis is described, and the specific functions of the occupational therapist's colleagues within the treatment team are outlined.

The role of the occupational therapist in the management of rheumatoid arthritis is then described in detail. Because the disease is extremely variable in its presentation and development, the occupational therapist will need to be flexible in her interventions and to be continually alert to the individual's changing situation. With this in mind, the chapter discusses the importance of ongoing assessment, with particular reference to self-maintenance, hand function and the performance of home, work and leisure activities. Elements of the occupational therapist's intervention are then outlined; these include guidance in performing daily living activities, instruction in the protection of joints, psychological support and hand therapy. The types and applications of orthoses for the rheumatoid hand are then described.

Throughout, the importance of the active involvement of the individual and his carers in the management of rheumatoid arthritis is stressed. The chapter concludes with a discussion of the ongoing need of carers for understanding and support.

RHEUMATOID ARTHRITIS

Rheumatoid arthritis is a chronic inflammatory disease of the synovium. It is a systemic disease primarily affecting the joints but may involve the lungs, heart and other organs.

History

Rheumatoid arthritis is considered to be a relatively new disease; there is no convincing evidence of it in prehistoric skeletal remains or in clinical descriptions dating from before the eighteenth century.

Incidence

The disease is no respecter of age or race, although the greatest incidence is among those aged 35 to 55 years. A higher incidence in females suggests that hormones may play a part in its development. It has been found to be familial but no direct hereditary factor has been identified.

Cause

The cause of the disease remains unknown but many theories have been put forward, including the possibility of infection or of abnormalities in immunological activity.

Patho

The syr
become
synovia
comes t
leads to
increase
laxity of
term ou
instabilit

Investig

Diagnosis
clinician's
ing stiffne
of the ha
fatigue. Ir
include b
anaemia a
showing e

IMPACT

Being a s
affects mar
be acknow
disease on
The areas c
headings of

- psycholo
- personal
- physical e
- functiona
- effects on

Psycholo

Much attent
physical effe
the psycholo
severe.

Individuals
titudes and al
controlling the
titudes may b
social factors.

varied, certain of these occur more frequently than others, and can have a direct effect on the therapist's involvement and on the outcome of rehabilitation.

Denial

Many people deny their disease as a way of protecting themselves from the pressures of reality. Denial may be identified by talking to the person and establishing how he perceives his disease and its effects on his daily life.

When coping with a person's denial it is important to first ascertain how much information he has about the disease. The therapist may be ill advised to try to make the person face 'reality' since this may only increase stress. It may be better to accept the person's response and adopt a positive approach in treatment and intervention. Practical advice and education may be more helpful in encouraging acceptance than attempting to change the person's perception per se.

Depression

It is important to establish the nature of any depression whenever possible, since many of the symptoms of systemic disease may be similar to those resulting from depression — for example, loss of appetite, fatigue, general malaise and loss of volition. The most common depression relates to the suppression of anger. This may be anger at having the disease, recognition of role loss, or anger at others' lack of sensitivity and recognition of the disease. Many people will often be able to explain their anger or depression through conversation and sensitive discussion. Depression can negatively affect the rehabilitation process, resulting in poor performance by the individual and sometimes frustration on the part of the therapist. A positive approach that highlights strengths and abilities and builds on these is often more successful than one that takes the person's limitations as a starting point; the latter approach may only serve to accentuate loss.

Acceptance

Though not easy to define, this best describes the attitude of a person who has experienced feelings of anger, sadness and helplessness, but is positive about those aspects of his life not affected by the disease and realistic about capabilities.

Personal effects

Self-image

Physical deformity resulting from rheumatoid arthritis can affect confidence and self-image. Whilst deformity of the hands, for example, may not always create extensive functional loss, the cosmetic impact can be embarrassing and lead to the desire to hide the hands from view.

The inability to 'keep up' with peers at work or in leisure activities can affect confidence and lead to demotivation at work and avoidance of social situations.

Sexuality

Disfigurement along with difficulty in the performance of sexual activity may make the individual feel less sexually attractive. Pain may result in avoidance of situations involving touch because 'even a hug hurts'. This may be frustrating to the individual who wishes to show and receive affection, and may be misconstrued by the partner as rejection.

Loss of role

The 'breadwinner' may find it extremely difficult to accept that he can no longer work at his trade and may now be confined to less demanding work and a reduced income. He may become home based, pursuing modest hobbies and relying on state benefits. In some instances this may lead to changes in role dominance in the home, further adding to possible relationship difficulties.

Physical effects

Joints

Pain and stiffness in the joints may reduce functional ability in the absence of physical signs. In the inflammatory stage of the disease the joints become hot and swollen and often exceedingly painful. Long-term joint damage frequently leads to instability and deformity, which may result in osteoarthritic changes in the joint.

Muscle

Pain may reduce the use of muscles, leading to restricted movement and stiffness. This may in turn lead to muscle wasting and weakness. For example, following prolonged sitting or bed-rest the quadriceps muscles in the legs weaken and thus reduce the ability to mobilise in transfers, walking and climbing stairs. Extensor muscles of the wrist are often weakened, affecting hand positioning for strong grip. Wasting of the small muscles of the hand affects power and pincer grip and opposition of the thumb to the fingers.

Tendons

Due to joint destruction and the laxity of the soft tissues around the joint, uneven tendon pull may further distort the joint into abnormal positions and create functional problems, especially in the hands. The extensor tendons to the fingers 'migrate' towards the grooves between the joints in an ulnar direction because of the loss of the restraining function of the proximal annular ligaments, which may have been weakened by synovitis. Similarly, damage affecting the metacarpophalangeal (MCP) and/or interphalangeal (IP) joints may result in abnormal tendon balance or alignment, leading to swan-neck or boutonnière deformities.

Nerves

Bony deformity or excessive swelling may cause pressure on nerves. The most common example is carpal tunnel syndrome, in which the median nerve is constricted as it passes beneath the flexor retinaculum. This causes unpleasant tingling and pain over the distribution of the median nerve in the hand, and if prolonged can result in weakness or loss of pincer grip and sensory loss. Vertebral damage, such as cervical spondylosis, or osteo-

phytes
the ner
result ir

Functi

These a
result fr
tion may
instabili
the syst
anaemia

Limite
impede
stability
stabilisin
reduce ac
ance of a
comfort i
actions.
resulting
sory awa
dexterity

Any or
ability,
arthritis
rently, tl
capabiliti
living is
distributi
the symp
abilities i
ing role d
Impairme
will partic
nipulative
volving li
ing the
effect upo

Effects
pursuits

Individuals
find that
tivies bec
disease. F

racquet sports such as squash, tennis or badminton, restrictions due to painful wrists, weakened grip or reduced mobility or fatigue may soon limit such activities. Similarly, active sports involving lower limb or whole body functions, for example football, running, canoeing or horseback riding, may soon become difficult.

Creative leisure pursuits such as sewing, knitting, woodwork or model building all require a considerable amount of dexterity and manipulative skill and, while these activities may be pursued for a longer time, they may eventually have to be relinquished because of increased impairment or because they threaten to cause further damage. For example, adopting the static grip position required by knitting for long periods of time may be contraindicated because of its effect on the MCP and wrist joints, which encourages ulnar drift and joint stiffness.

Severe impairments resulting from rheumatoid arthritis will significantly handicap the person in social activities, not only because of his physical limitations but also by virtue of the design of the environment. Many public buildings such as restaurants, pubs, cinemas, theatres, educational establishments and stately homes pose problems of accessibility, and do not provide parking, seating and toilet facilities for the disabled. Frequently, persons with severe disabilities are discouraged from undertaking activities outside of the home by a lack of information regarding access and facilities.

When considering the difficulties created by rheumatoid arthritis in all areas of living, professionals, carers and even disabled individuals themselves frequently emphasise and prioritise the areas of self-maintenance and role duties at the expense of social and leisure pursuits. However, it is important to achieve a balance of activities and to recognise the important role played by social and leisure pursuits in normal living. Suggestions for alternatives in the choice of leisure activities, and provision of information or supportive equipment may enable the person with rheumatoid arthritis to continue to enjoy healthy and enriching social and leisure pursuits. This will need organisation, planning and consideration of individual skills within the limits of the disease.

TREATMENT

Treatment may take place in the home or in hospital, depending on the severity of the condition, the home circumstances and support services available, and the particular treatment required. Traditionally, people with rheumatoid arthritis have been admitted to hospitals or specialist units during an 'acute' phase of the disease in order to receive intensive treatment by a team of doctors, nurses and therapists and to rest their joints from daily activity. Specialist units and teams with adequate facilities at their disposal have been able to provide home-based treatment, but much education of the family and carers is needed for this to be successful. Families and carers should have good access to information about the disease so that they can appreciate the needs of the individual, particularly during the active phase of the disease. Many people with rheumatoid arthritis experience considerable pain and fatigue; whilst these symptoms may not have physical manifestations, and may not be consistant with levels of deformity, they are significant in reducing the level of independence. This is sometimes difficult for carers and spouses to understand.

Chemotherapy

The most common complaint by people with rheumatoid arthritis is of constant pain, which requires ongoing analgesia; paracetamol is most frequently used for this purpose. Anti-inflammatory agents, such as aspirin, are also a mainstay of drug treatment for rheumatoid arthritis. When prescribed in small doses aspirin is an effective analgesic, and in higher doses it acts as a non-steroidal anti-inflammatory agent.

Steroids such as prednisolone are effective anti-inflammatory agents, but their undesirable side effects reduce their use in treating rheumatoid arthritis, except when other drugs have failed to control the inflammatory process.

Surgery

Surgery plays an important role in the treatment of severe rheumatoid arthritis. Although surgical

procedures may be undertaken for the sole purpose of pain relief, most surgical interventions are
undertaken with a view to correction or prevention
of deformity and improvement of function.

All members of the treatment team should contribute to the assessment of the individual's need
for surgery, where the proposed procedure will
have a direct effect on function. There are several
types of surgery in common use:

- Reconstructive surgery. Especially common is
  the repair of tendons, for example ruptured
  extensor tendons in the fingers
- Joint replacement. The most common joints
  to be replaced are:
  — the hips
  — the knees
  — the ankles
  — the MCP joints
  — the elbow joint
  — the shoulders.

Of these the hip replacement is the most common.

- Joint fusion arthrodesis. This involves fusing
  the joint to provide stability and eliminate
  pain. It may be necessary when a joint
  replacement has failed.

Selection for surgery

To be successful, any surgical procedure must be
appropriate for the individual concerned. The
decision to offer surgery, especially joint replacement, must take into account:

- the medical needs of the individual
- functional needs and wishes of the individual
- assessment by physicians, surgeons, therapists
  and carers
- functional potential following the procedure
- the level of understanding by the individual
  of the rehabilitation process after surgery.

Occupational therapists are responsible for functional assessment and for providing information on
the individual's abilities to the team. This assessment is important in highlighting patterns of usage
of joints in work activities, in the home, and in
leisure pursuits.

The t

The m
the dis
process
team as
be invo
thopaed
responsi
ease pro
among
interven
individu
cohesive

Nurses

Nursing
managen
hospital
environn
day-to-da
therapy a
particular
along wit
role in th

Nurses
and ways
ing prob
required
bed-rest
day-to-da
a person's
titudes or
and rehab
with relat
or on hom
regular co
the family
person's a
the family

Physioth

The aims o
son regard
disease and
cises, to
movement,

general mobility. The physiotherapist may also give instruction in pain management techniques and may provide orthoses and mobility equipment.

Many techniques employed by the physiotherapist interlink or overlap with those of the occupational therapist. Both professionals may be involved in providing information and advice on environmental and ergonomic considerations, working and resting positions, joint protection and the balance of activity in daily life.

Interventions specific to the physiotherapist include: hydrotherapy; the application of heat to relax muscles and ease pain; the use of ice packs to reduce inflammation and relieve pain; and the use of specific exercise techniques to maintain joint mobility and muscle strength.

Physiotherapy may be provided in the hospital or specialist unit but many people have home exercise programmes or receive physiotherapy in the home or community clinic, thus reducing the need to visit the hospital on an outpatient basis.

Social workers

The impact of arthritis on the pattern of daily life can be devastating. Loss of role, difficulties with maintaining home-based duties, constant pain, reduction in socialisation and problems with the demands of employment may all require specialist emotional and financial advice.

Many social workers are skilled counsellors who are trained in the assessment of family and social dynamics. Social workers are aware of support facilities available in the locality as well as the assistance and benefits to which the person or the family may be entitled.

Frequently it is the social worker who is involved in helping individuals to make major decisions in their lives such as whether to accept help or care, or whether to move to a more suitable living environment.

THE ROLE OF THE OCCUPATIONAL THERAPIST

The occupational therapist has a unique contribution to make in facilitating and promoting maximum function in daily activity. The therapist should encourage the individual to take responsibility for his own health. She should aim to facilitate educated, informed decision-making regarding treatment techniques and introduce ways of managing impairments and disabilities that minimise handicap in all aspects of daily living – at home, at work and at play.

Rosenbaum (1983) describes the individual's need to change from learned dependence to learned resourcefulness. This may involve education in joint protection principles, instruction on specific techniques to minimise or overcome impairments, or the identification of ways of managing disabilities in self-maintenance, role duties and leisure pursuits. The provision of advice to families and carers should be considered in the context of the person's role, daily needs and wishes, and the environment in which he lives.

The occupational therapist may be concerned with the restoration of specific anatomical function following a severe 'flare-up' of the disease or following surgery, particularly surgery to the hand.

Therapeutic intervention may extend over many years. It is frequently intermittent, responding to changing patterns of disability. Some people recover from the disease but many will require reappraisal of previous interventions and further adjustments or additions to care provision to meet the alterations in circumstances dictated by the disease process.

OCCUPATIONAL THERAPY APPROACHES

The most widely used approach for people with rheumatoid arthritis is the rehabilitative approach, which aims to enable people to compensate for limitation or loss of function.

A large variety of techniques, equipment, orthoses and adaptations have been developed specifically to overcome the limitations imposed by rheumatic diseases.

Some biomechanical principles may be employed to improve range of movement or restore muscle strength and activity tolerance following surgery or a severe exacerbation of the disease.

However, this approach accounts for a relatively small proportion of occupational therapy practice; in cases of rheumatoid arthritis it is most commonly applied to the restoration of hand function following surgery.

An educational approach is employed to promote joint protection techniques which will preserve the joints from undue stress or strain. This approach will equip the person to make informed choices as to how to perform actions and thereby to take some responsibility in avoiding future joint damage. While there is no evidence that joint protection techniques can halt or reverse the disease process, education in joint protection techniques may encourage behavioural changes which will *limit* joint damage in the person whose activity patterns have been consolidated over a number of years.

ASSESSMENT

Assessment of the person with rheumatoid arthritis should be an ongoing process, given the changing and often unpredictable pattern of the disease. Formal assessment, together with educated self-assessment, should be employed to ensure regular appraisal of abilities is maintained.

Initial assessment

This will establish a baseline for intervention. It usually takes the form of an interview together with observation of functional task performance. Specific measurements may be taken, depending on the nature of the referral.

The aim of the initial assessment is to produce a picture of strengths and deficits from which priorities can be determined and a strategy for intervention can be planned with the individual and his carers.

Review

Monitoring the effectiveness of intervention and changes in the process of the disease will help to ensure that treatment is both preventative and effective. For example, a person showing early symptoms of involvement of the knees in the dis-

ease w:
amount
of chair
of the j
be aime
and pro

Speci
nature
areas of
rheumat
related
tion; he
provisio

Self-m

Many pe
problem
These
manipul;
which a
and dre:
which n
or hoist
adaptatic

Specifi

- the pa
particu
are les
- the pa
may b
overco
assistiv
- the ex
stiffne
- the lev

Each a
presentin;
sessed. M
devised fc
standardis
score dail
related to
for peopl
setting wi
is less ap]
timed sel:

Robinson and Bashall for people with rheumatoid arthritis; this gives quantifiable measures against which individual performance can be compared. A considerable amount of research is required to develop and refine valid and reliable standardised daily living assessments for use with people suffering from rheumatoid arthritis.

Hand function assessment

Specific hand function assessment may form part of a fuller evaluation of function or may be particularly required in relation to the provision of orthoses or to a decision regarding surgery. The aim of hand assessment is to identify the nature and dynamics of hand function in relation to the signs and symptoms of the disease and the person's daily needs.

Particular attention should be paid to: the use of the hand in functional activities; hand dominance; occupations and task demands. Specific details regarding hand deformities, the rate of progress of the symptoms, levels of pain, oedema, grip strength and dexterity should all be noted. Any sensory deficit and loss of range of movement should be recorded. A number of functional and anatomical hand assessments are available (see Ch. 7). These should be chosen in accordance with the specific purpose of the evaluation and can be used to determine whether specific intervention in the form of orthoses, surgery, therapeutic hand activities or eduction in joint protection measures will improve hand function or prevent further deterioration. Monitoring of hand function before and after intervention will be necessary to determine the effectiveness of the therapeutic course taken.

Home assessment

This is a vital area of assessment for the person with a chronic rheumatic condition because of the extensive presentation and progressive nature of the disease. The aim of home assessment is to:

- establish the person's current level of abilities in the home
- identify the techniques the person is using in home-based activities

- evaluate the need for modifications of activity through altered techniques, the provision of equipment or services or adaptations to the home environment
- evaluate the 'realism' of the individual and his carers for present and future provision, i.e. is the person realistic about his present levels of capability or is he relying on a high level of support, which may or may not be in accordance with the wishes of the carer?
- evaluate the home environment (the cultural and environmental situation of the person's living circumstances), the type of home and neighbourhood and the local social support structure.

Observation of the techniques used to perform activities as well as the outcome of those activities will help to identify contraindicated practices. Assessment of socialisation and social activities is also important; the therapist should ascertain what social and leisure activities the person pursues and how these may affect the disease pattern.

As in all areas of disability, the person's psychological coping strategies are of paramount importance in determining the success of rehabilitation and adjustment. The presence of deformity and pain may negatively affect the person's attitudes, personality, morale and self-esteem and impede his motivation and drive to set and achieve personal goals or maintain interests. Some adverse psychological presentations may be linked to locus of control, while others may be the result of 'learned helplessness' (Sands 1988).

Assessing Physically Disabled People at Home by Kathleen Maczka is a useful text outlining procedures for home assessment.

Work assessment

Breaking down work activities into component parts enables the therapist to assess particular task requirements and identify problem areas. For people with rheumatoid arthritis who are employed in predominantly sedentary or desk work, the main problems may well be related to environmental needs; e.g. work surface heights may be inappropriate and adequate supportive seating may be lacking. People working in a secretarial capacity or with computers or word processors often find that this repetitive type of work causes pain over long periods if the hand and wrist joint are affected by the disease. Alterations to the work station design and the provision of support orthoses may be effective in reducing the strain on particular joints.

The broader issues of work should also be considered. Shift times may pose particular difficulties for those who suffer substantial early morning stiffness. It may be possible to renegotiate these times to take account of this. The length of the shift should also be considered in conjunction with levels of fatigue.

Mobility problems may pose difficulties with travel to and from work, either in relation to using public transport, particularly at busy times of day, or to driving a car. Alternative local transport should be investigated. The layout of the work environment, parking, steps and stairs, canteen and toilet facilities may also present difficulties for the person with severe chronic rheumatic disease.

For people employed in manual labour, many of the heavier tasks may cause severe strain on particular joints. If the person wishes to continue in his job, detailed analysis of such strains and exploration of alternatives will be necessary. Where changes in work practices are impossible, a change in employment may have to be considered. The Disablement Resettlement Officer (DRO) is skilled in negotiation with employers and is usually aware of local alternative employment opportunities. A social worker may also be valuable in ascertaining financial implications for continuing, changing or terminating employment in terms of benefits to which the person may be entitled.

With the expansion of modern technology and methods of communication, home-based employment may become a more realistic alternative to going out to work for many disabled people; this avenue should not be overlooked for the person with severe rheumatoid disease.

INTERVENTION

Occupational therapy intervention aims to remediate specific or global difficulties in the

person's

rheumat

out on a

The

rheumat

able. So

exacerba

fore the

from tha

gressive

physical

managen

cases.

For m

ease proc

well' for

ment for

progress

itial educ

of advice

further t

although

identifyin

Daily li

A program

the most

enable the

in accorda

Educati

in conjun

methods

tivities wi

include al

ing, sittin

as ironing

intricate fa

vantage of

any setting

son in a w

or home a

Howeve

such mear

modified c

to the env

visable.

Prescription of daily living equipment

The importance of accurate assessment for the provision of daily living equipment cannot be overstressed. An increasing variety of equipment is available in high street stores with little advice available for its use. While this availability is to be welcomed in the broader access it provides, care should be taken to ensure the equipment purchased is safe and suitable for the person's particular requirements.

The occupational therapist's assessment of the short- and long-term needs of the individual with rheumatoid arthritis will help to ensure the appropriate provision of equipment. Careful, individualised assessment is extremely important, as the needs of people with rheumatoid arthritis are particularly varied in light of the many deformities which may occur, and the variations in each person's environment and care provision.

Equipment should be as simple as possible and safe and easy to operate. Individuals and carers will frequently require instruction and practice in the use of different types of equipment before an accurate selection can be made. For this reason a range of equipment should be available for trial. Some equipment may require adaptation or modification to meet individual requirements.

Aid such as dressing sticks, long-handled shoe horns and grooming equipment may be especially useful for people with restricted joint range of movement. Adapted handles may be useful for those with poor grip or manual dexterity, particularly on items in regular use such as cutlery, crockery, writing implements and small kitchen tools. In addition, such equipment should be as lightweight as possible to reduce the strain on the joints of the hands.

Adapting equipment already in use may be preferable to providing new equipment in some cases. Offcuts of orthotic materials may be useful for extending combs, adapting keys to facilitate grip, or modifying knobs or handles. Velcro may be used to replace small buttons, laces and other difficult fastenings.

Chairs, wheelchairs or hoists and home adaptations may be needed to facilitate or maintain independence for the individual and his carers.

In arranging for the provision of equipment to facilitate bathing, toileting and mobility, the therapist should take into account the needs of carers as well as of the individual himself.

Disabled Living Centres are useful sources of information, particularly regarding equipment. The individual may be able to visit a Centre to try various items of equipment and evaluate the limitations and merits of specific models. The staff of these centres, many of whom are occupational therapists, may provide detailed assessments and give advice on available funding sources for equipment. In some centres, staff may make recommendations to social services or other providers on particular individual needs. Smaller pieces of equipment may be purchased directly from some centres.

The Department of Health Surveys of Equipment listed on pages 750 and 751 are valuable sources of information.

Home adaptations

Small adaptations to the home frequently make life much easier for the person with rheumatoid arthritis, particularly where the hands and upper limbs are affected. Alterations to environmental controls may be all that is required. Taps, door furniture, switches, plugs and heating controls may be difficult to operate either because of the fine manipulative skill required or because they are sited in places which are difficult to reach. Replacement with larger controls or resiting may overcome such difficulties. Larger adaptations inside the home are most frequently required in the bathroom or kitchen. Access to the toilet or bathing facilities may be eased by the provision of fixed rails in addition to support equipment. Some people may prefer to use a shower if bathing is difficult or impossible. In the kitchen, it may be necessary to adjust work surface heights and to reorganise storage so that equipment and supplies are easily reached by the person with limited joint range of movement.

For those with generalised mobility problems, home adaptations may be required to facilitate access to or within the home. These may include modification of steps or stairs to lessen the height of the risers and the installation of firm handrails on both sides to enable the person to remain ambulant with walking aids. Alternatives in the form of level or ramped access may be necessary for people using wheelchairs.

Major difficulties in internal mobility, particularly those caused by narrow doorways and by steps and stairs, may be overcome in a number of ways. Doors may be widened, steps may be ramped or reduced, and indoor lifts or stair lifts may be provided. The home may be adapted so that facilities are available on the ground floor for personal hygiene, toileting and sleeping. Alternatively, the person may prefer to consider moving to more ergonomically designed premises such as a flat or bungalow. This step should be considered carefully, especially where the person is in receipt of community support from friends, neighbours or relatives or where other members of the family have valuable local contacts. Proactive planning for future needs and regular review will ensure that modifications continue to meet the needs of the individual and his carers for as long as possible, despite changes in the pattern of disability as the disease progresses.

Other support

Many people with rheumatoid arthritis are able to fulfil their daily needs and duties with confidence once their home environment has been appropriately equipped and their day-to-day tasks organised.

However, for some people, particularly those who live alone and have other impairments, or those with severe chronic disease, additional help may be required. This is usually related to severe problems with transfers and mobility in the home and the community. The occupational therapist should be aware of the range of community support services available and, following the identification of need, discuss the options with the person and his carers. Referral to support agencies can then be made. Some examples of external supports which are frequently needed are Meals on Wheels, community nursing, bath attendants, home help services and community transport facilities.

Joint |

Melvin
joint pr(
involved
mation
structure
that join
most in(
own joi
reduce c
pattern (
tion tech
severity (

Princip|

1. *Adopt*
Each |
work/rest
pendence
working
fatigue.
The us
the mos
symptom;
identified
or week a
sential. B
therapist
grammes
minutes r(
becomes
and ignor(
a decrease
These
people wit
require l(
persons sl
hours' res
a minimu
2. *Resp*
Recogni
warning o
individual
pain-indu(
comfort m
if pain oc(

duration or techniques simplified so that stress on the particular joints which are painful is reduced.

3. *Reduce effort in daily activity.*

Energy conservation is an important aspect to consider in joint protection, as a reduction in effort lessens the stress on joints and may enable the individual to participate more fully in activities.

Melvin (1989) identifies nine principles of energy conservation:

- pre-plan and organise the proposed activity
- ascertain priorities
- eliminate unnecessary tasks
- take time, avoid rushing
- use good postures and body mechanics when performing the activity
- avoid unnecessary activity or energy expenditure
- organise the most ergonomic work environment
- use assistive tools or equipment where possible
- take frequent, planned rest periods.

4. *Avoid positions of deformity.*

Whether performing activity or resting, the individual should not strain joints or allow them to adopt positions of deformity. Performing actions which encourage MCP ulnar deviation, putting strain on IP joints by carrying handled objects using a 'hook' grip, straining the intervertebral joints through bending when lifting, or placing a pillow under the knees when resting (which encourages the development of flexion contractures at the hips or knees) should all be avoided. Problems may be overcome by education in alternative techniques to avoid such actions or by the provision of equipment to reduce strain. Examples of techniques to prevent joint deformity in the hands are given in Figure 30.1.

5. *Use larger, stronger joints for activity.*

Education in joint protection techniques should emphasise the importance of using the largest, strongest joints in the most stable anatomical positions when performing activities. For example, using the forearm or the palm of the hand when carrying flat objects is preferable to using a pincer or hook grip, and correct lifting practices which utilise the quadriceps and the hamstrings rather than placing stress on the vertebral column are recommended.

6. *Avoid static positions.*

Stress and fatigue result from maintaining or holding static postures. The person with rheumatoid arthritis should be discouraged from remaining in one position for long periods and should be advised to rest and change position at regular intervals. The optimum intervals may vary from person to person, but people should be encouraged to stretch, move or rest at least every twenty minutes.

7. *Avoid activities which cannot be halted.*

The person should be encouraged to plan ahead when preparing for activity and not to embark on an activity which cannot easily be stopped if it becomes too stressful. The build-up of stress on the joints may cause the onset of pain; such pain should be respected, and the activity terminated as soon as possible.

8. *Use equipment to assist in task performance.*

Many forms of assistive equipment are available, including normal labour-saving devices, specifically adapted tools to promote optimum functional performance with deformity, and orthoses to support joints when carrying out actions. In some situations these should be recommended as useful supports in the early stages of the disease that will prevent unnecessary strain which is likely to accelerate joint destruction; in other instances, they may be required once destruction has occurred to reduce further damage.

Equipment should aim to reduce the stress and strain on the joints but should not discourage the maintenance of joint range of motion and muscle tone, as this is likely to result in joint stiffness and muscle wasting. Such items of equipment as trolleys or perching stools, for example, are beneficial in that they reduce the need for carrying heavy items or for prolonged standing but do not completely replace carrying or standing activities.

Teaching methods

The principles of joint protection should be carefully explained to each individual. Opportunity should be provided for each person to practise

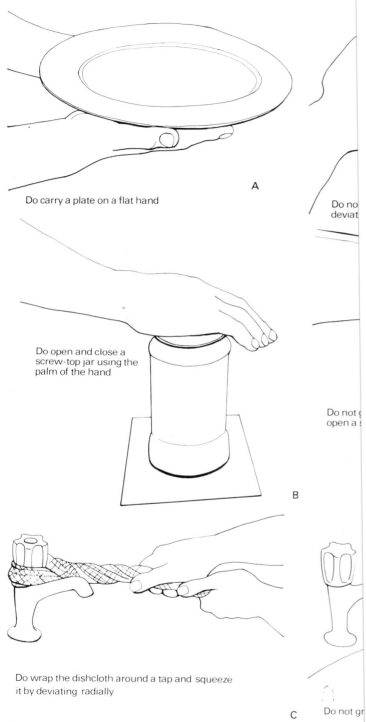

Do carry a plate on a flat hand

A

Do no
deviat

Do open and close a
screw-top jar using the
palm of the hand

Do not
open a

B

Do wrap the dishcloth around a tap and squeeze
it by deviating radially

C

Do not gr

Fig. 30.1 Hand joint protection techniques in rheumatoid arthritis. (A) Car
a dish cloth.

techniques under the guidance of the therapist. Simple leaflets with illustrations, many of which are designed by occupational therapists, are available for follow-up reference when personal guidance is no longer available.

Individuals and carers should be encouraged to extend their knowledge of joint care principles through the use of reference texts such as Brattstrom (1987), Dudley Hart (1982), Lorig and Fries (1983) and Melvin (1989) and through educational videos.

Learning may occur on a one-to-one basis with the therapist or may be in group or class situations similar to those used for people who suffer back pain. A group of people with similar problems may meet to discuss and practise activities at regular intervals over a period of weeks.

It should be considered that whilst it is important for the occupational therapist to provide information on joint protection techniques, adoption of alternative methods may involve considerable changes in some individuals' life-styles. The therapist must be flexible. She should advocate only those joint protection techniques of which the individual is physically capable and which are wholly appropriate to his situation. She must not impose a dogmatic regime, as this is likely either to result in total disregard for any of her suggestions or to raise the individual's anxieties about his ability to meet the requirements of the programme.

Psychological support

The unpredictable nature of rheumatoid arthritis, together with the lack of a cure and the diversity of its symptoms may have a profound, negative effect on the individual which can seriously impede the move towards self-responsibility and a positive problem-solving approach.

Recognition of psychological responses through discussion of feelings of anger, depression, helplessness and hopelessness in a supportive, caring environment may help the individual to face his situation. Depression related to loss of role may be alleviated by analysing the role with the individual and then planning and organising ways to maintain control over aspects of the role which are particularly important to him.

Many psychological reactions are linked to the person's perceived locus of control. Education about the nature of the disease, instruction in joint protection techniques, and the opportunity to discuss difficulties and practise solutions will enable the individual to more fully understand specific treatments and problem-solving strategies. The individual's active involvement in exploring possible solutions will promote a sense of responsibility and control over personal actions and life-style. Melvin (1989) refers to this as patient 'empowerment' while Sands (1988) equates it with a move towards 'learned resourcefulness'. Whatever the terminology used to describe this aspect of intervention, it is of vital importance to the individual's long-term acceptance of the disease and his development of positive coping strategies for the future.

One of the major factors affecting psychological behaviour is pain. Pain can be demoralising, frightening and demotivating. The protective postures which many people adopt as the result of pain produce muscle tension, which may further aggravate the pain and eventually result in contractures. Many members of the rehabilitative team may be involved with pain relief. Chemotherapy may have serious side effects if used over a long period. Education in joint protection to avoid pain-inducing situations is beneficial, but the occupational therapist may also be involved in pain management through education in the use of relaxation techniques. These aim to:

- create a better awareness of muscle tension and how to relieve it
- provide a method of releasing physical and emotional tension
- reduce pain
- reduce fatigue and promote sleep patterns.

A number of relaxation methods may be tried in order to identify which is most suitable for the particular person. Relaxation exercises increase awareness of muscle tension while soft talking and music are mentally diverting and aim to reduce both emotional and physical tension.

Education, counselling and support for carers and relatives can also help to promote greater understanding, more positive control and a more beneficial psychological approach to the future.

Hand therapy

Rheumatoid arthritis in the hands results in:

- inflammation of joint capsules and tendons (synovitis and tenosynovitis) with pain, swelling and raised temperature
- deformity and instability of joints — subluxation, dislocation and deviation
- long-term deformity with fixed positions and contractures
- secondary complications resulting from rupture of tendons or nerve compression
- skin changes, for example psoriasis and nodules, which may also restrict hand function.

Problems may occur at any of the joints, at the wrist or in the hand and the types of problems vary considerably from person to person. However, the following patterns of deformity are commonly seen:

- radial deviation and anterior subluxation at the wrist
- flexion of the MCP joint and hyperextension of the IP joint of the thumb
- MCP ulnar deviation of the fingers
- swan-neck or boutonnière deformities of the IP joints of the fingers.

These deformities are the result of a combination of damage to the periarticular tissues, which causes joint laxity and instability, together with tendon and ligament involvement, which may result in an inbalance in the dynamics of normal hand function (Melvin 1989). The occupational therapist may be involved in educating the person in joint protection to reduce further stress or strain, in the provision of orthoses to correct deformity or support weakened joints and in specific activity to improve functional performance of the hand.

Aims

- to in
  stres
- to m
  mov
- to m
- to in

Hand
but sho
effects
and the
the ind
hands r
tations.
realistic
the indi
requiren

Thera
part foll
ruptured
may be
physioth
surgeon
the rang
objective
following
limited
program
remedial
towards
duties an

Follow
necessita
resulted
increased
exercises
of mover

ORTH(

Orthoses
evaluated
process, b
value in
functiona
cated by
therapist

the individual, the skills of the team and the facilities available. The occupational therapist is most frequently involved in the manufacture of orthoses for the hands. In many instances, occupational therapists will be involved in monitoring the functional advantages gained by using an orthosis.

Aims

Orthoses for the rheumatoid hand are used:
- to rest joints in a position of function during the active phase of the disease
- to support joints in order to alleviate inflammation, oedema and pain
- to reduce pressure on nerves by maintaining a neutral position
- to support painful and unstable joints during activity in a functional position, while allowing movement to occur at the adjacent joints.

Types of hand orthoses

Volar forearm and hand resting orthosis (Fig. 30.2)

This is used overnight and when resting during the day. It extends over the palmar aspect of the hand and the volar aspect of the forearm and supports the hand and wrist in a functional position. Support may be provided for the thumb if necessary. A variety of materials may be used to fabricate this orthosis and it may be attached to the hand by straps or bandages. Where the problems are bilateral, orthoses are usually worn alternately on each hand, as the person is not able to use the hand for function when the orthosis is applied.

Wrist supports (Fig. 30.3)

These support the wrist during activity. They usually fully enclose the wrist joint but some may be applied only to the palmar aspect. They extend to the proximal palmar crease and up to two thirds of the length of the forearm. The wrist joint is usually positioned in slight extension to facilitate grip. A wide variety of materials may be used, depending on the needs of the individual and the nature of the activities to be performed. Some commercially manufactured wrist supports (for example, the Futuro) are available. Most of these orthoses are attached to the limb with straps.

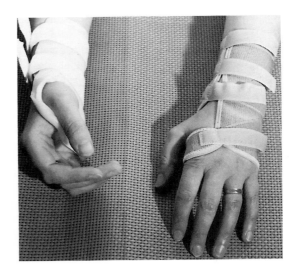

Fig. 30.3 Wrist supports.

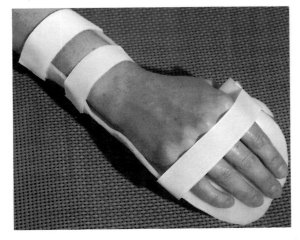

Fig. 30.2 Hand resting orthosis.

Dynamic extensor orthoses (Fig. 30.4)

These are used following MCP joint replacements, primarily to retain a correction of ulnar deviation.

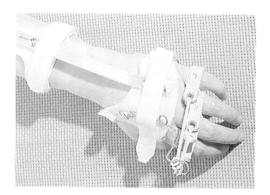

Fig. 30.4 Dynamic extensor orthosis.

Dynamic extensor orthoses may also be used to overcome extension lag at the same joints following extensor tendon repair. These orthoses are applied to the dorsal aspect of the forearm and hand and usually include outriggers to maintain digit extensor pull.

Corrective orthoses

These may be used to maintain correct alignment of joints post-operatively or may be required to support joints in a functional position for performance of hand activities. The condition of the joint should be known, for example by X-ray, and the nature of the deformity established. Fixed bony deformities cannot be corrected by the use of orthoses. If there is a substantial reduction in joint space or severe joint destruction, orthotic correction may be inadequate or contraindicated because of the risk of causing further damage to the joint.

Soft tissue deformities such as contractures of tendons or ligaments may be corrected by the use of orthoses. In addition to the enclosed wrist orthosis, which corrects radial deviation as well as providing support, orthoses may be used to restrict ulnar deviation and maintain alignment at the MCP joints or to correct swan-neck or boutonnière deformities of the digits (see Fig. 11.8). A variety of designs are available for such purposes and can be fabricated from a number of different materials in accordance with the extent of the deviation and the functional needs of the hand. If it is not possible to passively correct malalignment with the

first or
ively o
Therm
this pu
well as
contou

Thum

These
metaca
functio
held in
finger

Thu
port th
reduce

Thu
in ther
distal j
but wh
need t
free w
proble
necess
or sup

Fig. 30

Othe

The o
in the

some areas she may be responsible for the manufacture or monitoring of other forms of orthoses for the person with rheumatoid arthritis. These may include cervical collars, supportive orthoses for the lower limbs, foot orthoses and, in some instances, spinal jackets.

Manufacture of orthoses

A number of custom-made orthoses and patterns for manufacture are available. A trained orthotist may provide specific types of orthoses, particularly those which involve the moulding of high temperature materials or contain complex mechanical joints. The orthotist and the occupational therapist should work together to ensure that whatever orthosis is provided is functionally advantageous and that the person is familiar with its correct fitting and is able to put it on properly.

When the therapist is responsible for designing and manufacturing an orthosis she should be conversant with the design criteria, the functional dynamics and requirements for the joint or limb and the range of suitable options available. She should be able to design a pattern for the individual to meet his specific requirements in terms of the purpose of the orthosis, the times it is to be worn and the way it is to be applied and removed. She should be aware of the painful nature of the joints, any protrusions or nodules which may cause pressure points and the sensitivity of the skin. The siting and type of fastenings is crucial to independent fitting and removal of the orthosis for those people with limited reach or poor manual dexterity.

Whilst many orthotic materials require ovens or baths in order to be fabricated and moulded, some materials may be used in the community with a minimum of equipment, some of which may be easily transportable.

Review

It is important to review the orthosis regularly, particularly in the first week after application to ensure it retains its function and fit. The person should be informed of any possible risk areas and taught to check these. Particular risks are related to the dangers of pressure on protruding joints or sensitive skin. The person must be given advice on how to check for pressure points and whom to contact in the event of a problem. Any increase in pain, oedema or heat at the joint should also cause concern and should be checked to ensure the orthosis is not causing further aggravation to the joint.

There are instances where the person may find the orthosis does not provide the assistance anticipated or is intolerable to wear. In such cases the exact nature of the problem must be determined. If the difficulty is not the result of poor fabrication or inappropriate prescription the orthosis should be removed and alternative strategies considered.

SUPPORT FOR CARERS

Carers are often silent members of the community who have an extremely difficult task supporting their relatives for twenty-four hours a day. They may be frustrated by the lack of support services available or may be unaware of many of the resources to which they can turn for help.

When assessing the needs of individuals with rheumatoid arthritis it is important to also assess and respect the needs of carers and to ensure they have access to the support network which is available to them in their community.

Support should not only be viewed as practical help. Emotional and social needs are equally important. Respite care may be available to carers who are involved in continuous care of a person with a high level of disability. It is equally important to encourage carers to maintain a good quality of life, not only for those whom they look after but also for themselves. Carers should be encouraged to make use of the facilities available to them to retain and regain their strength to continue to look after their relative in the long term. Carers often need help in accepting respite care. Often they feel guilty about leaving a loved one in the care of others.

Some communities have self-help groups for carers which aim to provide support materially and emotionally in the form of a 'sitting' service, or just to provide the opportunity to discuss difficult situations and share problems with others. Many voluntary groups and charities also offer short relief visits to enable carers to go out and have a break. New faces may also offer stimulation and friendship to those in need of care. Local areas have different organisations which provide support, so it is vital for the therapist to be aware of what is available in the person's locality. National organisations such as the Arthritis and Rheumatism Council and Arthritis Care (see below) are also important sources of information and may have local groups which can provide support for the person and his carers. Additionally, many educational and social groups not specifically concerned with impairment may welcome people with disabilities. Provided the venue is accessible and suitable transport is available, attendance at such groups may provide valuable stimulation and support for the disabled person.

CONCLUSION

The treatment of people with rheumatoid arthritis is complex and varied and requires continuing review and evaluation. The therapist's role is to provide a service to the individual and his carers which includes assessment, treatment, education, the provision of advice and equipment, and specific therapeutic activity. People with rheumatic disease should be able to make informed decisions regarding treatment and the advice they accept.

Many
coping
Therap
refer tl
enhanc
therapi
advice

Wher
is invol
is vitall
tween h
therapis
ferred f
liaison b
treatmen
ensures
leagues t

It is i
couraged
confidenc
dent in a:
not only
from othe

Review
individual
point of v
ther supp
therapist r
interventic
dividual. 7
aware the t
their reque
confined t(

USEFUL ADDRESSES

Arthritis Care
6 Grosvenor Crescent
London SW1X 7ER

The Arthritis and Rheumatism Council
41 Eagle Street
London WC1R 4AR

The Disabled Living Centres Council
c/o The Disabled Living Foundation
380–384 Harrow Road
London W9 2HU

Department
Information
Health Publ
No. 2 Site,
Heywood, L
OL1D 2PZ

Surveys of E
include:

Assessment (

Assessment of car handbrake adaptations

Assessment of high stools and chairs for use in the kitchen or at a high workbench by disabled people

Assessment of long handled reachers

Assessment of lower limb dressing aids

Assessment of manual bed aids

Assessment of seat belt adaptations

Assessment of self rise chairs and cushions

Assessment of supplementary car mirrors

Assessment of writing aids

Easy chairs for the arthritic

Food preparation aids for rheumatoid arthritis patients
— Screw top jars and bottle openers, can openers, vegetable peelers and stabilisers
— 2A Kitchen knives and scissors
— 2B Food choppers, graters and food processors
— 3 Whisks, blenders and electric mixers

Office seating for the arthritic and low back pain patient

Report of an assessment of irons and ironing boards.

REFERENCES

Brattstrom M 1987 Joint protection and rehabilitation in chronic rheumatic disorders. Wolfe Medical Publications, London

Dudley Hart F 1982 Overcoming arthritis. A guide to stiff and aching joints. Martin Dunitz, London

Lorig K, Fries J F 1983 The arthritis handbook: what you can do for your arthritis. Souvenir Press, London

Melvin J L 1989 Rheumatic disease in the adult and the child: occupational therapy and rehabilitation. F A Davis, Philadelphia

Rosenbaum M 1983 Perspectives on behavioural therapy in the eighties. Springer-Verlag, New York

Sands J D (ed) 1988 A guide to arthritis. Home health care. Wiley, New York

FURTHER READING

Ball G V, Koopman W J 1986 Clinical rheumatology. W B Saunders, London

Banwell B F, Gall V (eds) 1988 Physical therapy: management of arthritis. Churchill Livingstone, New York

Berry H, Hamilton E, Goodwill J (eds) 1983 Rheumatology and rehabilitation: diagnosis and management. Croom Helm, London

Bird H A, le Gallez P, Hill J 1985 Combined care of the rheumatic patient. Springer-Verlag, Berlin

Boscheinen Morris J, Davey V, Bruce Connolly V 1985 The hand: fundamentals of therapy. Butterworth, London

Cailliet R 1982 Hand pain and impairment. F A Davis, Philadelphia

Clarke A K 1987 Rehabilitation in rheumatology: the team approach. Martin Dunitz, London

Currey H L F 1983 Essentials of rheumatology. Pitman Books, London

Golding D N (ed) 1979 Concise management of the common rheumatic disorders. J Wright & Sons, Bristol

Maczka K 1990 Assessing physically disabled people at home. Chapman & Hall, London

Moll J M H 1983 Management of rheumatic disorders. Chapman & Hall, London

Moll J M H 1987 Rheumatology in clinical practice. Blackwell Scientific Publications, London

Panayi G S 1980 Essential rheumatology for nurses and therapist. Baillière Tindall, London

Robinson H S, Bashall D A 1962 Functional assessment. Canadian Journal of Occupational Therapy 29: 123

Cardiology

31

Introduction to coronary care

Jenny C. King and Maryanne Cook

THE HEART AND CIRCULATORY SYSTEM

The heart is a hollow muscular organ slightly bigger than a clenched fist, situated behind and to the left of the sternum. Its vital role is to pump blood throughout the circulatory system, delivering oxygen and nutrients to the organs and tissues, and removing waste products. Blood also has a transport function, carrying protective agents (such as leucocytes and antibodies) and hormones (such as adrenaline).

The muscular wall of the heart is called the myocardium. It has an outer cover, the pericardium, and an inner lining, the endocardium. The myocardium forms two major chambers called ventricles which can pump the blood without tiring. The right ventricle pumps blood to the lungs for the removal of carbon dioxide and for oxygenation. The left ventricle then pumps the oxygenated blood to the organs and tissues (Fig. 31.1). Each ventricle has an atrium from which it draws blood. The atria are separated from the ventricles by valves which open to let blood in and then close to prevent backflow. The valve between the right atrium and ventricle is called the tricuspid valve and the valve between the left atrium and ventricle the mitral valve. Similarly, there are valves at the outlet of the ventricles: the

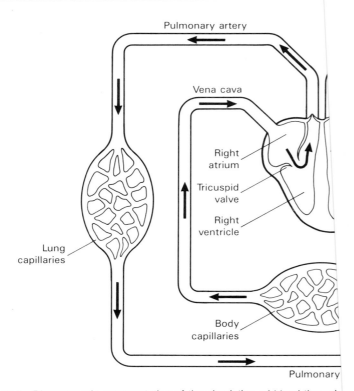

Pulmonary artery

Vena cava

Right atrium

Tricuspid valve

Right ventricle

Lung capillaries

Body capillaries

Pulmonary

Fig. 31.1 Diagrammatic representation of the circulation of blood through

pulmonary valve in the pulmonary trunk above the right ventricle to stop blood running back from the lungs, and the aortic valve between the left ventricle and the aorta (Fig. 31.2).

The myocardium, like all other living tissues, needs to be supplied with blood containing oxygen, nutrients and transported chemicals, and to have its waste products removed. This blood circulation comes from the two coronary arteries, the left main artery (with its left anterior descending and circumflex branches) and the right coronary artery. The blood flows through them in the diastolic pause between contractions of the heart.

CARDIAC CONTROL

The ability of the heart to adjust to the body's varying needs and to obtain its proper coronary flow is achieved through the regulatory systems which control the rate and force of the heart's pumping action, the blood pressure and the vari-

able resist
(periphera
beats is in
called the
the right
impulse w
electrical i
ventricles
of His) an
causes the
blood out

The peri
called syst
is known a
produces b
However, ii
the emotion
of discharg
pathetic ner
(hormones)
for example
fever, can al

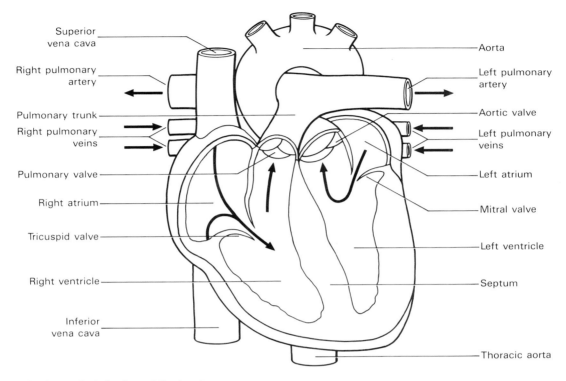

Fig. 31.2 Anatomical structure of the heart.

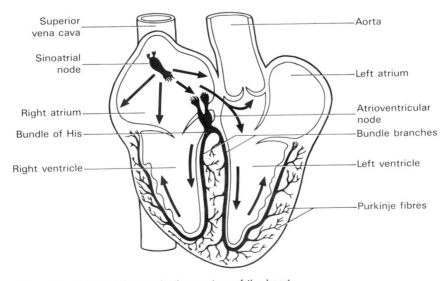

Fig. 31.3 Schematic representation of the conduction system of the heart.

Slowing of the heart is accomplished by reduction of stimulation and by direct parasympathetic nervous activity. If the parasympathetic system becomes overactive the heart rate can become slow enough to cause fainting.

Whereas adrenaline primarily speeds the heart rate (chronotropic action), the major effect of the other adrenal medullary hormone, noradrenaline, is to increase the force of the heart beat (inotropic action). The force of the heart beat also rises when there is an increased flow of blood into the ventricles: the increased return stretches the myocardial cells and stimulates a more forceful contraction. The blood pressure varies with the rate of the heart, the force of the heart beat, the volume of blood in the circulation and the resistance of the small peripheral blood vessels and tissue arterioles. It can fall with blood loss and vagal overactivity and rise with noradrenaline as in effort and anger.

Peripheral resistance refers to the state of tone in the small peripheral blood vessels and tissue arterioles. It provides a mechanism for controlling blood flow to the various tissues and organs, and ensures that the blood is appropriately supplied to the parts that need it, for example the gastrointestinal tract for digestion or the limb muscles for exercise. If there is an abnormally high state of tone, known as constriction, or if the blood vessel goes into spasm, a vital organ can be deprived of its proper blood supply.

The relationship between the cardiovascular system and the respiratory system is also an important regulator of the circulation. Failure of the heart and great overfilling of the veins can be caused when the carbon dioxide concentration of the blood is too high and the oxygen concentration too low. Conversely, overbreathing can cause an excess of adrenaline and great overactivity of the circulation, even during physical inactivity, and promote arterial constriction or spasm.

HEART DISORDERS

The disorders of the heart that reduce its capacity can be classified as structural (congenital and

acquire
two.

STRU

Cong

These
damage
man m
disorde
rowing
may be
atria an
valvar
remain
symptor
which n
Sometin
heart b
endocar
incompe

Some
surgical
two atri
Patent
tube des
open at
repairabl
of the b
counters
and take
lar septa
it to the
from cya
ing at t
to pass t
oxygenat

Other
transplan
means of

Acquir

These inc

- Inflam
  — of t
  — of t
  — of t

- Degenerative changes — for example alcoholic myopathy and vitamin deficiency (e.g. beri-beri)
- Valvar problems
  - inability of a valve to open properly (stenosis)
  - inability of a valve to close properly (incompetence)
- Cor pulmonale
  - failure of the heart from low oxygen and high carbon dioxide concentration as a result of chronic lung disease (such as emphysema)
- Hypertrophy
  - consequence of the need to pump against high resistance (pulmonary hypertension) or high pulmonary systemic resistance (systemic hypertension)
- Stiffness of the myocardium from fibrosis and scarring or tumour
- Ischaemic damage from acute coronary insufficiency (atheroma, spasm or clot) leading to stunning, infarction, hibernation, fibrosis or scarring and aneurysm of the myocardium
- Permanent rhythm disturbance
  - slower than normal (heart block)
  - faster than normal (e.g. atrial fibrillation from alcohol damage).

FUNCTIONAL DISORDERS

Transient disturbances of functions within the heart include:

- arrhythmia — loss of normal rhythm (for example 'extra' and 'dropped' beats from ectopic activity, irregularity from atrial fibrillation or regular fast beating from paroxysmal tachycardia)
- coronary artery spasm and constriction
- deconditioning (effort syndrome or Da Costa syndrome)
- side-effects of drugs such as betablockers and digitalis.

The diseased or disordered heart can more easily be loaded beyond its tolerance by factors such as:

- fever

- thyrotoxicosis
- anaemia
- extremes of temperature
- high humidity
- isometric effort and physical strain
- severe or prolonged emotional upset
- high altitude
- hyperventilation
- disorders of another system (e.g. a below-knee plaster could add 60% burden to the activities of daily living (ADL) and thereby increase the work of the heart).

SYMPTOMS OF CARDIAC DISORDER

Symptoms develop at varying rates; for example a woman with mitral stenosis might suffer mild symptoms for many years before a pregnancy led to atrial fibrillation and a sudden dramatic failure of the heart from the addition of arrhythmia to the organic valvar narrowing. In coronary heart disease, some people present with the sudden and dramatic symptoms of myocardial infarction, while others may describe a pattern of remission and recurrence of symptoms over a long period of time or suffer slowly progressive impairment.

When impairment is slow to develop, two groups of symptoms appear. The first group is caused by the heart failing to maintain an adequate supply of blood to the organs and tissues. It includes:

- abnormal fatigue and inability to sustain ADL
- weakness, fatigue and tiredness of the legs
- faintness when blood flow to the brain is inadequate for postural alterations (for example standing up quickly) and physical effort
- reduced renal function and fluid retention (oedema)
- cold hands and feet
- peripheral cyanosis (blue coloration of the hands, feet and in the cheekbones as in mitral disease).

The second group of symptoms occurs when the

heart cannot pump well enough to empty itself properly. It becomes overdistended and back pressure builds up. Symptoms may include:

- breathlessness on exertion
- pain or discomfort in the chest, throat or arms
- angina pectoris — this commonly occurs as a result of the work level outstripping the competence of the coronary system, but it can also be caused by constriction or spasm of a normal or near-normal coronary artery, tachycardia, bradycardia or anaemia
- breathlessness when lying flat — this is due to back pressure causing congestion of the lungs. It can easily be confused with asthma or hyperventilation
- disturbance of rhythm — the increase of back pressure in the atria may cause them to lose their normal rhythm and to flutter or fibrillate, or to undergo paroxysms of rapid beating. The ventricles often present extra beats (ectopics), and their fibrillating is a common cause of cardiac arrest.

INTERVENTION

Medical and surgical skills are aimed towards:

1. Allowing the heart to recover from the excessive demands put upon it by the use of rest, sedation and a modification of life-style
2. Reducing the volume of the blood and consequently the back pressure exerted upon the lungs by the use of drugs such as diuretics
3. Reducing the heart's demand for coronary blood flow by reducing nervous stimulation through beta blocking drugs
4. Improving coronary blood flow by the use of drugs such as coronary vasodilators and by surgery such as angioplasty and coronary artery bypass grafting
5. Treating clots by thrombolysis, or removing them by embolectomy
6. Opposing clot formation by the use of aspirin, heparin or anticoagulants.

PREV

In recer
in heal
public's
style fac
on the
primary
and sec
exist. U
have no
preventa
suffered
impairm
failure.
tinues to
for refe
Authorit
London

A com
must acc
disorders
Every in
and resp
psycholo
occupatic

OCCUF
CARDI
SURGE

Purpos

The purp
is:

- to achi
- to educ

Practic

The first
handicap
following

that might require special attention or additional resources for the success of rehabilitation:

- Functional capacity: ability to perform at the required level
- Social functioning: interaction with friends, family and the community
- Behavioural considerations: motivation, attitudes to self and others, expectations, a sense of autonomy and control, the ability to take responsibility for health
- Intellectual functioning: attention, mental alertness, memory recall and decision-making ability
- Emotional state: overall well-being and influences of anxiety, denial, depression, inadequacy, fear and rage
- Economic status and financial resources: for the duration of the illness and the possibility of unemployment.

The second step is agreement as to goals, and making practical and realistic plans for their achievement through occupation. If impairment of cardiovascular function prevents full restoration, the demands upon the heart must be reduced to an optimum level.

The third step is the provision by the occupational therapist of support, information and education as the plans to achieve goals are put into effect. Continuing assessment is necessary to review the success or failure of the plans and agreements.

The final step is the assessment of outcome, for quality assurance, audit and the improvement of practice.

CONCLUSION

The next two chapters address different aspects of the occupational therapist's role in cardiology. The first chapter considers those people who have functional disorders and organic impairment amenable to restoration and prevention through the process of rehabilitation. The second chapter describes the processes of adaptation and modification of the environment and lifestyle where the severity of the heart condition requires changes in the pattern of living.

It is advisable for the person to notify his insurance company of his illness, since failure of disclosure might be in breach of contract. There is usually no difficulty in maintaining cover, and most insurance companies will merely require a medical certificate stating the person is fit to drive.

Provided that the recovery has been uncomplicated, drivers are no longer required to inform the Driver and Vehicle Licensing Agency (DVLA, Swansea SA6 7JL) about the onset of a coronary condition. With regard to angina, driving should be stopped. The DVLA should be notified if the pain occurs during driving.

The law relating to professional drivers such as holders of heavy goods and public service vehicle licenses are stringent and licences will usually be withdrawn after myocardial infarction (Gold & Oliver 1990).

Going on holiday and flying

Many consider a holiday as a useful agent of recovery. Both the location and the type of holiday require consideration. The terrain should not be too hilly, nor the climate too hot or cold. The altitude should be below 6600 feet (2000 metres) in order to avoid hyperventilation, a physiological response to high altitude. Alcohol may be taken in moderation, but its effects will be increased by altitude and hyperventilation.

Travelling by coach or train is often less tiring than driving long distances. Car driving should be delegated or shared. Certainly the journey should be broken into easy stages and overnight stops planned to avoid fatigue.

Flying in a pressurised aircraft should not create any problems if the person is not put into anxiety or hyperventilation. The commonest hazards in practice are arriving late at the airport, carrying too much baggage (as judged by being unable to walk and talk at the same time), anxiety, hyperventilation (particularly during queuing), and loss of temper. Careful organisation is the best defence.

Airline staff are willing to do all they can to make the person's journey as hassle-free as possible, for example by providing wheel chair transport at airports if notice is given when the flight is booked. If the flight is made within 8 weeks of the myocardial infarction a certificate of fitness to fly from the family doctor might be demanded.

It is always wise to obtain adequate insurance cover against illness and cancellation and important to check the small print for exclusion criteria based on pre-existing illness, such as myocardial infarction.

Return to recreation and sport

Well-chosen physical exercise promotes a feeling of well-being, increases general mobility and stamina and serves to obtain the level of fitness required for reasonable recreation and sport.

For those who enjoy it, walking is a good choice of exercise. There is no 'correct' distance: it is what is right for each person on a given day that is important. The aim should be quietly to increase distance, promoting stamina rather than speed. Speed can be increased when distance has been achieved.

Common sense should prevail, for example:

• The person should not expect to be able to increase his ability if he neglects SABRES (Fig. 32.8)
• He should remember that there is always a return journey and not to wait for fatigue before deciding to turn back; 60–70% of what he thinks is his maximum — the level of activity that might be limited by symptoms — is about right. Observing the 60–70% rule also ensures that the person has enough reserves to cope with contingencies
• On a bad day, when he is grey and tired, or faced by adverse weather, he should accept the wisdom of backing off, that is staying in and resting or restricting exercise to a few gentle mobility exercises
• Exercise should not be taken after a large meal
• The vasoconstrictive effect of cold weather should be outwitted by warm clothing, breathing through a scarf and wearing gloves. A hat is important because about 25% of body heat is lost through the uncovered head.

Fitness training can be organised for those who

wish to return to sport. The warming-up phase must not be neglected.

The desirable training level of 60–70% of the person's maximum can be gauged from the pulse rate. A formula commonly used soon after myocardial infarction is to subtract 40 plus the person's age in years from 220. The result is called the 'target' or 'training heart rate'. This should be taken as the ceiling for 20 minutes of exercise 3 times per week (Nixon et al 1976b).

The safety and efficacy of this formula in an individual case should be checked by the doctor, who might exercise the person on a treadmill or bicycle ergometer to ensure that it does not create the risk of myocardial ischaemia.

Recreational activities or sports that put sudden severe demands upon the left ventricle, such as squash, should be discouraged, as well as those that depend upon isometric effort, particularly with exposure to cold, as in water-skiing. Going for 'the burn' as encouraged in some forms of aerobics is also inadvisable.

It is important for the person to be aware of the fact that competing with himself or with others is an invitation to defeat.

Those who enjoy sitting in the sauna should know that the heart rate will suddenly rise after a period and that they should move out before the onset of tachycardia.

Return to work

About 10 to 12 weeks from the time of the infarction or surgery most people begin to return to work.

Settling back into work is often accomplished more easily by returning to a three-day week, that is Mondays, Wednesdays and Fridays during the first month, keeping Tuesdays and Thursdays for rest and exercise, than by going back every day, even if the hours are reduced from 10 a.m. to 4 p.m.

Important influences upon the success of the return to work are the degree of control the person has over the effort of his work, and its effects upon the recreational, social and domestic needs of his life.

The place of work, the performance required,

the travelling entailed and the psychological factors involved must all be taken into account when the occupational therapist and the person plan strategies and consider whether the work itself, or the attitudes to it, might need modification.

Being compelled by the heart condition to change career, as in the case of heavy goods and public service vehicle drivers, puts a much heavier demand upon a person than going back to a familiar job with his old workmates and support groups.

FOLLOW-UP

It should be anticipated that at some point in his recovery the person will overtire himself, become anxious, hyperventilate and induce chest pain. When this occurs he should make an audit of his efficiency at SABRES (Fig. 32.8) by asking himself if he is:

- *sleeping* properly?
- too wound up (*aroused*) for his own good?
- *breathing* properly?
- keeping too busy, not balancing *rest* with *effort*, doing more than 60–70% maximum?
- feeling down and losing his *self-esteem* because he is taking on too much to be successful?

From the start of the illness to the time when she is no longer needed the occupational therapist should remain friendly and approachable, ready to give advice either formally by appointment or informally by telephone. This liaison provides not only continuous assessment and audit but also a valuable channel for communication between hospital, family doctor, community services and the person's domestic, social, recreational and work life. Through the occupational therapist's support and provision of information and education the individual learns how to recover healthy function and minimise the need for drugs and surgery.

Surgical intervention

It is taken as axiomatic that the occupational therapist is not asked to provide a programme of active rehabilitation where the person is in urgent need of surgical treatment. However, the occupational therapist might well be asked to act as the person's advocate and provide help where she can with such aspects of care as support, information, and assistance with relaxation and breathing techniques.

There are many cases where indications and contraindications for surgery are not clear cut. Here the occupational therapist might be asked to use the full remedial measures against the dynamic factors. If atherosclerotic factors precluded satisfactory progress most physicians recommend angiography to be carried out to help decision-making. This does not mean that the period of training with the occupational therapist is wasted: if surgery is recommended the surgeon is only too glad to find the person in a stable and orderly condition and well prepared to make a success of the operation. The informed person knows that coronary artery bypass grafting and angioplasty are not the cures for either atherosclerosis or the dynamic factors, and will continue to work with the occupational therapist after the operation.

CASE EXAMPLE 32.3

John, a 57-year-old clerical officer, had been tired and overstrained for two years. He had found that he was progressively limited in his capacity for daily activity and had begun to jettison activities such as his twice-weekly darts match. Before long he found he was falling asleep in front of the television. By day he would be brought to a standstill with discomfort in his chest on walking approximately half a mile or climbing a few flights of stairs, activities which formerly caused no difficulty.

On one especially busy day at work, when he had a deadline, John forced himself onwards, with the discomfort in his chest. As he ran up the stairs to the next floor he felt pain, diagnosed as angina by the company doctor, who referred him to the local cardiologist.

The cardiologist introduced John to the occupational therapist for assessment. She taught him about SABRES (Fig. 32.8) but this made little difference to his cardiac impairment. This was reported to the cardiologist, who then arranged for coronary arteriography and coronary artery bypass grafting, as the problem was found to be in the atheromatous occlusion of his coronary arteries. After surgery the occupational therapist restarted her work with him. She could now enable him to make a success of his recovery because the mechanical barrier, the rigid coronary arterial narrowings, had been bypassed.

CONCLUSION

Through the provision of support, information and guidance the occupational therapist helps the person to recover from the dynamic factors, to make the best possible adaptation to disease, and to choose realistic goals for rehabilitation. Psychological and social influences are interwoven intimately with physical factors, and none should be neglected.

The person needs to be taught to recognise and outwit the physical and psychosocial factors that led to his unhealthy state in the first place. The occupational therapist has an invaluable role to play in helping him to become more adept at recognising the signs of over-exertion and excessive arousal, and her continuing support will help him to adopt healthy patterns of behaviour so that he can resume his normal activities with confidence.

Together with other professionals, the occupational therapist must work cooperatively with the individual to overcome present hurdles and to prevent the recurrence of cardiovascular disorder in the future. The ultimate goal, of course, is for the individual to find an optimum level of independence and control in returning to normal life.

ACKNOWLEDGEMENT

I would like to thank Dr Peter Nixon FRCP, Consultant Cardiologist, Charing Cross Hospital, the Rayne Foundation and Smith's Charity for their support.

REFERENCES

Adam K, Oswald I 1984 Sleep helps healing. British Medical Journal 289: 1400–1401

Brindley D N, Rolland Y 1989 Possible connections between stress, diabetes, obesity, hypertension and altered lipoprotein metabolism that may result in atherosclerosis. Clinical Science 77: 453–461

Catford J, Parish R 1989 'Heartbeat Wales': new horizons for health promotion in the community — the philosophy and practice of Heartbeat Wales. In: Seedhouse D, Cribb A (eds) Changing ideas in health care. John Wiley, Chichester, ch 7, p 127–134

Dubos R 1980 Man adapting. Yale University Press, New Haven, p 256

Frankenhaeuser M 1986 A psychobiological framework for research on human stress and coping. In: Appley M H, Trumbull R (eds) Dynamics of stress. Plenum, New York, ch 6, p 101–113

Gold R, Oliver M 1990 Fitness to drive: updated guidance on cardiac conditions in holders of ordinary driving licences. Health Trends 22(1): 31–32

Henry J P 1983 Coronary heart disease and arousal of the adrenal cortical axis. In: Dembroski T M, Schmidt T H, Blumchen G (eds) Biobehavioral bases of coronary heart disease. Karger, Basel, ch 20, p 365–381

Henry J P 1986 Mechanisms by which stress can lead to coronary artery disease. Postgraduate Medical Journal 62: 687–693

King J C 1987 Coronary care. In: Turner A (ed) The practice of occupational therapy, 2nd edn. Churchill Livingstone, Edinburgh, ch 19, p 344–356

King J C 1988 Hyperventilation: a therapist's point of view. Journal of the Royal Society of Medicine 81: 532–536

King J C, Nixon P G F 1988 A system of cardiac rehabilitation: psychophysiological basis and practice. British Journal of Occupational Therapy 51: 378–384

Levine S A 1944 Some harmful effects of recumbency in the treatment of heart disease. Journal of the American Medical Association 126: 80

Levine S A, Lown B 1952 'Armchair' treatment of acute coronary thrombosis. Journal of the American Medical Association 148: 1365–1369

Nixon P G F 1973 Coronary heart disease and its emergencies. The Practitioner 35: 1–12

Nixon P G F 1976a The human function curve. The Practitioner 217: 765–769, 935–944

Nixon P G F, Carruthers M E, Taylor D J E, Bethell H J N, Grabau W 1976b British pilot study of exercise therapy: II patients with cardiovascular disease. British Journal of Sports Medicine 10: 54–61

Nixon P G F, Freeman L J 1988 The 'think test': a further technique to elicit hyperventilation. Journal of the Royal Society of Medicine 81: 277–79

Nixon P G F 1989 Human functions and the heart. In: Seedhouse D, Cribb A (eds) Changing ideas in health care. John Wiley, Chichester, ch 2: 31–65

FURTHER READING

Bloch G 1985 Body and self: elements of human biology, behavior and health. William Kaufmann, Los Altos

Buell J C, Eliot R S 1980 Psychological and behavioural influences in the pathogenesis of acquired cardiovascular disease. American Heart Journal 100: 723–740

Kagan A 1982 Introduction to the role of psychosocial stressors in ischaemic heart disease. In: Denolin H (ed) Psychological problems before and after myocardial infarction. Karger, Basel, ch 29; p 18–24

Lum L C 1976 The syndrome of habitual chronic hyperventilation. In: Hill O W (ed) Modern trends in psychosomatic medicine. Butterworths, London, vol 3: 196–230

Patel C 1987 Fighting heart disease. The British Holistic Medical Association, Dorling Kindersley, London

Sterling P, Eyer J 1988 Allostasis: a new paradigm to explain arousal pathology. In: Fisher S, Reason J (eds) Handbook of life stress, cognition and health. John Wiley, Chichester, pp 629–649

33

Chronic cardiac failure

Maryanne Cook

INTRODUCTION

The effects of chronic cardiac failure on a person and his family can be very dramatic and wide-reaching, involving major changes to life-style and routine. For many people 'old habits die hard', and for them it may be difficult to give up accustomed routines. However, it will be necessary for the individual, with the therapist's guidance, to examine his priorities and goals so that the demands of self-care, home-care, employment, leisure and family life can be brought into a healthy balance. Through her understanding of the nature of chronic heart disease and her careful assessment of the needs and limitations of the individual, the therapist can assist in the establishment of priorities for daily activity.

This chapter considers ways in which the occupational therapist can help the individual to manage his condition such that he is able to lead a full and satisfying life without over-taxing the diseased cardiovascular system. The basic principles of energy conservation and time management are set out, followed by specific suggestions for adaptations to the environment and to various activities. The impact of cardiac disease upon the individual's social and family life is also considered, together with the special needs of those who, as carers, must also adapt to the challenges and stresses of living with chronic heart disease.

HEART FAILURE

The various problems brought about by heart failure may depend on which side of the heart is affected. Heart failure can be classified into two types: left heart failure and right heart failure.

Left heart failure

In left heart failure the left ventricle becomes less able to perform adequately due to conditions such as hypertension (where a strain is put on the pump as too much blood returns too quickly to the left atrium), aortic valvular disease (backflow problems) or coronary artery disease (where the heart receives too little oxygen to function efficiently).

Symptoms of left heart failure include dyspnoea (or shortness of breath on exertion — SOBOE), sudden dyspnoea at night and cyanosis. Other diseases such as mitral valve disease (i.e. narrowing or stenosing of valves) can have further effects in reducing the efficiency of the left atrium. Also, with lack of use, the atruim wall atrophies, adding to the incompetence of the left side of the heart. Since the left side supplies freshly oxygenated blood to the body, other systems may be affected, causing additional medical problems such as renal failure, brain damage or transient ischaemic attack (TIA).

Right heart failure

This may occur as a result of left heart failure. It is characterised by general venous congestion occurring as a result of the inefficiency of the right side of the heart in dealing with blood returning from the body. In addition, any reduction in function of the right side of the heart leads to lack of efficiency in pumping blood out to the lungs for oxygenation. Pulmonary circulation is therefore affected, and this may lead to conditions such as emphysema and fibrosis of the lungs. Right ventricular failure may also result from the effort of forcing blood through obstructed or diseased pulmonary vessels (Sears 1979).

Early symptoms include cyanosis, coughing, haemoptysis and distended jugular veins. Later symptoms include enlarged liver and oedema. The resulting debilitation will be mainly due to symptoms such as lack of energy and stamina, fatigue, lightheadedness, disturbed sleep patterns and shortness of breath.

ROLE OF THE OCCUPATIONAL THERAPIST

The role of the occupational therapist is to facilitate management of the person's condition and to advise on environmental changes that may enhance this. She will be most likely to meet the person when he is at home and will normally work as part of a team, which may include social workers, home care managers, community physiotherapists, care attendants and the person's family. For individuals at home, her aim will be to reinforce any advice or guidelines offered during any spell of hospitalisation and to work towards an improved level of independence in the future. Everyone needs to be aware that, although the person may be less anxious at home than in hospital, he may still be concerned about the long-term consequences of leaving the protection of the health care environment. His situation needs to be monitored very carefully, with close liaison between all members of the team and the person to ensure a gradual upgrading of his level of activity.

GENERAL PRINCIPLES

Energy conservation and time management

For the individual with chronic heart failure, energy conservation entails the utilisation of techniques that ensure a measured level of activity without over-stressing the diseased heart and failing circulatory system. Performing activities whilst seated may help; a perching stool, for instance, might be used while cooking or ironing. Another example of energy conservation is to use a trolley to transport items around the house rather than carrying a tray. The work involved in tray carrying is static muscle work requiring high energy levels; pushing a trolley, however, provides the same service by use of isotonic muscle work, which is less demanding on the cardiovascular system. It is important to encourage the person to accept some help with 'heavier' tasks such as laundry, bedmaking or shopping. If the idea of getting help is presented in a sensitive way, it will not be seen as a sign of weakness, but as a sensible move to ensure that a certain level of activity is maintained. The amount of help given should be carefully assessed to prevent dependence whilst encouraging a gradual return to ADL; 'Little and Often' should be the person's motto in returning to activity without stress.

One of the main techniques that can be employed is time management, which can help to maximise the amount of activity the person can undertake. Advice can be given on adjustments to the daily life of the person and his family to allow activity and rest periods according to individual need. It is a good idea to set maximum activity times and spread these out during the day, without necessarily resorting to a strict minute-by-minute timetable. In this way, the person can gradually build up his tolerance and stamina for activity. It may be useful to keep a weekly chart or diary of activities, to reinforce timing of events and prevent over-commitment.

The following is an example of a daily schedule, allocating approximate times for regular activities:

- Morning
  - 1 hour: washing or taking bath/shower and getting dressed
  - $\frac{1}{2}$ hour: breakfast
  - $\frac{1}{2}$–1 hour: rest
  - 1 hour: medium-level activity such as a walk, some ironing or washing up breakfast and previous evening meal dishes
  - $\frac{1}{2}$ hour: rest
  - 1–2 hours: preparing and eating main mid-day meal and preparing light evening meal (perhaps with some help)

- Afternoon
  - 1–2 hours: rest
  - 1–2 hours: activity such as a walk, some local shopping, visiting or receiving visitors
- Evening
  - light evening meal followed by restful activity to relax before retiring (more stressful evening activities should be spread out through the week)

N.B 'Rest' does not necessarily mean sleep, but could take the form of relaxing with a book or the newspaper or seeing to some paperwork. A longer afternoon rest period in bed may suit some people, especially if their night sleep pattern is disturbed or shorter than usual.

Education

This is another major area where the occupational therapist will have a role. She will be involved in the following ways:

- *Establishing priorities.* The person will need help deciding which activities he will continue and which he will give up. The prospect of making such choices can be very daunting to someone who has always led a full and active life. It may be hard to give up the hustle and bustle of a busy schedule, particularly if to do so brings with it a sense of lessening status. A reduction in activity can be hard to accept, and needs careful handling with frank and honest discussion among all parties concerned.
- *Management of the condition.* Giving medical advice and prescribing medication is usually the responsibility of the general practitioner, but the person and his family may require additional information about coping with symptoms, and about supplementary treatments (such as relaxation techniques) or societies specialising in heart disease. As it is important for all concerned to be as well informed as possible, the occupational therapist should be prepared to give advice on local or national support agencies, to answer questions about the nature and treatment of the disease, and to respond to more general enquiries.

ASSESSMENT

The three main areas that need to be assessed by the occupational therapist concern function (self-care and home care), psychological well-being (cognitive and emotional) and life-style (employment and leisure). The aim of treatment will be either to return the person to as full a life as is feasible, or to make adjustments that will prevent recurrence of the acute cardiac state and reduce the symptoms of the chronic state. The final assessment and outcome, however, will vary with each individual according to his specific needs, wishes and level of ability.

Functional assessment and advice

Self-care

This is usually the main activity that a person wants to maintain control over. Cleanliness and hygiene are to be valued, but it should be remembered that individual standards are different and peoples' priorities vary. This area must be approached with sensitivity; the person's own priorities must be ascertained before any targets or goals can be set. However, in practice this may be difficult as feelings of general malaise and fatigue may lead to lack of self-awareness and neglect. Maintenance of good personal appearance will improve self-image and esteem, which will in turn help progress in other areas.

● *Washing*. The individual can minimise any breathlessness on exertion by remaining seated to wash, for example on the bed with a washbowl on a cantilever table along side, or on a perching stool beside the washbasin in the bathroom. In instances where the bath and basin are situated in close proximity, a bath board can be used as the seat.

● *Bathing*. This is a high-energy activity, requiring a degree of strength, balance, coordination and a tolerance to temperature change. The bathroom temperature should be warmer than normal to compensate for this, and the person encouraged to undress, bath, and dress again in the bathroom if space allows. If there is room for a chair or stool, or if a bath board is fitted, undressing, drying and dressing can be done whilst seated. The effort of washing in the bath can be reduced by using 'bubble bath' (without moisturiser or oil, to prevent slipping) or a liquid soap dispenser. Drying can be made easier by using a towelling robe rather than vigorously drying with towels.

However, most of the problems associated with bathing are related to difficulties in getting in and out of the bath (see p. 252). The following equipment may help in this regard (Fig. 33.1; see also Figs 29.6 and 35.5A):

— a bath board and seat with grab rails and non-slip mat for extra safety
— over-bath shower with or without bath board
— walk-in level floor shower used in conjunction with a seat
— Mangar/Aquajac/Bathability type bath board and seat combination.

The individual may also resort to the following strategies:

— having someone to assist, for example a relative, friend, neighbour, care attendant or a community care assistant arranged through the community nursing service
— not bathing at home at all, but having a wash-down and attending a day centre for a weekly assisted bath or going to a relative or friend with easier facilities.

● *Haircare*. This is an important activity that need not require much time or effort. Some suggestions are to keep an easy style, such as a short or 'permed' one, so that the hair can be washed separately or in the shower and left to dry. When professional hair care is required, some hairdressers will visit the home; alternatively, a visit to the hairdresser can be seen as a social event and included in the weekly activity plan.

● *Dressing*. If the time or energy needed by the person to dress himself is excessive, outweighing the advantage of being independent, help from a relative, care attendant or community care assistant may be appropriate. Advice can also be given about

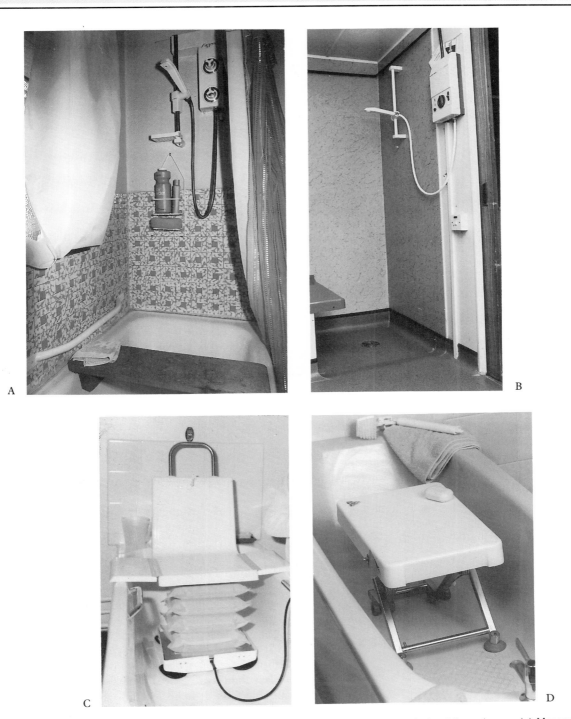

Fig. 33.1 Adaptations to the bath. (**a**) Over-bath shower with bath board. (**b**) Walk-in level floor shower. (**c**) Mangar bathlift. (**d**) Bathability bath seat. (Photographs (**a**)–(**b**) courtesy of Warwickshire County Council; photograph (**c**) courtesy of Mangar Aids Ltd; photograph (**d**) courtesy of Keep Able Ltd.)

which clothes to wear, such as those which are lightweight and easy to put on. Similarly, the individual needs to be reassured that it is not necessary to dress every day if he doesn't feel up to it. The person should dress seated if necessary, and wear as few garments as possible, for example a warm sweater rather than vest, shirt and pullover.

Home-care

- *Housework*. The traditional role of a housewife looking after her husband and family may be challenged by the effects of heart disease. If so, the person and her family need to understand that there is nothing wrong in making some adjustments to roles so that a spouse or carer assumes some responsibility for cooking and general housework. It is therefore important to tactfully check that carers have the skills and confidence to undertake all these new tasks. Priorities need to be established and, if required, domestic help (paid or otherwise) engaged. Mealtimes may have to be changed to when the person can cope best.

- *Kitchen work*. The kitchen should be arranged in a way that encourages energy conservation. Items required regularly (e.g. utensils, saucepans) should be placed to ensure the least number of trips across the kitchen. Everyday crockery and pans should be stored close to hand and everyday foods kept as close together as possible and in places which minimise bending, stooping, or stretching

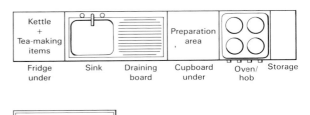

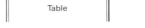

Fig. 33.3 An example of a linear layout kitchen.

(Fig. 33.2). Kitchens can be many shapes or sizes, with units placed in varying combinations, and this can complicate the task of reducing effort in kitchen activities. An example of a linear layout is shown in Figure 33.3. In a case such as this, items in regular use can be grouped together conveniently to prevent too many trips from one end to the other. If the milk is kept in the fridge then cups, coffee, tea, sugar and cutlery can be left ready on the worktop above along with the kettle. Similarly, saucepans and baking trays in regular use can be kept either under the cooker (if there is a storage area) or in the nearest available cupboard.

The layout of the kitchen area may not be easy to change, but there are some general principles that might be borne in mind when deciding where to position units and appliances if alterations are being made. The relative frequency of movements between fixed areas in the kitchen is shown in Figure 33.4. It can be seen that the most frequent trips are made between sink, cooker and preparation centre (Goldsmith 1984).

A perching stool may be used to prevent unnecessarily long standing times and may be moved easily around the kitchen to new work sites. Similarly, labour-saving devices such as food processors and microwaves can minimise effort. A larder or food store of tinned, dried or frozen food can be organised to ensure there is suitable food at hand for 'off-days'.

- *Shopping*. There are several alternatives to shopping trips that can reduce the effort required to acquire essential goods and services. Local shops are useful midway points for a walk

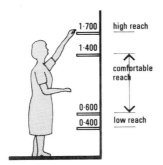

Fig. 33.2 Reach heights for elderly housewives. (From Goldsmith 1984, courtesy of RIBA Publications Ltd.)

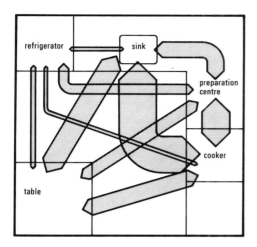

Fig. 33.4 Relative frequency of movements between fixed areas in the kitchen. (From Goldsmith 1984, courtesy of RIBA Publications Ltd.)

as part of an exercise programme, but there is the temptation of inducing too much effort by trying to carry items home on the return journey. Alternatives include:

—Home deliveries. Some shops offer a home delivery service, which means that goods can be ordered in the shop, or by telephone, and be delivered to the doorstep later in the day or week.
—Mobile shops. Although fewer in number these days, mobile shops still call in some areas. They usually sell mainly fruit and vegetables but these are the items that are bulky and heavy to carry.
—Catalogues. A wide variety of goods are now available by catalogue, for example shoes, clothes and household items. These can be ordered by telephone or post and returned if faulty or not suitable.
—Home help. Helpers can be employed either by the local social services department or privately. The service they offer usually includes shopping. Some home helps take the person to the shops or will do the shopping on his behalf (according to his wishes).

• *Laundry*. Washing machines and tumble driers (or use of a laundrette 'service wash')

greatly reduces the amount of time and effort required for the weekly wash. Washing and ironing can be kept to a minimum if leisure/track suits or clothes made from easy-care fabrics are worn. Alternatively, a home help may assist with laundering and ironing. Some areas offer a home collection laundry service which is particularly useful for bed linen and towels, which are heavy when wet and bulky to manage.

• *Cleaning*. Again, a home help may be available to assist with vacuuming, cleaning the kitchen and bathroom or dusting, but there will be activities that need doing in between, such as washing-up, bed-making and general tidying. These activities should be spread out during the day rather than compressed into one long session of housework.

• *Outdoor housework*. If the exterior of the house or garden falls into disrepair, this can cause worry and stress to the occupant. Windows must be clean, paintwork maintained and the garden kept tidy in order to protect the property. The occupant must understand, however, that it is more important to maintain his own standard of life than to worry what neighbours may think. Gardening may be carried out with the aid of tools that prevent stooping and kneeling. If possible, the help of another person (a neighbour, young relative or friend, or someone from a voluntary or private organisation) should be sought for heavy work such as digging, planting, and lawnmowing. In the long term, replacing annual plants and flowering borders with perennials, bushes and flowering shrubs will maintain colour in the garden while reducing work. For those reluctant to relinquish the pleasure of having bedding plants, hanging baskets, tubs or small raised beds may be substituted. To cut down on weeding the use of gravel, wood chips or ground-cover plants can be considered.

To minimise work even further, some areas of the garden may be paved or tiled, and then brightened up with tubs of flowers or shrubs. It may be possible for the individual to make an arrangement with someone who doesn't have a garden (or who would like to have a larger one) whereby that person would keep the garden tidy in exchange for produce or flowers.

● *Mobility.* General mobility of people with heart disease will vary tremendously. Some may manage at a level of activity close to that enjoyed previously, but many will be restricted in some areas. Stairs may be one area where help can be offered. An additional banister (see Fig. 35.5B), or in severe cases, a stair lift (particularly where the only toilet facilities are upstairs) may aid mobility within the home (Fig. 33.5). Failing this, a downstairs extension may be required for bathroom and bedroom facilities. Shopping and general outdoor exercise will be limited but the use of a wheelchair on these occasions may be helpful. An application for Mobility Allowance may be appropriate if walking is severely restricted and certain criteria are met. This money can then be used to buy or lease a car, electric wheelchair, or electric scooter (see p. 280).

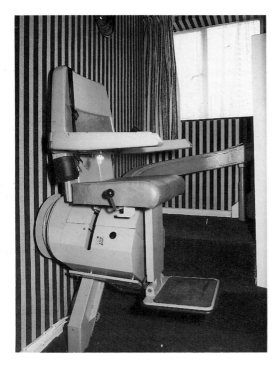

Fig. 33.5 An adaptation to aid mobility in the home: a stair lift. (Photograph courtesy of Warwickshire County Council.)

Psychological assessment and advice

The effects of an individual's chronic disease on his family can be devastating. Several problem areas may arise that require special intervention and a particularly caring attitude.

Relationships

A sense of rejection may occur between the individual and any of his closest contacts, particularly his spouse. This may not be an outright rejection but over-protection often presents itself as a convenient reason for lack of honesty, closeness or natural contact. The carer/spouse may need separate support from counselling or introduction to a support network or self-help group. Adequate information should be given to all concerned about the appropriate level of activity to be maintained in the individual to prevent the 'sick role' descending on the family, leading to isolation, depression and lack of motivation.

Feelings of fear and anxiety can only serve to exacerbate a situation already fraught with worries about health and perhaps finance. If these are apparent, they should be reduced as much as possible by putting such problems in perspective. The individual's fears may concern present issues (e.g. ability to cope with reduced function, lack of independence, or being a burden on the family) or the future prospects (e.g. of another attack or death). The occupational therapist must listen, encourage and allow the expression of feelings with the person and family concerned.

Sexuality is an area not readily discussed but tactful enquiries may bring a situation to light which can be helped. Over-protection is a common problem leading to lack of sexual activity for fear of harming the affected person or causing a heart attack. Uncertainties about abilities to satisfy each other or doubts about when to try can all add strain to a relationship, and an opportunity to voice these fears may be all that is necessary to get things going again. Fears of failure of frustration with the situation can be reduced by opening up the possibilities for constructive discussion and honesty.

An occupational therapist may or may not feel able to use her listening or counselling skills to the extent required to help with these sensitive issues. It will depend on her experience and knowledge of the particular concerns expressed. It is important to be aware that the following agencies are available if required (see also p. 789):

- Agencies involving other disciplines:
  — Psychological counselling service — this may be available at the local hospital or by referral from the General Practitioner
  — Specialist personnel in cardiac units
  — Sexual counsellors — e.g. Association to Aid the Sexual and Personal Relationships of People with a Disability (SPOD)
  — Social work service (where appropriate) to deal with any family problems or to clarify financial situations
  — RELATE (National Marriage Guidance).
- Self-help groups:
  — Self-help groups for sufferers and/or carers according to need. These groups usually provide contacts and exchange of information with people in similar situations.
  — Specific groups set up to provide information, advice and constructive ideas. These may be run on a course basis for a set number of sessions.
  — Local branch of Chest, Heart and Stroke Association (CHSA) for information and advice.

Life-style

As previously stated, the aim of occupational therapy is to assist the person to return to, or maintain, as full a life as possible. This is particularly relevant in areas of life-style such as employment or social and leisure activities. It is important to find out which activities the person was involved in before, as he may be able to return to them, even if in a slightly limited or altered capacity. Many sports and leisure activities can be done seated (for example, bowls, table tennis or darts) and some, such as gardening or athletics, can be modified to lessen exertion.

Employment

The reasons for working stretch far beyond the need for income. Going to work provides social contacts, status, self-esteem and job satisfaction. When a person has long-term sickness, it can be difficult for him to return to his job. If a person's health dictates a reduction in responsibility or work participation, it may still be possible for him to reduce stress levels whilst maintaining his position in the company. The amount of time spent at work is a great proportion of one's life, and can be sorely missed if it has to be given up. The occupational therapist may need to contact the employer and, along with the person carry out a job analysis to assess the demands of the job (physical, social and psychological) and possible ways of reducing effort. These may include returning to the same area but in a less demanding job, working part time, or moving to a new area of work.

If the job assessment shows that returning to or continuing work is not possible then other alternatives can be considered, such as:

- a complete career change if the person is young and fit enough
- retraining — in which case contact with the Disablement Resettlement Officer may be appropriate
- working from home
- early retirement.

If the person does not return to work at all, the occupational therapist can advise on the purposeful use of leisure time, such as attendance at day courses or involvement in voluntary organisations.

Social outings and entertaining

The relaxing, enjoyable, social side of life can be the first to suffer when illness such as heart failure affects the energy level and capacity for activity. When feeling generally unwell or less capable through weakness and fatigue, the person may find that the effort required to socialise becomes too much. Another reason for reduction in social contacts can be the fear of other peoples' reactions, and their natural tendency to over-protect and prevent full participation in activities. Maintenance of contacts with friends and neighbours can be a little easier, whereas meeting new acquaintances and explaining one's condition to them may be awkward at first. The more contacts that understand the situation, the easier future events will become. It is important to try to have some regular events that provide a focus for the week so that the person doesn't drift into lethargy or isolation, which can exacerbate the condition.

Hobbies

New hobbies can be taken up or old ones modified. Participation in clubs, committees and organisations of interest will provide a useful set of contacts and help to fill leisure time in a satisfying manner. Some examples of leisure activities, together with some ideas for their modifications are:

- *Gardening*. Planting seeds, taking cuttings, growing indoor plants and bulbs, and cultivating tray or bottle gardens can provide a rewarding alternative to the strenuous job of tending an allotment. Salad growing can be encouraged as an alternative to the heavy work involved in root vegetables.
- *Music*. Listening to music or playing a musical instrument individually or with a group can be a very relaxing and enjoyable pastime and can be modified according to the personal resources available.
- *Dance*. This can be good exercise whilst providing an opportunity for socialisation, and can also be modified to a suitable level according to physical tolerance; ballroom dancing, for instance, is less strenuous than styles such as Latin American or disco.
- *Pets*. Taking responsibility for a pet can ensure the owner also takes responsibility for himself. For example, shopping for the pet's food will entail an outing to get essential groceries, while walking a dog provides vital exercise. Choice of a new pet should obviously be made very carefully, taking into consideration food and care costs, the type of property that the individual lives in, and the space and exercise that the pet will need.
- *Sport*. Numerous sports activities provide a suitable level of exercise as well as social contacts, if carefully chosen and monitored for stress and energy levels. Competitive sports are generally more stressful and may be avoided, but activities such as swimming and walking can be retained as long as the length of time spent doing them is appropriate to the tolerance level of the person concerned.
- *Walking*. When walking any distance, it is good practice for the individual to take the local taxi firm's telephone number and money for the return journey, just in case it is needed. Other suggestions are to plan a route via friends' houses in case a rest-stop is needed, or to take transport out to a destination and walk back home. If a walk is planned along a bus route, then it is easy to catch a bus the rest of the way to the destination, or home. A voluntary driver or 'Dial-a-ride' scheme operates in some areas and can be used for lifts into shopping areas or to visit family and friends.
- *Arts*. Activities such as painting, writing, crafts, photography, video camera work and sewing can be rewarding and productive when more strenuous hobbies have to be given up. Attending at evening classes can be a good way of learning or continuing with an art subject, and of refreshing or renewing skills. As well as the social benefit of meeting with a group of people, there is the advantage of being able to continue the activity at home.
- *Holidays*. Restful periods away from home are essential to revitalise the carer/spouse as well as to provide a natural break from the usual routine. With regard to the person with heart disease, the only precaution is that air travel should not be undertaken until at least three months after an acute myocardial infarction, as the oxygen level in pressurised cabins is too low. Separate holidays for a couple may not seem appropriate, but a few days spent with another relative may give the spouse/carer a well-deserved break from the strain of being responsible for someone with a heart condition. The degree of stress felt by the carer cannot be overlooked and if respite care is tactfully put forward as a holiday for the patient, any fear of rejection or of being a burden can be reduced.

Travel agents will usually respond to any special needs if requested, and access guides are now available for many cities and towns and for other countries. These will give the reader an idea of places to stay that are accessible to wheelchairs, and therefore are likely to have few stairs, or a lift to rooms and services. The Winged Fellowship Trust provide a holiday service which includes the carer; their address, along with other ideas for holidays for people with particular needs can be found in *Holidays for the Physically Handicapped*, produced by RADAR, 25 Mortimer Street, London, W1N 8AB and available at major bookshops.

CONCLUSION

It is clear that chronic heart failure has the potential to affect virtually every aspect of an individual's life; the occupational therapist, therefore, has a challenging task before her in helping the individual to come to terms with his new limitations while maintaining an optimum level of independence. She must develop a sensitive understanding of the individual's particular needs and priorities in order to help him to set realistic goals and to view the future with optimism. This chapter has outlined the areas in which the occupational therapist will be able to offer practical advice and suggested various adaptive strategies that the the individual can apply to the activities of self- and home-care, employment, leisure, and family life. In addition to performing the roles of educator, assessor and advisor, the occupational therapist can provide vital liaison on the individual's behalf with family members, carers, and other members of the rehabilitation team. Further, her knowledge of other support agencies available within the community will open up additional channels of support and encouragement to individuals and families learning to cope with chronic cardiac disease.

USEFUL ADDRESSES

Bathability
Warren Hooker (UK) Ltd
Unit 20, Chalwyn Industrial Estate
St Clements Road
Parkstone, Poole
BH15 3PF

Coronary Prevention Group
60 Great Ormond Street
London
WC1N 3HR
071 833 3687

CHSA (Chest, Heart and Stroke Association)
123–127 White Cross
London EC1 78JJ
071 490 7999

Health Education Authority
Hamilton House
Mabledon
London WC1H 9TX
071 631 0930

Keep Able Ltd
Fleming Close
Park Farm
Wellingborough
Northants NN8 3UF

Mangar Bathlift
Mangar Aids Ltd
Presteigne Industrial Estate
Presteigne, Powys
0544 267674

RELATE (National Marriage Guidance)
Herbert Gray College
Little Church Street
Rugby CV21 3AP
0788 573241

SPOD (Association to Aid the Sexual and Personal Relationships of People with a Disability)
286 Camden Road
London N7 0VJ
071 607 8851

REFERENCES

Goldsmith S 1984 Designing for the disabled, 3rd edn.
   R.I.B.A. Publications Ltd, London
Sears W G, Winwood R S 1979 Medicine for nurses, 13th
   edn. Edward Arnold, London

FURTHER READING

Adapting kitchens for disabled people 1985 Kings Fund
Darnbrough A, Kinrade D 1981 Directory for the Disabled,
   published in association with R.A.D.A.R.
Equipment for the Disabled. Available from Mary
   Marlbrough Lodge, Nuffield Orthopaedic Centre,
   Headington, Oxford, OX3 7LP
Occupational Therapy Reference Book 1990, Parke Sutton
   Ltd., in association with the British Association of
   Occupational Therapists

34

Introduction to AIDS and cancer

Ann Turner

How can the light that burned so brightly
Suddenly burn so pale?

Mike Batt Bright Eyes

INTRODUCTION

A child born today can expect to live until the age of 70 if a boy and 76 if a girl. Although we all die, most of us in Western society do so at a relatively advanced age. Also, most of us are not bereaved until adult life and, therefore, for the majority, the experience of death is unfamiliar. When faced with death, therefore, be it one's own or that of another, many people have little relevant experience to bring to the event.

Whilst receiving a diagnosis of AIDS or cancer does not necessarily mean that one is going to die within a fixed time period, the experience of receiving such a diagnosis is inevitably followed by a period of shock, change and adjustment. Whilst for some the diagnosis may mean that death will definitely occur at an earlier than anticipated time, for others it begins a time of uncertainty about whether they will die early or be cured; many in the latter group fluctuate between believing one prognosis or the other.

This introduction, therefore, aims to look at the

needs of people who are aware that their lifetime may be limited and at what the occupational therapist may have to offer them during this period of serious and/or terminal illness.

THE EXPERIENCE OF LOSS

Throughout life we experience loss. Some losses may be of things that assume great importance to us — as in the loss of a job, the failure of a relationship, a divorce, the thwarting of an ambition because of exam failure, the loss of freedom through a prison sentence or of independence through the demands of a young family. Other losses may assume less importance, as in the case of a lost or stolen item, the loss of daily contact with a friend or community because of moving house, or the loss of money through a 'bad' buy. All these occasions involve change and adjustment to a new situation. The experience of loss brings with it memories of old ways and forces us to begin again with the new. It has many similarities to the situation in which the terminally ill person may find himself and, whilst he may have no direct experience of death, he may well benefit from the opportunity to draw similarities between previous occasions of loss and his present situation. To realise that he has experience, even if it is limited, of losing a familiar situation and having to face a new one may help him draw on past strategies and use them to his advantage.

A FRAMEWORK FOR THINKING

When working in such circumstances the occupational therapist should bear in mind that she, too, has needs. Work with the terminally ill can be emotionally draining and at times even harrowing. Whilst this work is not without its joys and successes the therapist must examine the effect it has on her and create a system of support for herself and any assistants. Similarly, because of the diverse and sometimes physically intangible nature of the work it is vital that the therapist base her intervention on sound theoretical principles. These will provide guidance for her own input and will help her, as part of a team, to recognise the boundaries within which she is functioning.

The occupational therapist's needs may be summarised as follows:

- A sound knowledge of the process of dying and bereavement and of the medical procedures and philosophical viewpoints applied by the unit in which she is working
- A support system for herself and other members of the occupational therapy team in which there is the opportunity to express feelings, discuss ideas and gain emotional support
- A knowledge of the services, both voluntary and statutory, which are available in her area
- Self-knowledge: an awareness of her own attitudes, prejudices, fears, strengths and weaknesses and a clear view of her own areas of experience and inexperience
- An ability to work as part of a team and to listen and communicate well within it
- A conceptual framework on which to base her intervention.

With regard to this last point, many 'conceptual frameworks' could be used (see Ch. 12). The therapist must use the framework that she is most comfortable with — the one that she feels is the most meaningful and that best meets the individual's needs. This framework should also fit in with the philosophy of the unit in which she is working. The Reed and Sanderson model (1980), for example, has provided a framework for one unit working in the field of HIV/AIDS (see Ch. 35). For others, models and theories postulated by theorists such as Mosey or Keilhofner may seem more appropriate. This introduction, however, will use Abraham Maslow's 'hierarchy of needs' as a basis for thinking. (This theory is also discussed in Ch. 3.)

MASLOW'S HIERARCHY OF NEEDS

In 1954 Abraham Maslow (1970) postulated a hierarchy of human needs that he felt motivated human action. He saw our basic needs as physiological ones and felt that these were the strongest drives that had to be satisfied before other, higher needs could be fulfilled (Fig. 34.1). Thus, higher needs, such as fulfilling one's am-

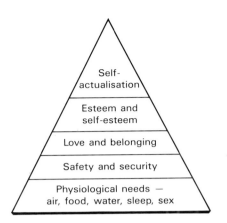

Fig. 34.1 Maslow's hierarchy of needs. (After Dworetzky 1988.)

bitions, can be interfered with by disturbances of needs at lower levels. For example, one might argue that a person is unlikely to feel good about himself (self-esteem) if he does not feel loved by others (love and belonging) or, on a more vernacular note, that he will not be able to concentrate on an exquisite piece of music at a concert if he needs to visit the toilet!

Whilst Maslow's hierarchy has been developed since it was first postulated, this chapter will use the five-layer version (Dworetzky 1988) as a basis for illustration. In using this version of the hierarchy as a background the occupational therapist could consider her intervention within the categories described below.

Physiological needs

These are seen as the strongest drives and the ones that need fulfilment before an individual can consider other needs. These physiological needs encompass basic bodily drives such as for food, drink, air, sleep and sex.

The ability to meet these independently is a basic need for most people. The loss of dignity and control which comes from being fed or taken to the toilet can increase feelings of helplessness and non-worth. The occupational therapist can discuss and explain methods, techniques and equipment available to enable the person to continue to look after himself for as long as is feasible. Establishing

priorities, however, is equally important in enabling both physical and emotional energy to be used most effectively. Looking at standards and discussing how some things cannot be as they have always been may help alleviate feelings of guilt about not coping. Thus, the role of the occupational therapist at this stage is to help the person accept that some tasks will gradually have to be given over to others. This may be done by encouraging the individual and his family to talk about and organise such tasks. By helping to create an environment that allows the person to conserve energy, the therapist helps to ensure that he will be able to care for his basic needs for as long as possible (see also Ch. 33). Assisting with mobility problems through the provision of a wheelchair, chair raises, grab rails, a hoist or other equipment or methods, will also help the person in this way.

People who experience difficulties with breathing and/or sleeping, as a direct result of their condition and/or because of increased anxiety related to their diagnosis, may benefit from the use of relaxation techniques, yoga, anxiety management skills or biofeedback techniques. People who are relaxed are more likely to be able to reduce or cope with pain, which is often a feature of cancer, and to fall asleep more easily.

Other physical symptoms such as vomiting and incontinence can cause great distress to both the individual and his carers and the persistence of these can make progress in other areas impossible. They also draw attention to the increasing lack of control the person has over his body. Whilst control of these symptoms is not within the province of the therapist, she may be involved in helping the person to cope practically with them by arranging for the provision of laundry services and/or equipment, and by offering the person and his carers the opportunity to express their feelings of guilt, disgust and despair.

Sexual needs may be overlooked, either because of embarrassment or, in times of high emotion and distress, a reduction of libido. The person (or his lover) may find his body unattractive because of the physical changes brought about by the illness. Expressions of love through hugs, kisses, presents and treats, rather than full sexual activity, can provide comfort and give great support. Morris (1980) found that a year after surgery 25% to 33% of women who had had a simple mastectomy still had sexual and relationship problems as well as disrupted working lives and depression. He found that people suffer high levels of anxiety and depression during their illness and that these feelings were often exacerbated by such treatment as chemotherapy and radiotherapy, which made them feel extremely ill, affecting their self-image, confidence and relationships. In other words, because of their illness and its treatment people found difficulty in fulfilling even their most basic needs; the fulfilment of higher needs was consequently disrupted.

Safety and security

According to Maslow, the need for safety and security is, after physiological needs, the strongest basic motivator. A feeling of safety derives from being able to operate from a firm, stable base. This can be seen both as a 'physical' base, e.g. one's familiar home and surroundings, as well as a 'psychological' base, that is, the security gained from familiar roles, routines and customs.

When familiar routines and roles are disrupted for whatever reason there is strain on both the individual and those close to him. Where illness causes an inability to perform familiar roles and routines, the person may need help to adjust to this changed situation (see Ch. 13). The occupational therapist's knowledge of the individual's roles and duties within the home and family, at work and during leisure time can provide a basis for helping to reduce stress. By assisting him to prioritise routines, in terms of role demands, perceived needs and leisure interests, she can help him retain those that are most important to him. Familiar routines such as coping with a daily shower and styling hair are vital to some people's self-image and form a high priority in their need to be 'themselves'. For others such activities may be less important; whilst walking the dog, attending church, writing letters, going to work or meeting friends for a drink on Friday night may be the ones they are reluctant to relinquish. By helping the individual to explore and prioritise his activities, relinquishing those

that are less personally important and maintaining the others for as long as possible, the occupational therapist can help him to feel 'himself' for as long as possible.

It is also important to discuss the need to give a structure to the days and weeks as old and familiar routines disappear. Loss of habits that give a framework to a person's life can leave him feeling unmotivated to undertake even the smallest task. Setting a focus to each day, be it a regular phonecall to a friend, a trip to the hairdresser or attending an evening class, helps the individual plan his time purposefully around the event and to look forward to it the next time. Establishing new routines in place of those which have gone can also bring satisfaction. The person may find that he now has time to do things that he could not do before, such as embarking on a course of study or attending local community meetings, and may gain much pleasure from doing so.

Maintaining his role, and role duties, also helps the person to retain a feeling of security in that which is familiar. Too much change all at once can increase anxiety and insecurity, especially when accompanied by changes to the body brought about by the condition. The individual needs to consider how he will maintain those roles that are most important to him. The therapist can help him reflect on how he sees his roles, and the importance they hold for him. His role as a breadwinner may assume great importance. Discussion with his employer as to the possibility of viable alternative arrangements, negotiations with his bank and other financial institutions to rationalise his financial situation and make practical arrangements, and making a will or paying off his mortgage may help him feel he has done the best for his dependents for the future.

In his role as a homemaker the person should be encouraged to learn energy-saving techniques, to continue to make decisions about how the home is run, and to relinquish those role duties that can be taken over by others.

The person may be tempted to relinquish social and leisure roles very early in order to continue with others that seem more important, but remaining in contact with friends and acquaintances will help him to keep as many aspects of his life intact as possible. If he is no longer able to bowl for his local cricket team or play a game of football, his knowledge and experience may be of use in keeping club books or helping to organise social events.

A person's role as a partner or lover should not be overlooked. His ability to give support and pleasure to his 'other half' remains important if the relationship is not to become one of constant giving by one person and receiving by the other. Whilst an imbalance of this kind may be to a certain extent inevitable during the course of the illness, the person's ability to fulfil the physical and emotional needs of his relationship is vital both to himself and to his partner. Similarly, the person may see his role as a parent as one of the most important parts of his life and he may need help in working through how he will remain 'a parent' to his children even though he can no longer do with them those things he has done before.

Safety, the other element of this level of Maslow's hierarchy, is also found in working within one's physical and emotional capacity. Safety within the home environment can be enhanced by adaptations and equipment and by working within one's physical capacity. Tricks of the trade are useful, and remembering well-tried advice (e.g. 'If the bedroom's a mess, make the bed; if the kitchen's a mess, wash up; if the garden's a mess, mow the lawn; If you're a mess, take a bath') can save much energy and worry.

In reflecting that safety stems, to an extent, from remaining in control it is clear that the individual may need help to accept the changes that are happening to him. He should be encouraged not to pretend that nothing has happened, or that nothing will change, but should address these changes and make positive decisions *around* them, rather than reluctant changes *because* of them.

Love and belonging

In Maslow's view, when the two previous basic needs are satisfied, the need for love, affection and belonging becomes the strongest drive. A person will feel the need to be part of a group or family and, without this, will feel lonely, rootless and ostracised. He may also feel an especial need to regain or strengthen ties with a wider group — his home town and old school friends for example, if he has moved away from these, or his religious, cultural or ethnic roots if he is apart from them.

All human beings have a need to love and be loved and to belong within a family and social group, and many anxieties and sadnesses can be created for an individual and his family when they fear they will lose this love.

People also have the need to actively 'let go', to say goodbye and to 'put their house in order' when faced with the possibility that life will not continue as anticipated. Much anxiety can be reduced by sorting out what will happen and how things will change. Putting one's house in order may mean different things to different people. Some may need help and information to make a will; others may wish to discuss their faith and the afterlife if this is important to them. To be able to teach carers new skills and to watch these being acquired can bring comfort during this period of letting go and may also lessen guilt and help the person to relinquish his roles more positively.

Some people may need encouragement to seek help for problems they cannot overcome themselves. For example, a man relinquishing his role as a father, breadwinner and husband may feel enormous guilt at the stress and burden he is causing his partner, and despair at not seeing his children grow up. The opportunity to express these feelings along with other deep emotions may help him let go of some of the 'emotional luggage' which he might feel is overwhelming him at times. The inability to express fears, either because of concern for the worry and distress this may cause his family, or because such fears may betray weakness or seem 'trivial', can greatly hinder communication between loved ones at a time when this is extremely important. Fears often revolve around the unknown and may relate to the process of dying or of losing one's identity and body image as the illness progresses. The individual may also have fears of loneliness, pain, suffering, loss of dignity and self-control, and, as his illness progresses and his world diminishes, he may fear isolation and rejection as he becomes physically and emotionally less able (Fig. 34.2).

'Cones of Awareness'

How the dying person's view of the world may change

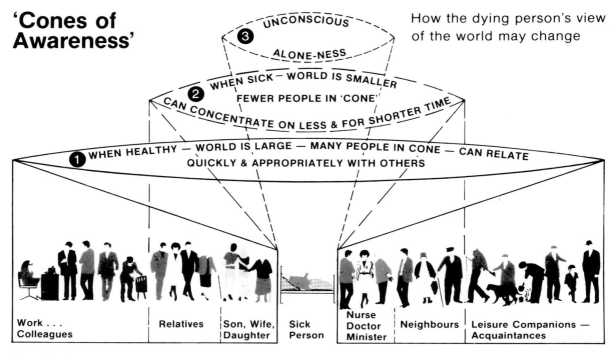

Fig. 34.2 Cones of awareness. How a person's view of the world changes as his condition deteriorates. (Reproduced from Ainsworth-Smith & Speck 1982 by kind permission of SPCK, London.)

The opportunity and encouragement to express these fears can help reduce the person's anxieties about them. He may need 'permission' to be frightened and sad. To facilitate communication, partners and families need to make conscious opportunities to talk. Wining and dining with each other, going for walks together, reviewing family albums, reminiscing on anniversaries, taking 'away-days' and second honeymoons may all be ways in which these opportunities can be created. The occupational therapist may encourage the person's expression of feelings through the use of reminiscence, drama, and other creative and expressive techniques. Education and understanding of the processes of bereavement and dying and an understanding of the disease and treatment processes and their consequences can help reduce fear of the unknown.

Anticipatory grief, which follows from the awareness of what is to come, affords the individual and his family the opportunity to reminisce on both good and bad aspects of the past, to 'bury the hatchet' or 'clear the air' if need be, and to express disappointment about what will not be. Garfield (1980) and Worden (1986) consider that gradual loss is easier for relatives to accept than sudden bereavement. However, such a process can cause problems if the family or individual withdraw from one another in anticipation of the event. The maximum period during which the anticipation of loss may have some benefit is seen as six months; after this time problems such as withdrawal begin to occur.

Making the most of the present with those he loves, within the circles to which he belongs, should be a goal for the person at this time. Where changes and illness bring unsolvable problems, seeking a viable, albeit imperfect, alternative rather than dwelling on the unattainable will help reduce stress and enhance a feeling of belonging and caring.

Esteem and self-esteem

All people, according to Maslow, have a need or desire for a stable, firmly based and (usually) high evaluation of themselves. This need is, first, a desire for achievement, competence, independence and freedom and, secondly, a desire for status, recognition and dignity. Those who satisfy their self-esteem needs feel confident and useful. These positive feelings are of particular importance to a person who is terminally ill in order that he can see personal purpose and worth in his remaining life. When such needs are thwarted, feelings of inferiority and helplessness result; this will particularly impede the person's ability to cope with his condition and its often unpleasant side effects.

Loss of normal appearance and familiar bodily functions can lead to diminishing self-esteem, loss of ability, energy and roles, and increased feelings of helplessness and uselessness.

The individual should be encouraged to pursue activities and goals that help him to feel more positive about himself. Opportunities to 'give' to others, especially through articles related to the person himself, will help him feel that something of himself can still give lasting pleasure to others. Creating a life history album for children or grandchildren, researching and producing an illustrated family tree, passing on a skill, growing a cutting from a prized plant, or making a gift of home-made preserves, wine or confectionery can give the person a long- or short-term project which will result in an end product that he feels is very much part of himself.

The individual should be encouraged to continue to make decisions and to be in control. He should be listened to and consulted and should not be made to feel that he is being 'written off' because he is no longer physically able to carry decisions through. Taking part in everyday decisions as he has always done — for example: what to eat for lunch, and when and where to eat it; what to watch on television; whether to turn on the central heating; what vegetables to plant in the allotment — is all-important in maintaining one's self-worth. Being involved in long-term decisions that will affect events in the future is equally im-

portant. Which model of car to buy, which wallpaper to use, and whether or not to have the house painted outside this year or to wait until next year are decisions for which the person's experience, opinion and knowledge can still be sought.

Help with improving or maintaining personal appearance is also important, as is support in retaining special skills which particularly reflect the individual's self-image. If a person has always enjoyed and been good at playing the piano or taking photograghs, for example, continuing these skills for as long as possible will help him feel good about himself.

Self-actualisation

Maslow (1970) describes self-actualisation as 'a tendency toward fulfilment, toward actualisation, toward the maintenance and enhancement of the organism'. Self-actualisation entails developing one's potential to the fullest. It involves the quest to do what one is fitted for. Maslow writes:

> A musician must make music, an artist must paint, a poet must write, if he is to be ultimately at peace with himself. What a man *can* be, he *must* be. He must be true to his own nature.

As this is the highest level of the hierarchy, Maslow considers it to be somewhat fragile and easily interfered with by lower needs. He also describes the experience of 'transient self-actualisation' which, he considers, is felt by many people during 'peak experiences' — times of happiness and fulfilment that may occur in a variety of contexts. Transient self-actualisation may indeed be the state that a terminally ill person should seek if true self-actualisation eludes him.

According to Owens and Naylor (1989), coming to terms with oneself and 'getting on with living' are two gains that the terminally ill person might derive from his situation.

The ability to retain control of one's physical self for as long as possible has been discussed earlier. Remaining one's 'own person' emotionally stems from self-knowledge and self-esteem and a positive attitude to the time ahead.

'Getting on with living', therefore, reflects the

ability to express and pursue one's own hopes, dreams and ambitions in accordance with this self-knowledge. Long-standing ambitions may now be realised, past dreams fulfilled or hopes satisfied. The chance to carry out activities that satisfy the soul, spirit and emotions can help the person gain joy and peace. He should be encouraged to use his time in a way that is positive and meaningful to him — doing what he wants to do, rather than what his roles and duties have compelled him to, enjoying being lazy, or keeping busy in activities that bring personal pleasure and have special significance. Whilst some people seem to 'fulfil a mission' by raising money for special medical equipment, visiting Lourdes or writing a book, others talk of fulfilling ambitions such as learning to ride a horse, travelling in a helicopter, visiting South America or undertaking a course of study.

For some, self-actualisation comes on a more modest scale. By continuing with or restarting activities that make life meaningful, the individual can continue to live his life positively rather than 'wait for death', and this he should be encouraged and helped to do in the most practical and feasible ways possible.

The therapist must be aware, however, of the pitfalls involved in encouraging the person to set goals that he may not be able to achieve, either because they are beyond his physical, financial or emotional means or because his condition is deteriorating to the point where he can no longer pursue them. It is important to consider the person's risk of failure against his right to choose his goals and his right to fail to achieve them.

CONCLUSION

The therapist working with people whose life span may be shortened needs to have a clear theoretical framework upon which to base her intervention. Many frameworks may be considered and this chapter has discussed how Maslow's hierarchy of needs can be used.

Whilst working with this, or any other, theoretical framework the therapist must be aware that people will not conveniently fit within it in the order in which it is discussed. Neither, indeed, does everybody the therapist works with require help in all, or any, of the stages mentioned. Frameworks, therefore, must be used as a guide to thinking rather than as fool-proof recipes for intervention.

This chapter has also discussed how the therapist herself will need support when working in this field and how the family of the individual forms an integral part of the work with that person.

ACKNOWLEDGEMENT

My thanks are extended to Dr Marie Midgley for her criticisms and to Chris Maddison, DipCOT, whose finalist paper on the role of the occupational therapist working with terminally ill people gave impetus to the structure of this chapter.

REFERENCES

Ainsworth-Smith I, Speck P 1982 Letting go. SPCK, London

Dworetzky J P 1988 Psychology, 3rd edn. West Publishing, St Paul

Garfield C A 1980 Emotional aspects of death and dying. In: Twycross R G, Ventrafridda V (eds) The continuing care of terminal cancer patients. Pergamon Press, Oxford, pp 43–56

Maslow A H 1970 Motivation and personality, 2nd edn. Harper & Row, New York

Morris T 1979 Psychological adjustment to mastectomy. Cancer Treatment Review 6: 41–6

Reed K, Sanderson S 1980 Concepts of occupational therapy. Williams & Wilkins, Baltimore

Owens R G, Naylor F 1989 Living with the dying. Thorsons, Wellingborough

Worden I W 1986 Grief counselling and grief therapy. Tavistock Publications, London

FURTHER READING

Broome A K 1989 Health Psychology. Chapman & Hall, London

Griffiths D 1981 Psychology and medicine. British Psychological Society and Macmillan Press, London

Hinton J 1982 Dying. Pelican, Harmondsworth

Kubler-Ross E 1970 On death and dying. Tavistock, London

35

HIV disease and AIDS

Louise Cusack and Louise Phillips

INTRODUCTION

By the end of September 1989 the cumulative total of cases of acquired immune deficiency syndrome (AIDS) in the UK was 2649, with 1388 deaths. There were 11 218 reportings of Human Immunodeficiency Virus (HIV) (Lancet 1989). There may be many more unknown and non-reported cases.

AIDS was first recognised in 1981 and brought to attention in Los Angeles, California when 5 men were admitted to hospital with an unusual form of pneumonia, known as *Pneumocystis carinii* pneumonia (PCP). This had previously been seen only in patients with severe combined immune deficiency syndrome (SCID), which had affected kidney, heart and liver transplant patients, leukaemia sufferers and persons receiving chemotherapy. At the same time, in New York, there was a further report of Kaposi's sarcoma (KS), a malignant skin lesion rarely seen in the United States. The only link between these reports was the fact that the people affected had a marked impairment of the cellular immune response (Miller et al, 1986).

By 1981, all were reported to have 'related immunodeficiency' due to an unknown cause. The condition was characterised by the occurrence of unusual infections not normally seen in previously healthy individuals. The condition was called AIDS. It is now known to be caused by a virus, which was identified in 1983 by Montagmer and colleagues at the Pasteur Institute in Paris, France.

The virus has been given various names, including Human T-cell Lymphotrophic Virus Type III by the Americans and Lymphadenopathy Associated Virus by the French, but is now universally known as Human Immunodeficiency Virus (HIV). It is transmitted through blood or blood products.

The first death caused by AIDS in the United Kingdom occurred in 1981 at a London teaching hospital. In 1982, in Britain, a surveillance scheme was set up to moniter AIDS based on reports by genitourinary physicians, the incidence of opportunistic infections and death certifications of AIDS and KS (Daniels 1987).

Rapid research, study and surveillance has meant that we have learnt much about the virus in a very short space of time, particularly in relation to immunology, virology, venereology and the clinical management of persons with HIV infection and AIDS.

The management of individuals' psychological well-being has also gone through rapid reappraisal. Counselling and educational services, in a still somewhat sensitive and stigmatised area, have been set up.

AIDS has come to be recognised as one of the century's major threats to public health in this country. In early 1985 the British Government took measures to try to stop the spread of AIDS and began to screen all blood donations for HIV antibodies. In January 1987 a £20 million publicity campaign was introduced on television, in cinemas, and through other media. As part of the campaign, information leaflets were sent to 23 million households.

In this chapter, the transmission, clinical manifestations and psychosocial implications of HIV disease and AIDS are discussed. The psychological impact of HIV antibody testing and of a positive diagnosis of AIDS is then examined. Individuals found to have AIDS are likely to undergo a process of psychological adjustment to the loss of their former health and life-style (and indeed to the imminence of death) that mirrors the stages of grief described by Parkes (1972). The stages in this process are described, along with the supportive role that can be adopted by the occupational therapist in helping the individual and those close to him to come to terms with feelings of helplessness and grief.

The 'Human Occupation Model' constructed by Reed and Sanderson (1988) is then presented as a useful framework for the occupational therapist's work with individuals with AIDS or HIV disease. Following this model, the therapist can assess the evolving practical and social needs of each person as he carries out occupations of self-maintenance, productivity and leisure. The motor, sensory, cognitive, intrapersonal and interpersonal skills needed by the individual in everyday life are considered, together with interventions on the part of the occupational therapist which will help the person to retain maximum independence and an optimum quality of life as the disease progresses. Throughout the chapter, the ongoing nature of the occupational therapist's involvment is stressed, along with her importance as the individual's advocate, who provides vital liaison on his behalf with various professionals, support groups, family members and friends.

THE AIDS EPIDEMIC AND HIV INFECTION

WHAT IS AIDS?

AIDS is the acronym for acquired immune deficiency syndrome. A person who contracts the Human Immunodeficiency Virus (HIV) is known as HIV antibody positive. While antibodies normally protect a person against invading pathogens, this is not so in HIV disease and AIDS. It is believed that infection, when acquired, persists for life and that infected persons remain potentially infectious to others (Fig. 35.1).

It is important to realise that many people with HIV infection are symptomless: one of the features of the condition is that people may remain perfectly fit for many years, even though infected.

HOW IS HIV TRANSMITTED?

Despite the inexorable spread of the HIV infection and AIDS globally, the three main routes of transmission described below remain the only ones demonstrated to be important. (See Fig. 35.2.)

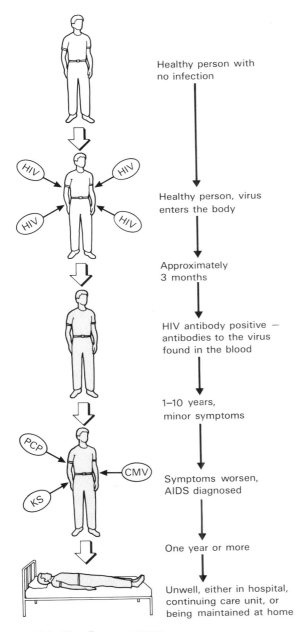

Fig. 35.1 The disease process.

Healthy person with no infection

↓

Healthy person, virus enters the body

Approximately 3 months

↓

HIV antibody positive — antibodies to the virus found in the blood

↓

1–10 years, minor symptoms

↓

Symptoms worsen, AIDS diagnosed

↓

One year or more

↓

Unwell, either in hospital, continuing care unit, or being maintained at home

Known routes of transmission

- *Inoculation of blood.* This includes:
  - transfusion of blood and blood products
  - needle sharing among drug users
  - injection with unsterile needles
- *Sexual*
  - homosexual, between gay men
  - heterosexual, from men to women and vice versa
- *Perinatal.* This may be:
  - intrauterine
  - peripartum.

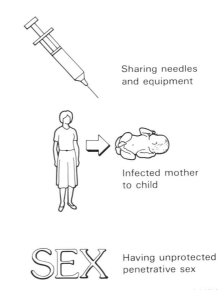

Sharing needles and equipment

Infected mother to child

SEX Having unprotected penetrative sex

Fig. 35.2 Known routes of transmission of HIV infection.

Routes investigated and not shown to be involved in transmission include:

- close personal contact
- household environment, e.g. laundry
- health care work without exposure to blood
- insects.

CLINICAL MANIFESTATIONS OF HIV DISEASE

While it is but a few years since the causal agent

of AIDS — the Human Immunodeficiency Virus — was isolated, an enormous amount is known about it. However, our knowledge is far from complete and new manifestations of HIV infection and AIDS are constantly being recognised. It is beyond the scope of this section to describe all but the most common, and further information can be obtained elsewhere (Adler 1987).

PGL: persistent generalised lymphadenopathy

Presenting as enlarged glands due to no known cause, this condition is a sign of relatively early HIV infection. Usually this is associated with tiredness and symptoms are intermittent.

ARC: AIDS-related complex

AIDS-related complex represents in people a moderate impediment of immune function and results in many common but easily treatable opportunistic infections. ARC is more serious than PGL but not as serious as AIDS.

AIDS

This is the most serious manifestation of HIV infection and represents a severe impairment of the cellular immune system, leaving the body vulnerable to multiple opportunistic infections and enabling tumours to proliferate. Certain specific tumours and infections confer on people a diagnosis of AIDS. In Great Britain two thirds of people found to have AIDS have either PCP or KS — these two diagnoses are the commonest ones which result in a diagnosis of AIDS (Office of Health Economics 1988).

PROGNOSIS

Survival figures of persons with AIDS present a gloomy picture. The survival of these persons largely depends on the presenting diagnosis. Survival ranges from 1 year or more for those with PCP and up to 21 months for people with KS.

With the advent of specific antiviral treatment (AZT/Zidovudine) and with increasing clinical experience of this polymorphous condition, survival rates have undoubtedly improved, though to what extent is not known.

HIV and the nervous system

Finally, HIV is thought to be neurotropic: that is, it actively seeks out, infects, and ultimately impairs the intricate workings of the nervous system. There is evidence that central nervous system involvement is common and presents AIDS care with the ultimate challenge. Only further research and study can clarify this aspect of AIDS. The effects of HIV brain disease are often debilitating and progressive, offering little or no hope of amelioration.

PSYCHOSOCIAL IMPLICATIONS OF AIDS

Death, dying, loss, bereavement, sexuality, homosexuality, drug addiction and prostitution are all terms that are accompanied with stigma in our society today. People try to change the subject very quickly when these areas are mentioned, or avoid answering questions altogether. The subject of AIDS envelops all these terms.

If occupational therapists are to attempt to meet the needs of someone with HIV infection, or indeed AIDS, they first must have a sound basic knowledge of the syndrome and its associated medical effects. As carers we are dealing mainly with a well-informed group of young people; therefore, the therapist's feelings, attitudes and prejudices may be challenged. The therapist must therefore examine these feelings and begin to come to terms with her own sexuality, 'hang ups' and ambivalence.

PSYCHOLOGICAL FACTORS RELATED TO HIV ANTIBODY TESTING

A person's psychological adjustment to being informed of his antibody status should be dealt with even before the HIV antibody test is taken.

A person should receive 'pre-test counselling' covering a wide range of issues. The pre-test counsellor must first highlight the total confidentiality of testing. The counselling relationship must offer such confidentiality as well, if a rapport is to be built and very personal details shared, aired and addressed.

An explanation of the HIV antibody test must be given, with particular reference to: the difference between HIV and AIDS; what the test will indicate (this being the presence of or lack of antibodies to the virus in the blood); and the fact that antibodies may take up to a year after infection to show. The test which is most commonly used is the enzyme-linked immunosorbent assay (ELISA). Other techniques may be radio immunoassays (RIA), membrane immunofluorescence, fixed-cell immunofluorescence and western blotting.

People need to be informed of how the virus is transmitted and made aware of 'risk' behaviour. Regardless of a positive or negative test result, people may need to change their behaviour and be given guidance on 'safer sex'.

The consequences of seeking an HIV antibody test may need to be considered when life insurance and a mortgage are a possibility for the future. Having the test will be important when facing a major decision; therefore, support networks need to be established early on. The result may take up to two weeks and it is standard practice for it not to be given over the phone. It would be up to the person to return to the clinic for the result.

On a negative result it may be necessary for retesting to be carried out in 3 months, and for clear guidance on safer sex and safer drug usage, if appropriate, to be given. If a result is positive the result needs to be communicated clearly, allowing time for the result to be digested and absorbed. The most important thing that a counsellor may offer at this stage is time: time for the person to express his feelings. It is extremely important to check the support networks again and find out who the person is going to confide in and who would immediately readily support him. It may be necessary to give telephone numbers of support agencies and organisations that assist newly diagnosed HIV persons. Quite often it is necessary to follow up a newly diagnosed person, as the reaction of shock to such news may be delayed. Issues relating to work, diet, alcohol, smoking, medical follow-up and treatments can be explored when felt appropriate.

If a person has continuing difficulty with coming to terms with his diagnosis, referral to a social worker or other health care worker for ongoing support should be made possible. This support might include counselling or training in areas such as anxiety management, relaxation, life skills and social integration.

When a person is aware of his HIV status he should be offered regular medical health checks on an outpatient basis and encouraged to have a general practitioner (GP) to assist in his health care. Regular follow-ups should monitor psychological factors such as mood, appetite, sexual libido, self-esteem, guilt, anxiety and fatigue as well as medical issues. Abnormal reactions have been found to be more common in people at the extremes of the age range, in those lacking a partner, and in those living in a rural environment (Seidlot 1989).

At present there is no evidence for severe and persistent psychological problems at the time of testing. The large majority of problems are dealt with successfully by doctors and counsellors and only a minority of persons appear to develop disorders which require referral to mental health specialists (Catalan 1988).

PSYCHOLOGICAL IMPLICATIONS OF AN AIDS DIAGNOSIS

Bereavement and grief

Bereavement is the involuntary loss of someone or something that is precious to the individual. Grief is the emotion precipitated by that loss, and mourning is the process by which grief is coped with (see p. 43). Parkes (1972) summarises the conventional stages of mourning as:

- shock
- denial, self-isolation
- guilt, anger, fear
- new life-style, healthier living
- altruism

- sadness
- continued depression and/or anxiety
- acceptance
- resignation.

He compares these stages with those typical of the mourning process in HIV disease, which he identifies as:

- alarm
- realisation
- anger, guilt
- search for health
- identity with loss
- feeling of loss
- pathological grief
- acceptance
- resignation.

It is a misconception that bereavement is experienced only by the family and friends of a person when he has died. With HIV and AIDS, bereavement begins as soon as diagnosis is made. A person given a positive HIV antibody status experiences a sense of great loss of life, control, health, relationships, sexuality, job, income, support, friends and life-expectancy. This list is by no means complete. Other areas and aspects may become evident once the therapist works with and gets to know the person.

Around 60% of people with AIDS become aware of their AIDS diagnosis after admission to hospital following a period of ill health. Having an AIDS diagnosis, as one would expect, presents a profound set of psychosocial difficulties which have to be dealt with and reviewed by a person and his partner, relatives, friends and colleagues. It demands straight talking and 'no-jargon' explanations by the health care team, who, at the same time, must show sensitivity and care. As yet there is no cure for AIDS; therefore, having an AIDS diagnosis may present the person with the realisation of what lies ahead. Commonly, the person has had a partner or friends who have died of an AIDS-related illness, or been in an environment where others are very ill with AIDS. A person may experience extreme isolation and stigmatisation because of the disease and its implications. His self-esteem may completely collapse under the strain of rejection by family and friends and their complete denial of the issues raised.

Quite often, this is the first time the person has revealed his homosexuality to friends and family, and this may be greeted with shock, denial and anger. Even though a person may have been unwell for a period of time, and may have had his suspicions, such a diagnosis will still be a shock, no matter how well prepared he is thought to be. It may, however, come as a relief to some to have their suspicions confirmed, so that they know what they are up against. People with AIDS usually experience overwhelming changes, both psychologically and physically. A person's life may alter considerably; health, social life, leisure, income and finances may all be affected.

Once an AIDS diagnosis is given, it will take time for its implications to be digested and for the person to feel able to question or respond. It is therefore important for the team to visit regularly following diagnosis so that the questions that will inevitably be asked can be responded to, and so that support can be given at this difficult stage. Some people may not have known their HIV antibody status prior to becoming unwell; for them, receiving such a diagnosis will have been a great shock, causing denial and numbness. A person may be heard to say 'I just can't believe it, it can't be me.' The person's reaction may be overlaid with anger and guilt; the anger may be directed towards himself, his partners or his close friends. One of the greatest difficulties in coming to terms with an AIDS diagnosis is the uncertainty — uncertainty about the course of the disease, about how people will react, and about how the individual's sexuality, life-style and independence will be affected. The reaction to the AIDS diagnosis may well mirror the mourning process (see p. 43) as the person will be grieving for the loss of his previous healthy life and will be coming to terms with a new state of uncertainty and ill health. The reaction may be shown in the following ways (Parkes 1972):

- *shock* at the diagnosis and the possibility of death
- *anxiety* related to uncertainty about the
  — prognosis and course of illness
  — effects of medication and treatment

— status of lovers and the lovers' ability to cope
— reactions of others (family, friends, etc.)
— loss of cognitive, physical, social and occupational abilities
— risk of infection from others and to others
- *depression* stemming from
  — feelings of helplessness in the face of changed circumstances
  — the perception that the virus is in control
  — reduced quality of life in all spheres
  — the prospect of a gloomy and possibly a painful, uncomfortable and disfiguring future
  — self-blame and recriminations for past 'indiscretions'
  — reduced social and sexual acceptability and isolation
- *anger* about
  — past, high-risk life-style and activities
  — the inability to overcome the virus
  — new and involuntary life-style restrictions
- *guilt* about
  — being homosexual
  — being a drug user
  — having the 'unacceptability' of homosexuality confirmed via illness

- *obsessions*. These may show as over-activity related to:
  — a relentless searching for explanations
  — a relentless searching for new diagnostic evidence on one's body
  — the inevitability of decline and death
  — a faddism over health and diets.

The length of time needed for an individual to adjust to an AIDS diagnosis and its implications ranges from days to months. At this time follow-up by the counsellor or health care worker may be needed to monitor, support and assist the person in resolving issues and solving problems.

THE CONTINUING MANAGEMENT OF AIDS

In the continuing care of a person with AIDS it may be important to introduce him to a counsellor or long-term support network, to continue discussion with partners and friends, and to give information about support agencies, both voluntary and statutory. The occupational therapist is

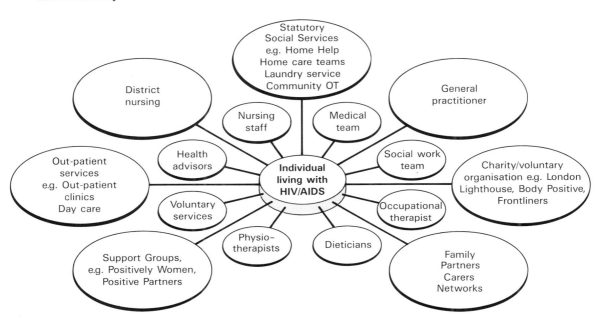

Fig. 35.3 The multidisciplinary team.

but one part of a multidisciplinary team (Fig. 35.3).

It will be up to the individual how involved he wishes his partner, carer or family to be in this process. However, it would be usual to involve the partner at the earliest opportunity, as he or she too will experience the bereavement process and will need to adjust. Commonly counselling time is offered to partners either alone or with the individual.

It is at this time that spouses, brothers and sisters, other relatives, lovers and friends become far more important than perhaps ever before. Many people, in the absence of parents or family, develop a very close network of friends who provide practical support and friendship, especially during difficult times. As the family and friends also experience the 'bereavement reaction' to the news of a friend or relative with AIDS, they may be able to take initiatives by engaging appropriate resources and finances. Buying groceries or putting the heating on before the discharge of the person may seem small errands but will help that person greatly. The person's partner or family may also need to be directed towards appropriate agencies.

Many groups have evolved through a wide range of organisations to provide a safe and useful support mechanism for people with AIDS as well as for friends and families. Support groups have almost become an intrinsic part of the treatment of people with AIDS, providing opportunities to share concerns, problems and pleasures, and helping people with AIDS to develop friendships and, perhaps, reach a point of acceptance of their diagnosis and illness.

As a person's disease progresses such that specific treatments are required and hospitalisations become frequent, normal daily routines and patterns become more disrupted and sometimes more difficult. The strain may be intense and cause anxiety and fear of losing loved ones. Intimacy, love, affection and expression of sexuality are needed towards the later stages of the disease. Many people during this stage may seek pastoral or spiritual support. Some look to other faiths such as Zen Buddhism or Christian Science.

Towards the later stages of the disease, people living with AIDS should be given the opportunity to state where they wish to die, whether this be at home or elsewhere, and whom they would like to have near them. Many choose home, fully supported by partners, friends and family where possible. Health care workers should strive to facilitate and respect this decision, which is one that may be difficult for the carers to cope with. The health carer's or therapist's work may not end when someone dies. She must take care not to cut herself off from relatives and partners and disappear out of the carers' lives like their relative has done. It is important to meet with the 'survivors' in order to share, support and facilitate their grief. Roles may need to be identified, taken up or rejected. 'Even if there is ample warning of an incipient death it is not easy to prepare adequately for bereavement' (Saunders 1973).

What most people who are bereaved need is a friend, whether it be a nurse, chaplain, social worker or next-door neighbour who will try to understand their needs and be a 'good-listener', allowing them time to talk through and share their feelings. As Elizabeth Kubler-Ross (1986) says, 'Death is the final stage of growth in this life.'

There are no rules about how people should cope or how partners and family should deal with the issues that arise, but people can be gently assisted and guided in order to have as full a life as possible with AIDS and to die with dignity.

OCCUPATIONAL THERAPY INTERVENTION

HIV disease can manifest itself in many ways and a person can present with a wide variety of problems and differing degrees of disability. A person may present to the occupational therapy service at any stage of illness. A person who is HIV positive and well, but has associated maladaptive coping mechanisms, or a person living with AIDS with central nervous system (CNS) involvement such as paraplegia, may benefit from the therapist's input, but intervention and treatment aims will be very different. The occupational therapist will find that each person has differing assessment and treatment needs and that long-term goals may require amending as the disease progresses and the level of debility, or the person's needs, change. As in any specialty, interventions and goals must be jointly contracted between the person and therapist, respecting the former's wishes.

THEORETICAL BASIS FOR PRACTICE

Reed and Sanderson's 'Human Occupations Model' (Fig. 35.4), was one of the occupational therapy models developed to provide a theoretical and scientific background to the practice of occupational therapy (Reed & Sanderson 1988). Within this framework an 'occupation' is defined as any activity which engages a person's resources of time and energy and which involves the application of skills and values — 'skill' being understood as a learned behaviour and 'value' as a belief that something is good or desirable. Occupations may be classified as relating to 'self-maintenance', 'productivity', or 'leisure'. To carry out a given occupation, a person must have competence in the particular performance components that it requires. These performance components may be described under the following headings: motor, sensory, cognitive, intrapersonal and interpersonal.

Definitions
Performance components

- Motor skills — the level, quality and/or degree of range of motion, gross muscle strength, muscle tone, endurance, fine motor skills and functional use
- Sensory skills — refers to skills and performance in perceiving and differentiating external and internal stimuli
- Cognitive skills — the level, quality and/or degree of comprehension, communication, concentration, problem-solving, time management, conceptualisation, integration of learning, judgement and time/place/person orientation
- Intrapersonal skills — the level, quality and/or degree of self-identity, self-concept and coping skills
- Interpersonal skills — the level, quality and/or degree of dyadic and group interaction skills.

Occupational components

- Self-maintenance occupations — those activities or tasks which are done routinely to maintain the person's health and well-being in the environment such as dressing or eating
- Productivity occupations — those activities or tasks which are done to enable the person to provide support to the self, family and society
- Leisure occupations — those activities or tasks done for the enjoyment and renewal that the activity or task brings to the person. They may contribute to the promotion of health and well-being, e.g. bowling or collecting antiques.

In applying the 'Human Occupations Model', the occupational therapist aims to help the person to enhance his quality of life and to maintain

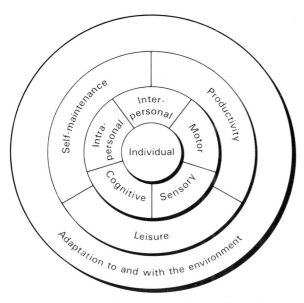

Fig. 35.4 Reed and Sanderson's Human Occupations Model (an adaptation).

maximum independence within his chosen environments. In doing so, the therapist uses a 'client-centred' and 'problem-oriented' approach.

ASSESSMENT

The occupational therapist may learn about the person with HIV disease/AIDS from a variety of different sources — nursing staff, the medical team, social services departments, or from the person himself.

Gaining accurate information about the person is essential in order that needs can be determined and a treatment plan established. Information must be specific to the individual at his particular stage of function and can be obtained from a variety of sources, including medical notes, multidisciplinary team meetings and, of course, from the person himself.

The first meeting should be carried out with sensitivity, bearing in mind that the person may still be in a state of shock about his condition and may have difficulty articulating his feelings, fears and needs. As well as ascertaining his level of physical function the therapist can observe the person's attitudes, knowledge and appearance during the interview.

Following an initial meeting, further specific assessments will need to be carried out in order to pinpoint specific areas and levels of difficulty. Once these have been identified the individual and the therapist should establish jointly a treatment programme based upon perceived and objective needs.

METHODS OF INTERVENTION

PERFORMANCE COMPONENTS

Motor

As mobility is often reduced because of muscle

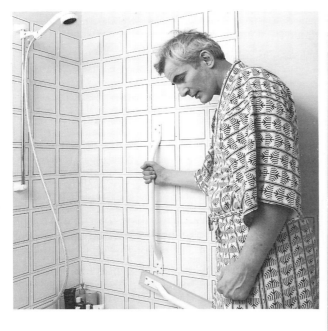
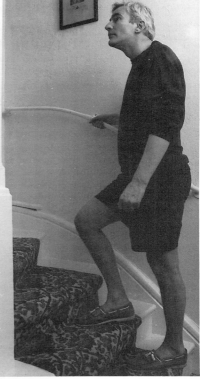

Fig. 35.5 Provision of handrails can facilitate independence and safety at home.

weakness or decreased exercise tolerance, the occupational therapist may need to assess for an appropriate wheelchair. A chair may be required for occasional indoor use and over longer distances outdoors, and for this purpose a model 8 chair, which provides a folding frame, removable armrests and a folding backrest for easier transportation, is usually appropriate. Pneumatic tyres make a more comfortable ride on rough outdoor ground! (See p. 279.) Cushioning should also be considered and ordered along with the wheelchair. Specialist cushioning is often required for pressure relief, prevention of pressure sores and to ease discomfort when sitting elsewhere — for example, in the bath. This again needs thorough assessment and the appropriate seating system should be ordered and provided.

Transfer practice and activities aimed at increasing mobility in areas affected can be incorporated into the therapist's treatment programme along with liaison and referral to the physiotherapist. Safety when moving outdoors and crossing roads as well as safety within the home should be considered (Fig. 35.5). Often a person may be weak and have reduced range of movement and so the appropriate use of remedial activities can be made, according to the person's interests and needs.

Energy conservation is also important to this group of people, who already may be prone to profound weakness and lethargy. In order to help save energy the person can be advised to:

- Use labour-saving equipment such as electric tin openers, microwave cookers, perching stools, intercom systems and stair lifts
- Always sit rather than stand
- Never start a large task during which he cannot take rests or stop
- Pace himself and take frequent rests during quiet moments of the day
- Plan his day's activities and reserve his energy for the priorities in his life, for example time spent with loved ones and leisure activities. (See p. 796.)

Sensory

Sensory disturbance may affect external sensory appreciation, including vision, and/or proprioception. Pain may also be present.

Vision

Cytomegalovirus (CMV) manifests itself systemically and affects the eyes, causing partial loss of vision and, at times, blindness. This, of course, causes varying degrees of disability. Coping with poor vision can be stressful and tiring and takes a great deal of determination to overcome. But relatively small and simple occupational therapy interventions can do much to enhance a person's life-style.

Lighting and colours are important. A room should be well lit and small knobs and switches can be highlighted by the use of bright contrasting colours. Strips of coloured paper can be used to mark temperature controls, dials and knobs on cookers, microwaves and washing machines. Telephones can be highlighted in the same way or fitted with a large numbered dial by British Telecom. The edge of steps can be marked with a white line and bannisters can be installed. Magnifying glasses and sheets are available to facilitate reading and writing. A talking-book library and large-print books are available from the Royal National Institute for the Blind (RNIB). Most local libraries also carry large-print books. Talking clocks and watches are useful as well.

The ability to move around the home and perform self-maintenance skills safely should also be assessed if necessary. Advice can be given on how best to organise the home and workplace and carry out activities so that the effect of visual loss can be minimised.

Pain

If a person complains of pain, assessment of pain should be requested and suitable measures for its relief taken. If appropriate a therapist may contribute to this by demonstrating and encouraging good posture, arranging for the provision of supportive seating, mattressing and cushioning, or by splinting for correct positioning of joints. Relaxation may also be appropriate. Referral can also be made to complementary therapists such as acupuncturists, aromatherapists or reflex zone therapists according to the person's wishes. It is every person's right to live and die free from pain. Remember, the therapist is often the person's advocate.

Sensory appreciation

When the person loses all or some of his ability to appreciate sensation, either from his external environment or his body, he will find difficulty in carrying out safely his normal, everyday activities. He should be made aware of the need to take care with hot and cold items such as saucepans, bath or shower water and packets of frozen food and take precautions by using protective gloves or asking another person to check water for temperature. Sharp objects may scratch or cut without him noticing and he needs to check regularly for cuts and abrasions.

Loss of proprioception may affect the way he moves, as he is unable to receive information about the position of his body. He may find he stumbles more easily, and so should take care over rough ground, on stairs, in crowded places and on public transport. He may also experience trouble when driving because of reduced appreciation of the position of his feet on the pedals, or with activities done without visual feedback, such as touch-typing.

Cognitive

Within HIV disease varying degrees of memory impairment may occur. Depending on the cause, the deficits may improve with rehabilitation and medical treatment or, unfortunately, may deteriorate so that the person requires longer term care. Whatever the prognosis the occupational therapist has a vital part to play in helping the person to improve and adapt life skills. Through assessment the therapist will have established the person's level of cognitive impairment and, as a result, will have set up a rehabilitation programme around the person's needs and his normal day-to-day activities.

At the beginning of a treatment session, the therapist may need to highlight who she is and establish the day, date and year, the surroundings, and the events taking place that day. If possible this can all be written down so the person is left with a visual cue. Self-maintenance skills such as washing and dressing (if possible using the person's own clothes) can be practised at the appropriate time of day, and a programme of activities for the day can be settled upon.

Tasks should be set which lend purpose to getting washed and dressed, such as going to the local shops to buy a newspaper or magazine. This can serve as an opportunity for further assessment in areas such as money handling and safety awareness, and can enhance community orientation.

Participation by hospitalised persons in ward activities such as drop-in groups, tea parties and current affairs groups is also important, as it provides vital contact with other people and staff, who may also give cues and prompts to the disorientated. Depending on future placement, domestic activities, leisure skills, community networking, home assessment and liaison with appropriate agencies, partners and carers can all be incorporated into the treatment plan.

Communication, comprehension, concentration and organisational skills should also be taken into consideration. For example, is the person able to follow and understand a written recipe, organise the required tasks in a logical order and then carry them out?

Treatment sessions should be of increasing duration — with graded activities that have easily achieved goals.

Intrapersonal

A person diagnosed as being HIV antibody positive or having AIDS may experience periods of tension, anxiety and panic. If this tension reaches a level where it disrupts his life-style or prevents him carrying out everyday activities, anxiety management and relaxation techniques may need to be taught. The causes of anxiety should be identified and the person's reaction to these situations established to help recognise the symptoms of stress. A normal pattern of breathing can be facilitated by deep-breathing exercises, followed by a variety of relaxation techniques. A person

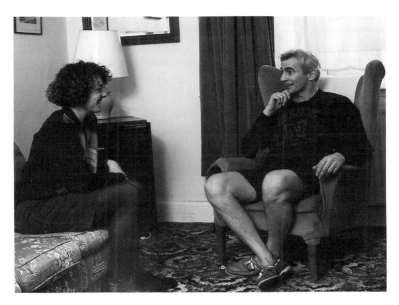

Fig. 35.6   Giving time to listen and offer support.

may often achieve a state of relaxation more easily by one particular method, so several different techniques should be tried initially. A person should be encouraged to practise regularly at home and in anxiety-provoking situations.

Throughout all stages of illness it is vital that the person receive adequate psychological support. A therapist should make time to offer this and should have good listening and communication skills (Fig. 35.6). If the therapist feels inadequately skilled, referral should be made to an appropriate professional, such as a counsellor or social worker, to give the person the opportunity to explore and fully understand his feelings.

Hospitalisation often reduces motivation and initiative, as all daily tasks can be carried out by the caring staff. It offers a sheltered, protective environment, thus encouraging institutionalisation and inhibiting decision-making and action. Occupational therapists can encourage a person to be a 'doing body' rather than having everything done for him. By supporting him in all areas, the occupational therapist can help the person to retain his autonomy and remain 'his own person' rather than become just another 'drug treatment' or 'admission'. For example, a 55-year-old man was

admitted to hospital with PCP, this being a new AIDS diagnosis. He became very withdrawn, taking to his bed, and became increasingly dependent on the nursing staff. The occupational therapist, devising graded activities of self-maintenance and setting goals of increasing difficulty for productive occupations, facilitated this man's return to home and work with minimal community support.

Interpersonal

Group work can be an important and effective tool in the treatment of people with HIV disease and AIDS. A person is given the opportunity to share and communicate ideas and feelings clearly and accurately, within a safe environment. An effective group enhances interpersonal skills, providing understanding, building trust and giving constructive feedback.

Groups have unique properties as a whole, which make them an advantageous treatment medium. Therapists may become involved in self-help groups, such as personal growth groups, where the goal is to increase awareness of self and others and to build skills. Other psychosocial groups might include 'current affairs' and 'lunch cookery'.

Group work involves sensitivity and understanding from the leader or facilitator, as many different and difficult interpersonal problems may arise when so many are responding at once. Environmental factors can influence proceedings and need to be considered when groups are initiated. For example, rooms, lighting, seating and the possibility of noise must all be considered prior to embarking on group work. Sociological and demographic characteristics influencing group dynamics include sex, race, age, culture, social class, occupational/religious subgroups, and coalitions among group members.

OCCUPATIONAL COMPONENTS

Self-maintenance

Personal ADL include washing, dressing, grooming/hygiene, drinking and eating as well as domestic activities such as meal planning and preparation, cleaning, laundry and shopping. These areas may be affected for a variety of different reasons and intervention must therefore take into account the underlying cause. Lack of independence may be caused by:

- neurological problems such as peripheral neuropathy or hemiplegia
- psychological difficulties, including lack of motivation or depression
- lethargy and weakness caused, for example, by tuberculosis (TB) or anaemia
- memory loss from HIV encephalopathy or persistent multifocal leucoencephalopathy (PML).

It is not possible to cover all aspects of self-maintenance here, nor to give solutions to all the different problems which may arise, but thorough assessment of the person's abilities is vital in order to form a baseline for planning treatment and services. The therapist will then be able to apply her learned skills and knowledge to design a treatment programme which aims to improve deficits and function in response to the underlying cause. This programme may include:

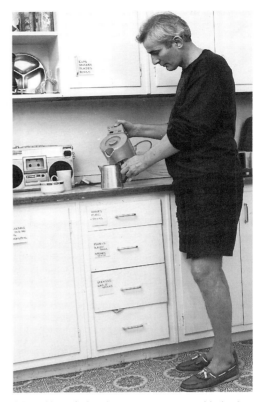

Fig. 35.7 Use of visual cues as memory aids in the person's home.

- graded exposure to self-maintenance activities to increase tolerance and strength
- supervised practice and experiential learning
- the use of adaptive equipment, energy conservation techniques
- discussion around what assistance is available and appropriate from outside statutory and voluntary agencies.

Productivity

Despite having HIV disease, people do and can work. The person is under no obligation to inform his employer about his condition and has statutory rights against unfair dismissal which are not reduced because he is infected.

By working, the person can maintain his role as a wage-earner and keep contact with colleagues. If his job becomes too difficult or tiring to carry out, alternative employment can be sought; part-time work or a transfer to a less physically demanding job, such as a supervisory or administrative position, can be considered. Adaptive and energy-saving equipment can also be provided by social services or charitable funding. Retraining, if appropriate, may be a possibility.

Some larger companies do encourage their staff to inform them of their health status, the benefits being a more sympathetic attitude to sick leave, alternative working methods, and pension and retirement schemes.

Many voluntary agencies are looking for people who have time to spare to work as volunteers. These roles vary, requiring different levels of ability, and might be considered by a person who is not in paid employment.

A person should be encouraged to look at his various roles. For example, an HIV positive mother with two children has the role of child carer, homemaker and provider. Housework, laundry and parentcraft are the necessary productive activities and tasks in which the woman engages to maintain this role. The occupational therapist must be aware of the wide variety of cultural and social roles a person may be required to perform within his life. (See p. 28.)

Leisure

Because a person may have given up work due to fluctuating ill health, he may often find he has much time on his hands, during which he is not satisfied by watching endless hours of television. Part of the occupational therapist's role is to encourage and support the person in structuring leisure time, helping him to seek new interests and to make use of new opportunities (Fig. 35.8).

The therapist must be aware of the groups and centres that exist locally and of what events take place and when. If transport is a problem there may be a Taxicard scheme in place or a voluntary service which would be prepared to assist a person with mobility problems. The onus is on the therapist initially to seek out and explore what is available so at least she has the background information to impart. If in fact there is little available, what is to stop the therapist from creating and

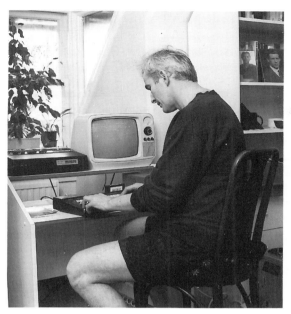

Fig. 35.8 Using a computer as a new interest.

starting a leisure interests group specifically for people living with HIV disease? In London, for example, there are gardening and swimming groups which meet weekly. As it becomes easier for the person to structure his time, he can perhaps begin to create his own opportunities and develop the group further. Voluntary agencies may be able to supply additional helpers to assist in facilitating a group.

The therapist can also ease integration into existing groups or centres by accompanying the individual on his first visits if he wishes, and gradually withdrawing input as he feels more confident and at ease with his new-found interest.

ADAPTATION TO THE ENVIRONMENT

A person's environment is all-encompassing and therefore there is a need for him to feel able, and to be able, to function at an optimum level within varying surroundings, such as home, work and school. One area in which the occupational therapist's skills are often called for is within the person's home.

During all stages of treatment a person's wishes must be respected: this applies, for example, to the person's preference as to where he is to be cared for in the future or after hospital admission. If a person wishes to return to, or die, at home this avenue must be fully explored and the resources to enable him to do so must be researched and discussed. Other persons who will be involved as carers must be liaised with. It may be necessary to carry out a home assessment prior to discharge, during which both the individual and his primary carers are present. Further home visits after discharge may also be required. A home assessment may be necessary in order to:

- establish the person's abilities within his own environment
- assess the need for adaptive equipment or alterations (Fig. 35.9)
- assess for the provision of support services
- discuss the person's impending return with primary carers within the home setting.

During the resettlement period from hospital to home, regular contact should be kept and support

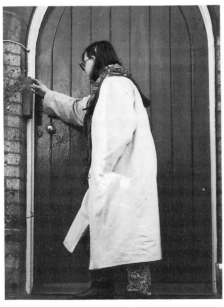

Fig. 35.9 Intercom system enables a person to allow easy access to the home for visitors.

offered in this often difficult transition. Follow-up visits may be necessary for reassessment if circumstances change; because of the nature of HIV disease, prompt response is required from the therapist.

If the person chooses not to die at home the alternatives have to be considered. If there is a choice of residential settings available, the person should be given the opportunity to visit and spend some time at each and be given time to choose where he would like to end his days. This may at times be difficult for him, so the therapist should help him explore his options and be supportive in his final decision. The person may, in fact, remain in his current setting, where the therapist can maintain contact.

CONCLUSION

Working with people who have HIV disease or AIDS presents the occupational therapist with exciting new challenges and a range of opportunities to develop her skills, as she addresses both psychosocial and physical problems in endeavouring to enhance a person's quality of life.

As a member of a multidisciplinary team, the occupational therapist must work closely with other professionals, giving the opportunity for 'shared care' and support, and making best use of others' expertise and resources.

The need for support for the occupational therapist working in this field must be recognised and acted upon. This is an area that should not be overlooked, especially with regard to therapists entering this area of work for the first time.

Many agencies, both voluntary and statutory, have evolved with the AIDS epidemic, offering a wide range of services from 'befriending' to 'home care'; these may be useful in assisting with care with this client group. (See Useful Addresses, p. 819). Whatever the therapist feels she is able to offer, it is of paramount importance to remember that her efforts must be client centred, respecting the rights and wishes of this expanding and knowledgeable group of people.

ACKNOWLEDGEMENT

The authors extend their thanks to Beth Hunter, Medical Photographer at Westminster Hospital; Mr Christopher Keegan for his patience; Miss Sally Westwick, Senior Occupational Therapist, National Hospital for Neurology and Neurosurgery and all the staff working at the HIV Services Unit at Westminster Hospital and St Stephens Clinic.

USEFUL ADDRESSES

AIDS Care Education and Training (AECT)
Bramount House
71 Uxbridge Road
London W5
081 840 7879
(A church-based AIDS charity which aims to provide:
—a home care network: 400 volunteers; practical support; nursing and medical support
—hospice care: accommodation; terminal care; day care
—financial grants: equipment; clothing; services
—education and training: professionals and volunteers; schools; churches; organisations.)

Body Positive
P.O. Box 493
London W14 0TH
071 373 9124 (daily 7–10 p.m.)
(Services include hospital visiting, counselling, a support group for people who are HIV positive, a nightly telephone helpline, a support group for heterosexual people with HIV, a fortnightly newsletter. There is also a Daycentre at 51B Philbeach Gardens, London SW5 (071 835 1045), which offers various groups, networking, and drop-in facilities.)

Haemophilia Society
123 Westminster Bridge Road
London SW1 7HR
071 928 2020
(Offers advice, support and counselling as well as financial assistance for people with haemophilia. Contact: AIDS Officer.)

Health Education Council
73 New Oxford Street
London WC1
(Offers literature, references and information on all aspects of HIV and AIDS.)

Immunity
BM Immunity
London WC1N 3XX
071 837 0749
(Promotes and organises research and education on all aspects of HIV infection. Immunity also provides a legal service for all people affected by AIDS.)

Landmark
47A Tulse Hill
Brixton
SW2 2TN
081 678 6687
(A social centre for people living with HIV or AIDS. It is also intended for people who are partners, carers, lovers or friends of people with HIV or AIDS. Operates on a drop-in basis. Was set up by Lambeth AIDS Action, a group of local people concerned about HIV and AIDS.)

London Lighthouse
111–117 Lancaster Road
London W11 1QU
071 792 1200
(Offers a range of integrated services, including a social centre, counselling, health programmes, home support, respite and terminal care. Also provides support to the partners and friends of people affected by AIDS and runs training courses for statutory, private and voluntary organisations and for individuals concerned with AIDS-related issues.)

National AIDS Trust
Room 1403, Euston Tower
286 Euston Road
London NW1 3DM
(Offers information, updates, newsletters and advice on HIV and AIDS issues.)

PACE
London Lesbian & Gay Centre
67–69 Cowcross Street
London EC1M 6BP
(Offers free individual, couple and group counselling as well as a weekly clinic for one-off crisis counselling by appointment.)

Terrence Higgins Trust
BM AIDS
London WC1N 3XX
071 831 0330
Helpline: 071 242 1010 (7–10 p.m. weekdays, 3–10 p.m. weekends)
(The largest AIDS charity set up to inform, advise and help people with AIDS and related conditions.)

REFERENCES

Adler Michael W 1987 ABC of AIDS. BMA, Taylor & Francis, UK
Catalan J 1988 Psychosocial and neuropsychiatric aspects of HIV infection: review of their extent and implications for psychiatry. Journal of Psychosomatic Research 32(3): 37–248
Daniels V J 1987 AIDS: the acquired immune deficiency syndrome, 4th edn. MTP Press, Lancaster
Kubler-Ross, E (ed) 1986 Death: the final stage of growth. Simon & Schuster, New York
Lancet 1989 Latest AIDS figures. 11: 1055
Miller D, Webber J, Green J 1986 The Management of AIDS patients. Macmillan, London
Parkes, Colin M 1972 Studies of grief in adult life: bereavement. Tavistock Publications, London
Reed K, Sanderson S 1988 Concepts of occupational therapy, 2nd edn. Williams & Wilkins, Baltimore
Saunders C (ed) 1978 The management of terminal disease. Edward Arnold, London
Seidl O, Goebel F D 1987 Psychosomatic reactions of homosexuals and drug addicts to the knowledge of a positive HIV test result. AIDS-Forschung 2(4): 181–187
Wells N, Taylor D 1988 HIV and AIDS in the United Kingdom. OHE briefing, 1988(23) Office of Health Economics, London

FURTHER READING

AIDS Project Los Angeles 1987 AIDS: a self care manual IBS Press, Santa Monica
Cusack L, Phillips L, Singh S 1990 The role of the occupational therapist in HIV disease and AIDS. British Journal of Occupational Therapy 53(5): 181–183
Farthing C F 1986 A colour atlas of AIDS. Wolfe Medical Publications, London
Green J, McCreaner A 1989 Counselling in HIV infection and AIDS. Blackwell Scientific Publications, Oxford
Helber M, Pinching T, Brewster K 1987 Living with AIDS: a guide to survival by people with AIDS. Frontliners UK, London
Kirkpatrick B 1988 AIDS — sharing the pain. Darton, Longman & Todd, London
Kubler-Ross E 1970 On death and dying. Tavistock Publications, London
Miller C 1987 Living with AIDS and HIV. Macmillan, London
Miller R, Bar R 1987 AIDS — a guide to clinical counselling. Science Press, London
Pratt R 1987 AIDS — A strategy for nursing care. Edward Arnold, London
Richardson D 1987 Women and the AIDS crisis. Pandora Press, Routledge, Chapman & Hall, New York
Royal Society of Medicine. The AIDS Letter. (Available from 1 Wimpole Street, London WIM BAE)
Scott P 1989 National AIDS manual. National AIDS Manual, London
Tatchell P 1987 AIDS — A guide to survival. Gay Men's Press, London
Wilkinson, G 1987 Working with gay men with AIDS. Sussex Helpline, Brighton

36

Cancer

Susan Beresford

INTRODUCTION

Having cancer is a very lonely and frightening position to be in, people are embarrassed and frightened if you talk about it. It is far easier to say you feel well and are coping, than to tell the truth about how frightened you are, about the pain and dying and the fears that beset you. (Maggie Hoult, quoted in Foreman & Hobbs 1988.)

Despite an increasing awareness of the disease and its treatments, cancer is still perceived by most people to be a terrifying illness. It requires people to think about many feelings that they are uncomfortable with, and which they would often rather ignore. It is, however, a subject that most health care professionals will have to consider at some point in their working lives.

Oncology can be defined as the study or science of cancer, a disease that has been known about for over 2000 years. More money is spent on research into causes of and cures for cancer than on research into any other medical condition, but sufferers still have to deal with the misguided attitudes of family and friends.

This chapter discusses the role of the occupational therapist in helping the cancer sufferer to cope with his illness, to maintain the maximum independence possible and to gain satisfaction from life regardless of the prognosis of his disease. The chapter begins with an introduction into the causes, pathology and clinical features of cancer, and describes the physical and psychological problems that are likely to be faced by the person with cancer. The various forms of medical treatment that are available for cancer are also outlined.

The chapter then turns to the philosophy of care adopted by many professionals in their interventions with cancer sufferers. This philosophy places the unique needs of each individual at the centre of treatment, and recognises that these needs will be emotional and spiritual as well as physical. The occupational therapist taking this approach will include the individual's family and loved ones within her 'unit of care', offering her support and advice to them as well as to the individual. As in other areas of treatment, the occupational therapist will work as part of a multidisciplinary team. Her communication skills will be of paramount importance as she assesses the needs and desires of the individual and his carers and strives, with her team colleagues, to provide comprehensive and cohesive care.

The chapter next turns to more specific aspects of the therapist's intervention with cancer sufferers, describing her varied role in the areas of 'prevention', 'restoration', 'support' and 'palliation'. Particular attention is given to the practical assistance and advice she may offer in regard to life skills such as personal care and mobility, as well as to the support she can offer as the individual adjusts emotionally and psychologically to the effects and implications of his disease. The importance of social and leisure activities is also stressed, and the therapist's vital role in helping the individual to maintain his involvement in productive activity is discussed.

The final section of the chapter describes the occupational therapist's role in the individual's resettlement at home following treatment in hospital. As always, her support will extend to family members, and her intervention will be carried out in cooperation with the other members of the rehabilitation team.

CAUSES OF CANCER

'Cancer' is a general term that refers to a malig-

nant growth of tissue in any part of the body. The growth is parasitic, non-functional and invasive. One in three people are likely to develop cancer at some stage in their lives and one in five will die as a result of the disease. Much is now known about the disease — many of the 200 or more forms of it respond to treatment and 40% of sufferers can expect to be cured. It is thought that cancer can be caused by external agents which, in some susceptible people, result in malignant disease. The list of implicated agents grows as new carcinogens are discovered through research. Many forms of cancer (up to 70%) are known to be preventable and emphasis is now being placed on health education in an effort to encourage people to adopt a healthier way of life (Fig. 36.1).

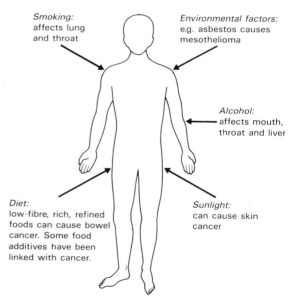

Fig. 36.1 Some causes of cancer.

PATHOLOGY

A tumour, or neoplasm, is an abnormal overgrowth of cells. Tumours fall into two main categories:

- *Benign*. These tumours are made up of normal cells which resemble the host tissue.

Primary site	Risk of metastases	Common sites of spread	Favourable prognostic factors	Poor prognostic factors	Appropriate investigations
Gynaecological Ovary	***	Peritoneal cavity Direct extension Lung Liver	Stage 1 Low grade histology	Advanced stage High grade histology	Abdominal CT scan or ultrasound
Uterus	*	Direct extension Lymph nodes Lung	Stage 1 (tumour confined to corpus) Low grade No myometrial invasion	Tumour spread beyond corpus Large uterine cavity High grade histology Myometrial invasion	Chest x-ray
Cervix	**	Direct extension Lymph nodes	No parametrial/pelvic extension	Advanced stage	IVP Lymphogram
Urological Kidney	**	Direct extension Lymph nodes Lung Bone	Tumour confined to kidney – capsule intact	Extra-renal spread Positive lymph nodes Renal vein invasion	Chest x-ray Abdominal CT scan or ultrasound Bone scan
Bladder	**	Direct extension Lymph nodes	Low grade Papillary tumour Early stage	High grade Deep muscle invasion Squamous histology	IVP Lymphogram CT scan
Prostate	***	Direct extension Lymph nodes Bone	Small nodule Low grade histology	Extracapsular spread High grade histology	Acid phosphatase IVP Lymphogram Bone scan
Head and neck	*	Direct extension Lymph nodes	Localised tumour	Advanced stage Bulky nodes	CT scan/x-ray tomography Skull x-rays (special projections) e.g. SMV
Melanoma	**	Direct extension Lymph nodes Liver Lung Brain	Superficial lesions (Clark I and II) Negative nodes	Large primary Infiltrating lesions (Clark III–V) Positive nodes	Chest x-ray Liver scan/ultrasound Bone scan Brain scan
Thyroid Papillary and follicular	*	Lymph nodes Lung	Young patients Primary < 5cm Negative nodes	Older patients Large primary	Chest x-ray ¹³¹I Body scan
Medullary	**	Lymph nodes Lung Liver Bone	Normal calcitonin following surgery Negative nodes	Persistently raised calcitonin Positive nodes	Chest x-ray Bone scan Liver scan Serum calcitonin
Anaplastic	***	Lymph nodes Lung Liver Bone		Any anaplastic histology	Chest x-ray Liver scan Bone scan

Fig. 36.2 (cont'd overleaf)

Primary site	Risk of metastases	Common sites of spread	Favourable prognostic factors	Poor prognostic factors	Appropriate investigations
Breast	***	Lymph nodes Bone Liver Lung	Small primary tumour Low grade histology Negative axillary nodes	Large primary tumour High grade histology Positive nodes Family history	Chest x-ray Bone scan Liver scan/ultrasound (contralateral mammogram)
Bronchus	***	Lymph nodes Liver Brain Bone/bone marrow	Resectable lesion (except small cell type) Negative nodes	Non-small cell history Lymph node/blood vessel invasion Extra-thoracic spread	Liver scan/ultrasound Bone scan Brain scan
Gastro-intestinal Stomach	***	Direct extension Lymph nodes Liver Lung Bone	Small lesion Low grade histology Confined to muscularis mucosa Negative nodes	High grade histology Extension through wall Positive nodes	Gastroscopy Barium studies Liver scan/ultrasound
Pancreas	***	Direct extension Lymph nodes Head lesion – liver Tail lesion – liver, lungs, bone		Any pancreatic cancer	CT scan/ultrasound of abdomen
Colon and rectum	**	Direct extension Lymph nodes Liver	Duke's stage A and B Low grade histology	Dukes C_1 and C_2 Positive nodes High grade histology	Liver scan/ultrasound
Hodgkins disease	**	Contiguous nodes Spleen Liver/Bone marrow	Early stage < 4 node groups involved No 'B' symptoms	Advanced stage Mediastinal involvement 'B' symptoms Lymphocyte depletion	Chest x-ray + tomography Lymphogram + IVP CT scan abdomen Bone marrow trephine Exploratory laparotomy
Non-Hodgkins lymphoma	***	Non-contiguous lymph nodes Liver Bone marrow CNS Extranodal sites	Nodular histology (all stages) Stage I disease (diffuse/mixed histology)	Diffuse histology Advanced stage	Chest x-ray ENT examination Lymphogram Bone marrow trephine Liver ultrasound/biopsy CSF cytology (diffuse)

Fig. 36.2 Patterns of metastases. (Reproduced by kind permission of Farmitalia Carlo Erba Ltd.)

They are slow-growing, encapsulated and do not produce secondary deposits (metastases). They may be cysts (filled with fluid), adenomata (glandular tissue) fibromata (fibrous tissue) or lipomata (fatty tissue). Whilst they are not usually life threatening, they may encroach upon and compress other tissue, thus potentially causing very serious problems, or, if left untreated, may develop into something more grave.

- *Malignant*. These tumours are fast-growing cells, abnormal to the host area, which spread, if left untreated, via the lymphatic and circulatory systems. This spread results in metastases forming away from the primary tumour. Many primary tumours have a predictable line of spread (Fig. 36.2) and since many of them have few initial signs and symptoms, they may not be detected until they have formed metastases. There has been an increase in health education in this area to encourage people to have any unusual lumps investigated promptly.

CLINICAL FEATURES

Many tumours have very few initial signs and symptoms, but are detected at routine examinations, which include self-examination and body scanning techniques such as mammography. Certain symptoms, described below, are common to many types of tumour.

Fatigue and weight loss

These symptoms will often prompt a person to see his general practitioner. They are insidious in onset and the person tends to feel foolish about bothering his physician over something so trivial. By the time he has sought advice, however, it is not unusual for a person to have lost up to 2 stone in weight. The general practitioner is unlikely to make a diagnosis of cancer on these symptoms alone, but will refer the person to a specialist so that further investigation can be made.

Pain

Seventy per cent of people suffering from cancer experience some form of pain. The chronic pain of cancer is different from the acute pain that accompanies a fracture or an infection such as appendicitis. Whereas the individual will expect acute pain to decrease as health is restored, he may see chronic pain as meaningless and unending. The majority of sufferers have more than one site of pain. The treatment of chronic pain is complex and requires specialist knowledge. It is important to diagnose accurately the cause of the pain. Regular analgesia, of the correct strength, should be provided to prevent the pain returning before the next dose is due. This medication should be closely monitored and adjusted according to the severity of the pain. As well as the cognitive aspect (actual perception of the pain), there is also an affective aspect (how the person responds emotionally to the pain). This can vary, not only from one person to another, but in the same person from day to day or even hour to hour. Medication is only part of the overall management of pain and consideration needs to be given to the psychological aspect of pain. This is an area where occupational therapy can make a valuable contribution.

Besides medication, there are other forms of pain control that may be considered; these include nerve blocks, transcutaneous electrical nerve stimulation (TENS) and radiotherapy. Some surgical procedures are also useful and may be indicated.

Nerve stimulation (acupuncture) has been used to relieve pain for thousands of years. Its effectiveness in relieving the pain of cancer has not been proven, but it may be helpful for some individuals.

Constipation

This may be drug induced, a symptom of bowel cancer or a combination of the two. The strong analgesics, particularly the opiate drugs, used in the treatment of cancer pain have a very constipating effect. If this constipation is left untreated, it can cause pain and discomfort, anorexia, vomiting or confusion. For this reason, aperients should be prescribed routinely for people taking pain-killers of this type.

Nausea and vomiting

These symptoms, which may be accompanied by anorexia, may be due to medication (morphine often causes nausea when first taken) or to an intestinal blockage. They may also be side effects of radiotherapy or chemotherapy. Once the cause has been discovered they can be treated effectively with antiemetic drugs and careful dietary management. Depression can often be associated with nausea and vomiting.

Respiratory symptoms

Dyspnoea can be frightening to the sufferer, although it is not necessarily related to the severity of the disease. It brings a fear of suffocation; consequently, it is important to attend to environmental factors by providing good ventilation or a cooling fan. Anxiety often accompanies breathing problems and this should be treated along with any physical causes such as pleural effusion or chest infection. Physiotherapy can reduce dyspnoea by encouraging the use of breathing exercises and relaxation techniques to reduce anxiety.

Lymphoedema

When this occurs in conjunction with cancer, it is caused by a blockage in the lymphatic system, usually as a result of surgery or radiotherapy damage. The build-up of fluid in the affected area causes the limb to swell, reducing mobility and increasing pain. Lymphoedema often occurs in the arm following mastectomy.

The condition is treatable in most cases, requiring the use of compression pumps and, in more severe cases, a course of compression bandaging. Following this treatment, it will be necessary for the person to wear a pressure garment on the affected limb to prevent the return of the swelling.

The reduction of lymphoedema is usually the province of the physiotherapist; however, any loss of mobility and strength resulting from the condition can be treated by occupational therapy.

Neurological symptoms

Mood changes, confusion, hemiparesis, headaches, ataxia and dysphasia can all be symptomatic of cerebral tumours. As intracranial pressure fluctuates, these symptoms can vary in severity. Tumours growing close to the spinal cord can result in cord compression, which in turn can cause paraplegia and incontinence.

People who develop paraplegia and hemiplegia will almost certainly be referred to the occupational therapist for help. The main consideration in these cases is that the medical condition is unstable and that the person's disability will change accordingly. Nevertheless, treatment should be offered in the usual way.

The control and management of symptoms is very important, whether a person is receiving treatment and can be expected to recover or if the disease has progressed beyond this stage. It can mean the difference between 'living' and 'existing'. Most symptoms can now be controlled, not only by medication but also by a variety of other means.

MEDICAL TREATMENT

Certain tumours respond well to specific interventions. The three main types of treatment offered to people who have been diagnosed as having cancer are:

1. Surgery. This is most often indicated if there are no signs that the tumour has spread.
2. Radiotherapy. This can be very effective in the treatment of Hodgkin's disease.
3. Chemotherapy. This is efficient in treating leukaemia.

Surgical intervention

There are three main types of surgical treatment in cancer care:

Explorative

Much diagnostic work is now done using X-rays and body scanners. However, these machines cannot tell if a tumour is malignant. This still requires the removal of part or all of the tumour for subjection to pathological tests.

Curative

Surgery is usually performed if the tumour is small, well defined and sited away from any vital organs. Such surgery may necessitate the use of deep X-ray treatment (DXT) and chemotherapy to ensure that all the malignant cells have been removed. For example, when a breast tumour is removed, the use of DXT and/or chemotherapy can eliminate the need to perform a complete mastectomy.

Palliative

Removal of part of a tumour may be necessary if the tumour is threatening one or more of the vital organs. This type of surgery may involve procedures such as forming a colostomy to bypass an intestinal obstruction.

Radiotherapy

Radiotherapy aims to shrink the tumour by killing the cancer cells using gamma- or X-rays. Cancer cells are more sensitive than normal cells and are less able to repair damage. Since normal cells can be affected by radiotherapy, courses of this type of treatment are carefully planned to give maximum exposure to the tumour and cause minimum damage to normal tissue.

The skin over the treated area may become red and sore. Since DXT affects the fast-dividing tissue of a tumour, it can also affect normal fast-dividing tissue, as in the alimentary tract. If the radiation is close to this type of sensitive tissue, it can give rise to the more common side effects such as tiredness, mouth ulcers, nausea, vomiting and loss of appetite.

Chemotherapy

This form of treatment uses cytotoxic drugs which are very toxic (poisonous) to cancer cells, but, fortunately, are not so toxic to normal cells. There are many different drugs used, in combination, during chemotherapy. Four of the main groups are:

- alkylating agents
- cytotoxic antibiotics
- antimetabolites
- Vinca alkaloids.

The choice of drug depends on the nature of the tumour. It may be necessary to use 3, 4 or 5 drugs in combination to attack some tumours. Administration may be by:

- mouth
- subcutaneous or intramuscular injection
- intravenous drip.

Chemotherapy is usually given for several days, followed by a rest period before the next course is started. Treatment usually continues whilst a response is gained and the tumour shrinks, and may last many months.

As with DXT, chemotherapy affects the cells which reproduce rapidly. These include the cells of the alimentary tract, the mouth and the bone marrow. Side effects, if any, are likely to be nausea, vomiting and mouth ulcers; if the first two are severe and troublesome, antiemetic drugs can be prescribed. As the blood cells are produced in the bone marrow, tiredness may occur as a result of decreased production of red blood cells. Moreover, the decreased production of white blood cells can lead to the loss of immunity to infection. Sometimes the cells of the scalp are affected, resulting in hair loss, but the hair will regrow after treatment has ceased.

PHILOSOPHY OF CARE

You matter because you are you. You matter to the last moment of your life and we will do all we can, not only to help you die peacefully, but also to live until you die.

(Dame Cicely Saunders, cited in Zora & Zora 1981)

This philosophy of care is based upon the hospice philosophy, a set of ideas and attitudes on the care of a person suffering from a life-threatening disease such as cancer. The practice of hospice care need not be confined to an institute and is just as relevant in the home as in the hospital setting.

Whilst it would be inappropriate to recreate the total hospice philosophy in a hospital setting, many of its features could and should be incorporated into the care of cancer sufferers wherever they receive treatment. The principles of this philosophy are summarised below.

CARE AND EMPATHY

These qualities underpin this type of work. Even if the disease is curable, a diagnosis of cancer can be very frightening and brings the person face to face with his own mortality. This is an area that many people avoid, so any health care professional working in this field must be able to listen to these fears and not be afraid of them. She may not have all the answers, but to care is often enough. Although this type of care requires the therapist to give of herself, its rewards can be immense.

NEEDS OF PEOPLE (Fig. 36.3)

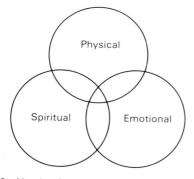

Fig. 36.3 Needs of people.

Three-dimensional perspective

People are 'three dimensional' — that is to say, they have needs which can be identified as physical, emotional and spiritual and, as Figure 36.3 shows, these needs are interconnected. In order

that a person remains healthy, all these aspects need attention. The person who suffers pain which no amount of analgesia can control often has deep anxieties and fears which need consideration. Whilst most people accept they have physical and emotional needs, many find difficulty accepting their spiritual needs. Coping with a potentially life-threatening situation can necessitate consideration of a person's spirituality. The chaplain or other spiritual minister is an important member of the multidisciplinary team and people receiving treatment should be aware of his availability.

The acknowledgement of physical, emotional and spiritual needs is equally important for the members of the treatment team themselves. They should give consideration to their own needs if they are to remain effective in helping others identify theirs.

It is important to find out what the individual person needs. Something which may seem like an insurmountable problem to one person may be unimportant to another. It is necessary to take time to listen to each individual and gain a sensitive understanding of his priorities and needs.

Unit of care (Fig. 36.4)

People do not live in isolation. When a disease such as cancer strikes, it affects the family or others with whom the person lives. Close family members will probably become the main carers and will need help and support in their task. It is worth bearing this in mind from the start, and to aim to involve the family as much as possible.

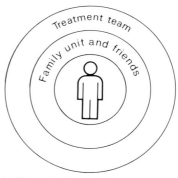

Fig. 36.4 The unit of care. The treatment team must consider the needs of the individual and his family unit.

Grief reaction

Kubler-Ross (1970) has described the five emotional stages through which people pass on being told they have a life-threatening disease. These are: denial and isolation, anger, bargaining, depression and acceptance (see Ch. 3). Although not all people pass through these stages in order, and many shift back and forth between two stages for a while, Kubler-Ross's model is generally accepted. Throughout this emotional journey it is important to preserve a sense of hope, which must be distinguished from denial. Hope is demonstrated, for example, by the usually realistic person who talks openly of his prognosis but also occasionally expresses a hope for the future. This is the kind of optimism that keeps life bearable.

COMMUNICATION

This is a skill that can be learned. The heart of good communication lies in the ability to listen creatively, hear what is being said, and respond accordingly.

By listening attentively to the person as he expresses his needs the therapist affirms that he is important and deserving of respect. She helps to restore his self-esteem and supports him in solving some of his problems. As well as providing a solid foundation for her relationship with the individual, careful listening may offer the therapist insight into how she might help with the other problems.

TEAM WORK

Just as people do not live in isolation, neither do they work in isolation. A good team, working together, cannot be bettered. The team of people working in this field can be quite extensive. The roles of individual members frequently overlap and boundaries of responsibility may become blurred. It may be helpful for each member of the team to have his or her own exclusive care responsibility. This helps to identify each member's role and affords him or her the freedom to operate with maximum effectiveness in the other area of work.

An occupational therapist working predominantly within the field of oncology must be ma-

ture and secure. It can be very lonely to be the only member of a particular professional group in a team, without the back-up of other occupational therapy staff.

The team usually comprises a consultant, ward doctor, physiotherapist, occupational therapist, chaplain, social worker, dietitian, speech therapist, and radiographer, as well as nurses (including Macmillan nurses) and technicians. Other disciplines may be represented as necessary.

Macmillan nurses are registered general nurses with a district nurse qualification who have been specially trained to advise on pain relief and symptom control. They work as part of the primary health care team with general practitioners, district nurses, and hospital and hospice staff. They provide emotional support to cancer sufferers and their families, which continues through bereavement. They are an education and teaching resource for the district in which they work and enable many people who would otherwise be hospitalised to remain at home.

In some instances, the number of people involved in caring for a family can become very large. It can be advantageous to nominate a key worker within the team to coordinate the different services. This role often falls to the Macmillan nurse, but may equally be undertaken by any other member of the team if he or she is better acquainted with the family and their needs.

Staff support

Working with people who suffer from a life-threatening illness can be emotionally as well as physically draining. Staff support varies widely. Some people favour formal support groups, run by a member of the team, whilst others see the need to employ a counsellor who is not directly involved or working within the team to provide support. It is necessary that all team members are supported by one another on a daily basis in addition to having access to formal support.

CARE OF THE BEREAVED

Grieving is a normal process. It is experienced by people who have lost a loved one and begins at the time they are told that the loved one will not recover. It is important, therefore, having been told the prognosis, that a person be given the opportunity to return and discuss his worries and feelings as they occur. Since the unit of care is identified as the whole family, there needs to be provision for bereavement counselling, both before and after death. This may be done on an individual or group basis. (Bereaved people often find group support by other people in the same position most effective.)

It is important to help the person to live his life as fully as possible, throughout the duration of his illness, whether his life expectancy is 10 days or 10 years.

CANCER REHABILITATION

The overall aim of cancer rehabilitation can be defined as endeavouring 'to improve the quality of survival of cancer patients so that during their period of survival they will be able to lead as independent and productive a life as possible at the minimum level of dependency, regardless of life expectancy' (Dietz 1981). Dietz further identifies four stages on the way to rehabilitation:

- Prevention. Potential disability is lessened by training and education (i.e. people learn about causes of cancer and how they can adjust their life-style to prevent this).
- Restoration. The disease is reduced or eliminated by treatment.

- Support. The disease cannot be eliminated but treatment can reduce the impact of disability.
- Palliation. The progress of the disease causes increasing problems but treatment can improve the quality of life.

At present, oncology rehabilitation is carried out in the community, in district general hospitals, in oncology/radiotherapy units and in hospices. Fig. 36.5 shows these settings in relation to Dietz's stages of cancer readaptation.

Hammond (1988) shows that more work with cancer sufferers is undertaken by occupational therapists working in radiotherapy units and hospices than by those working in other settings and feels that this may be either the result of doctors' lack of awareness of the scope of the occupational therapy service, and therefore this type of patient does not get referred, or by a shortage of staff with sufficient training to carry out this work in general hospitals or the community.

THE ROLE OF THE OCCUPATIONAL THERAPIST

The contribution by occupational therapists to oncology rehabilitation is still developing. It is a new and exciting area of work that requires a blending of traditional skills and new ideas to form a complete concept of care.

In Chapter 34, Maslow's hierarchy of needs was used to illustrate how occupational therapy inter-

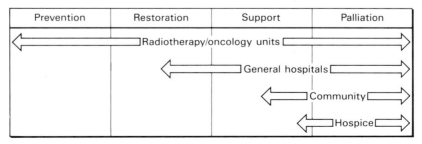

Fig. 36.5 Involvement of adult oncology settings in relation to Dietz 1980. Stages of cancer re-adaptation. Reproduced by kind permission of Weston Park Hospital, Sheffield.

vention can improve a person's self-esteem and quality of life. It was also shown that cancer sufferers commonly feel that they have lost control over their lives. It is essential that as much control as possible is given back to the individual for as long as he is able to exercise it. To this end, any treatment offered should be centred around the person and not decided upon on his behalf.

Another area that should be addressed is that of communicating bad news and discussing painful emotions. Unfortunately, there is still a tendency to question whether a person should be told of the severity of his illness. Even in cases where the relatives are told it is often felt that the individual will not be able to cope with the seriousness of his condition. Sadly, where this situation occurs the person has often guessed what is wrong and has therefore been denied the opportunity to share his fears and anxieties with those closest to him. By sensitive handling of such a situation it should be possible to inform the individual of his situation whilst still allowing hope to remain.

Whilst it is not appropriate for the occupational therapist to impart such information it is necessary for her to find out what the person has been told before she begins to assess his needs.

If, during treatment, the person raises the question of his prognosis, this is usually an indication that he wishes to discuss his fears and anxieties rather than merely to obtain factual answers to his questions. Such discussion can be promoted by indicating a readiness to listen and by allowing these fears to be expressed. There are many techniques that the therapist can learn to help her deal with difficult emotional situations. However, spontaneity in listening and responding is invaluable, for it is unlikely that the individual will confide his feelings in accordance with a predictable timetable.

The following section identifies areas of need that are common to many people with cancer. Some of these fall directly within the sphere of occupational therapy, whilst others may equally be performed by a physiotherapist, social worker or Macmillan nurse. In any event it is important that each task is undertaken by the person best qualified to perform it.

REFERRALS

The method of referral depends largely on the area in which the work is carried out. Ideally, a blanket referral system should be adopted as this has the benefit of allowing the occupational therapist to screen her case load and provide appropriate intervention at the right time. Clearly, such a system can only be successful in a defined work area such as a unit or ward. Where this is not possible, for example in the community, problems may arise when referrals arrive too late for a good service to be provided. Under such circumstances the therapist may consider instituting an education programme to increase appropriate referrals.

ASSESSMENT

Whilst, as with any assessment, this should cover the person's physical, psychological, emotional and social needs the therapist must also become aware of any goals or ambitions that are particularly important to the individual. Additionally, as the person's condition and circumstances are likely to fluctuate, evaluation during treatment is essential.

It can be helpful to use a problem-orientated assessment and record-keeping method such as POMR (Problem Orientated Medical Records). These can separate findings into those areas which are 'active' and can be solved, for example a person's inability to get dressed, and those which are 'inactive' and cannot be 'solved' as such, but none the less require the awareness and attention of team members. Examples of the latter might be the fact that the person is diabetic, or pregnant. If such records are available for all team members any one of them may add comments as appropriate.

INTERVENTION

The treatment programme begins to be formulated during assessment and the direction it takes will depend on the stage at which the person is referred. Someone referred following successful medical treatment, for example, will require different kinds of help from the person who has been told that his condition can be controlled for the moment, but not cured. As with all treatment planning it is important for the therapist and the individual to consider treatment aims together, in order that a meaningful series of priorities can be worked out.

Generally, however, the treatment plan must be flexible and capable of frequent alteration if the person's needs change. It is important in planning treatment to remember that the person's medical condition will not remain stable. A series of short-term goals should enable the person to achieve good results, thus improving morale and increasing self-esteem.

Areas of intervention may include the following:

Provision of information

Whilst team members may have concerns regarding the amount of information a person can accept about his condition, the individual will often be quite clear about the level he can accept. One man, for example, on being asked how much he knew of his condition, replied 'I know as much as I want to know and I will learn the rest as I go along.' Another woman arrived for her clinic appointment saying 'Don't you go telling me anything I don't want to hear!' Both these people made their feelings quite obvious and, clearly, such feelings must be respected.

If, however, the signals are not so clear, it is important to answer questions accurately without giving too much detail, thus leaving the way open for further questions. In this way the person can find out the information he requires at the time and can control the amount he has to cope with.

Some of the information a person requires will be painful for him to hear and will take time to assimilate. For this reason a person may ask the same question many times, of different team members, before he is able to accept the implications of the answer. It is important to remember this so that team members can be sure that answers are consistent and that they do not become irritated by being asked the same question many times.

In this field of work the information available is vast; clearly, no one person can know all the answers. Whilst it is essential to admit this it is also vital to know where to look, or who to ask, to get information. For example, the therapist should be aware of national and local organisations with information and education resources.

Life skills

Personal and home care

Although the emphasis will depend upon the level at which the person is functioning, this area of intervention will need to include self-care and home care advice and practice as well as the provision of equipment to help overcome disability. Equipment, where necessary, should be loaned if at all possible so that it may be easily changed if the need arises.

In cases where dramatic changes have occurred, such as amputation of a limb or compression of nervous tissue resulting in paraplegia, the presenting condition will obviously require practical consideration along with the other concerns of particular relevance to the individual. Attention to body image changes will also be necessary (see below) as will regard to the instability of the condition.

If the condition is well advanced it may be necessary to teach energy conservation techniques (see Chs 33 & 34). The therapist may also need to work with the person and his carers in helping the former to come to terms with being 'cared for', especially in circumstances where the individual has been the key homemaker.

Enabling a person to become independent in daily living activities following a period of dependency can improve self-esteem and achieve goals far in excess of those expected.

Mobility

Encouraging purposeful activity to improve mobility can increase stamina and generally enable a person to lead a more active life. A person who has been inactive through fear of exacerbating symptoms such as pain can often regain high levels of activity once his symptoms are controlled by correct medication and he has gained the confidence to begin activities again.

In some cases it may become obvious that full

mobility will not be achievable. However, the person may be reluctant to entertain the idea of using a wheelchair and it will be necessary to introduce the subject with sensitivity. Where stamina is low the use of a wheelchair can greatly improve a person's sphere of activity. It may, for example, enable him to visit the shops or a club after he has been confined to the house for some time. The ultimate decision as to whether to use a wheelchair or not, however, must remain with the individual, as he may still prefer to remain less mobile rather than use a wheelchair, even after all the advantages of the latter have been explained.

If the disease has progressed to the point where extensive metastases have weakened bone tissue, pathological fractures may occur. In such instances, and in others where mobility is not possible, full assessment for a permanent wheelchair, appropriate seating and other accessories will be necessary. The person will then require training in the use of the chair and in transfer techniques (see Ch. 10).

Emotional aspects

People who have cancer will obviously suffer considerable emotional stress. Whilst the degree of this may fluctuate, an individual will find it very difficult to pursue an active and productive life if he is continuously hampered by negative emotions. Under these circumstances the therapist can do much to help him, and his carers, by acknowledging the presence of these feelings and offering techniques and strategies which may help him come to terms with them. Some of the techniques outlined below may form the basis of this help.

Relaxation

Tension can both increase pain and decrease the effects of medication. One way of helping to dispel tension is through the use of relaxation techniques. People who teach relaxation often develop preferred methods, most of which evolve from one of the following techniques. However, whilst the therapist may have a preference for a particular method she must be flexible in her use of different techniques to suit varying needs.

- Progressive relaxation. This approach involves the individual becoming aware of different muscle groups and areas of the body in turn and learning to tense and relax them.
- Autogenic training. This involves relaxation of each part of the body in turn, e.g. hand, wrist, forearm, whilst imagining each part becoming warm and heavy.
- Imagining. Here the power of imagination is used to visualise a story or an activity, for example walking through a warm, sunny meadow or along a peaceful beach.

These, or any other techniques, can be used in conjunction with breathing exercises in order to help the person gain maximum benefit.

Whilst relaxation sessions are normally initiated by the therapist it is possible to obtain taped cassettes of exercises for those who wish to continue relaxation at home. In this way the person can learn to reduce tension as and when it occurs, rather than just during therapy sessions.

When considering different relaxation methods the therapist should remember that the method should be as simple and short as possible, whilst still being effective, especially to begin with. As the person becomes more proficient it may be possible to increase sessions in length and complexity.

Body image adjustment

Some medical treatments used in cancer management can lead to disfigurement. Where this occurs the occupational therapist, with her knowledge of adapted clothing and her ability to create individual solutions to individual problems, can offer much help. She may, for example, be involved in arranging the supply of a wig for someone suffering the effects of chemotherapy, or she may make an arm support for a person with lymphoedema. Alternatively she may be involved in helping a person alter her clothing following a radical mastectomy or the onset of paraplegia, or helping another come to terms with an altered body image following limb loss. Hairdressing and beauty care are important, especially for women, as is the ability to retain an accustomed level and mode of dress for all.

When a person suffers physical disfigurement the attitudes of people around them are very important. Acceptance of a person as he is, however he may look, can be difficult for some if disfigurement is severe, and some individuals may need help just to come out of their room and meet others if they feel they are physically unacceptable. Tact and sensitivity are vital in such situations and helping the person initially to simply be in the same room as others, without having to interact with them, can help build his self-esteem. As confidence grows, activities that involve communication with one, then later several others, can be used before the person is helped to meet people outside the unit, perhaps through a trip to the hospital shop and then outside the confines of the institution.

Reminiscence work

The importance of reminiscence work is discussed in Chapter 34. Whilst such work may take various forms, either in a group or on a one-to-one basis, this section will outline the format used in Cynthia Spencer House, Northampton. This is a Macmillan Continuing Care Unit built with locally raised funds and staffed by NHS and voluntary personnel. In this unit one element of reminiscence work takes the form of a tape-recorded interview which is later transcribed and given to the interviewee to keep. Whilst this technique is not strictly a 'therapy', those who choose to be interviewed find the experience worthwhile and rewarding. It can be pleasant to talk to an interested listener and to reflect upon the past. A project based on work of this type has been running in Northampton since 1987 and two booklets of excerpts from these transcriptions have been published to date. Examples are given in Box 36.1.

Creative writing forms another part of this work. Jane Eisenhaur (1989), a writer, has used this activity in her work at St Joseph's Hospice in London. Because it takes some effort to put pen to paper a person who is less well may need a scribe to put his ideas onto paper for him.

Box 36.1 Illustrations of creative writing by people with cancer. Reproduced from *Slices of Life* (Foreman & Hobbs 1988) and *Life at Work* (Forman 1989)

I sold my business, retired and bought a small van and done a little bit of, not wholesaling like I done before, but retailing. I used to do bags of potatoes, polythene bags, and I used to go up the club or the pub or anywhere and get rid of thirty or forty bags. I was always doing something. I kept that up until . . . almost 'til this [present illness] come along.

Well, I've enjoyed life. That's one good thing. And I've made a fair bit of cash. That's another thing. So I've got nothing to grumble at, have I?

Harry Saunders (born 1900)

Beauty can be found
In oh, so many things.
Amongst the most amazing:
A pair of insect wings

A filigree of colour
Of every shade and hue,
And movements quite
Incredible to folks
Like me and you.

Pat Groot

We used to go to Harlestone Firs. We used to go up there and take a bottle of drink with us. Usually landed up with cold tea! [laughs] And some sandwiches. We used to eat that then go back for tea. Just friends, like, several friends. It was a happy childhood really.

June Baucutt (born 1925)

Support

The amount of support required by cancer sufferers and their carers varies widely and will, therefore, have to be tailored to suit the individual. Support may be given by anyone on the team; often, each member contributes in his or her own way. Support can take many forms, which include the following:

● *Emotional support.* In order that the occupational therapist can offer professional counselling it will be necessary for her to undertake postgraduate training in order to develop her skills. However, it is quite possible for her to help in complementary ways by using the skills she has already learned during her training.

The occupational therapist's skill in problem-solving can be helpful both emotionally and physically. When a person has developed a major physical problem, for example, the occupational therapist may be involved in assessing his future needs. This will involve working with both the person and his carers, who may need a great deal of emotional support as they consider various options and come to terms with the fact that solutions may not suit everyone or, indeed, that a satisfactory solution is not possible.

If the disease has progressed past the restoration stage, carers will need both physical and emotional support. Many people want to care for their loved one at home for as long as possible and may, indeed, wish for them to die at home rather than in hospital. In order for this to be possible, practical help in the form of equipment, advice on lifting and general nursing care will be essential. The individual may also need respite care, possibly for a week or two or perhaps just for an afternoon to enable his carers to go shopping.

● *Self-help groups.* Many cancer sufferers have much to offer in the way of support. Self-help groups are run locally throughout the country by cancer sufferers for others in the same position. There may be input from professionals such as Macmillan nurses but these professionals are not the key figures within the group. Groups offer a meeting place for the individual and his carers where they can discuss problems and help each other find solutions.

The occupational therapist should be aware of self-help groups in her area. She may, indeed, be asked by such groups for help and advice.

● *Charities.* Many national and local charities have been established to help people who are suffering from cancer (see p. 838). Some of these offer financial assistance whilst others offer practical help. It is important for the therapist to be aware of these charities and of the type of help they offer.

● *Carers' support groups.* Whilst emotional support for carers can be offered on an individual basis by team members it may be appropriate for the occupational therapist and/or social worker to establish a support group for them where carers can meet and draw support from others in the same situation, as well as gaining further access to professional advice.

● *Bereavement support.* Bereavement counselling is another area where, if the occupational therapist wishes to become involved she must first seek further training. It is, however, possible to offer support to people coping with grief through the relationship that has developed between the therapist and the individual's carers. The opportunity to talk to someone who has known their loved one, and the occasion to share information can be very comforting at this time.

Grieving is a normal process (see Ch. 3) and most people, if allowed, will cope well with bereavement with the sensitive help of friends and relatives. It is helpful, however, for the occupational therapist to be able to spot the development of any problems and to be aware of counselling facilities in her area.

Anyone offering support needs to achieve warm, friendly relationship with the individual and his carers whilst retaining a measure of objectivity and professionalism. It is important not to take personally the unpleasant feelings that may be exhibited during and after a long, distressing illness and to maintain a sense of proportion at all times.

Social and leisure activities

People's attitudes to cancer can vary enormously; consequently, it can be a daunting prospect for a person suffering from cancer to get out and about following treatment for his disease. He may feel rejected by friends who find his condition hard to cope with or talk about, or he may feel he wishes to tell everyone about his experiences, thus creating fears and barriers within relationships. Alternatively, he may feel he cannot cope with an excessive curiosity on the part of colleagues and friends, or by their apparent lack of interest, which may stem from their discomfort at not knowing what to say. Allowing time for discussion of these feelings, therefore, may be valuable.

Large gatherings and crowds may be equally daunting for a person who does not feel very well. Keeping outings short, and restricting them to places where the person feels comfortable, and which he can leave early if he feels the need, can help him retain his social life.

Where the disease has reached an advanced stage it may be difficult for the person to get out. In some areas, units have access to adapted vehicles; alternatively, charities and local organisations may offer to help. Where this cannot be arranged it is important to 'take the mountain to Mohammed' by encouraging visits, phone calls and letters so that the person does not feel isolated from his family, friends and colleagues. Where a day centre facility is available for cancer sufferers this can provide not only company and support for the individual but also support and relief for his carers.

Specific therapeutic activity

Whilst there has been an apparent move away from the use of certain therapeutic activities by occupational therapists in recent years, such activities do have a place in the treatment of people suffering from cancer, particularly in the later stages of the illness.

Although it would be arrogant to presume to divert the person's attention from his situation a person suffering from cancer, especially in the later stages, is facing events and circumstances with which he has to come to terms. As it is neither possible nor desirable for him to dwell upon these continuously, time set aside for discussion of these worries can be interspersed with activities and hobbies which provide much-needed light relief and interest.

If a person is in pain and, possibly, waiting for medication to take effect, concentrating on an activity in which he is interested can relieve tension and shift his focus of attention away from his pain.

The later stages of the disease may also be the time for the person to participate in hobbies he has previously not had time for. Activities should be easy to start and put down, to be completed later, and should also be quick to finish.

When a person suffers from a disease like cancer there is a temptation to think he needs to have a lot done for him. Whilst this may be so, it is also important for him to feel useful and productive; activities can be selected with this in mind. For example, articles can be made for fund-raising events or as presents to give away. Such presents are especially important as they serve as a lasting reminder of a person even after his death.

Whilst it may be tempting to encourage a person to continue with an interest he has had in the past this can prove unsatisfactory as he may no longer be able to perform it as well as he used to. For this reason it may be wiser to encourage a totally new interest.

Other therapies

A person with cancer may feel the need to find a way of complementing the treatment he is receiving via orthodox medicine. He may, indeed, feel that the conventional treatment he is receiving does not meet his needs and he might, therefore, look to alternative therapy. Many alternative therapies are available and he may choose, for example, to be helped by aromatherapy (massage using aromatic oils), homeopathy, visualisation (relaxation combined with visualising the growth as being weak as it is attacked and destroyed by the body's immune system), and so on. The basis for many of these therapies is positive thinking and attitude and the realisation that the effort to get better has to come from within. There has been little documented work on the effectiveness of these therapies but many people who have used them feel they have derived benefit from doing so. However, the person may feel a failure if he is not cured, as he may feel that he did not work hard enough at his treatment.

Resettlement

While a person is being cared for in hospital it is hoped that he will regain much of his independence. However, until he returns home he still relies on physical and emotional support from staff. Most skills involved in helping a person with cancer to return home are no different from those used in resettling any other person being discharged from hospital, but there are one or two points that need particular consideration, especially if the person concerned is quite unwell.

As has been stated, most people suffering from cancer are not medically stable; consequently, consideration needs to be given to each individual's expectations. If it is felt that the person will continue to improve following treatment and discharge, any action to be taken is usually reasonably easy to determine on a home visit. However, if expectations are not so high, it may be necessary for two or more members of the team to undertake a home visit. This will afford the opportunity for team members and carers to talk together in the carers' own environment and to bring to light the carers' areas of concern. There may also be times when the health care team have reservations about the appropriateness of a person returning home; whilst they clearly do not have the right to prevent him from doing so, observing him in his own home can give them a basis for open discussion about their concerns.

There will often be discussion concerning whether the carers, as well as the individual, feel they can cope once the person is at home. Sometimes this may serve to crystallise feelings of fear and anxiety and can lead to the realisation that, no matter how much help and support is provided, the carers will be unable to cope and a different solution must be sought. In fact, it is not unknown for a home visit to be necessary in order to allow a person to come to this conclusion and to give him 'permission' not to return home.

Following the home visit there will often be problems to solve before discharge. Solutions need to be realistic and if alterations are to be made it will be necessary to choose those which take the least time whilst affording maximum benefit to the person. Prognosis is often very difficult to assess and it is essential to keep a positive attitude once a decision has been taken to help a person return home.

Once the person has returned home, he and his carers may encounter further difficulties. It is important to encourage carers to accept help before they reach a state of exhaustion. If a day care facility is available this can provide time off for carers as well as new interests, social contact and support for the individual. If this is not available, or in some cases of severe illness, agencies such as Crossroads can offer a sitting service to allow carers to take a break.

In some areas the occupational therapist may be the main link between the hospital and the community. In such cases it is important for her to arrange for the continuation of support links in accordance with the person's needs.

CONCLUSION

Oncology rehabilitation is an area that has been developing rapidly in recent years. There is much that can be done to help a person and his carers cope with the possibility of a devastating crisis in their lives. There is no magical formula for this help, only the implementation of good, caring practice. Neither are there any right or wrong answers; what must be sought are the solutions that seem best for a particular person at a particular time.

The occupational therapist working in this field will find herself having to call on nearly all the skills learned in her basic training as she helps the person and his carers in the physical, emotional and social aspects of their lives. However, her practice will also be enriched by additional training in specific areas such as counselling and relaxation techniques.

ACKNOWLEDGEMENT

Grateful acknowledgement is made to Dr Nigel Bird, Clinical Assistant, Cynthia Spencer House; Jackie Phillips, Senior Clinical Nurse, Cynthia Spencer House; Martin Eagle, Farmitalia; Alison Hammond, Occupational Therapist, Derby School of Occupational Therapy; and to Dr Peter Kaye and all the staff at Cynthia Spencer House, Northampton, and our patients, past and present, who are a constant source of inspiration to us all.

USEFUL ADDRESSES

Association of Carers
1st floor, 21–3 New Road
Chatham
Kent ME4 4JQ

BACUP (British Association of Cancer United Patients)
121–123 Charterhouse Street
London EC1M 6AA

British Association for Counselling
37a Sheep Street
Rugby
Warwickshire CV21 3BX

Cancer Aftercare & Rehabilitation Society (CARE)
21 Zetland Road
Redland
Bristol BS6 7AH

Cancer Relief (National Society for Cancer Relief)
Anchor House
15/19 Britten Street
London SW3 3TZ

Cancer Research Campaign
2 Carlton House Terrace
London SW1V 5AR

Crossroads (Association of Crossroads Care Attendant Scheme)
94 Coton Road
Rugby
Warwickshire CV21 4LN

CRUSE (National organisation for bereaved people)
Cruse House
126 Sheen Road
Richmond TW9 1UR

Disabled Living Foundation
380–384 Harrow Road
London W9 2HU

Help the Hospices
BMA House
Tavistock Square
London WC1H 9JP

Hospice Information Service
St Christopher's Hospice
51–9 Lawrie Park Road
London SE26 6DZ

Institute for Complementary Medicine
21 Portland Place
London W1N 3AF

Marie Curie Memorial Foundation
28 Belgrave Square
London SW1X 8OQ

Lisa Sainsbury Foundation
8–10 Crown Hill
Croydon
Surrey CR0 1RY
(Provides videos, tapes and book references and organises workshops)

There are many more relevant charities, some are set up to help people suffering from particular forms of cancer. Their addresses are published annually by:

Family Welfare Association
501–503 Kingsland Road
Dalston
London E8 4UA

REFERENCES

Bryan J, Lyall J 1987 Living with cancer. Penguin, Harmondsworth
Buckman R 1988 I don't know what to say. Papermac, London
Dietz J H, Jnr 1981 Rehabilitation oncology. Wiley & Sons, New York
Eisenhaur J (ed) 1989 Traveller's tales: poetry from hospice. Marshall Pickering, London
Foreman R (ed) 1989 Life at work. (Compilation of reminiscences.) Copies available from Cynthia Spencer House, Kettering Road, Northampton NN3 1AD
Foreman R. Hobbs L (eds) 1988 Slices of life. (Compilation

of reminiscences.) Cynthia Spencer House, Northampton

Hammond A 1988 The role of the occupational therapist in oncology. (Unpublished MSc thesis. Copies obtainable from the author, Derby School of Occupational Therapy, Highfield, 403 Burton Road, Derby DE3 6AN.)

Kubler-Ross E 1970 On death and dying. Tavistock Publications, London

Lamerton R 1985 Care of the dying, rev. edn. Pelican, Harmondsworth

Lewis M 1989 Tears and smiles: the hospice handbook. O'Mara Books, London

Regnard C, Davies A 1986 A guide to symptom relief in advanced cancer, 2nd edn. Haigh & Hochland, Manchester

Sampson J 1987 The courage to hope. Scripture Union, London

Souhami R, Tobais J 1986 Cancer and its management. Blackwell, Oxford

Strong J 1987 Occupational therapy and cancer rehabilitation. British Journal of Occupational Therapy 50(1): 4–6

Tigges K 1980 Occupational therapy for the person with terminal cancer. Sabbatical Report to the Department of Occupational Therapy, State University of New York at Buffalo, unpublished

Whitehouse J M A 1986 Chemotherapy: a guide for patients. Farmitalia, St Albans, Herts

Zora R, Zora V 1981 A way to die. Sphere Books, London

FURTHER READING

Boston S, Trezise R 1987 Merely mortal. Methuen Paperbacks, London

DuBoulay S 1984 Cicely Saunders. Hodder Christian Paperbacks, London

Brearley G, Birchley P 1986 Introducing counselling skills and techniques. Faber & Faber, London

Chave-Jones M 1982 The gift of helping. Inter-varsity Press, Leicester

Downie P 1976 Cancer rehabilitation. Faber & Faber, London

Hinton J 1967 Dying. Pelican, Harmondsworth

Kopp R 1980 Encounter with terminal illness. Lion Publishing, Tring, Herts

Kopp R 1986 When someone you love is dying. Lion Publishing, Tring, Herts

Kushner H 1981 When bad things happen to good people. Pan, London

Kushner H 1986 When all you've ever wanted isn't enough. Pan, London

Lewis C S 1940 The problem of pain. Collins, Glasgow

Lewis C S 1966 A grief observed. Faber & Faber, London

Munro E, Manthei R, Small J 1976 Counselling: a skills approach. Methuen, London

Parkes C M 1976 Bereavement. Penguin, Harmondsworth

Part 4
Appendix
Index

Appendix

Common abbreviations, prefixes and suffixes

RELATED TO PEOPLE, MEMBERSHIP, QUALIFICATIONS

CE	Chief executive
CN	Community nurse
DipCOT	Diploma of the College of Occupational Therapists
DN	District nurse
DNO	District Nursing Officer
DNS	Director of Nursing Services
DPH	Director of Public Health
DRO	Disablement Resettlement Officer
DSS	Director of Social Services
FRCP	Fellow of the Royal College of Physicians
FRCS	Fellow of the Royal College of Surgeons
GAA	General administrative assistant
GM	General manager
GP	General practitioner
HCO	Higher clerical officer, Home care organiser
HO	House officer
HV	Health visitor
MCSP	Member of the Chartered Society of Physiotherapy
MPS	Member of the Pharmaceutical Society

MRCP	Member of the Royal College of Physicians
MRCS	Member of the Royal College of Surgeons
NO	Nursing Officer
OT	Occupational therapist
PA	Personal assistant
PAM	Professions allied to medicine
PRO	Public relations officer
Pt	Patient
PT	Physiotherapist
RN	Registered Nurse
SHO	Senior house officer
SN	Senior nurse
SR	Senior registrar
SRCh	State Registered Chiropodist
SRD	State Registered Dietitian
SROT	State Registered Occupational Therapist
SRP	State Registered Physiotherapist
SW	Social worker
VSO	Voluntary services organiser
WTE	Whole time equivalent

RELATED TO DEPARTMENTS/ORGANISATIONS

ACAS	Advisory, Conciliation and Arbitration Service
ACHCEW	Association of Community Health Councils for England and Wales
ADSS	Association of Directors of Social Services
A & E	Accident and Emergency
AMA	Association of Metropolitan Authorities
ASH	Action on Smoking and Health
ASTMS	Association of Scientific, Technical and Managerial Staffs
BAOT	British Association of Occupational Therapists
BDA	British Dietetic Association

BJOT	British Journal of Occupational Therapy
BMA	British Medical Association
BMJ	British Medical Journal
BNF	British National Formulary
BOS	British Orthoptic Society
BUPA	British United Provident Association
CC	County Council
CEH	Centre on the Environment for the Handicapped
CCETSW	Central Council for Education and Training in Social Work
CHC	Community Health Council
CIPFA	Chartered Institute of Public Finance and Accountancy
COHSE	Confederation of Health Service Employees
COSLA	Convention of Scottish Local Authorities
COT	College of Occupational Therapists
CPAG	Child Poverty Action Group
CPSM	Council for Professions Supplementary to Medicine
CSP	Chartered Society of Physiotherapy
CSSD	Central Sterile Supply Department
DES	Department of Education and Science
DGH	District General Hospital
D of H	Department of Health
DHA	District Health Authority
DMU	Directly Managed Unit
DSC	Disablement Services Centre
DSS	Department of Social Security
ENB	English National Board (Nursing)
EOC	Equal Opportunities Commission
FHSA	Family Health Services Authority
FIS	Family Income Supplement
FPO	Federation of Professional Organisations
GMC	General Medical Council

GMWU	General and Municipal Workers Union	NPU	National Pharmaceutical Union
HA	Health Authority	NUPE	National Union of Public Employees
HAS	Health Advisory Service	O & M	Organisation and Methods
HCSA	Hospital Consultants and Specialists Association	OH	Occupational Health
		OME	Office of Manpower Economics
HEA	Health Education Authority	OPD	Outpatients Department
HMSO	Her Majesty's Stationery Office	OR	Operational Research
HSC	Health Service Commissioner (Ombudsman)	OU	Open University
		OPCS	Office of Population and Censuses and Surveys
HSE	Health and Safety Executive	P & T	Professional and Technical (Whitley Council)
IHSM	Institute of Health Services Management	RADAR	Royal Association for Disability and Rehabilitation
IPM	Institute of Personnel Managers/Management	R & D	Research and Development
JCC	Joint Consultative Committee	RCM	Royal College of Midwives
JCPT	Joint Care Planning Team	RCN	Royal College of Nurses
JLC	Joint Liaison Committee	RCGP	Royal College of General Practitioners
LA	Local Authority		
LASS	Local Authority Social Services	RCP	Royal College of Physicians
LBC	London Borough Council	RCS	Royal College of Surgeons
MDC	Metropolitan District Council	REMAP	Rehabilitation Engineering Movement Advisory Panel
MEDLARS	Medical Literature Analysis and Retrieval System	RHA	Regional Health Authority
MIMS	Monthly Index of Medical Supplies	RIBA	Royal Institution of British Architects
MPU	Medical Practitioners Union	RICS	Royal Institute of Chartered Surveyors
MRC	Medical Research Council		
MSC	Manpower Services Commission	RSH	Royal Society of Health
		SED	Scottish Education Department
NAB	National Advisory Board	SGT	Self Governing Trust
NAHAT	National Association of Health Authorities and Trusts (England and Wales)	SHAS	Scottish Health Advisory Service
NAIDEX	National Aids for the Disabled Exhibition	SHHD	Scottish Home and Health Department
NALGO	National Association of Local Government Officers	SI	International System of Units
		SIFT	Service Instrument for Teaching (Medical and Dental)
NAFTE	National Association of Teachers in Further Education	SMA	Socialist Medical Association
NAO	National Audit Office	SSD	Social Service Department
NBTS	National Blood Transfusion Service	SSI	Social Services Inspectorate
		TGWU	Transport and General Workers Union
NHS	National Health Service		
NJC	National Joint Council	TSSU(D)	Theatre Sterile Supply Unit (Department)
NMC	Nurses and Midwives (Whitley) Council	TUC	Trades Union Congress

UGC	University Grants Committee
VSO	Voluntary Service Overseas
WFOT	World Federation of Occupational Therapists
WHO	World Health Organization
WO	Welsh Office
WRVS	Womens Royal Voluntary Service

RELATED TO FACTS RECORDED DURING THE EXAMINATION OF A PATIENT

BP	Blood pressure
CNS	Central nervous system
C/o	Complained of
CVP	Central venous pressure
CVS	Cardiovascular system
DA	Doctor's appointment
D & V	Diarrhoea and vomiting
DNA	Did not attend
DOA	Date of admission, dead on arrival
DOB	Date of birth
FH	Family history
GI	Gastrointestinal
GU	Genitourinary
ISQ	No change (in status quo)
KUB	Kidneys, ureter, bladder
NAD	Nothing abnormal discovered
NAI	Non-accidental injury
NFA	No further appointment
NYD	Not yet diagnosed
O/A	On admission
OE	On examination
PH	Past history
ROM	Range of movement
RS	Respiratory system
RTA	Road traffic accident
SOB	Shortness of breath
SOL	Space-occupying lesion
TCI	To come in
UG	Urogenital
WNL	Within normal limits
△	Diagnosis

RELATED TO TESTS PERFORMED TO AID DIAGNOSIS

A and P	Anterior and posterior (X-ray view)
AER	Auditory evoked response
BMR	Basal metabolic rate
BSR	Basal sedimentation rate
CSF	Cerebrospinal fluid
CT	Computerised tomography
ECG	Electrocardiograph
EEG	Electro-encephalograph
EMG	Electro-myelograph
ESR	Erythrocyte sedimentation rate
FBC	Full blood count
Hb	Haemoglobin
IVP	Intravenous pylography (kidney function)
LP	Lumbar Puncture
VER	Visual evoked response
WR	Wassermann reaction
XR	X-ray

EXAMPLES RELATED TO SPECIFIC DIAGNOSIS

AIDS	Acquired Immune Deficiency Syndrome
APM	Anterior poliomyelitis
BI	Bony injury
Ca	Cancer
CCF	Congestive cardiac failure, Chronic cardiac failure
CDH	Congenital dislocation of the hip
COAD	Chronic Obstructive Airways Disease
CP	Cerebral palsy
CVA	Cerebral vascular accident
DU	Duodenal Ulcer
DVT	Deep vein thrombosis
GOK	'God only knows'
GU	Gastric ulcer
HI	Head injury

IDK	Internal derangement of the knee joint
LVF	Left ventricular failure
MD	Muscular dystrophy
MI	Myocardial infarction, mitral incompetence
MND	Motor neurone disease
MS	Multiple sclerosis, mitral stenosis
OA	Osteoarthritis
PD	Parkinson's disease
PE	Pulmonary embolism
PID	Prolapsed intervertebral disc
PNL	Peripheral nerve lesion
PUO	Pyrexia of unknown origin
RA	Rheumatoid arthritis
RDS	Respiratory distress syndrome
RVF	Right ventricular failure
SI	Spinal injury
TIA	Transient ischaemic attack
UTI	Urinary tract infection

RELATED TO TREATMENT

AOF 5G	Wheelchair prescription form
CAPE	Clifton Assessment Procedures for the Elderly
DXR	Deep X-ray
EUA	Examination under anaesthetic
GA	General anaesthetic
MUA	Manipulation under anaesthetic
POP	Plaster of Paris
RT	Radiotherapy
THR	Total hip replacement
TLC	Tender loving care

RELATED TO DRUG THERAPY

AC	Before meals (ante cibos)
BD or bd	Twice a day (bis in die)
IM	Intramuscular
IV	Intravenous
MAOI	Monoamine oxidase inhibitor

Nocte	At night
NSAID	Non-steroidal anti-inflammatory drug
OD	Once a day (omni die)
PC	After meals (post cibos)
PRN	As required (pro re nata)
QDS	Four times a day (quater in die sumendum)
SC	Subcutaneous
TID or TDS	Three times a day (ter in die sumendum)

RELATED TO LIMBS

AK	Above knee
BK	Below knee
CMP	Carpometacarpal (joint)
DIP	Distal interphalangeal (joint)
FWB	Full weight-bearing
LL	Lower limb
NWB	Non weight-bearing
PIP	Proximal interphalangeal (joint)
PWB	Partial weight-bearing
SLR	Straight leg-raising
UL	Upper limb

PREFIXES

Prefix	Meaning	Example
a	without	aphasia (without language)
ab	away from	abduction (move away from median plane)
ad	towards	adduction (move towards median plane)
an	absence of	anaesthesia (absence of sensation)
ante	preceding, before	anteorbital (in front of the eyes)

Prefix	Meaning	Example	Prefix	Meaning	Example
anti	preventing, opposed to	anti-coagulant (agent that prevents clotting of blood)	gen	referring to birth, production, reproduction	genitalia (reproductive organs)
arthro	joint	arthritis, arthrosis (articulation)	gyn	female	gynaecology (study of women's diseases)
auto	self	autograft (graft taken from one part of body and implanted elsewhere in body of same person)	haem	blood	haemorrhage (bleeding)
			hemi	half	hemiplegia (paralysis of one side of the body)
baro	pressure	barotrauma (injury due to pressure)	hetero	other, differing	heterogenous (of differing type)
bi	two	bilateral (on both sides)	homo	same, common	homogenize (reduce material to uniform consistency)
bio	life	biopsy (visual examination of tissue from living person)	hydro	water, accumulation of fluid	hydrotherapy (treatment in water)
brady	slow	bradycardia (slow heart beat)			hydrocephalus (accumulation of CSF in ventricles)
calc	calcium	calcification (deposition of calcium salts in tissues)	hyper	excess, high	hypertension (raised blood pressure)
cardio	heart	cardiovascular system (circulatory system)	hypo	lack of, below	hypotension; hypothermia (lowered body heat)
chondro	cartilage	chondroblast (cell-producing matrix of cartilage)	in	in	inverted (turned inwards, upside down)
con	together with	congenital (present at birth)	infra	below	infraclavicular (below the clavicle)
dys	impaired, difficult	dysarthria (difficulty with articulation)	inter	between	intervertebral disc
			intra	within, inside	intravenous (into a vein)
e	out	evert (turn outwards)	iso	same, equality, similarity	isotonic (describing muscles with equal tonicity)
end/ endo	inside, inner	endothelium (inner lining of various body structures)			
epi	outside	epidermis (on the skin/outer layer of skin)	macro	large	macrocephaly (abnormal largeness of head)
extra	outside	extra-cellular (outside cell walls)	mal	bad	malunited (badly united)

Prefix	Meaning	Example	Prefix	Meaning	Example
micro	small	microcephaly (abnormal smallness of head)	pre	before	prefrontal lobe (region of brain at very front of each cerebral hemisphere)
multi	many	multifactorial (believed to have resulted from interaction of factors, e.g. genetic, environmental)	pro	in front, before	prodrome (symptom indicating onset of a disease)
my/myo	muscle	myocardium (heart muscle)	pseudo	false	pseudoplegia (paralysis of limbs not associated with organic abnormalities)
neo	new	neoplasm (new growth)			
neuro	nerves	neurology (study of structure, function and diseases of nervous system)	py	pus	pyelitis (inflammation of the pelvis of the kidney)
osteo	bone	osteoblast (cell producing bone)	quadri	four	quadriplegia (paralysis of all four limbs)
ortho	straight, normal	orthopaedics (science/practice of correcting deformities caused by trauma/disease to bones/joints)	radio	radiation	radiography (technique of examining the body by X-ray)
para	near, partial, beside	parasthesia (spontaneous abnormal tingling sensations)	retro	backward, behind	retropulsion (tendency to walk backwards)
per	through, complete	perforation (creation of hole in tissue/organ)	sub	below	subdural (below the dura mater)
peri	around, enclosing	pericardium (membrane surrounding the heart)	super	above, extreme	superficial (in anatomy situated at/close to the surface)
pneumo	air, lung	pneumonia (inflammation of the lung)	supra	above, upon	suprarenal (above the kidney)
poly	many	polyneuritis (any disorder involving all peripheral nerves)	syn	with, union	syndrome (combination of signs and/or symptoms forming a distinct clinical picture of a particular disorder)
post	after	posterior (situated at or near the back of the body/an organ)	tetra	four	tetraplegia (as quadriplegia)
			tri	three	triceps (muscle with three heads of origin)

Prefix	Meaning	Example
ultra	beyond	ultrasound (sound waves of extremely high frequency inaudible to human ear)
uni	one	unilateral (on one side)

SUFFIXES

Suffix	Meaning	Example
. . . aemia	blood	anaemia (reduction of haemoglobin in the blood)
. . . algia	pain	neuralgia (severe stabbing/burning pain following course of a nerve)
. . . cardial	heart	myocardial (pertaining to heart muscle)
. . . derm	skin	epidermis (outer layer of skin)
. . . ectomy	removal, cutting out	appendectomy (removal of appendix)
. . . esis	action, process	arthrodesis (surgical fusion of bones across joint space)
. . . genic	producing	pathogenic (producing disease)
. . . graphy	recording	radiography (recording by radiation i.e. X-ray)
. . . itis	inflammation	arthritis (inflammation of joint(s))
. . . kinesia	movement	bradykinesia (slowness of movement)
. . . oid	like	osteoid (like bone)
. . . ology	science	neurology (see prefix 'neuro-')

Suffix	Meaning	Example
. . . oma	tumour	neuroma (benign tumour growing from peripheral nerve fibrous coverings)
. . . opia	eye	hemianopia (absence of half normal field of vision)
. . . osis	condition	diagnosis; spondylosis (degenerative spinal disorder)
. . . ostomy	to form an opening	colostomy (opening in colon to form artificial anus)
. . . otomy	cutting	osteotomy (cutting through bone, usually for realignment)
. . . paresis	weakness	hemiparesis (weakness in one side of the body)
. . . pathy	disease	myopathy (any disease of muscles)
. . . plasty	to form, mould	arthroplasty (to make a new joint)
. . . plegia	paralysis	paraplegia (paralysis of lower limbs)
. . . pnoea	breath	dyspnoea (difficulty in breathing)
. . . sclerosis	hardening	arteriosclerosis (hardening of arteries)
. . . therapy	treatment	occupational therapy
. . . trophy	nourishment, growth	atrophy (wasting of normally developed organ/tissue)
. . . uria	urine	albuminuria (albumen in the urine)

MISCELLANY

EL	Executive letter
GNP	Gross national product
HC	Health circular
HN	Health notice
IPR	Individual performance review
IT	Information technology
LAC	Local authority circular
PM	Personnel memorandum
PRP	Performance related pay
QA	Quality assurance
RSG	Rate support grant
VDU	Visual display unit

Index